CLINICAL GYNECOLOGIC UROLOGY

CLINICAL GYNECOLOGIC UROLOGY

Edited by

Stuart L. Stanton, F.R.C.S., M.R.C.O.G.

Senior Lecturer,
Department of Obstetrics and Gynecology,
St. George's Hospital Medical School,
Cranmer Terrace, London;
Consultant Obstetrician and Gynecologist,
St. Helier Hospital,
Carshalton, Surrey, United Kingdom

with 450 illustrations

THE C. V. MOSBY COMPANY

St. Louis   Toronto   1984

MOSBY

A TRADITION OF PUBLISHING EXCELLENCE

Editor: Karen Berger
Assistant editor: Terry Van Schaik
Manuscript editor: Judi Wolken
Book design: Jeanne Bush
Cover design: Suzanne J. Oberholtzer
Production: Linda R. Stalnaker, Teresa Breckwoldt, Kathleen L. Teal

Printed in the United States of America

The C.V. Mosby Company
11830 Westline Industrial Drive, St. Louis, Missouri 63146

Library of Congress Cataloging in Publication Data
Main entry under title:
Clinical gynecologic urology.
    Includes bibliographical references and index.
        1. Urinary organs—Diseases. 2. Generative organs,
Female—Diseases. I. Stanton, Stuart L. [DNLM:
1. Urologic diseases. 2. Urinary tract—Anatomy and
histology. 3. Urinary tract—Physiology. 4. Genital
diseases, Female. 5. Urination disorders. WJ 190 C641]
RG484.C55 1984   616.6   83-19452
ISBN 0-8016-4755-X

GW/MV/MV 9 8 7 6 5 4 3 2 1   02/D/255

In memory of my late father, Michael A. Stanton,

and

father-in-law, Mac Goldsmith

Contributors

Paul Abrams, M.D., F.R.C.S.

Clinical Tutor in Urology, Department of Urology, University of Bristol, Bristol, United Kingdom; Consultant Urologist, Department of Urology, Southmead General Hospital, Westbury-on-Trym, Bristol, United Kingdom

Linda Cardozo, M.D., M.R.C.O.G.

Senior Registrar, Obstetrics and Gynaecology, Kings College Hospital, Denmark Hill, London, United Kingdom

William Ross Cattell, M.D., F.R.C.P., F.R.C.P.(Ed.)

Lecturer and Recognised Teacher, University of London; Department of Medicine and Nephrology, The College of St. Bartholomew's Hospital; Consultant Physician and Senior Nephrologist, Department of Medicine and Nephrology, St. Bartholomew's Hospital, London, United Kingdom

B.L.R.A. Coolsaet

Professor and Chairman, Department of Urology, Academic Hospital Utrecht, Utrecht, The Netherlands

John Malcolm Davison, B.Sc. M.D., M.Sc., M.R.C.O.G.

Scientific Staff, Medical Research Council, Human Reproduction Group, Princess Mary Maternity Hospital; Consultant Obstetrician and Gynaecologist, Newcastle District Health Authority, Newcastle-Upon-Tyne, United Kingdom

Professor Sir John Dewhurst, M.B., F.R.C.O.C., F.R.C.S. (Ed.), Hon. D.Sc., M.D., F.A.C.O.G.

Professor of Obstetrics and Gynaecology, Institute of Obstetrics, Gynaecology, University of London; Queen Charlotte's Hospital for Women, London, United Kingdom

John Arthur Gosling, M.B., Ch.B., M.D.

Professor of Anatomy, University of Manchester Medical School, Manchester, United Kingdom

Derek John Griffiths, B.A., Ph.D.

Doctor, Department of Urology and Department of Biological and Medical Physics, Erasmus University Rotterdam, Rotterdam, The Netherlands

Tage Hald, M.D., D.M.Sc.

Associate Professor of Surgery, Faculty of Medicine, University of Copenhagen; Chief Urologist, Department of Urology, Herlev Hospital, Denmark

Paul Hilton, M.D., M.R.C.O.G.

Senior Lecturer and Consultant, Department of Obstetrics and Gynaecology, University of Newcastle-Upon-Tyne; Princess Mary Maternity Hospital, Newcastle-Upon-Tyne, United Kingdom

John R. Hindmarsh, M.D., F.R.C.S.

Senior Lecturer, Institute of Urology, University of London; Honorary Consultant Urologist, St. Peter's Hospital, London, United Kingdom

Prof. Dr. Udo Jonas

Professor and Chairman, Department of Urology, University of Leiden, Medical Faculty; Professor Doctor, Department of Urology, Academisch Ziekenhuis, Leiden, The Netherlands

Richard H.G. Kerr-Wilson, F.R.C.S. (Ed.), M.R.C.O.G.

Senior Obstetrical and Gynaecological Registrar, Simpson Maternity Memorial Pavilion, Royal Infirmary of Edinburgh, Edinburgh, United Kingdom

Robert J. Krane, M.D.

Professor and Chairman, Department of Urology, Boston University School of Medicine; Chairman, Department of Urology, University Hospital, Boston, Massachusetts

Dorothy A. Mandelstam, M.C.S.P., Dip. Soc. Sc.

Incontinence Advisor, Disabled Living Foundation and Royal Free Hospital, London, United Kingdom

Peter Henry Millard, M.B., B.S., (Hons.) F.R.C.P.

Eleanor Peel Professor of Geriatric Medicine, Department of Geriatric Teaching and Research; Professor of Geriatric Medicine, Department of Geriatric Medicine, St. George's Hospital Medical School, London, United Kingdom

Christine Norton, M.A. (Cantab.), S.R.N.

Sister and Incontinence Advisor, Incontinence Clinic, St. Pancras Hospital, London, United Kingdom

Kingsley R.W. Norton, M.A. (Cantab.), M.B., B.Chir., M.R.C. Psych.

Lecturer, Academic Department of Psychiatry, St. George's Hospital Medical School; Honorary Senior Registrar, Department of Psychiatry, St. George's Hospital, London, United Kingdom

Donald R. Ostergard, M.D.

Professor of Obstetrics and Gynecology, Department of Obstetrics and Gynecology, University of California at Irvine, California College of Medicine, Orange, California; Chief, Division of Gynecologic Urology, Associate Medical Director of Gynecology, Department of Obstetrics and Gynecology, Women's Hospital, Memorial Hospital Medical Center, Long Beach, California

Dr. med. Eckhard Petri, M.D.

Department of Gynecology and Obstetrics, University of Mainz, Medical School, Mainz, Federal Republic of Germany

Stanislav Plevnik, D.Sc.

Senior Research Associate, Department of Biocybernetics, Automatics and Robotics, J. Stefan Institute, "E.Kardelj" University, Ljubljana, Ljubljana, Yugoslavia

Margaret Patricia Ramage, SR.N., RS.CN.

Senior Instructor in Human Sexuality, Department of Psychology, St. George's Hospital Medical School; Sexual Therapist, Adult Psychiatry (Sexual Dysfunction Clinic), St. George's Hospital, London, United Kingdom

Jack R. Robertson, M.D.

Clinical Professor, Department of Obstetrics and Gynecology, University of California at Irvine, Orange, California; Staff Member, Department of Obstetrics and Gynecology, Marian Medical Center, Santa Maria, California

Mike B. Siroky, M.D.

Associate Professor of Urology, Department of Urology, Boston University School of Medicine; Attending Physician, Department of Urology, University Hospital, Boston, Massachusetts

Elizabeth Margaret Gordon Stanley, M.R.C.S., L.R.C.P.

Senior Lecturer in Human Sexuality, Departments of Obstetrics and Gynecology and of Psychiatry, St. George's Hospital Medical School, London, United Kingdom

Stuart L. Stanton, F.R.C.S., M.R.C.O.G.

Senior Lecturer, Department of Obstetrics and Gynecology, St. George's Hospital Medical School, Cranmer Terrace, London; Consultant Obstetrician and Gynecologist, St. Helier Hospital, Carshalton, Surrey, United Kingdom

Dr. Thelma M. Thomas, M.R.C.P.

Member of MRC Clinical Scientific Staff, MRC Epidemiology and Medical Care Unit, Northwick Park Hospital, Harrow, Middlesex, United Kingdom

Michael John Torrens, M. Phil. Ch.M., F.R.C.S.

Consultant Neurological Surgeon to the Southwest Regional Health Authority, Frenchay Hospital, Bristol, United Kingdom

Professor Richard R. Trussell, O.B.E., M.B., Ch.M. F.R.C.O.G.

Professor Emeritus, Department of Obstetrics and Gynaecology, St. George's Hospital Medical School, London, United Kingdom

Mrs. T. Rashmi Varma, F.R.C.S., F.R.C.O.G., Ph.D.

Senior Lecturer, Department of Obstetrics and Gynaecology, St. George's Hospital Medical School; Consultant Obstetrician and Gynaecologist, Department of Obstetrics and Gynaecology, St. George's Hospital, London, United Kingdom

Alan J. Wein, M.D.

Chairman, Division of Urology, University of Pennsylvania School of Medicine; Chief, Division of Urology, Hospital of the University of Pennsylvania, Philadelphia, Pennsylvania

Hugh N. Whitfield, M.A., M.Chir., F.R.C.S.

Consultant Urological Surgeon, Department of Urology, St. Bartholomew's Hospital, London, United Kingdom

Peter H.L. Worth, M.A., M.B., B. Chir., F.R.C.S.

Honorary Lecturer, Institute of Urology and Faculty of Clinical Science, University College, London; Consultant Surgeon, University College Hospital and St. Peter's Hospitals, London, United Kingdom

Preface

Gynecological urology concerns the function and disorders of the lower urinary and genital tracts. There are close anatomical and functional links between the two, and diseases that affect one also commonly affect the other. In this era of subspecialization of the main branches of medicine, many obstetricians and gynecologists on both sides of the Atlantic feel that gynecological urology should be considered a subspeciality of obstetrics and gynecology. Implicit in this, however, is the belief that gynecological urologists should continue to understand and treat the patient as a whole.

It seems appropriate, therefore, to edit a book that brings together experts in gynecology, urology, and many other disciplines, who have a common interest in this subject, to present the varied facets that can be considered to be germaine to gynecological urology today.

I would like to acknowledge and thank all the authors who have gallantly agreed to contribute to this book. I would also like to thank consultant colleagues at St. George's and St. Helier Hospitals and many others who have referred clinical problems and who have acted as a stimulus for this book. My special thanks go to my past research fellows, Linda Cardozo, Paul Hilton, and Keith Hertogs, who have been a source of encouragement and provocative ideas. I have enjoyed the collaboration and support of Dr. John Williams, Director of Radiology, and his staff in the Department of Radiology at St. George's Hospital. Many of the illustrations and photographs have been expertly prepared by Stephen Norton, Educational Technology Unit at St. George's Hospital, and photographed by Andrew Rolland and Kenneth Cook, Department of Medical Photography at St. George's Hospital, and Brian Rice of St. Helier Hospital. I would also like to thank Sue Fomin, Julie Norwood, and Pauline Sharrocks for their painstaking efforts and patience in the typing and collation of the manuscript.

I would like to acknowledge and thank Karen Berger and Terry Van Schaik of The C.V. Mosby Company, whose professional advice and support for a rather errant author were always present.

Finally, I am grateful to my wife Ann and my daughters Claire, Talia, and Joanna, who have all helped in the preparation of this book. I hope that they will feel that the end product is worth the time I had to spend away from them.

Stuart L. Stanton

Contents

CLINICAL
GYNECOLOGIC
UROLOGY

part ONE

BASIC SCIENCE

chapter 1

Anatomy

JOHN ARTHUR GOSLING

EMBRYOLOGY
Formation of cloaca and external genitalia

In the presomite stage of human development the embryonic plate is composed initially of two layers of cells, the ectoderm and the endoderm. Approximately 15 days after fertilization, cells in the vicinity of the primitive streak differentiate and migrate between the other two layers. This intermediate layer forms the intraembryonic or secondary mesoderm and, in most regions, converts the bilaminar embryonic plate into a trilaminar structure. However, in the caudal part of the embryo adjacent to the attachment of the connecting stalk, the mesoderm fails to excavate between the ectoderm and endoderm. The persistence of this bilaminar region results in the formation of the cloacal membrane (Figure 1.1). (NOTE: A similar bilaminar arrangement persists cranially, forming the buccopharyngeal membrane.)

During the later presomite stage (17 to 19 days after fertilization) an endodermal outgrowth (the allantois) derived from the yolk sac adjacent to the cloacal membrane extends into the connecting stalk. As somites appear, the cranial and caudal extremities of the embryo bend ventrally to form the head and tail folds. During these changes part of the endoderm lining the yolk sac is carried into the cranial and caudal folds to form the foregut and the hindgut respectively. As the tail fold continues to enlarge, the connecting stalk and contained allantois are displaced onto the ventral aspect of the embryo. Similar positional changes affect the cloacal membrane, which moves from its original dorsal position to a ventral location at the base of the tail fold and connecting stalk. As a consequence of these growth changes, part of the endoderm of the newly developed hindgut forms the inner layer of the cloacal membrane. The hindgut undergoes slight dilatation and receives the termination of the allantois. At this stage of development, the cloaca can be defined as the part of the hindgut that lies caudal to the attachment of the allantois. Mesoderm that borders the cloacal membrane produces bilateral elevations, the urethral folds. The cranial ends of these folds form a midline elevation (the genital tubercle) that lies immediately ventral to the cloacal membrane (Figure 1.2). Subsequent growth of the urethral folds and genital tubercle leads to the formation of the labia minora and clitoris respectively.

Partition of cloaca

At about the time the mesonephric (wolffian) ducts reach the ventral part of the cloacal wall (28

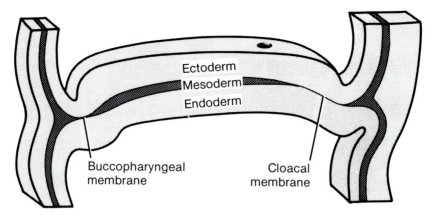

Figure 1.1 Embryonic plate approximately 1 day after fertilization. Ectoderm and endoderm are separated from each other by mesoderm except in region of buccopharyngeal and cloacal membranes. (Courtesy of Professor J.A. Gosling, Dr. J. Dixon, and Dr. J.R. Humpherson from Functional anatomy of the urinary tract, © Gower Medical Publishing, Ltd., 1982. London.)

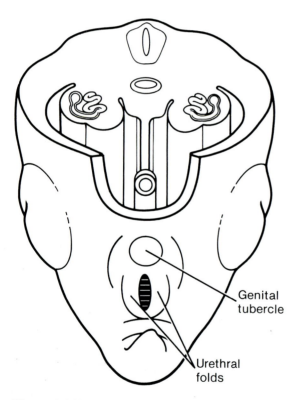

Figure 1.2 Ventral view of lower part of embryo. Relationship between genital tubercle, urethral folds, and cloacal membrane (crosshatched) is illustrated. (Courtesy of Professor J.A. Gosling, Dr. J. Dixon, and Dr. J.R. Humpherson from Functional anatomy of the urinary tract, © Gower Medical Publishing, Ltd., 1982. London.)

days, 4.5 mm crown-rump length), the cloaca begins to be partitioned into smaller dorsal and larger ventral compartments. This process is produced by the growth of a spur of tissue lying in the angle between the allantois and the cloacal opening of the hindgut. This septum, the urorectal septum, grows caudally into the lumen of the cloaca parallel to its dorsal wall (Figure 1.3). As the urorectal septum extends toward the cloacal membrane, the growth of the lateral attachments of the septum to the side walls of the cloaca outstrips its central part. Thus the caudal part of the septum forms a free margin, the concave edge of which is directed toward the cloacal membrane. Immediately before complete septation, a channel connecting the rectum and primitive urogenital sinus lies on the cranial aspect of the cloacal membrane. Persistence of this interconnection (called the cloacal duct) because of failure of further growth by the urorectal septum will result in a permanent fistula between the definitive rectum and urethra. On reaching the cloacal membrane, the urorectal septum divides it into a ventral urogenital membrane and a dorsal anal membrane. The urogenital opening (vestibule) is formed by the independent involution of the urogenital membrane, a process that is usually complete as early as the 18 mm crown-rump length stage. As indicated previously, the mesonephric ducts open into the ventral part of the lateral cloacal wall. The line of growth of the urorectal septum lies dorsal to these openings so that by the 8 mm crown-rump length stage, the ducts already ter-

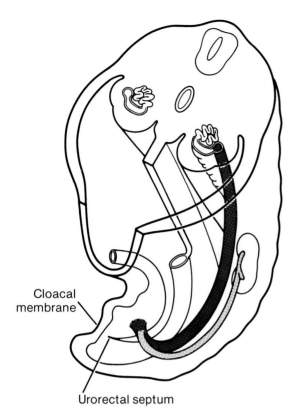

Cloacal
membrane

Urorectal septum

Figure 1.3 Embryo approximately 32 days (8 mm crown-rump length) after fertilization. Definitive ureter and mesonephric duct share a common opening into partially divided cloaca. Cloacal membrane and urorectal septum are indicated. Note that ureter has induced formation of kidney from metanephrogenic blastema. (Courtesy of Professor J.A. Gosling, Dr. J. Dixon, and Dr. J.R. Humpherson from Functional anatomy of the urinary tract, © Gower Medical Publishing, Ltd., 1982. London.)

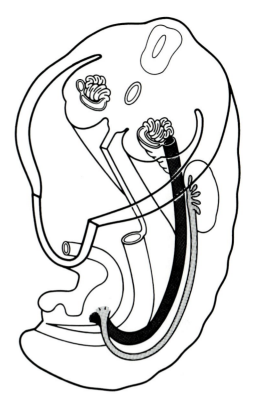

Figure 1.4 Further growth of urorectal septum has almost divided primitive cloaca in this diagram of embryo 34 days (11 mm crown-rump length) after fertilization. Ureteric and mesonephric ducts have just begun to separate. (Courtesy of Professor J.A. Gosling, Dr. J. Dixon, and Dr. J.R. Humpherson from Functional anatomy of the urinary tract, © Gower Medical Publishing, Ltd., 1982. London.)

minate in the urogenital sinus portion of the partially divided cloaca (Figure 1.3).

Formation of bladder and urethra

The primitive urogenital sinus receives the allantois and the terminal parts of the mesonephric ducts and is limited caudally by the urogenital membrane (Figure 1.4). These attachments in effect anchor the urogenital sinus so that, as the position of each structure changes with respect to the other, the sinus is caused to undergo corresponding changes in size and shape. Initially, the membrane lies at the root of the connecting stalk, and subsequent growth causes these two structures to separate from one another as the anterior abdominal wall develops. Since the urogenital sinus is fixed to the connecting stalk by the allantois, the ventral wall of the sinus must increase to accommodate

these positional changes. Failure of this process will give rise, after breakdown of the urogenital membrane, to the condition bladder exstrophy. As the posterior abdominal wall elongates, the mesonephric ducts draw the adjacent parts of the primitive urogenital sinus in a dorsal direction. That portion lying between the terminations of the mesonephric ducts and the allantois undergoes dilatation and forms the vesicourethral canal. It is from this structure that the female urinary bladder and urethra develop; the vestibule is formed solely from the remainder of the urogenital sinus.

Development of upper urinary tract

The ureter arises as an outgrowth of cells from the dorsomedial aspect of the mesonephric duct. As development proceeds, the mesonephric duct shortens because of the absorption of its distal extremity into the wall of the vesicourethral canal. The latter process continues with the result that the ureter opens separately into the vesicourethral canal through an orifice placed lateral to that of the mesonephric duct. Continued resorption results in further separation of the ureters and mesonephric ducts (Figure 1.5), and by 17 mm crown-rump length, a well-defined trigone can be distinguished. The ureters open into the bladder at the craniolateral angles of the trigone, whereas the mesonephric ducts, which remain closely apposed to each other, open into the definitive urethra (Figure 1.6). The terminal parts of the mesonephric ducts open on either side of a midline elevation (müllerian tubercle) produced by the fused paramesonephric ducts (see p. 8). In the absence of actively secreting testes, the mesonephric ducts regress to form the vestigial Gartner's ducts.

It is well known that ectopic ureters frequently open into the genital tract—an association attributable to the juxtaposition of these organ systems.

The free cranial end of the ureter grows first in a dorsal direction and then, at about 30 days (7.5 mm crown-rump length), it turns cranially and begins to excavate the caudal end of the nephrogenic cord. As it invades the cord, the ureter induces condensation of the constituent mesoderm to form the metanephrogenic blastema around the ureteric bud (Figure 1.3). The presence of the developing ureter is essential for this differentiation, and absence of the outgrowth is invariably associated with renal agenesis. Once formed, the metanephrogenic blastema in its turn induces changes in the ureter, causing it to expand and subdivide at its cranial end. During the period from 32 to 37 days (10 to 14 mm crown-rump length), continued growth of the ureter causes the metanephrogenic blastema to ascend dorsal to the mesonephros. The first partial division of the expanded cranial end of each ureteric bud occurs at 33 to 35 days (11 mm crown-rump length) and gives rise to two approximately equal branches (Figure 1.7). These branches undergo further subdivision, a process that continues until the time of birth and ultimately results in the formation of the renal pelvis, major and minor calyces, and the collecting ducts of approximately 1 million nephrons per kidney. The remaining parts of each nephron are derived from the mesoderm of the metanephrogenic blastema.

Development of ovary and genital tract

During the fifth week genital ridges make their appearance as thickenings of celomic epithelium

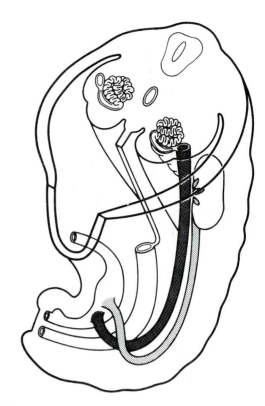

Figure 1.5 By thirty-seventh day (14 mm crown-rump length) cloaca has been divided into ventral urogenital and dorsal alimentary parts. In addition, kidney has continued to ascend and undergo medial rotation. (Courtesy of Professor J.A. Gosling, Dr. J. Dixon, and Dr. J.R. Humpherson from Functional anatomy of the urinary tract, © Gower Medical Publishing, Ltd., 1982. London.)

on the medial side of each mesonephros. These thickenings, together with the mesonephros, constitute the urogenital ridge (Figure 1.8). In developing from the undifferenitated gonad, the primordial germ cells of the ovary remain in a cortical position close to the epithelium covering the genital ridge. The primitive sex cords and the mesonephric tubules usually regress, leaving remnants, the epoophoron and the paroophoron.

During the eighth to the twentieth weeks the primordial germ cells undergo repeated divisions to provide the adult complement of oogonia. During this differentiation and growth the ovary gradually projects further into the celomic cavity and displaces the regressing mesonephros in a dorsolateral direction (Figure 1.4). The original attachment of the ovary to the mesonephros becomes reduced to a mesentery, the mesovarium. The displaced mesonephros consists of a dorsolateral portion with regressing tubules and a ventrolateral tubal part containing the mesonephric and paramesonephric (müllerian) ducts.

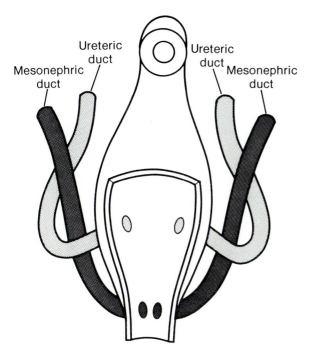

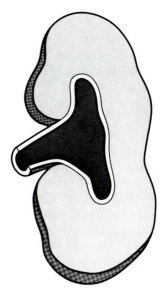

Figure 1.6 Urogenital sinus and associated ducts approximately 40 days (17 mm crown-rump length) after fertilization. Trigone lies between separated ureteric and mesonephric ducts. (Courtesy of Professor J.A. Gosling, Dr. J. Dixon, and Dr. J.R. Humpherson from Functional anatomy of the urinary tract, © Gower Medical Publishing, Ltd., 1982. London.)

Figure 1.7 First division of ureter into two approximately equal parts within mesoderm of metanephrogenic blastema. (Courtesy of Professor J.A. Gosling, Dr. J. Dixon, and Dr. J.R. Humpherson from Functional anatomy of the urinary tract, © Gower Medical Publishing, Ltd., 1982. London.)

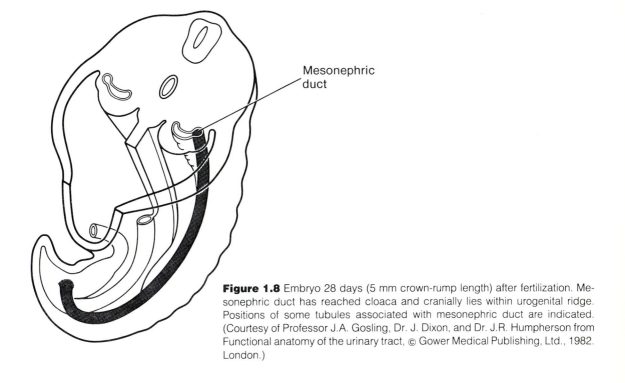

Figure 1.8 Embryo 28 days (5 mm crown-rump length) after fertilization. Mesonephric duct has reached cloaca and cranially lies within urogenital ridge. Positions of some tubules associated with mesonephric duct are indicated. (Courtesy of Professor J.A. Gosling, Dr. J. Dixon, and Dr. J.R. Humpherson from Functional anatomy of the urinary tract, © Gower Medical Publishing, Ltd., 1982. London.)

From the caudal end of the ovary a band of mesoderm extends across the abdominal wall into the inguinal region. This continues into the labia majora through the future inguinal canal and forms the gubernaculum. As the uterus develops, the gubernaculum becomes attached to the junction between the body of the uterus and the uterine tube. The cranial portion of the gubernaculum forms the ovarian ligament; the caudal part becomes the round ligament of the uterus.

Uterine tubes and uterus

During the sixth week the paramesonephric ducts develop as groovelike invaginations of the celomic epithelium. Each invagination extends caudally as a solid rod growing parallel to the mesonephric duct. The rod of epithelial cells acquires a lumen from the cranial end; the opening into the celomic cavity persists as the ostium of the uterine tube.

Each paramesonephric duct extends toward the midline and continues growing in a caudomedial direction to fuse with its contralateral counterpart. The caudal end of the fused ducts contacts the dorsal wall of the urogenital sinus to form an elevation, the müllerian tubercle. The fused paramesonephric ducts form the uterovaginal canal. Initially a septum divides the cavity, and this normally disappears during the twelfth week. The cranial part of the uterovaginal canal forms the uterus, the unfused portions of the paramesonephric ducts forming the uterine tubes (Figure 1.9). Many uterine abnormalities can be explained in terms of incomplete fusion of the paired paramesonephric ducts. The uterovaginal canal contacts the dorsal wall of the urogenital sinus at the müllerian tubercle and induces the formation of the distal portion of the vagina. Hence the proximal three quarters of the vaginal epithelium is derived from the mesoderm of the uterovaginal canal and the remainder from the endoderm of the urogenital sinus.

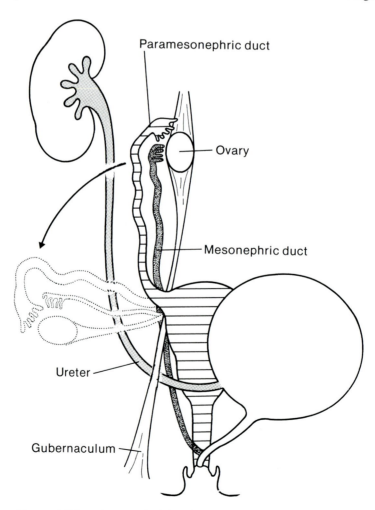

Figure 1.9 Developmental origins of definitive female urogenital organs.

FUNCTIONAL ANATOMY OF LOWER URINARY TRACT

The urinary bladder performs a dual function, acting at times as a passive reservoir allowing fluid to accumulate within its lumen and at others as a contractile organ actively expelling its contents into the urethra. In the following paragraphs the tissue components and, where appropriate, their neurological control are considered in each of these physiological states. Emphasis has been given to those aspects of structure and function that have particular importance in the clinical evaluation of the lower urinary tract.

Continence of urine

During continence the bladder acts as a reservoir and retains fluid as the result of forces acting on the urethra that produce an intraurethral pressure greater than the bladder pressure. From an anatomical standpoint the relatively short urethra, devoid of the passive elastic resistance offered by the prostate, places the female at a disadvantage. Nevertheless, several tissue components play a part in generating urethral resistance in the female and make either an active or a passive contribution. These components can best be described on a regional basis beginning at the bladder neck.

Bladder neck and proximal urethra. The role played by the bladder neck and adjoining urethra in the maintenance of continence has been the subject of considerable controversy. Recent data have, however, helped to dispel some previously held theories. Detrusor muscle does not extend into the proximal urethra (Figure 1.10) and cannot therefore play any part in apposing the walls of this part of the urinary tract. In the bladder neck region the smooth muscle is arranged so that most fibers are orientated longitudinally, and a so-called internal sphincter (analogous to the clearly defined male preprostatic sphincter) cannot be anatomically recognized. Consequently, it seems most unlikely that active smooth muscle contraction in the female bladder neck region can be considered an important factor in the continence of urine. Other than for a few fibers on the anterolateral aspect of its wall, the proximal urethra is also devoid of striated muscle cells. Furthermore, although the urethral epithelium is richly supplied with blood vessels, their

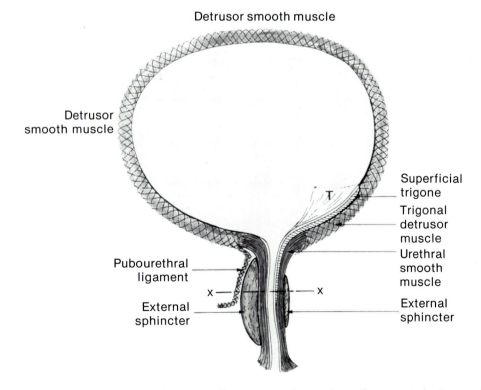

Detrusor smooth muscle

Detrusor smooth muscle

Superficial trigone

Trigonal detrusor muscle

Urethral smooth muscle

Pubourethral ligament

External sphincter

External sphincter

Figure 1.10 Adult female lower urinary tract. Detrusor smooth muscle continues posterior to superficial trigone and forms trigonal detrusor muscle. In bladder neck region detrusor is replaced by urethral smooth muscle, which extends throughout length of urethra. Pubourethral ligament extends toward pubis and lies anterior to urethral striated muscle of external sphincter. Plane of section illustrated in Figure 1.11 is shown x----x.

arrangement does not present any unusual or specialized features, and it seems doubtful that a vascular component contributes significantly to urethral resistance. However, the walls of the bladder neck and proximal urethra possess innumerable elastic fibers that are probably of particular importance in producing passive occlusion of the urethral lumen (Lapides, 1958). Consequently, these morphological findings considered in relation to urethral pressure measurements support the view that the passive elastic resistance offered by the urethral wall (in conjunction with intraabdominal pressures transmitted to the urethra) is the most important factor responsible for the closure of the bladder neck and proximal urethra in the continent female.

External urethral sphincter. The urethra contains within its walls striated muscle forming the external urethral sphincter. This muscle sphincter is thickest in the middle third of the urethra (Figure 1.11), corresponding to the zone where maximum urethral closure pressures are normally recorded. In this region striated muscle completely surrounds the urethra, although the posterior portion lying between the urethra and vagina is relatively thin. The striated muscle extends into the anterior wall of both the proximal and distal thirds of the urethra but is deficient posteriorly in these regions. The constituent striated fibers of the external sphincter are anatomically separate from periurethral muscle, are of small diameter (one third to one quarter of that of periurethral muscle), and are physiologically slow twitch (Gosling et al., 1981). In addition, the sphincter does not possess muscle spindles. Clearly, therefore, this striated muscle is well adapted to maintain tone over relatively long periods without fatigue and plays the most important active role in producing urethral occlusion at rest. This tonus is probably assisted by passive elastic forces similar to those occurring in the wall of the bladder neck and proximal urethra. However, it is not known whether the force exerted by the sphincter is maximum at all times between two consecutive acts of micturition or whether additional motor units are recruited during such actions as coughing and sneezing to enhance the occlusive force on the urethra during these events.

Periurethral muscle (levator ani). The medial parts of the levator ani muscles (sphincter vaginae) are related to (but structurally separate from) the urethral wall. These periurethral fibers consist of an admixture of large-diameter fast- and slow-

twitch fibers, together with numerous muscle spindles. Therefore, unlike the external sphincter, periurethral muscle possesses morphological features that are similar to other "typical" voluntary muscles. The levator ani plays an important part in urinary continence by providing an additional occlusive force on the urethral wall, particularly during events that are associated with an increase in intraabdominal pressure, such as coughing and sneezing. This urethral occlusive force in the female is maximum at a level immediately distal to the maximum urethral pressure generated by the external urethral sphincter. Thus, in addition to providing support for the pelvic viscera, the periurethral parts of the levator ani also play an important active role in the urethral mechanisms that maintain continence of urine.

Innervation of external sphincter and levator ani. The motor cell bodies of the nerves supplying the external urethral sphincter lie in the intermediolateral columns of the second, third, and fourth sacral segments of the spinal cord. The nerve fibers travel via the pelvic splanchnic nerves (Gil Vernet, 1968) (Figure 1.12) and *not* the pudendal nerves as often described. The clinical relevance of this arrangement is that pudendal blockade or neurectomy performed to reduce urethral resistance may not achieve the desired effect, since the motor innervation of the striated sphincter remains unaffected by these procedures. Furthermore, since the innervation of the levator ani is provided by the pudendal nerve, electromyogram (EMG) recordings obtained from this muscle should not be assumed to represent the activity of the adjacent less accessible and differently innervated striated muscle of the external sphincter. Accurate EMG evaluation of the external urethral sphincter can only be obtained by direct measurement of the activity of its constituent fibers.

Micturition

To enable fluid to flow along the urethra, it is necessary for the pressure in the urinary bladder to exceed that within the urethral lumen. Under normal circumstances, to initiate micturition a fall in urethral resistance immediately precedes a rise in pressure within the lumen of the bladder. This pressure rise is usually produced by active contraction of detrusor smooth muscle at the onset of micturition—an indication of the low resistance to flow offered by the relaxed urethra in normal individuals.

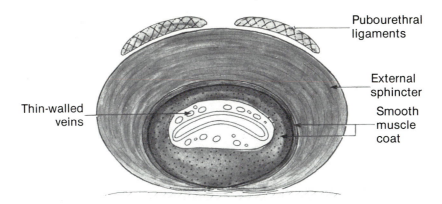

Figure 1.11 Horizontal section of female urethra in plane x----x shown in Figure 1.10. Pubourethral ligaments lie anterior to striated urethral muscle, which forms external sphincter. Smooth muscle coat consists of relatively minor outer circular part and much thicker inner longitudinal component. Lamina propria contains numerous prominent thin-walled veins.

Detrusor smooth muscle. The detrusor muscle coat consists of numerous interlacing bundles that form a complex meshwork of smooth muscle. This arrangement can be considered a functional syncytium and is ideally suited to cause reduction in all dimensions of the bladder on contraction of the intramural muscle coat. Thus the detrusor muscle is collectively involved during bladder contraction, and it is unnecessary to attach special significance to the precise orientation of individual bundles within the wall of the viscus.

Neurological control of detrusor smooth muscle. The cell bodies of preganglionic autonomic neurons involved in producing bladder contraction are located in the intermediolateral columns of the second, third, and fourth sacral segments of the spinal cord. These fibers travel in the pelvic splanchnic nerves (Figure 1.12) before synapsing on parasympathetic presumptive cholinergic neurons located within the vesical part of the pelvic plexuses and the wall of the bladder. These peripheral neurons supply numerous ''cholinergic'' nerve fibers that ramify throughout the thickness of the detrusor smooth muscle coat. Such is the extent of this innervation that most smooth muscle cells are individually supplied by cholinergic nerves. The profuse distribution of these motor nerves emphasizes the importance of the autonomic nervous system in initiating and sustaining bladder contraction during micturition.

Bladder neck and trigone. Detrusor smooth muscle is replaced in the bladder neck region by urethral smooth muscle, which possesses quite different histological, histochemical, and pharmacological properties. Such an arrangement throws

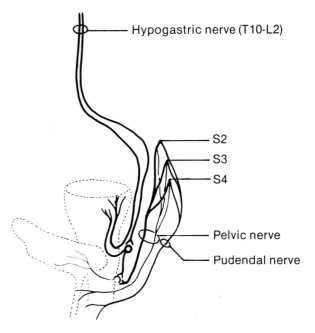

Figure 1.12 Peripheral autonomic innervation of female lower urinary tract and uterus. Note that pelvic nerve carries preganglionic fibers to pelvic plexus together with motor nerves that innervate striated muscle of external urethral sphincter.

considerable doubt on the concept that the bladder neck is actively opened by detrusor muscle passing in continuity through this region into the wall of the urethra (Wesson, 1920). Trigonal muscle has also been implicated in previous theories on the mechanism of bladder neck opening (Hutch, 1972). Although it extends through the bladder neck into the urethra, trigonal muscle forms only a minor component of the total muscle mass of this region.

Consequently, the part played by trigonal muscle in actively opening the bladder neck and proximal urethra is probably inconsequential. In view of the absence of any specialized anatomical arrangement, it is likely that the rise in vesical pressure at the onset of micturition is sufficient to overcome the passive resistance offered by the bladder neck and proximal urethra. In other words, fluid flow occurs when the pressure differential between the bladder and urethra is sufficient to overcome the elastic resistance of the bladder neck.

Pubourethral ligaments. Close to the midline a pair of fibromuscular ligaments firmly anchor the anterior aspect of the urethra to the posteroinferior surface of the symphysis pubis (Figure 1.10). These so-called pubourethral ligaments are continuous superiorly with the pubovesical ligaments. In addition to many collagen fibers, the pubourethral ligaments contain smooth muscle bundles (Zacharin, 1972). As with detrusor muscle proper, the muscle cells of the pubourethral ligaments receive a rich presumptive cholinergic innervation. From a functional standpoint these ligaments provide an important supportive role for the bladder neck and anterior aspect of the urethral wall. In addition, the smooth muscle component of the pubourethral ligaments may contract simultaneously with the detrusor muscle, thereby maintaining the position of the urethra relative to the pubis at the time of micturition.

External urethral sphincter. As previously noted, the external urethral sphincter is of particular importance in the mechanisms that maintain urinary continence. Immediately before the onset of micturition, the active tonus of the sphincter is reduced by central inhibition of its motor neurons. This inhibition is mediated by descending spinal pathways originating in higher centers of the central nervous system. Concomitantly, other descending pathways activate (either directly or via sacral interneurons) the preganglionic parasympathetic motor outflow to the urinary bladder. This central integration of the nervous system of the bladder and urethra is essential for normal micturition—it is well known that incoordination of bladder and urethral function is a frequent complication following lesions of the spinal cord.

REFERENCES

Gil Vernet, S. 1968. Morphology and function of vesico-prostato-urethral musculature. Treviso, Italy. Canova.

Gosling, J.A., et al. 1981. A comparative study of the human external sphincter and periurethral levator ani muscles. Brit. J. Urol. **53**:35-41.

Hutch, J.A. 1972. Anatomy and physiology of the bladder, trigone and urethra. London. Butterworth.

Lapides, J. 1958. Structure and function of the internal vesical sphincter. J. Urol. **50**:341-353.

Wesson, M.B. 1920. Anatomical, embryological and physiological studies of the trigone and neck of the bladder. J. Urol. **9**:279-317.

Zacharin, R.F. 1972. Stress incontinence of urine. New York. Harper & Row, Publishers, Inc.

chapter 2

Neurophysiology

MICHAEL JOHN TORRENS

Most forms of incontinence are due to a disturbance of neuromuscular function. Following many years of structurally based theories of the genesis of incontinence, this may seem an extreme view. However, it is becoming more and more realistic.

An understanding of physiology is of paramount importance in this field, but it is not easy to acquire. Much of the recorded information is related to animal experimentation, and the extrapolation from this to the human situation has led to a number of preconceptions that do not "hold water." Equally, the repeated quotation of the numerous reflexes that may be related to micturition, originally cited by Barrington (1914, 1931) and later by Kuru (1965), does little to aid understanding in the clinical context. It is better to observe and measure the activity of the human lower urinary tract and relate these observations to pathological situations. This chapter is designed as a simple, practical guide to the significance of the nervous system in incontinence. It is in no way a comprehensive treatise on neurophysiology.

MICTURITION CYCLE

Bladder filling and voiding may be represented as a pressure—volume loop (Figure 2.1). It can be divided into various components as described in the legend to the figure. In addition, the urethra goes through a related, reciprocal cycle of activity, remaining closed during bladder filling and opening during voiding.

The most important physiological properties of the lower urinary tract are to contract and relax at the right times. Abnormal function is best described in terms of the observed overactivity or underactivity of the appropriate parts of the system. Certain passive or mechanical factors may be relevant, but they are relatively less important.

Filling phase

The normal bladder fills without much significant rise in intravesical pressure. It has been suggested that during the collecting phase the bladder behaves as if it were a hollow sphere of passive viscoelastic material (Griffiths, 1980). This is an admittedly mechanical analogy. The process of ac-

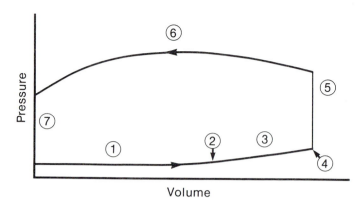

Figure 2.1 Micturition cycle represented as pressure/volume loop. Various phases, indicated by numbers, are as follows. *1*, Accommodation—partly because of intrinsic properties of bladder wall and partly because of unconscious nerve-mediated inhibition. *2*, First conscious sensation—mediated by tension receptors, since no rise in detrusor pressure is necessary. *3*, Postponement—cortical function, lost in certain cerebral lesions. *4*, Initiation of voiding—coordinated by pontine micturition centers. *5*, Isometric detrusor contraction—phase before flow starts, usually short in female. *6*, Sustained detrusor contraction—phase in which detrusor pressure remains relatively constant throughout voiding. *7*, Relaxation phase—majority of which occurs after voiding has ended. In some cases detrusor pressure may rise as bladder neck closes (isometric "aftercontraction").

commodation (Figure 2.1) to increasing volume may be related in part to the physical properties of the bladder wall, but it is also influenced by the intrinsic tone of the smooth muscle and by the extent of nerve-mediated inhibition.

The pressure/volume relationship during filling is usually observed by a cystometrogram. Under these circumstances the relationship is best described in terms of compliance. Compliance is defined as the change in volume for a given change in pressure and as a measurement is not subject to terminological confusion. The normal bladder is highly compliant over the usual volume range, and low compliance is abnormal.

Tone, or tonus, is a physiological concept that is best avoided in clinical practice. It is generally regarded as entirely myogenic, being uninfluenced by anesthesia or ganglionic blockade (Ruch, 1960). It cannot be assessed without inducing such an artificial paralysis of the detrusor. Tone contributes to compliance but is *not* equivalent to it. Terms such as hypertonic and hypotonic should not be used.

The urethra remains closed during the filling phase, the intraurethral pressure being greater than the intravesical pressure. Often, although not always, the electromyographic activity of the pelvic floor muscles increases as the bladder fills. It is assumed that the striated muscle of the urethral sphincter behaves similarly.

Voiding phase

The filling and voiding phases should always be considered together when classifying function. Toward the end of the filling phase the sensation of bladder fullness is consciously appreciated (during an artificial cystometrogram this may occur earlier). This sensation leads to the voluntary postponement of micturition, and sometime later an appropriate place and position for voiding is chosen. This is a function of the cerebral hemispheres.

A normal person should be able to initiate a void regardless of the volume in the bladder. The sequence of events is said to be a relaxation of the pelvic floor with descent of the bladder base and reduction of intraurethral pressure, followed by contraction of the bladder. In fact, the events are probably initiated at the same time, the bladder taking longer to respond. The bladder neck opens as the intravesical pressure exceeds the intraurethral pressure. Further than this, the control of bladder neck function in the female has not been identified.

The voiding contraction should be sustained until the bladder is empty. The intravesical pressure during voiding, which should be more or less constant, depends on the rate at which the urine can be discharged. In females with a high urine flow rate the pressure may be low. In some cases it may hardly change from the resting level, but this does not

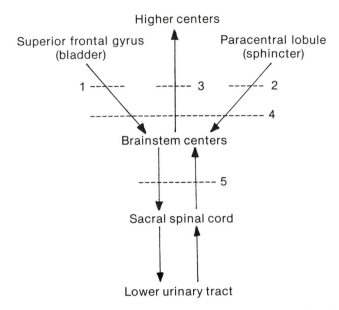

Figure 2.2 Simplified scheme of interaction of various levels of nervous system in micturition. Location of certain possible nervous lesions are denoted by numbers and explained in the following. *1,* Lesions isolating superior frontal gyrus prevent voluntary postponement of voiding. If sensation is intact, this produces urge incontinence. If lesion is large and destroys more of frontal lobe, there will be loss of social concern about incontinence. *2,* Lesions isolating paracentral lobule, often with hemiparesis, will cause spasticity of urethral sphincter and retention. This will be painless if sensation is also abolished. *3,* Pathways of sensation are not known accurately. In theory, isolated lesion of sensation above brainstem would lead to unconscious incontinence. Defective conduction of sensory information would explain enuresis. *4,* Lesions above brainstem centers lead to involuntary voiding that is coordinated with sphincter relaxation. *5,* Lesions below brainstem centers but above sacral spinal cord lead, after period of bladder paralysis, to involuntary "reflex" voiding that is not coordinated with sphincter relaxation (detrusor/sphincter dyssynergia).

mean that the bladder is acontractile, as will be discussed later.

The compliance of the urethra can be defined in a similar way to that of the bladder, as a function of the intraurethral pressure and urethral diameter. It is not a parameter that can be measured easily, but it is a useful concept. Urethral compliance during voiding depends on normal relaxation of the urethral sphincter muscle and on normal urethral distensibility. Decreased compliance may produce urethral obstruction, rare in the female. Increased compliance, producing a "baggy" urethra, may be relatively common. The pathological significance of this latter condition has not been fully appreciated.

CENTRAL NERVOUS SYSTEM INFLUENCES

The most important coordination centers for micturition are situated in the brainstem, especially the reticular formation of the pons. Various adjacent areas may have slightly differing functions, but the net effect is that the reticular formation contains the origin of the final common path for coordinated bladder and sphincter activity (Figure 2.2). The effects of neurological lesions are explained in the legend. The organization of the central nervous system in relation to micturition has been reviewed by Nathan (1976) and by Fletcher and Bradley (1978).

Sensation

Specialized sensory endings have not been identified peripherally in the lower urinary tract. Sensory nerves cannot be detected morphologically unless the dorsal root ganglia are ablated experimentally. It is likely that enteroceptive (pain, temperature, touch) sensation arises from unspecialized submucosal endings. Sensation is more acute in the urethra than in the bladder. Proprioceptive sensation from the bladder arises from receptors in the bladder wall whose discharge is proportional to the intramural tension (Iggo, 1955). Pacinian corpuscles have been found in the bladder of animals but not in humans. Proprioception from intramural urethral muscle must be mediated by unspecialized ending, since no muscle spindles have been seen. Spindles do exist normally in peri-urethral striated muscles of the pelvic floor.

Sensation is difficult to assess objectively. The integrity of sensory pathways can be checked by monitoring responses evoked from bladder or urethra (Rockswold and Bradley, 1977). An attempt has been made to quantitate the urethral sensory threshold by Powell and Feneley (1980). For the particular bipolar stimulating catheter that they used, the normal sensory threshold was between 4 and 8 mA. Abnormal thresholds correlated well with pathological states.

Clinical studies confirm that discriminatory sensation, both proprioceptive and enteroceptive, is mediated by the sacral roots S2 to S4. A vague sensation of pressure or discomfort can still be felt after complete cauda equina lesions or complete sacral anesthetic block. It is presumed that afferent nerves with the sympathetic component of the thoracolumbar nerves produce this poorly localized feeling.

There is some disagreement as to the exact location of sensory pathways centripetally in the spinal cord. Most of the information has been obtained from patients who have undergone anterolateral spinothalamic tractotomy. Nathan (1976) considers that all the intrinsic sensation from the bladder and urethra ascends in the spinothalamic tracts. Following section of these tracts, the only sensation retained by the patient is that of the imminence of micturition. This sensation arises from the posterior urethra and the pelvic floor and is mediated by the posterior columns. Some workers (Hitchcock, Newsome, and Salama, 1974) have shown that bladder sensation may be preserved after spinothalamic tractotomy even in the presence of bilateral sacral anesthesia. Some experiments in animals (Kuru, 1965) suggest that a proportion of a bladder's afferent nerves ascends in the medial part of the posterior column, but in general the spinothalamic tract is the most important conduit, and anterior spinal artery thrombosis will usually abolish bladder sensation.

Brain centers

Analysis of the effects of ablation, stimulation, and tumor growth in humans, reinforced by stimulation studies in animals, has revealed areas in the brain with an influence on micturition.

The cortical control of the lower autonomous centers has developed in proportion to the social significance of micturition in animals and humans. The cortical areas involved in humans are the superior frontal gyrus and the adjacent anterior cingulate gyrus. Lesions in these areas reduce or abolish both the conscious and unconscious inhibition of the micturition reflex. The bladder tends to empty at a low functional capacity. Sometimes the patient is aware of the sensation of urgency, and sometimes micturition may be entirely unconscious. The lesions may not, however, abolish the social distress caused by incontinence. These areas are supplied by the anterior cerebral and pericallosal arteries, spasm or occlusion of which produces incontinence. Similar symptoms occur in more generalized cerebral disorders such as atrophy and hydrocephalus. Localized lesions rather more posteriorly in the frontal regions, in the paracentral lobule, may produce retention rather than incontinence because of a combination of impaired sensation and spasticity of the pelvic floor.

Many areas of the subcortical brain have been described as influencing micturition. The highest autonomous centers probably exist in the septal and preoptic areas (Nathan, 1976) and project to the reticular formation of the brainstem, especially the pons, where neuronal activity has been found to be associated with detrusor contraction (Fletcher and Bradley, 1978). Other areas may also influence this pathway (Figure 2.3). Although it is tempting to localize brain function topographically into specific areas, this is manifestly not the way the brain works. Rather, there is a continuous interaction of inhibitory and facilitatory activity that finally summates to produce discharge of the appropriate motor neurons.

Efferent tracts

The descending influences from the reticular formation of the brainstem pass caudally in the reticulospinal tracts. Their location in humans is not entirely clear. The fibers may be laterally close to the insertion of the dentate ligaments (Hitchcock, Newsome, and Salama, 1974) or more medially between the lateral corticospinal tract and the intermediolateral gray matter of the spinal cord (Nathan, 1976). Kuru (1965) suggests that the fibers causing detrusor contraction and detrusor relaxation are separated into the lateral and ventral retic-

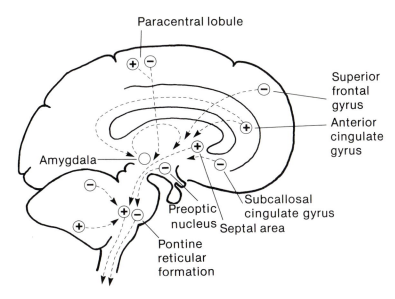

Figure 2.3 Simplified representation of cerebral areas involved in micturition. Multiplicity of interactions makes it easy to appreciate why subject should be left to the research physiologist. +, Facilitation; −, inhibition. (From Torrens, M.J., and Feneley, R.C.L. 1982. Rehabilitation and management of the neuropathic bladder. In Illis, L.S., Sedgwick, E.M., and Glanville, H.J., editors. Rehabilitation of the neurological patient. Oxford. Blackwell Scientific Publications.)

ulospinal tracts respectively, and in a similar way fibers activating and inhibiting the urethral sphincter mechanism may travel separately in the ventral and medial reticulospinal tracts.

Sacral micturition center

It is generally considered that the motor neurons supplying both the bladder and the sphincter mechanism are located in the gray matter of the sacral spinal cord. Certainly stimulation of this area can evoke a bladder contraction. Unlike the centers in the brain, this area cannot coordinate parasympathetic, sympathetic, and somatic activity. When it is disconnected from the brain, there is a tendency for bladder and sphincter contraction to occur together. This uncoordinated contraction is described as *dyssynergia*.

The initial effect of spinal transection is detrusor paralysis or areflexia. After a variable time, reflex detrusor contraction develops. This delay emphasizes the importance of supraspinal control of the sacral neurons. Transection presumably causes many synaptic sites of these neurons to be vacated, and the cells cannot discharge again until the sites have been reoccupied.

The parasympathetic preganglionic cell bodies innervating the bladder are found at the lateral edge of the anterior horn of the spinal cord. The cell bodies of the somatic efferent neurons to the urethral sphincter mechanism are situated anteromedially in a group in the anterior horn of the spinal cord. These cells seem to be relatively unaffected in, for example, motor neuron disease. They also seem to continue to function soon after spinal cord injury. The cells innervating the sphincter are located about one cord segment higher than those that supply the bladder.

PERIPHERAL INNERVATION

The possible organization of the peripheral nervous system in relation to the lower urinary tract is summarized in Figure 2.4 and explained in the legend. It is likely that this interpretation will require modification as knowledge advances.

Innervation of detrusor

The parasympathetic fibers in the anterior sacral roots (S2 to S4) are the principal motor supply to the detrusor. Shishito (1961) has demonstrated a few efferent fibers in the posterior roots. These preganglionic parasympathetic nerves run out through the sacral and pelvic plexuses to the autonomic ganglia lying both outside and inside the wall of the bladder. Here the majority of the final interaction between the sympathetic and parasympathetic systems occurs.

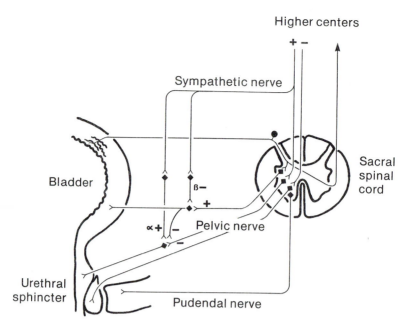

Figure 2.4 Summary of possible organization for peripheral nervous supply to lower urinary tract. Preganglionic parasympathetic fibers and postganglionic sympathetic fibers both synapse with ganglion cells close to, and within, bladder wall. Arrangement in relation to urethra may be morphologically similar but functionally different. Somatic nerve supply to intramural urethral striated muscle runs with pelvic nerve (and is vulnerable during pelvic surgery).

The human detrusor muscle is richly supplied with presumed cholinergic nerve fibers, the density of the innervation being such that the majority of muscle cells are individually supplied with nerves (Gosling, 1979). The density of this innervation may well be related to the fact that the detrusor is under direct nervous control, in many ways more like striated muscle than like the smooth muscle of the intestine. Because the ganglia from which these nerves arise are located close to the bladder, it is technically almost impossible to denervate the organ. The section of preganglionic nerve fibers will only "decentralize" the detrusor.

Unlike certain experimental animals, the human detrusor does not contain many noradrenergic nerves. Those that do exist are mainly around the bladder base. If the sympathetic nervous system does have a significant effect on the detrusor, this effect must take place at the ganglia, where a profuse sympathetic innervation has been observed.

Because sympathectomy caused no demonstrable difference in bladder function, the sympathetic nervous system was dismissed by some earlier workers as being responsible only for vasomotor activity. Learmonth (1931) showed that stimulation of the presacral nerve was followed by contraction of the region of the bladder neck and trigone. He also allowed himself to be injected with epinephrine (Adrenalin), which he noted caused a prolonged bladder relaxation. Sundin and Dahlstrom (1973) developed a technique for measuring bladder relaxation and showed that sympathetic (hypogastric nerve) stimulation produced an initial contraction that was followed by a prolonged relaxation of the bladder. The initial contraction could be reduced to one third by the administration of α-adrenergic blocking drugs, and the subsequent bladder relaxation was entirely abolished by β-adrenergic blocking drugs. In theory, therefore, there may be peripheral sympathetic inhibition of the bladder, which assists urine storage by accommodation. However, it is indisputably true that extensive lumbar sympathectomy in the human does not interfere with continence or obviously affect the ability to store urine, although retrograde ejaculation is well documented. It therefore appears that central inhibition is more important for accommodation than are the activities of the sympathetic nervous system.

Stimulation of parasympathetic fibers in the sacral nerves produces sustained detrusor contraction. The threshold for this response is higher than

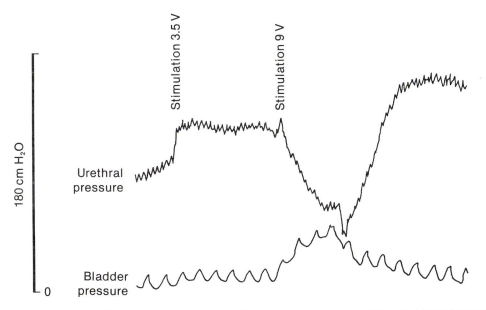

Figure 2.5 Urethral and bladder pressure responses to sacral nerve stimulation in female. Urethral response has two components, contraction at low voltage and relaxation at higher voltage. (From Torrens, M.J. 1978. Urol. Int. **33:**22-26.)

that required for an effect on the striated urethral sphincter (Figure 2.5), perhaps because the nerve fibers involved are of a smaller caliber. Conversely, section or ablation of sacral nerves will temporarily abolish activity of the detrusor. Activity tends to return, and the rate and extent of recovery are greater the more proximal the denervation and the less extensive the damage. It is also more likely for normal function to return if part of the nerve supply has been completely damaged (for example, single level sacral nerve ablation) than when all of the nerve supply has been partly damaged (for example, central prolapsed disk).

The physiological response to nerve damage depends on whether motor or sensory fibers are involved. If sensory fibers only are ablated, there is impairment of detrusor contractility, but the bladder pressure remains low. If motor fibers alone or motor and sensory fibers together are involved, the effect is a decrease in detrusor contractility but an increase in the bladder pressure with time. An explanation for this increased bladder pressure, and consequently decreased compliance, has been suggested by Norlen et al. (1976). Parasympathetic denervation leads (at least in the cat) to a very marked increase in the adrenergic innervation of

the bladder. This results in the conversion of the normal relaxation (β) response to hypogastric stimulation into a contractile (α) effect. Although no profuse vesical adrenergic innervation exists in humans, it is possible that a similar effect could occur at the peripheral ganglia.

Innervation of urethra

Noradrenergic sympathetic nerve fibers have been identified in relation to the male preprostatic urethra but are not common in the female urethra at all. In contrast, the dominant innervation of the longitudinal urethral smooth muscle in the female is cholinergic. Despite this discrepancy the majority of the measurable resting urethral pressure in both sexes can be abolished by the use of α-sympathetic blocking drugs. This has led to the conclusion that the functional innervation of the urethral smooth muscle is adrenergic, despite the fact that in the midurethra there is no significant adrenergic innervation demonstrable morphologically.

All this serves to emphasize how far apart the morphological and physiological studies are at present. It may be that there are α-adrenergic receptors on the urethral smooth muscle but no nerves to produce the transmitter. On the other hand, α-adrenergic effects may occur at the level of the pelvic ganglia. It is also likely that α-adrenergic blocking drugs have effects on neuromuscular transmission that are not conventionally recognized. Phenoxybenzamine (Dibenzyline) in particular is not a "clean" drug.

There are two groups of striated muscle fibers in relation to the urethra that Gosling (1979) calls intramural and periurethral. The intramural striated muscle is supplied by myelinated fibers from S2 to S4 that run with the pelvic nerve. This explains why it is not affected by pudendal block or pudendal neurectomy. The periurethral striated muscle is part of the pelvic floor and is supplied by the pudendal nerve, also S2 to S4.

The effect of stimulation on the urethra depends on the voltage applied (Figure 2.5). Experiments in humans (Torrens, 1978) have shown that the response to a low voltage is one of sphincter contraction. As the voltage is increased and another population of fibers perhaps stimulated, the urethra relaxes. This is a peripherally integrated and specific effect, since it occurs on stimulation of the distal end of a cut nerve and does not require any contemporaneous bladder contraction.

Transection of the sacral nerves, including parasympathetic and somatic fibers, reduces the voluntary contractility of the urethral sphincter but does not reduce the resting pressure unless the denervation is very extensive. It is further evidence for the importance of a sympathetic nervous effect.

NEUROTRANSMITTERS

It was shown in the previous section that some confusion exists when the functions of nerves and receptors are compared. The understanding of this aspect of physiology is very much in evolution. Some of the reasons why progress is slow in this field are given in the following list:

1. Individual nerves may produce more than one neurotransmitter.
2. Neurotransmitters may act on more than one type of receptor, producing different actions.
3. Neurotransmitters may act in different ways at the same receptor site according to their concentration.
4. Neurotransmitters may interact with one another.
5. There are considerable species differences in both neurotransmitters and receptors.

An example of fundamental controversy is the question of the principal neurotransmitter to the detrusor muscle. The postganglionic parasympathetic fibers are presumed to be cholinergic in that they are associated with identifiable acetylcholinesterase. However, if the transmitter is acetylcholine, it should be blocked by atropine. Although some species are atropine sensitive, perhaps the majority are not. This has led to the suggestion that another substance may be the principal neurotransmitter, or alternatively the receptors on bladder muscle may have more nicotinic than muscarinic characteristics, or perhaps some receptors are not accessible to freely circulating atropine. Suggestions for alternative transmitters include 5-hydroxytryptamine, purine nucleotides such as adenosine 5′-triphosphate (ATP), and prostaglandins. The problem has been reassessed recently by Nergardh (1981), who used field stimulation to activate muscle strips in vitro. As far as the cat bladder is concerned, it would appear that atropine does not inhibit contraction but rather enhances it, which makes acetylcholine an improbable neuromuscular transmitter. Quinidine, which is said to block receptors to ATP, had no effect, which suggests that purinergic nerves in the cat bladder are unlikely to be significant. On the other hand, indomethacin, which blocks prostaglandin synthetase, inhibited the effect of field stimulation. Selective antagonists of 5-hydroxytryptamine also produced inhibition of contraction. A great deal of parallel work is currently being performed on human muscle preparations, and a more reliable understanding of bladder neuropharmacology should soon emerge. Meanwhile, the unpredictable response to the pharmacotherapy of detrusor overactivity becomes less surprising.

DETRUSOR CONTRACTILITY

Detrusor muscle is a functional syncytium and also has an intramural nerve plexus. There are thus two ways in which the stimulus to contract can be propagated throughout the bladder wall. In some species a pacemaker center exists from which depolarization can spread. In humans there is no evidence for the existence of such a pacemaker. Observations of the response to direct electrical stimulation and the existence of the high density of innervation described earlier suggest that contraction is likely to be initiated at much the same time throughout the organ.

Differential contraction of the various areas of the bladder, especially around the base, has sometimes been postulated to explain the opening of the bladder neck. Such a phenomenon could be due to neuropharmacological effects. There may be no need to look for a morphological explanation. However, very little evidence has yet been collected, and this whole area remains obscure.

Bladder contraction depends both on an intact nerve supply and on the characteristics of the muscle. In a clinical context the bladder may be normal, overactive, or underactive. The typical manifestation of detrusor overactivity is the appearance of frequent, involuntary, but otherwise characteristic bladder contractions. These are associated typically with either a disturbance of nervous control or with an obstructed outflow tract. Conversely, detrusor underactivity is characterized by delayed, poorly sustained, or absent contraction, associated with neural depletion or muscle damage.

The contractility of detrusor muscle is judged usually from the pressure it can generate during voiding. However, this pressure depends not only on the integrity of nerve and muscle but also on the potential flow rate of urine. The higher the flow, the lower the pressure. Only if flow is zero is the pressure directly proportional to the strength of muscle contraction, which is then *isometric*. Griffiths (1980) has classified detrusor contractions as strong or weak (on the basis of the isometric detrusor contraction pressure) and as fast or slow (on the basis of the speed of shortening of muscle, extrapolated from a flow-related coefficient).

In clinical practice the more useful concept is that of the isometric detrusor contraction pressure (P_{det}iso). This can be measured by sudden occlusion of the urethra during micturition. Not all females may be able to contract the urethral sphincter voluntarily to achieve this. Mechanical pressure may be necessary. The detrusor pressure should rise when flow stops. If no such rise occurs, it may mean that a bladder has relatively impaired contractility, and retention will be more likely after any operation that raises urethral resistance.

REFERENCES

Barrington, F.J.F. 1914. The nervous mechanism of micturition. Q. J. Exp. Physiol. **8**:33-71.

Barrington, F.J.F. 1931. The component reflexes of micturition in the cat. Brain **54**:177-188.

Fletcher, T.F., and Bradley, W.E. 1978. Neuroanatomy of the bladder/urethra. J. Urol. **119**:153-160.

Gosling, J.A. 1979. The structure of the bladder and urethra in relation to function. In Turner-Warwick, R., and Whiteside C.G., editors. Symposium on clinical urodynamics. Urol. Clin. North Am. **6**:31-38.

Griffiths, D.J. 1980. Urodynamics. Bristol. Hilger.

Hitchcock, E., Newsome, D., and Salama, M. 1974. The somatotopic representation of the micturition pathways in the cervical cord of man. Br. J. Surg. **61**:395-401.

Iggo, A. 1955. Tension receptors in the stomach and urinary bladder. J. Physiol. **128**:593-607.

Kuru, M. 1965. Nervous control of micturition. Physiol. Rev. **45**:425-494.

Learmonth, J.R. 1931. A contribution to the neurophysiology of the urinary bladder in man. Brain **54**:147-176.

Nathan, P.W. 1976. The central nervous connections of the bladder. In Williams, D.I., and Chisholm, G., editors. The scientific foundations of urology. London. Heinemann Medical Books.

Nergardh, A. 1981. Neuromuscular transmission in the corpus-fundus of the urinary bladder. Scand. J. Urol. Nephrol. **15**:103-108.

Norlen, L., et al. 1976. The adrenergic innervation and adrenergic receptor activity of the feline urinary bladder and urethra in the normal state and after hypogastric and/or parasympathetic denervation. Scand. J. Urol. Nephrol. **10**:177-184.

Powell, P.H., and Feneley, R.C.L. 1980. The role of urethral sensation in clinical urology. Br. J. Urol. **52**:539-541.

Rockswold, G.L., and Bradley, W.E. 1977. The use of evoked electromyographic responses in diagnosing lesions of the cauda equina. J. Urol. **118**:629-631.

Ruch, T.C., 1960. Central control of the bladder. In Handbook of physiology. vol. 2, Washington, D.C., American Physiological Society.

Shishito, S. 1961. Experimental studies on the innervation of the urinary bladder. Urol. Int. **12**:254-269.

Sundin, T., and Dahlstrom, A. 1973. The sympathetic innervation of the urinary bladder and urethra in the normal state and after parasympathetic denervation at the spinal root level. Scand. J. Urol. Nephrol. **7**:131-149.

Torrens, M.J. 1978. Urethral sphincteric resources to stimulation of the sacral nerves in the human female. Urol. Int. **33**:22-26.

Torrens, M.J., and Feneley, F.C.L. 1982. Rehabilitation and management of the neuropathic bladder. In Illis, L.S., Sedgwick, E.M., and Glanville, H.J., editors. Rehabilitation of the neurological patient. Oxford. Blackwell Scientific Publications.

chapter 3

Mechanism of continence

TAGE HALD

Continence of urine is generally thought of by nonmedical people and also by many physicians as a simple, natural function. When studying incontinent patients, however, one quickly learns that urinary continence is a complex matter and that the mechanisms of continence are only partly understood.

The prerequisite of urinary continence is the existence of a higher intraurethral pressure than bladder pressure, or to put it slightly differently, the urethral closure pressure must be positive between voidings. To function properly, the lower urinary tract must be an intact local anatomy. Equally important, however, is the integrity of the centers and pathways in the nervous system that coordinate the action of smooth and striated muscle in the lower urinary tract and pelvic floor.

Such a complex system can best be described by breaking it down into factors known to affect continence. The reader must realize that in the normal individual continence factors act in concert, although they are probably not a equal importance and are certainly not all operative at the same time. The continence factors to be described here are (1)

the bladder factors, comprising bladder capacity and detrusor reflex control; (2) the bladder neck factor with its intrinsic and extrinsic elements; (3) the urethral smooth muscle factor; (4) the external sphincter factor; (5) the inner urethral factor; (6) the pressure transmission factor; (7) the pelvic floor factor; and (8) the coordination taking place in the central nervous system.

BLADDER FACTORS

There are two interrelated aspects of bladder storage function that are important to continence—bladder wall distensibility and detrusor reflex control. Both factors influence bladder capacity.

Wall distensibility

With a daily diuresis of 1200 ml, for example, the functional bladder capacity must be 300 ml to allow the person to get along with only four voidings a day. Capacity may be reduced by a change in the *viscoelasticity* of the bladder wall (Coolsaet et al., 1975), for example in tuberculosis, radiation, and interstitial cystitis. With progressive shrinking, frequency occurs, and in the terminal stage frequency may be so pronounced that a true incontinence situation is established. Shrinking of the bladder causes bladder wall tension to increase abnormally on filling. Frequently, such patients therefore also have a problem of detrusor hyperreflexia, which contributes further to the frequency-urgency situation. The functional bladder capacity may also be reduced by the presence of large amounts of residual urine. This situation is always a sign of detrusor insufficiency, which again may be due to obstructive or neurological disease.

Detrusor reflex control

Detrusor reflex control depends on intact frontal cortical centers; an intact bladder stem center; intact inputs from the cerebellum, thalamus, limbic system, and several other areas; and also undamaged pathways between these centers and the bladder. Detrusor reflex control is partly involuntary and partly voluntary. The reflex is best described as consisting of a neural loop extending from the bladder wall sensory receptors through the pelvic nerves and spinal cord to the brainstem reticular formation, and from there back through the spinal cord, the intermediolateral cell masses in the sacral cord, and the parasympathetic nerve fibers in the

pelvic plexus to the detrusor muscle cells. The adequate stimulus is stretch of the bladder wall (proprioception) (Figure 3.1). This loop is again under the control of a supraspinal loop (actually several loops [Bradley et al., 1976]) (Figure 3.2), the net effect of which is inhibitory to the detrusor. The loops mature between 2 and 4 years, and the persistence of infantile uncontrolled bladder function beyond the age of 5 years is termed enuresis.

The bladder proprioceptive input is influenced by exteroceptive impulses from the urinary tract itself (cystitis, urethritis), the genital tract (vaginitis), and the skin (for example, cold exposure). The general effect is enhancement of the detrusor reflex with a tendency to instability. Damage to the suprasacral part of the nervous system usually causes detrusor hyperreflexia (detrusor instability) and therefore often the symptoms of frequency, urgency, and urge incontinence. Damage to the infrasacral part of the detrusor reflex loops causes areflexia with a tendency toward retention and overflow incontinence, voiding being dependent on an increase in abdominal pressure.

The cause of the frequency-urgency urge incontinence syndrome is often obscure. This is especially the case in many adult women. The most

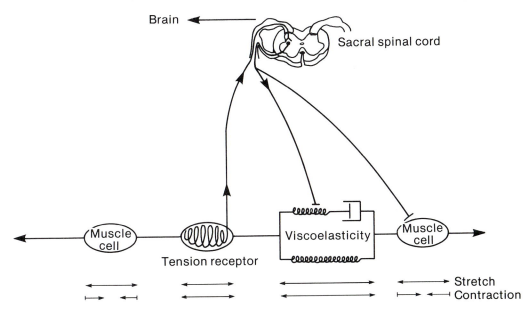

Figure 3.1 Bladder wall elements are interrelated. Muscle cells are connected in series with tension receptors, which are therefore stimulated both by passive stretch of bladder wall and by active contraction of detrusor. Detrusor muscle cells are also part of viscoelastic elements of bladder, and their contractile state influences stiffness—distensibility—of organ and also perception of desire to void via tension receptors. Interdependence of contractility, proprioception, and viscoelasticity explains some features of both hyper- and hypoactive bladder conditions.

Loop 1

Loop 2

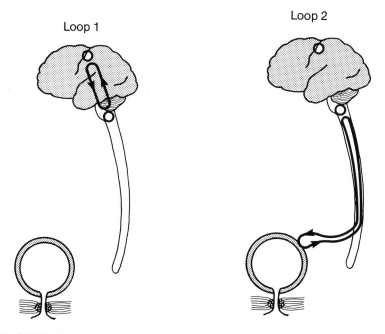

Figure 3.2 Bradley's loop *1* controls loop *2*. Both are essential for detrusor reflex control.

Inhibition

Stimulation

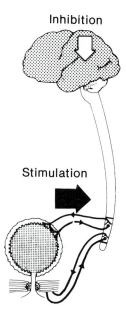

Figure 3.3 Detrusor instability may be due to either increased sensory input from bladder (possibly also urethra, vagina, and pelvic floor) or defective cerebral inhibition.

striking finding is detrusor instability (motor urgency), whereas the finding of a stable detrusor is less frequent (sensory urgency). The most plausible cause of idopathic detrusor instability is a disturbed balance between the sensory input to the central nervous system and the supraspinal inhibition (Figure 3.3). An increased sensory input may be present with local inflammatory and degenerative urogenital organ changes, but in most cases this cannot be confirmed by a clinical investigation. Some authors believe that the influx of urine into the proximal urethra during abdominal straining may set up the reflex.

A defective supraspinal inhibition is probably more often in question. This hypothesis seems to be supported by the frequently beneficial effect of psychotherapy, bladder training, and biofeedback therapy. Patients with detrusor instability may be able to influence detrusor activity by contracting the pelvic floor and striated sphincter and thus stay dry. This negative feedback from pudendal to pelvic nerve innervation is, however, often lost when the supraspinal innervation is damaged.

Detrusor areflexia is often associated with an incontinence manifesting itself when the patients exercise physically (because of increase in abdominal pressure), or it may be continuous (because of a simultaneous urethral ''denervation''). Such patients also have a capacity problem caused by re-

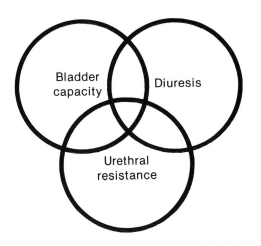

Figure 3.4 Three important factors in geriatric incontinence.

sidual urine that occupies most of the cystometric capacity, leaving the functional capacity quite small.

With increased age the bladder factors may suffer, especially because of the development of detrusor hyperreflexia, but it should be borne in mind that numerous elderly people have an inverse diuresis caused by the nocturnal excretion of fluid retained during the daytime. This may be the cause for nocturia and nocturnal incontinence, and the situation is aggravated when detrusor hyperreflexia and urethral incompetence are also present (Figure 3.4).

The importance of the detrusor reflex makes the cholinergic transmission in the pelvic ganglia and the neuromuscular junction crucial. Transmission may be blocked by anticholinergics, but oral administration is often inadequate in this respect. Other transmitters like norepinephrine (noradrenaline), prostaglandins, vasoactive intestinal peptide, and substance P may play a role but are as yet not fully investigated.

BLADDER NECK FACTORS

Continence is normally maintained at the bladder neck level. This is true in both sexes even under the most massive abdominal straining. The urethral closure pressure profile seems to contradict this, but measurements of intraurethral pressure during straining (Constantinou and Gowan, 1981) and radiography (Olesen and Walter, 1977) point unequivocally to the bladder neck as the physical barrier of most importance. The bladder neck factor is a complex one, consisting of intrinsic and extrinsic elements.

Intrinsic elements

The bladder neck opens in response to detrusor contraction because of traction by the detrusor muscle fibers (Lapides, 1958). Passive closure seems to be due to an interplay between abundant elastic connective tissue and bladder neck smooth muscle. In the male a circular α-adrenergic innervated preprostatic sphincter can be localized, but this has not been observed in the female (Gosling, 1979). Therefore the muscular element seems to play a minor role in the female.

Extrinsic elements

The bladder neck is suspended by ligaments attached to the pubic bone and the levator fascia (see Pelvic Floor Factor). They keep the bladder neck in a high position, thereby creating ideal circumstances for the abdominal pressure to be transferred to the urethral lumen (see Pressure Transmission Factor). These extrinsic elements of the bladder neck closure mechanisms play extremely important roles in the maintenance of continence.

URETHRAL SMOOTH MUSCLE

Urethral closure pressure profilometry, with blocking and stimulation with drugs active on the urethral smooth muscle, has shown that intraurethral pressure depends on a stimulatory α-adrenergic innervation. Patients with Shy-Drager syndrome have a tendency toward a low urethral closure pressure and genuine stress incontinence, indicating the importance of the sympathetic innervation. Also, prostaglandin $F_{2\alpha}$ and estrogens seem to enhance urethral closure. The exact importance of the urethral smooth muscle can hardly be ascertained by pharmacological studies alone. If the bladder neck mechanism is intact, urethral smooth muscle should play a minor role. The results of treating genuine stress incontinence in the female with, for example, α-adrenergic stimulating agents (Ek, 1977) seem to support this hypothesis, since the effect is marginal.

EXTERNAL SPHINCTER

The striated urethral sphincter participates in passive as well as active urinary continence. Massive curarization in the experimental animal and pudendal nerve resection in the human result in a reduction of urethral closure pressure by approximately one third. It is therefore fair to conclude that the striated sphincter, even in the female, contributes to passive, unconscious urethral closure, although its most important function is its immediate reflex contraction in response to increased abdominal pressure. It may—by a conscious or unconscious contraction—prevent leakage when the detrusor contracts, and it may also be an aid when the bladder neck mechanism fails. In up to 85% of urge-incontinent females the normal protection by the external sphincter is lost, since it relaxes in response to detrusor contraction. This is also true in many patients with supraspinal disease (for example, cerebrovascular disease and multiple sclerosis). In this context the urge-incontinent situation is actually the equivalent of a coordinated voiding act that is released at an inappropriate time. The external sphincter may have a more complex innervation than previously believed, a portion being innervated through the pelvic plexus and another through the pudendal nerves. A contrary view is expressed by Gosling (see Chapter 1), who believes that the pudendal nerve plays no part in this innervation. It is also possible that presynaptic α-adrenergic innervation plays a role in its function. The external sphincter is hardly crucial to the maintenance of continence in the female, but if other continence factors are lost, it may be of extreme importance. In the male the external sphincter along with infraprostatic smooth muscle constitutes the distal sphincter mechanism (Turner-Warwick and Whiteside, 1970), which is essential to continence after prostatic surgery. Lesions of both the smooth and the striated elements may be responsible for genuine stress incontinence developing after prostatectomy.

INNER URETHRAL FACTOR

For a tube to occlude perfectly it is important that the inner walls be soft and compressible (Zinner, Sterling, and Ritter, 1980). The urethral mucosa and the subepithelial vascular bed act to provide these conditions. Both are dependent on estrogens for their trophic state. This fact may explain why genuine stress incontinence so often becomes clinically manifest at the time around the menopause. Whenever a postclimacteric woman exhibits signs of vaginal atrophy, there is reason to believe that the urethral mucosa and vascular bed suffer the same fate.

PRESSURE TRANSMISSION FACTOR

When a person raises the intraabdominal pressure by coughing, sneezing, lifting, and the like, the intravesical pressure also rises. To maintain a pressure gradient between the bladder and urethral lumen, the intraurethral pressure must rise proportionally. In the healthy person this is always the case. This function can only be effective when the bladder neck is within the abdominal pressure zone, that is, is suspended sufficiently high (see Pelvic Floor Factor). When the urethra and bladder neck are infiltrated with fibrous tissue, as after multiple surgical procedures, the pressure transmission may fail. It is difficult to separate the effects of direct pressure transmission and those of a reflex external sphincter or pelvic floor contraction, but there is no doubt that pressure transmission is jeopardized when the bladder neck slides down either anteriorly or posteriorly and thereby out of the abdominal pressure zone (Enhörning, 1961). The results of bladder neck relocation surgery indicate that pressure transmission is indeed of extreme importance to continence. This is especially the case when retropubic surgery is employed, because no attempt is being made to reconstruct the pelvic floor or the urethra with such methods.

PELVIC FLOOR FACTOR

The bladder neck mechanism and also the pressure transmission factor cannot be operative when the pelvic floor and its ligamentous system is slackened. The bladder neck is suspended by two ligamentous slings that tend to keep it within the abdominal pressure zone (Olesen and Gray, 1976).

One sling is composed of the pubourethral ligaments running from the posterior aspect of the pubic symphysis to the fibromuscular nodes lateral to the bladder neck and uniting behind the vagina.

The other is of less substance, but it is evident on dissection of the pelvic floor. It appears as ligamentous strands in the levator fascia, extending into the fibromuscular nodes lateral to the bladder neck, which are again united by the precervical arc, a fibrous network located at the anterior bladder neck. The backward-upward pull exerted by this loop is easily seen on lateral voiding cystourethrograms as a marked anterior shelf. Disappearance of this shelf gives an 85% chance of the patient's having genuine stress incontinence (Figure 3.5).

The posterior suspension defects produce a variety of symptoms, notably voiding difficulties with the use of abdominal strain and also urge and stress incontinence. These are two distinctly different types of posterior suspension defects. The trigonocele denotes a herniation of the bladder base be-

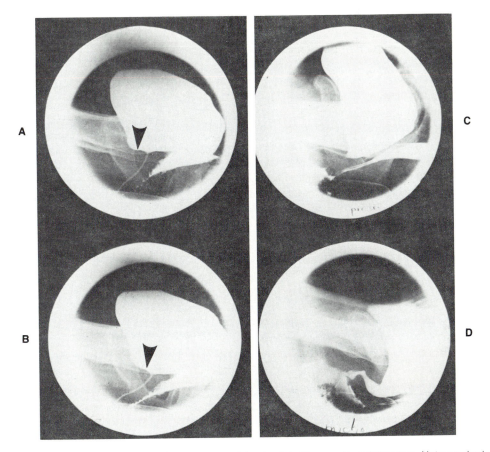

Figure 3.5 A, Normal bladder neck as seen on lateral micturition cystourethrograms. Note marked anterior shelf *(arrow)*. **B,** Bladder neck disappears during coughing. Typical case of anterior suspension defect of bladder neck. **C,** Case of trigonocele. Bladder base herniation between urethra and vagina is pronounced. **D,** Typical teapot deformity as seen in posterior bladder descent.

tween the two levators, the bladder neck being in place (Figure 3.5, *C*). Obstructive symptoms are prominent. The posterior bladder descent is seen as the typical teapot deformity on the lateral voiding cystourethrogram (Figure 3.5, *D*). Mixed incontinence and obstruction dominate, most patients voiding by abdominal straining. Since the ligamentous bladder neck apparatus is intimately related to the levator muscles, it is not surprising that pelvic floor exercises can be effective in relieving genuine stress incontinence in some patients.

CENTRAL NERVOUS SYSTEM COORDINATION

The preceding sections described the local factors important to urinary continence, but it has been emphasized constantly that central coordination is important (see Innervation of Detrusor in Chap-

ter 2). The supraspinal innervation secures voluntary coordinated voiding. Lesions at this level (for example, multiple sclerosis and cerebral hemorrhage) tend to produce detrusor hyperreflexia, often with inappropriate relaxation of the pelvic floor, resulting in massive incontinence. The spinal innervation is the target in cord lesions. Detrusor hyperreflexia associated with involuntary external sphincter contraction is customary, giving rise to reflex incontinence when the sphincteric contraction gives way during relaxation of the detrusor.

Lesions of the peripheral detrusor motor and sensory innervation result in detrusor areflexia with accumulation of residual urine. Such lesions dissociate the lower urinary tract from the central nervous system. The detrusor and urethra are hypersensitive to transmitter substances like cholinesters and norepinephrine. The typical examples are patients who have had radical hysterectomy and lymph node dissection and also patients who have had abdominoperineal excision of the rectum. Lesions of the peripheral pelvic floor and striated sphincter innervation produce a situation that favors decreasing resistance and therefore also a tendency to genuine stress incontinence.

However, few neurological lesions are exactly alike, and some features may differ. There is still insufficient experience to predict exactly what the urinary problem will be with a specific lesion. Such a development awaits further refined studies, and the picture will hardly be easier to comprehend but will rather prompt the development of a subspeciality: neurourology.

REFERENCES

Bradley, W.E., et al. 1976. Neurology of micturition, J. Urol. **115**:481-486.

Constantinou, C.E., and Gowan, D.E. 1981. Contribution and timing of transmitted and generated pressure components in the female urethra. In Zinner, N., and Sterling, A. Female incontinence. New York. Alan R. Liss.

Coolsaet, B.L.R.A., et al. 1975. Viscoelastic properties of the bladder wall. Urol. Int. **30**:16-26.

Ek, A. 1977. Innervation and receptor functions of the human urethra. Thesis. Studentlitteratur. Lund.

Enhörning, G. 1961. Simultaneous recording of intravesical and intraurethral pressure: a study of urethral closure in normal and stress incontinent women. Acta Chir. Scand. Suppl. **276**:1-68.

Gosling, J. 1979. The structure of the bladder and urethra in relation to function. Urol. Clin. North Am. **6**:31-38.

Lapides, J. 1958. Structure and function of the internal vesical sphincter. J. Urol. **80**:341-353.

Olesen, K.P., and Grau, V. 1976. The suspensory apparatus of the female bladder neck. Urol. Int. **31**:33-37.

Olesen, K.P., and Walter, S. 1977. Colpocystourethrography. Dan. Med. Bull. **24**:96-101.

Turner-Warwick, R.T., and Whiteside, C.G. 1970. Investigation and management of bladder neck dysfunction. In Riches, Sir E., editor: Modern trends in urology. London. Butterworth.

Zinner, N.R., Sterling, A.M., and Ritter, R.C. 1980. Role of inner urethral softness in urinary incontinence. Urology **16**:115-117.

ACKNOWLEDGMENT

Professor A.M. Sterling, Ph.D., provided useful criticism of this manuscript.

chapter 4

Pharmacology: theory

DONALD R. OSTERGARD

The clinical importance of pharmacology in gynecological urology has only recently been recognized. Drugs that affect the neuromuscular junctions of both smooth and skeletal muscles or the muscles directly now assume considerable value for the clinician who wishes to pharmacologically treat the lower urinary tract. Comprehensive clinical application of basic pharmacological principles is the goal of any practitioner who deals with the incontinent female. Alteration of the type of drugs or the dosages used for medical indications may cure or decrease a patient's incontinence, so that unnecessary surgery may be avoided. It is the goal of this chapter to review the basic pharmacological theory that pertains to the use of drugs to alter lower urinary tract function in the female.

NEUROTRANSMITTERS OF AUTONOMIC NERVOUS SYSTEM

In the ganglia of the autonomic nervous system, acetylcholine is the neurotransmitter for both the sympathetic (adrenergic) and the parasympathetic (cholinergic) nervous systems. This agent is the product of the combination of choline with acetate in the presence of coenzyme A and choline transferase. It is stored in clear vesicles in the terminal buttons of the neurons. The excitatory impulse in the preganglionic neuron or the postganglionic cholinergic neuron causes an increase in the membrane permeability for calcium, which causes calcium influx into the nerve ending. Acetylcholine is then liberated into the synaptic cleft by exocytosis. During this process the acetylcholine vesicle moves to the cell membrane, which opens to free the neurotransmitter into the synaptic cleft. After crossing the cleft, it alters the membrane potential of the opposite neuron and causes its excitation. Its effect is very short lived because of the almost instantaneous hydrolysis of acetylcholine by acetylcholinesterase to choline plus acetate.

The neurotransmitter for the postganglionic sympathetic neuron is norepinephrine (noradrenaline). Its production is more complicated and involves the hydroxylation of tyrosine to form dopa that is then decarboxylated to form dopamine. Dopamine is subsequently hydroxylated to form norepinephrine. Its destruction is accomplished by several routes. Most is absorbed by the nerve fiber itself. Some diffuses into the circulatory system, and some is enzymatically destroyed.

Both acetylcholine and norepinephrine react with a cell membrane receptor substance. The exact character of the receptor is not resolved, but it is probably a protein or lipoprotein. It alters the permeability of the cell wall and thereby changes the membrane potential. Generally conduction is only in one direction.

SMOOTH MUSCLE CHARACTERISTICS

Smooth muscle is unique in several aspects. It has the capacity to contract when stretched in the absence of any extrinsic nervous impulses. The actual stretching causes an alteration in membrane potential that increases the tone of the muscle. This tone gradually decreases until the actual muscle tension may be less than it was originally before stretching. This property of smooth muscle makes it impossible to correlate tension with length, since there is no resting length, just varying degrees of tone and inherent plasticity.

Smooth muscle also has the capability of undergoing a stress-induced relaxation or, as in the case of the urinary bladder, a volume-induced relaxation. This is due to the capacity of smooth muscle to change length without much change in tension of the muscle fibers. If the process is gradual enough, no intraluminal pressure increase occurs, as is seen with antegrade or retrograde fill cystometry.

EFFECTS OF STIMULANTS ON SMOOTH MUSCLE

Smooth muscle is basically of two types with regard to action potentials. There are those that generate action potentials and those that normally do not (Figure 4.1). The stimulant substance initially combines with the receptor in the cell membrane of the smooth muscle. Several events may follow to cause an alteration in the action potential of the smooth muscle membrane. The effect may be direct and cause alteration in the membrane without any intermediary action (pathway 1). It may induce various biochemical changes that then cause the opening of receptor-operated channels for calcium (pathway 2). The influx of calcium into the cell then alters the partial pressure of calcium and also its ionic concentration within the cell (pathway 3). The altered calcium composition within the cell then causes an increase in the tension of the intracellular contractile proteins either directly (pathway 3) or in a previous depolarization of the membrane (pathway 4). Alternative routes for affecting the tension of the contractile proteins involves the release of receptor-bound calcium and other biochemical changes (pathway 5). In the case of those smooth muscles that do not normally generate action potentials, changes in metabolism then occur. For those smooth muscles that usually generate action potentials, an increase in the frequency of action potentials may occur (pathway 6) in addition to a direct effect of the calcium influx on the contractile protein tension (pathway 3 on the left). This causes an increase in the frequency of contractions. Pathways 1, 3, and 6 ultimately display changes in metabolism resulting from the stimulated muscle contraction.

Although a variety of mechanisms may be ultimately responsible for the contraction of a smooth muscle cell, the effects of calcium influx predominate in the process. Alterations in sodium concentrations by changes in cell membrane permeability are probably also important, but this is less clearly understood.

CONTRIBUTION OF CALCIUM TO SMOOTH MUSCLE CONTRACTION

The calcium that is important in the genesis of a smooth muscle contraction is derived from several sources through several mechanisms (Figure 4.2). As discussed previously (see Figure 4.1), the receptors for the stimulant substances directly act on their specific receptor-operated ion channels (route II) to allow calcium influx through the cell membrane. The stimulant drug molecule attaches to its specific receptor site to accomplish this event. Its attachment to the receptor may also cause the intracellular release of calcium that has been bound to the intracellular side of the receptor. This calcium influx or release then causes increased tension of the contractile protein and muscle contraction without the need for actual depolarization of the cell membrane. As anticipated, the greater the intracellular concentration of stimulant drug molecules, the greater the number of occupied receptors. The more occupied receptors, the greater the number of open receptor-operated ion channels and the more pronounced the calcium influx. The greater the concentration of intracellular calcium, the more intense the muscle contraction will be.

The second major route for calcium influx is the action potential–sensitive ion channel (route I). This ion channel opens in response to a change in the membrane potential induced by stimulant substances causing membrane depolarization. The decreased membrane potential opens these channels and allows calcium influx to occur, which increases the intracellular ionized calcium concentration. The result is contraction of the contractile proteins.

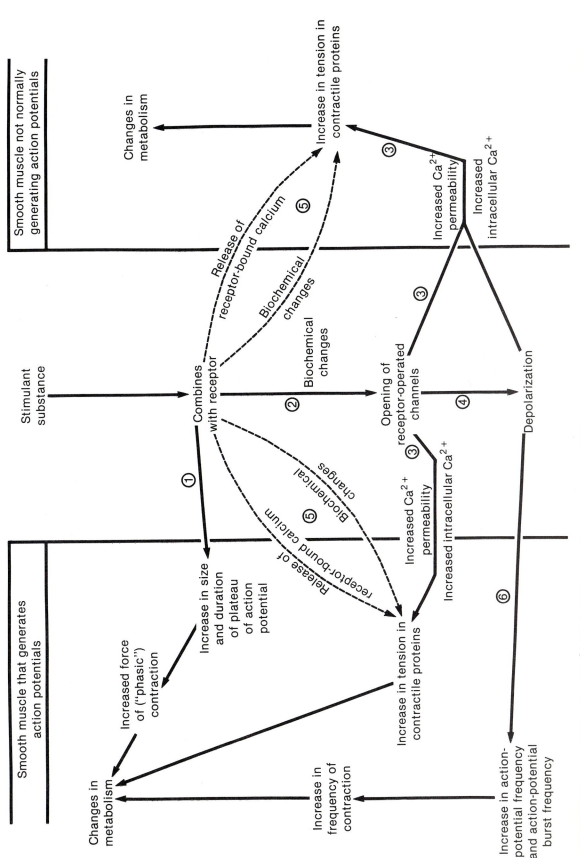

Figure 4.1 Two smooth muscle types. Stimulant substance produces changes in cellular metabolism by two different routes depending on whether the smooth muscle does or does not generate action potentials. (Modified and redrawn from Bolton, T.B. 1979. Physiol. Rev. **659**:606-718.)

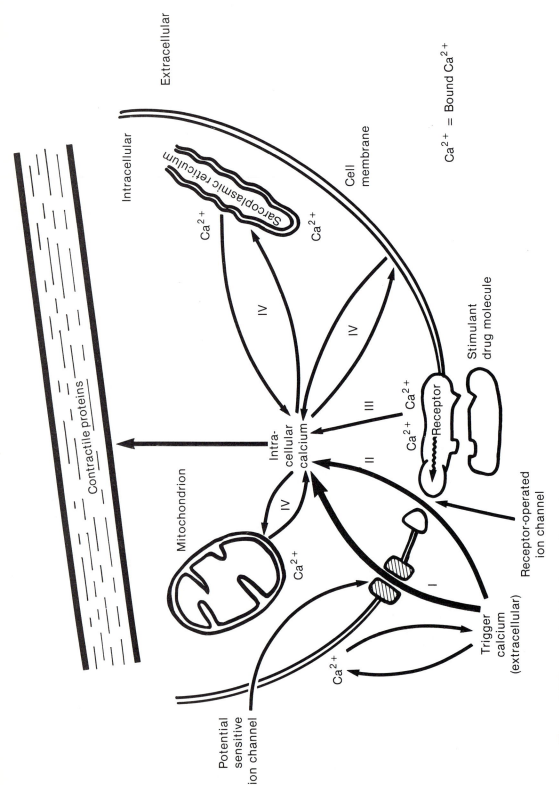

Figure 4.2 Sources of calcium in smooth muscle metabolism. (Modified and redrawn from Bolton, T.B. 1979. Physiol. Rev. **659**:606-718.)

Additional sources of increased intracellular ionized calcium include that calcium bound to endoplasmic reticulum, mitochondria, and the cell membrane, as well as to the nucleus and the nuclear membrane. Release from these sites follows the calcium influx because of decrease in membrane potential and the opening of action potential–sensitive ion channels.

Probably most of the calcium that is ultimately available to cause contraction of the intracellular contractile proteins is derived from the intracellular stores discussed previously. However, for this calcium to be released, a trigger calcium is required. The trigger calcium probably is that calcium derived from the extracellular space that enters the cell in response to the opening of action potential–sensitive ion channels or receptor-operated ion channels.

The four major sources of increased calcium concentration are (1) the trigger calcium from the extracellular space, (2) the internal stores, (3) the calcium bound to the intracellular surface of the receptor sites, and (4) the calcium released from the endoplasmic reticulum, the inner surface of the cell membrane, and possibly also the mitochondria.

The effect of drugs and endogenous neurotransmitters is mediated by the receptor sites present on the extracellular surface of the smooth muscle cell. The intensity of the effect is directly proportional to the concentration of stimulant substance and its ability to open ion channels in the cell membrane.

SPECIFIC EFFECTS OF NEUROTRANSMITTERS

Acetylcholine is the neurotransmitter for all preganglionic neurons of the autonomic nervous system and for postganglionic cholinergic (parasympathetic) neurons. It combines with the muscarinic receptor located on or within the membrane of the smooth muscle cell. Its usual effect is depolarization. Although its effects are generally blocked by atropine, the human bladder has a relative atropine resistance. Since the bladder does not always respond in the anticipated manner, it is postulated that other transmitters are involved in the cholinergic nerve endings present in the bladder. The exact nature of these other transmitters is currently unknown. Various substances have been explored, for example catecholamines, 5-hydroxytryptamine, adenosine 3′-5′ monophosphate (cyclic AMP), histamine, and γ-aminobutyric acid. Prostaglandins may be involved, since

they are known to modify the spontaneous release of neurotransmitters from smooth muscle cells. They may also act directly on the smooth muscle cell with or without the intermediary of a specific receptor site.

A purine nucleotide, adenosine 5′-triphosphate (ATP), seemed a possible transmitter and was found to fulfil the criteria necessary to qualify as a neurotransmitter, and the purinergic nerve hypothesis was formulated (Burnstock, 1971). Later findings suggested that it was unlikely that all nonadrenergic, noncholinergic nerves had a single transmitter. Electron microscopy revealed up to nine morphologically distinguishable neurons in the enteric plexuses that contained a complex mixture of vesicles, suggesting that these may contain more than one transmitter.

Concepts are now being developed that there are nerve cells that may liberate more than one transmitter (Burnstock, 1981). There is evidence that ATP is stored together with norepinephrine and acetylcholine in autonomic nerve terminals, probably in vesicles. It may be released together with catecholamines from the adrenal medullary vesicles in perfused adrenal glands. In certain in vitro conditions a single sympathetic neuron may at different times release norepinephrine, acetylcholine, or a mixture of the two (Hill et al., 1976).

α-Adrenergic neurons release the neurotransmitter norepinephrine. This neurotransmitter increases the permeability of the cell membrane to potassium, sodium, and chloride. As potassium crosses the cell membrane, hyperpolarization and relaxation result. If potassium is accompanied by sodium or chloride, depolarization and contraction result. Its specific effects on calcium are variable. β-Adrenergic neurons invariably cause relaxation of smooth muscle. The mechanism by which this occurs is currently obscure. Cyclic AMP may be involved.

ORGANIZATION OF AUTONOMIC NERVOUS SYSTEM IN LOWER URINARY TRACT

The parasympathetic nervous system is stimulatory to vesical and urethral smooth muscle. Vesical contraction overshadows the weaker urethral stimulatory effect. The α-adrenergic nervous system is stimulatory to the urethral and trigonal smooth muscle where its receptors are concentrated. The effect on vesical smooth muscle is minimal, since there are very few α-receptors located in other parts of the bladder wall. The β-adrenergic nervous system relaxes urethral and vesical smooth muscle. Most of the β-receptors are concentrated in the bladder dome, with very few in the trigone and urethra. The predominant effect of the β-component is to relax the bladder during its filling phase.

OTHER DRUG EFFECTS ON LOWER URINARY TRACT

Prostaglandins have already been discussed. Their effects on the lower urinary tract cause urethral relaxation and vesical contraction. Therapeutic usefulness of these properties is currently under investigation.

Angiotensin II usually causes a contraction of smooth muscle by causing an increase in action-potential discharges. Histamine has a variable effect on smooth muscle. If contraction results, it is usually associated with depolarization and increased action-potential discharge. Bradykinin also has variable effects on smooth muscle. Relaxation by this agent is blocked by prostaglandin inhibitors, indicating a possible role of this agent as an intermediary in its effects.

Caffeine causes contraction of smooth muscle. This seems to be the result of release of intracellularly bound calcium. The role of caffeine in the genesis of irritative lower urinary tract symptoms in women is well known.

Nifedipine is a unique agent with a strong potential for therapeutic usefulness. It relaxes smooth muscle when the initial contraction is calcium dependent. Its specific effect is to block intracellular calcium migration caused by the opening of ion channels. It accomplishes this by alteration in the membrane action potential. It may also act closer to the contractile protein itself to block its tension generation.

SUMMARY

The relevance of the pharmacology of the lower urinary tract to the treatment of various disorders of the bladder and the urethra is now recognized. Clinical investigation with a variety of pharmacological agents is now going on. This chapter indicates that those drugs affecting calcium uptake by the muscle cell or the exchange of potassium and sodium and other ions from intra- to extracellular or vice versa will provide pharmacological therapy of the bladder and the urethra in the future. Other drugs that interfere with specific receptor sites on the effects of activation of a receptor site will also be important. A further classification of drugs that includes those that have their effects on the contractile proteins themselves will also assume prominence in pharmacological research.

REFERENCES

Bolton, T.B. Mechanisms of action of transmitters and other substances on smooth muscle. Physiol. Rev. **59:**606-718.

Burnstock, G. 1971. Neural nomenclature. Nature **229:**282-283.

Burnstock, G. 1981. Nueortransmitters and trophic factors in the autonomic nervous system. J. Physiol. **313:**1-35.

Hill, C., et al. 1976. Specificity of innervation of iris musculature by sympathetic nerve fibers in tissue culture. Pfluegers Arch. **361:**127-134.

chapter 5

Epidemiology of micturition disorders

THELMA M. THOMAS

Most information about micturition disorders has so far been based on studies of patients coming to hospital clinics. However, such studies give an incomplete picture of the morbidity caused by these disorders because some patients with symptoms of equal severity do not seek medical advice. Prevalence studies must include all cases in the total population at risk.

Estimates of prevalence have little meaning unless a clear definition of the symptom or disease in question is stated. Without this it will be impossible either to interpret individual studies or to make comparisons between different studies. The definition may be derived arbitrarily before embarking on a study. This is a valid method provided the definition is clearly specified and rigidly adhered to throughout the study. An alternative approach is to use a population survey to arrive at a definition. This definition, based on the formal data collected, can then be used in future studies. An example of this method of establishing a definition is the study of Osborne (1976), who asked a group of 600 working women aged 35 to 60 to complete questionnaires about bladder habits. Likewise, Wolin (1971) asked over 4000 American nursing students to complete a questionnaire about their bladder habits. However, there is still not much information about normal voiding patterns in the general population.

The agreed definition must, for epidemiological purposes, be one that can be easily applied on a large scale. It therefore needs to be simple and unambiguous and should not depend on the results of hospital-based or invasive diagnostic techniques. Although such additional measures may be used later to validate results, attempts to include them in surveys will seriously limit response rates and provide biased results based only on largely self-selected groups of the population.

Prevalence (the proportion of a defined population with the symptom or disorder in question) is the most commonly used measure for chronic conditions. *Incidence rates* (or the number of new cases over a given time) may be more appropriate than prevalence for short-lived symptoms such as frequency and dysuria caused by cystitis or "urethral syndrome." However, if these attacks are considered part of an ongoing process with intermittent bacteriuria (Smith, 1981), prevalence may once again be the more appropriate measure, though difficult to establish without a persisting marker of the condition.

PREVALENCE OF MICTURITION DISORDERS
Urinary symptoms other than incontinence

Relatively little information about micturition disorders can be gained from routine statistics. In the National Morbidity Survey Report (Office of

35

Population Censuses and Surveys, 1974) general practice consultation rates per 1000 for women (all ages) were:

Acute cystitis	32.7
Chronic cystitis	1.2
Incontinence of urine	1.3
Frequency of micturition	4.6
Polyuria	0.1
Hematuria	0.8

Acute attacks of dysuria are common in women of childbearing age, and medical help is not always sought. Walker, Heady, and Shaper (1981) carried out a postal survey of 7700 women aged 20 to 54 years in four London general practices. Of the 4100 who replied, 52% had had symptoms of acute dysuria at some time in their lives—20% in the previous year. Also, 10% had had more than one episode in the last 12 months. In a study of women of childbearing age, Rees (1978) showed that 35.6% had had symptoms definitely suggestive of cystitis and a further 23% had had possible attacks.

Milne et al. (1972) found that 23% of a random sample of 200 women aged between 62 and 90 living in a defined area of Edinburgh had noticed that they passed urine more often than they did in the past. At the time of questioning, 3% of the women had pain on passing urine, and a further 21% reported that they had had pain in the past. Nocturia was reported by 58% of the women, and 10% reported getting up more than twice. In a general practice–based study of 375 women aged 65 and over, Brocklehurst et al. (1971) reported that 61% had nocturia, 32% precipitancy, 23% urinary incontinence, 13% scalding, and 3% difficulty in passing urine.

Urinary incontinence

The prevalence of urinary incontinence in women has been determined in a number of studies, some of which are listed in Tables 5.1 and 5.2. The estimates obtained in the different studies appear to show quite wide variations. This is probably due both to the different methods used to obtain the data and to the different definitions of incontinence. The studies confirm that urinary incontinence of some degree is common. One or more episodes of stress incontinence, defined as urine loss with coughing, laughing, sneezing, or excitement, seems to be a fairly general experience even for young women. However, the suggestion that 16% of 421 American nursing students were incontinent daily (Wolin, 1969) has not been repli-

cated in other studies. Incontinence is most common in certain groups with disabilities such as reduced mobility, cerebrovascular disease, or neurological disease (Table 5.2).

The study by the Medical Research Council Epidemiology and Medical Care Unit on the prevalence and health service implications of urinary incontinence was based on the definition of "regular" urinary incontinence as "involuntary excretion or leakage of urine in inappropriate places or at inappropriate times twice or more a month, regardless of the quantity of urine lost" (Thomas et al., 1980). Urinary incontinence was considered as either "recognized" or "unrecognized." The study of "recognized" urinary incontinence was carried out in two London boroughs. Agencies (for example, community nursing, old people's homes) likely to be in touch with incontinent patients were provided with the survey definition and asked to give details of patients under their care. The study of "unrecognized" urinary incontinence was based on postal questionnaires sent to those aged 5 and over on the practice lists of 12 general practitioners in England and Wales. The questions were worded so that answers could be interpreted in terms of the survey definition. To provide some details on urge and stress incontinence, as well as on bed-wetting and wetting at other times, two of the questions were:

1. Do you ever wet yourself if you cannot get to the toilet as soon as you need to pass water?
2. Do you ever wet yourself when you cough, sneeze, laugh, or lift something?

Replies were received from 18,084 (89%) of the 20,398 patients approached. In two of the practices, those who gave answers indicating "regular" urinary incontinence were then interviewed to establish the prevalence of different degrees of incontinence. Four categories were defined:

Minimal—No extra laundry; no pads or expenses; no restriction in activities

Slight—Very small amount of extra laundry; pads worn only occasionally; no restriction in activities

Moderate—Extra laundry, pads, expenses; some restriction in activities

Severe—Laundry, pads, and expenses; activities restricted; requires assistance from others

Of the girls aged 5 to 14, 5.1% were "regularly" incontinent of urine, of whom only 60% were bed wetters, the remainder having mainly urge incontinence. In contrast, 90% of the 6.9% of the boys

TABLE 5.1 Studies of the prevalence of the urinary incontinence in women living at home

Authors	Study group	Method	Prevalence
Brocklehurst, J.C., et al., 1971.	375 women aged 65 or over from a general practice population	Nurse interview questionnaire	23% including stress 12% stress only
Brocklehurst, J.C., et al., 1972.	454 women aged 45-64 from a general practice population	Nurse interview questionnaire	57% stress incontinence
Crist, T., Shingleton, H.M., and Koch, G.G., 1972.	1008 hospital staff, students, and nongynecological patients	Questionnaire on accidental urine loss	2% frequently 7% infrequently 25% rarely
Milne, J.S., et al., 1972.	272 Edinburgh women aged 62-90	Doctor interview questionnaire "mild" incontinence—stress or urgency "Severe"—night wetting or other wetting	5% severe 38% mild
Nemir, A., and Middleton, R.P., 1954.	1327 nulliparous American students	Self-administered questionnaire on urine loss with coughing, laughing, sneezing, or excitement	5% frequently 47% occasionally
Osborne, J.L., 1976.	600 working women aged 35-60	Questionnaire on "troublesome" or "clinically significant" stress incontinence	26% stress incontinence
Scott, J.C., 1969.	349 nulliparous student nurses aged 17-25	Self-administered questionnaire on involuntary urine loss	40% stress incontinence
Thomas, T.M., et al., 1980.	7767 women aged 15 years or over	Postal questionnaire	10% incontinent twice or more a month 18% incontinent less often
Van Zonneveld, R.J., 1959.	1450 inhabitants of a Dutch town aged 65 or over	Interviews by medical students	2% incontinent
Wolin, L.H., 1969.	4211 American nursing students	Self-administered questionnaire on urine loss with coughing, laughing, sneezing, or excitement	16% daily 35% occasionally
Yarnell J.W.G., et al., 1981.	1000 women in South Wales aged 18 or over	Interviews	30% less than weekly 8% weekly or more 5% daily or continuous

TABLE 5.2 Studies of the prevalence of urinary incontinence in women living in institutions and in other selected groups

Authors	Study group	Prevalence
Beck, R.P., 1979.	1000 premenopausal gynecological out-patients in Alberta, Canada	31% stress incontinence
Hald, T., 1975.	Estimates using existing data about illnesses associated with incontinence	2% of Danish population have urinary incontinence
Isaacs, B., and Walkey, F.A., 1964.	248 elderly women in a geriatric hospital	43%
Knox, J.D.E., 1979.	30 general practitioners' records of patients (male and female) with "major degrees of dribbling incontinence known to them"	0.2%
McLaren, S.M., et al., 1981.	121 female psychogeriatric patients	91% incontinent at least once in 3 weeks
Masterson, G., Holloway, E.M., and Timbury, G.C., 1980.	404 male and female residents of 11 Scottish local authority old people's homes	17% severe 19% occasional
Miller, H., Simpson, C.A., and Yeates, W.K., 1965.	297 male and female patients with multiple sclerosis	36% urge incontinence 10% unconscious incontinence
Shepherd, A., 1974.	250 patients attending gynecological outpatient clinics in London	32% stress incontinence
Thomas T.M., et al., 1978.	210 women who had had pelvic floor surgery up to 7 years earlier	35% incontinent twice or more a month (11% with socially disabling urinary incontinence)
Thomas, T.M., et al., 1980.	Population of two London boroughs; those with incontinence and known to health and social service sources; incontinence twice or more a month	0.2% in women 15-64 2.5% in women 65 and over (including those in institutions)
Thomas, T.M., et al., 1981.	Geriatric patients (male and female) General wards (male and female)	29% incontinent 10% incontinent twice or more a month

aged 5 to 14 who were "regularly" incontinent were bed wetters.

Age. Figure 5.1 shows the prevalence of urinary incontinence by 10-year age groups in women aged 15 and over and the proportion of each age group reporting urge incontinence only, stress incontinence only, and combined urge and stress incontinence. Prevalence in women changed little between the ages of 35 and 64 but fell in those aged 65 to 74 and rose in those aged 75 and over. The lower prevalence in the 65 to 74 age group was consistent in all the practices surveyed and seems to be accounted for by the less frequent occurrence of stress incontinence in the older age groups. This

was previously also noted by Brocklehurst et al. (1971). The prevalence of urge incontinence alone was similar between the ages of 15 and 54 but increased after this age.

Parity. Figure 5.2 shows the results by parity in those aged 15 or over. Even in this large survey, the numbers with subcategories of urinary incontinence in different parity groups are sometimes small, and some caution is therefore necessary in interpreting the results. Urge incontinence may be a little more common in parous than in nulliparous women, but within parous women there is no obvious increase in the prevalence of urge incontinence with increasing parity. The rise in the prev-

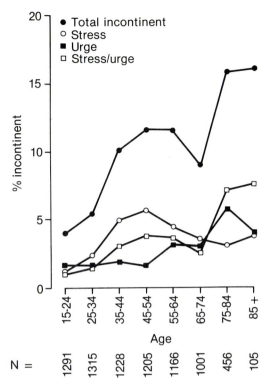

Figure 5.1 Prevalence of stress, urge, and stress/urge incontinence in women by age.

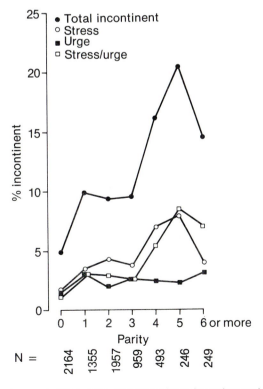

Figure 5.2 Prevalence of stress, urge, and stress/urge incontinence in women by parity.

alence of incontinence with parity is due to a rise in the prevalence of stress (and stress/urge) incontinence. The effects of parity on the prevalence of urinary incontinence are independent of the effects of age.

At the interview, questions were asked about bladder symptoms other than incontinence. Of the women between 15 and 64 who had reported only stress incontinence on the postal survey form, at the interview 79% reported urgency or nocturia as well. Stress incontinence alone, without symptoms suggestive of bladder instability, was thus reported by only 8% of the women aged 15 to 64 with "regular" urinary incontinence and was even less common above this age.

Nocturnal enuresis. Epidemiological studies of bed-wetting and associated symptoms in children have provided useful information about the natural history of enuresis (De Jong, 1973; Forsythe and Redmond, 1974; Miller et al., 1974; and Essen and Peckham, 1976), but relatively little is known about the natural history of urinary incontinence in younger and middle-aged adults. There are no data available, retrospective or prospective, to throw light on the hypothesis that persistent childhood bed wetters are more likely to be incontinent in old age than those dry early (Willington, 1976). Urinary incontinence has been reported to be transient in up to a third of incontinent elderly patients (Willington, 1969; Milne, Hope, and Williamson, 1970; and Yarnell and St. Leger, 1979). This was not confirmed by findings of the Medical Research Council Epidemiology and Medical Care Unit study, where only one in nine of those aged 65 and over were dry at a follow-up interview after 1 year. This difference may be due to the different definitions used in the different studies.

There are no international comparisons of indices of urinary incontinence based on clearly defined and comparable criteria. Anecdotal accounts suggest that urinary incontinence may not be a common problem among people who squat to void and need to be able to direct their stream accurately (Shepherd, 1980). The effect that varying approaches to "toilet training" in childhood may have on the prevalence of urinary incontinence in later life has not been determined.

SERVICE IMPLICATIONS

Knowledge of the prevalence and severity of micturition symptoms, especially incontinence, establishes a baseline for the planning and assessment of services.

Yarnell et al. (1981) estimated that between 3% and 7% of women in the general population have "significant" urinary incontinence, of whom only a small proportion seek medical help. In the study by Thomas et al. (1980), about 2% of women were found to have urinary incontinence of a moderate or severe degree (see earlier definition). About a third of this group were receiving little if any help from health or social services. A further 7% of women had regular urinary incontinence of a minimum or slight degree. Although most of these women did not consider themselves to have problems warranting medical intervention, a few would certainly have welcomed more active management than they were receiving. About 90% of the incontinent women had been so for longer than a year. Less then 20% had had any investigation other than examination of a midstream urine specimen. For those in receipt of services, there was nevertheless evidence of considerable room for improvement (Thomas et al., 1981), which is a finding reported from other areas (Slack, 1981).

Ideally, the effectiveness of management methods—whether by nursing, medical, or surgical means—should be assessed by randomized controlled trials using clearly defined outcome measures. The advantages of using an objective urodynamic outcome measure must be weighed against those of a subjective clinical assessment. Whatever measure is used, it should be made "blind"—that is, without knowledge of which treatment the patient has had. Subjective assessments of the outcome of surgical treatments should therefore be made by someone other than the surgeon who carried out the treatment.

However, not all topics are amenable to conventional randomized controlled trials, even assuming that such trials are otherwise feasible. For example, many features determine the most appropriate type of management in incontinent patients with multiple sclerosis—such as mobility or impairment of hand control or vision. Assessments of distinct regimes such as self-catheterization, for example, will thus often be inappropriate, since only a small subgroup of patients will be eligible. Trials could, however, be based on the value of a "flexible package" in which treatment is tailored in detail to the needs of the individual and a comparison made with patients whose management is dealt with on a more routine basis.

Investigations such as urodynamic measurements should only be carried out routinely when there is a clear understanding of their value in improving diagnosis and management (Cardozo and Stanton, 1980; Jarvis et al., 1980). Hilton and Stanton (1981) have suggested that invasive investigation of urinary incontinence could be avoided in a proportion of incontinent elderly women (60% in their series) if an algorithmic method of assessment is used. The use of randomized controlled trials in assessing the indications for urodynamics has not been sufficiently exploited.

The evaluation of equipment for the management of incontinence is based largely on subjective measures such as acceptability, comfort, and efficiency. Costs should also be included in the evaluation, since choices may have to be made between providing a comprehensive service for a few or providing a less detailed service for a large number (Tam, Know, and Adamson, 1978; Shepherd and Blannin, 1980; Watson, 1980; and Townsend et al., 1981). Once the size of the problem in institutions or in other groups is measured, it should be possible to assess both the costs and the potential impact of active management campaigns such as those advocated by Brocklehurst (1976), Clay (1978), and King (1979).

REFERENCES

Beck, R.P. 1979. Urinary stress incontinence reviewed. In Stallworthy, J., and Bourne, G., editors. Recent advances in obstetrics and gynaecology. Vol. 13. Edinburgh. Churchill Livingstone.

Brocklehurst, J.C. 1976. Incontinence in the elderly: the majority can be cured. Mod. Geriatr. **6**:19-22.

Brocklehurst, J.C., et al. 1971. Dysuria in old age. J. Am. Geriatr. Soc. **19**:582-592.

Brocklehurst, J.C., et al. 1972. Urinary infection and symptoms of dysuria in women aged 45-64 years: their relevance to similar findings in the elderly. Age Ageing **1**:41-47.

Cardozo, L.D., and Stanton, S.L. 1980. Genuine stress incontinence and detrusor instability: a review of 200 patients. Br. J. Obstet. Gynaecol. **87**:184-190.

Clay, E.C. 1978. Incontinence of urine. Nurs. Mirror, pp. 36-38.

Crist, T., Shingleton, H.M., and Koch, G.G. 1972. Stress incontinence in the nulliparous patient. Obstet. Gynecol. **40**:13-17.

De Jonge, G.A. 1973. Epidemiology of enuresis. In Kolvin, I., MacKeith, R.C., and Meadow, S.R., editors. Bladder control and enuresis: clinics in developmental medicine. 48/49. London. Heinemann Medical Books.

Essen, J., and Peckham, C. 1976. Nocturnal enuresis in childhood. Dev. Med. Child Neurol. **19**:577-589.

Forsythe, W.I., and Redmond, A. 1974. Enuresis and spontaneous cure rate study. Arch. Dis. Child. **49**:259-263.

Hald, T. 1975. Number of people with urinary incontinence in Denmark, Ugeskr. Laeger **137**:3001-3003.

Hilton, P., and Stanton, S.L. 1981. Algorithmic method for assessing urinary incontinence in elderly women. Br. Med. J. **282**:940-942.

Isaacs, B., and Walkey, F.A. 1964. A survey of incontinence in elderly hospital patients. Gerontology **6**:367-376.

Jarvis, G.J., et al. 1980. An assessment of urodynamic examination in incontinent women. Br. J. Obstet. Gynaecol. **87**:893-896.

King, M.R. 1979. A study on incontinence in a psychiatric hospital. Nurs. Times **75**:1133-1135.

Knox, J.D.E. 1979. Ambulant incontinent patients in general practice. Nurs. Times **75**:1683.

Masterson, G., Holloway, E.M., and Timbury, G.C. 1980. The prevalence of incontinence in local authority homes for the elderly. Health Bull. **38**:62-64.

McLaren, S.M., et al. 1981. Prevalence and severity of incontinence among hospitalised female psychogeriatric patients. Health Bull. **39**:157-161.

Miller, F.J.W., et al. 1974. The school years in Newcastle on Tyne. Oxford. Oxford University Press.

Miller, H., Simpson, C.A., and Yeates, W.K. 1965. Bladder dysfunction in multiple sclerosis. Br. Med. J. **1**:1265-1269.

Milne, J.S., Hope, K., and Williamson, J. 1970. Variability in replies to a questionnaire on symptoms of physical illness. J. Chronic Dis. **22**:805-810.

Milne, J.S., et al. 1972. Urinary symptoms in older people. Mod. Geriatr. **2**:198-212.

Nemir, A., and Middleton, R.P. 1954. Stress incontinence in young nulliparous women. Am. J. Obstet. Gynecol. **68**:1166-1168.

Office of Population Censuses and Surveys. 1974. Morbidity statistics from general practice second national study: studies on medical and population subjects. No. 36. London.

Osborne, J.L. 1976. Post-menopausal changes in micturition habits and in urine flow and urethral pressure studies. In Campbell, S., editor. The management of the menopause and postmenopausal years. Lancaster, England. MTP.

Rees, D.L.P. 1978. Urinary tract infection. In Stanton, S.L., editor. Gynaecological urology: clinics in obstetrics and gynaecology. Vol. 5.1. Eastbourne, England. Saunders.

Scott, J.C. 1969. Stress incontinence in nulliparous women. J. Reprod. Med. **2**:96-97.

Shepherd, A. 1974. Personal communication.

Shepherd, A. 1980. Re-education of the muscles of the pelvic floor. In Mandelstam, D., editor. Incontinence and its management. London. Croom Helm.

Shepherd, A.M., and Blannin, J.P. 1980. A clinical trial of pants and pads used for urinary incontinence. Nurs. Times **76**:1015-1016.

Slack, P. 1981. Hidden handicaps: incontinence—a forward look. Nurs. Times **77**(suppl.):14-19.

Smith, P. 1981. The urethral syndrome. In Fisher, A. Gynaecological enigmas: clinics in obstetrics and gynaecology. vol. 8. No. 1. Eastbourne, England. Saunders.

Tam, G., Knox, J.G., and Adamson, M. 1978. A cost-effectiveness trial of incontinence pads. Nurs. Times **74**:1198-1200.

Thomas, T.M., et al. 1978. Urinary incontinence before and after pelvic floor surgery. Eighth meeting of the International Continence Society. Oxford. Pergamon Press.

Thomas, T.M., et al. 1980. Prevalence of urinary incontinence. Br. Med. J. **281**:1243-1245.

Thomas, T., et al. 1981. Incontinence in patients in two District General Hospitals. Unpublished data.

Townsend, J., et al. 1981. Cost of incontinence to families with severely handicapped children. Community Med. **3**:119-122.

Van Zonneveld, R.J. 1959. Some data on the genito urinary system as found in old age surveys in the Netherlands. Gerontology **1:**167-173.

Walker, M., Heady, J.A., and Shaper, A.G. 1981. Prevalence of urinary tract infection symptoms in women. J. Epidemiol. Community Health **35:**152.

Watson, A.C. 1980. Incontinence: a trial of Mölnlycke pants and diapers. Nursing Times **76:**1017-1019.

Willington, F.L. 1969. Problems in urinary incontinence in the aged. Gerontology **11:**330-356.

Willington, F.L., editor. 1976. Incontinence in the elderly. London. Academic Press.

Wolin, L.H. 1969. Stress incontinence in young healthy nulliparous female subjects. J. Urol. **101:**545-549.

Wolin, L.H. 1971. Voiding patterns in young healthy women. J. Urol. **106:**923-926.

Yarnell, J.W.G., and St. Leger, A.L. 1979. The prevalence, severity and factors associated with urinary incontinence in a random sample of the elderly. Age Ageing **8:**81-85.

Yarnell, J.W.G., et al. 1981. The prevalence and severity of urinary incontinence in women. J. Epidemiol. Community Health **35:**71-74.

part TWO

INVESTIGATION

chapter 6

Principles of investigation

STUART L. STANTON

The management of a woman with a lower urinary tract disorder has become increasingly complicated over the last decade. Investigations are more informative and more invasive so that the physician assumes an even greater responsibility to ensure that the patient is protected from overzealous investigations and that only those that are likely to directly benefit the patient are carried out.

The history and physical examination still remain the basis for diagnosis. The history indicates the condition, its extent or severity, and its duration. The question that cannot always be answered is what factor in the evolution of the disease has finally prompted the patient to seek medical advice. Many patients are greatly embarrassed by their symptoms and are unwilling to discuss certain taboo areas with their physicians. Improvements in health education of the public and the greater awareness among the medical and nursing professions should overcome this. It is important that the history take into account the effects of the disorder on the patient's social and domestic life. The clinical examination may confirm signs of bladder and urethral disorder and will detect any related or unrelated pathological condition elsewhere in the body.

The bladder is known to be an unreliable witness, and some objective assessment therefore is necessary to make a diagnosis. Jarvis et al. (1980) and other authors have shown the need for basic urodynamic investigations to confirm the clinical diagnosis. The range of investigations available will depend on the size of the hospital, more resources being concentrated in departments or urodynamic units that specialize in these disorders. Since invasive studies carry a small risk of urinary tract infection (2% according to Walter and Vejlsgaard [1978]), care must be exercised to carry them out in as sterile a manner as possible. It would seem that a midstream specimen of urine for culture and sensitivity, twin-channel subtracted cystometry, and uroflowmetry are the minimum basic investigations for any patient complaining of incontinence, especially if surgery is contemplated. Complex cases may require the addition of videocystourethrography, urethral pressure measurements, or electromyography.

REFERENCES

Jarvis, G.J., et al. 1980. An assessment of urodynamic examination in incontinent women. Br. J. Obstet. Gynaecol. **87:**893-896.

Walter, S., and Vejlsgaard, R. 1978. Diagnostic catheterization and bacteriuria in women with urinary incontinence. Br. J. Urol. **50:**106-108.

chapter 7

History and examination

STUART L. STANTON

Early description of disease relied much on the ability of the clinician to accurately record the history and clinical examination; confirmatory investigations were rudimentary, most information being provided by histological specimens either removed during the operation or at a postmortem examination. Complex and sophisticated investigations have gradually evolved, but we still rely on the history and examination to provide the framework for diagnosis, although these have also undergone change.

HISTORY

Most history taking still uses the patient's own words and is written in prose (usually neither as lengthy nor as literate as in the past). More use is made now of the structured questionnaire—designed for the condition being studied and computer coded for easy data collation and analysis. This method has the following advantages:

Questioning is consistent without omission of data. This is especially important before an operative procedure, since frequently the patient's recall of symptoms is incomplete.

Different physicians can produce similar data, ensuring consistency of recording within the department.

The history is legible and is an efficient and rapid method of dealing with a large patient throughput (Cardozo, Stanton, and Bennett, 1978).

A variety of questionnaires have been developed (Hodgkinson, 1963, and Robertson, 1974). Reliance on simple questions and examination is nowadays considered too inaccurate. This is because the bladder is an unreliable witness. Bates, Loose, and Stanton (1973), studying a group of patients following bladder repair, demonstrated that stress incontinence was a complaint of 50% of the patients with detrusor instability. Jarvis et al. (1980) showed that clinical diagnosis was accurate only in 65% of cases. Cardozo and Stanton (1980) found that stress incontinence and urge incontinence were complaints of 55% of patients with urethral sphincter incompetence and by 35% of patients with detrusor instability. Symptom analysis, or the use of symptom complexes when groups of symptoms are linked, is more accurate, reaching 96% accuracy in the diagnosis of some conditions (Farrar et al., 1975). Some clinicians nevertheless feel that the history still only gives a guide to the degree of disability experienced by the patient (Warrell, 1965, and Susset et al., 1976).

Our own questionnaire (Cardozo, Stanton, and

ST. GEORGE'S HOSPITAL

| | | | Card No. | 1 |

URODYNAMIC DATA 1   Surname   Hosp. No. _____

2 5 □□□□

Unit No. .... (2 5)

Ref. Consult./G.P. ....   First Names   (10 15) Date of Birth

6 9 □□□□

Date of Consultation .... (6 9)   Sex

PRESENT CONDITION   (9 = No Data)   Age: ....

10 15 □□□□□

| | Main Complaints | Duration |

16 18

19 21

22 24

1) ....

2) ....

3) ....

Duration: $0 = < \frac{1}{12}$, $1 = \frac{1\ 6}{12}$, $2 = \frac{7\ 12}{12}$, $3 = \frac{13}{12}$ 2yrs, 4 = 3 5yrs, 5 = 5 10yrs, 6 = >10yrs.

Frequency Day: $<$ Hourly   No. of times . $0 = No$, $1 = \{\frac{1/2\ 1}{10+}$, $2 = \{\frac{2}{7\ 9}$, $3 = \{\frac{3}{5\ 6}$, $4 = \{\frac{4}{4}$, $5 = \{\frac{5}{3\ 4}$, $6 = \{\frac{6}{3}$, $7 = \{\frac{7}{2\ 3}$, $8 = \{\frac{8}{2}$,

25 □

26 □

Night: No. of times · 0 = None, 1 2 3 4 5 6 7 8+ 9 = No Data

Other Symptoms 0 = No   1 = Yes occasionally   2 = Yes frequently   3 = Not applicable

Stress Incontinence (27)	Urgency (28)	27 □ 28 □
Urgency Incontinence (29)	Wet at rest (30)	29 □ 30 □
Wet on standing up (31)	Wet at night (32)	31 □ 32 □
Ability to interrupt flow (33)	Complete emptying (34)	33 □ 34 □
Post micturition dribble (35)	Good stream (36)	35 □ 36 □
Straining to void (37)	Retention of urine (38)	37 □ 38 □
Dysuria (39)	Aware of full bladder (40)	39 □ 40 □
Aware of being wet (41)	Aware of prolapse/dragging (42)	41 □ 42 □
Protective underwear (43)	Dyspareunia (44)	43 □ 44 □
Rectal soiling (45)	Weakness of legs (46)	45 □ 46 □
Cough (47)	Constipation (48)	47 □ 48 □

Other symptoms   1) ....

49 50 □□

2) ....

51 52 □□

53 □

Periods   1 = Premen., 2 = Menopausal, 3 = Postmen., 4 = Hysterectomy +/-BSO

O.C.Pill. .... Cycle. .... LMP. ....

Heavy/Normal .... Irreg. Bleeding Yes/No

Effect of a period on a main symptom   0 = No Effect   2 = Aggravated   3 = Better

9 = No Data or No periods

54 □

Diabetes Mellitus   0 = No   1 = Yes   9 = No Data

55 □

Neurological disorder · 0 = None 1 = UMN lesion 2 = LMN lesion 3 = Mixed 4 = Unspecified

5 = MS 9 = No Data

56 □

Psychological disorder   0 = None 1 = Schizophrenia 2 = Other Psychosis 3 = Neurosis

57 □

Other Disorders   1) ....

58 59 □□

2) ....

60 61 □□

Present Medication	**Name**	**Success**	**Duration**
1)			62 66 □□□□□
2)			67 71 □□□□□
3)			72 76 □□□□□

Success: 0 = No success   1 = Improved 2 = Cured 3 = Irrelevant 9 = No Data

Other   1) ....

77 78 □□

2) ....

79 80 □□

Figure 7.1 Urodynamic questionnaire used at St. George's Hospital, London. First sheet contains current history, second sheet contains past history and examination findings, and third sheet contains results of investigations. Follow-up visits are tabulated on fourth sheet. *Continued.*

ST. GEORGE'S HOSPITAL

URODYNAMIC DATA 2

Surname	Hosp. No. _____ ____.

Unit No..(2.5)

Ref. Consult./G.P...

Date of Consultation.......................(6.9)

First Names

Date of Birth

Sex

Card No. | 2

2·5 | | | | |

6·9 | | | | |

Past History   (9 = No Data)

Surgical/Medical	Date	Success	Duration
1).............................			
2).............................			
3).............................			
4).............................			
5).............................			

10·14

15·19

20·24

25·29

30·34

00000 = No operation. Success · 0 = No Success 1 = Improved 2 = Cured 3 = Irrelevant
9 = No Data

Duration: $0 = <\frac{1}{12}$, $1 = \frac{1\cdot6}{12}$, $2 = \frac{7\cdot12}{12}$, $3 = \frac{13}{12}$ · 2yrs, $4 = 3\cdot5yrs$, $5 = 5\cdot10yrs$, $6 = >10yrs$.

Drug Name	Success	Duration of Therapy
1).............................		
2).............................		
3).............................		

35·39

40·44

45·49

Parity   0   1   2   3   4   5   6   7   8+   9 = No Data   50

Birth weight of heaviest infant (kg)   00 = None/No Data   51·52

Enuresis   0 = No 1 = Yes 9 = No Data   Until......................years.   53

Retention   0 = No 1 = Yes 9 = No Data   54

Urinary Tract infection   (attacks in last 2 years) 0 = None   1   2   3   4   5   6   7+   55
8 = chronic infection 9 = No Data

Examination   (9 = No Data)

Breasts..Height (cms.)..(56·58)   56·58

Abdo..Weight (kg.)..(59·61)   59·61

Neuropathy   · 0 = None   1=mild / 2=severe > UMN   3=mild / 4=severe > LMN   5=mild / 6=severe > Mixed   62

Congenital lesions   · 0 = None 1 = Ectopic Ureter 2 = Epispadias 3 = Spina Bifida (overt)   63
4 = Spina Bifida (occult) 5 = other

Anterior Wall prolapse · 0 = None   1=slight / 2=marked > Cystourethrocoele   3=slight / 4=marked > Cystocoele   64

Rectocoele   · 0 = None   1 = slight   2 = marked   65

Enterocoele   · 0 = None   1 = slight   2 = marked   66

Uterine/Vault Descent · 0=None 1=1° 2=2° 3=3° 4=slight vault descent 5=marked vault descent   67

Uterine Size   · 0=Normal, 1=$<\frac{12}{52}$ 2=$\frac{12+}{52}$ 8= No uterus   68

Stress incontinence   · 0= No 1 = Yes   69

Other pelvic pathology 0= No 1 = Yes   70

Anal Sphincter tone   · 0= Normal I = Decreased 2 = No tone   71

$S_{2, 3, 4}$ Outflow   0 = Normal   1=Dec. / 2=Inc. > Motor   3=Dec. / 4=Inc. > Sensory   5=Dec. / 6=Inc. > Both   72

Other   1)...   73·74
2)...   75·76

Figure 7.1, cont'd. For legend see p. 47.

ST. GEORGE'S HOSPITAL

URODYNAMIC DATA 3

Surname	Hosp. No. _____

Unit No..(2 5)

Ref. Consult./G.P...

Date of Consultation........................(6.9)

First names	Date of Birth
	Sex

Card No. 3

2 5

6 9

INVESTIGATIONS (9 = No Data)

M. S. U. Date:...0 = Sterile, 1 = E.Coli, 2 = Proteus, 3 = Strept. faecalis
4 = Staph. albus, 5 = Pseudomonas, 6 = Klebsiella, 7 = Candida, 8 = Mixed/Other

I. V. U. Date:..0 = Normal, 1 = Ureteric fistula, 2 = Pyelonephritis
3 = Hydronephrosis &/or Hydroureter, 4 = Congenital anomaly, 5 = Combination

10

11

UROFLOWMETRY Date:................................

Peak flow rate......................................

Volume voided......................................

Sensation of fullness 1 = full, 2 = almost full, 3 = half full, 4 = Not full

12 13

14 17

18

URETHRAL PRESSURE PROFILE Date:................................

Urethral pressure · rest................................

Urethral pressure · squeeze............................

Ext. Urethral Sphincter E.M.G. 0 = normal, 1 = diminished, 2 = increased

19 21

22 24

25

VIDEOCYSTOURETHROGRAPHY Date:................................

Residual (ml)......................................

First sensation (ml).................................

Capacity (ml)......................................

Pressure rise on filling (PR_1) (cm H_2O) ....

Pressure rise on standing (PR_2) (cm H_2O) ....

Stress Incontinence   0 = no, 1 = slight, 2 = marked

Descent of Bladder Base   0 = no, 1 = slight, 2 = marked

Milkback complete   0 = no, 1 = yes, 2 = unable to void

Interrupt stream   0 = no, 1 = yes, 2 = unable to void

Maximum voiding pressure (cm H_2O).................................

Peak flow rate (ml/sec)......................................

Residual (ml)   0 = no, 1 = slight, 2 = marked

Other   1 = reflux, 2 = fistula, 3 = other

26 29

30 32

33 36

37 38

39 40

41

42

43

44

45 46

47 48

49

50

CYSTOMETRY   Date:................................

Residual (ml)......................................

First sensation (ml).................................

Capacity (ml)......................................

Pressure rise on filling (PR_1) (cm H_2O)............................

Effect of   1).........................   0 = None 1 = PR < 10 2 = PR > 10 3 = other

            2).........................   0 = None 1 = PR < 10 2 = PR > 10 3 = other

51 54

55 57

58 61

62 63

64

65

66 67

OTHER 1)...

         2)...

CYSTOSCOPY Date ....

Residual (ml)......................................

Muscosa 0 = normal 1 = papilloma 2 = inflammation 3 = ulceration 4 = calculus 5 = slight
trabeculation 6 = marked trabeculation 7 = other

Ureteric Orifices · 0 = normal 1 = ectopic 2 = other abnormality

Capacity (ml)......................................

URILOS Date:...............................   0 = No leak 1 = Cough 2 = Tap 3 = Urge 1.
4 = Walk 5 = Drink 6 = Change of position 7 = Jump 8 = Combination

OTHER 1)...

68 71

72

73

74 77

78

79 80

Figure 7.1, cont'd. For legend see p. 47.

Bennett, 1978) was designed after close scrutiny of many excellent questionnaires already available and has now been used for over 3000 patients (Figure 7.1). It is computer coded, with an initial space for the patient's history in her own words and then a series of questions with graded answers (one to three or one to nine). The questionnaire is printed on self-carbonating paper, so that one copy is filed in the patient's case notes and the other is retained in the unit (invaluable for retrieving data, since the notes never leave the department). Alternatively, the notes can be entered directly onto a computer and stored on magnetic tape or disk, with speedy retrieval for insertion of additional information as the patient's investigations and treatment proceed.

In some departments the history is completed by the patient alone or aided by a nurse. We think this is disadvantageous and prefer a physician to be responsible for history taking so that dubious questions may be enlarged on. The history is divided into urological, neurological, gynecological, and medical sections, followed by psychiatric, drug, and past history sections.

Urological history

Incontinence. The most common initial symptom is incontinence, and it needs careful evaluation. At the outset, I should state that stress incontinence is regarded as a symptom and sign and not as a diagnosis. It must be distinguished from urgency leading to urge incontinence. The following qualifying questions should be answered: Is it intermittent or continuous? Is it precipitated by effort or is it present at rest or on physical stress, giggling, seeing running water, putting the key in the door, intercourse, or orgasm? Does it occur after micturition as the patient stands up (postmicturition dribble)? How severe is the incontinence, and how often does it require a change of pants or incontinence pads? Does incontinence occur at night?

Urethral sphincter incompetence is likely to cause stress incontinence alone but often there is urge incontinence. Detrusor instability usually causes urge incontinence, but some patients also have stress incontinence; incontinence can occur on giggling, seeing running water, and putting the key in the front door. Both conditions can cause incontinence at night; the former, however, is usually associated with some physical effort, whereas the latter may appear as nocturnal enuresis. Post-

TABLE 7.1 Causes of urgency, urge incontinence, and frequency	
Urgency/urge incontinence and frequency	**Additional causes of frequency**
Urinary tract infection	Increased fluid intake
Upper motor neuron lesion	Impaired renal function
	Reduced bladder capacity
Irritative mucosal lesion	Pelvic mass
	Chronic residual urine
Urethral syndrome	Diabetes insipidus
Detrusor instability	Diabetes mellitus
Habit	Increased age
	Diuretic therapy
	Hypothyroidism
	Hypercalcemia
	Hypokalemia

micturition dribble may be due to a urethral diverticulum. Continuous incontinence may be associated with congenital anomaly (ectopic ureter or epispadias), a urinary fistula, or retention with overflow.

Urgency. The sudden desire to void, if uncontrolled or unfulfilled, may result in urge incontinence. Urgency on its own is a commonplace symptom. Bungay, Vessey, and McPherson (1980) studied fit women between 30 and 64 years old and found that approximately 20% had urgency. The common causes are indicated in Table 7.1.

Frequency. Voiding more than seven times a day is defined as frequency, whereas nocturnal frequency is arousal from sleep twice or more a night. Its common causes are also indicated in Table 7.1. Urgency and frequency are often linked, and it is tempting to think that sometimes a vicious circle of frequency → urgency → frequency exists. Certainly we have shown that operative cure of one is associated with cure of another (Stanton, Williams, and Ritchie, 1976).

The actual incidence can be charted by a patient using a urinary diary or frequency volume chart (Figure 7.2) that records input and output volumes and allows a subjective assessment also of the volume of urine lost together with episodes of urgency and leakage.

Voiding difficulty. Most women are completely unaware of their voiding ability and potential; they have no concept of stream velocity or cast distance.

TIME	INTAKE (ml)	OUTPUT (ml)	LEAKAGE			
			ACTIVITY	Amount	Urge	Wet Bed

DAY: THURSDAY 22. 4. 82

TIME	INTAKE (ml)	OUTPUT (ml)	ACTIVITY	Amount	Urge	Wet Bed
01.10		120cc			Yes	
02.50		120cc			Yes	
05.10		120cc			Yes	
07.35		90cc			Yes	
08.35	240cc	60cc			Yes	
09.25		60cc			Yes	
10.30			Sneezed	Soaked Underwear		
10.55	240cc					
11.30		90cc			Yes	
12.50		90cc			Yes	
1.00	240cc					
2.15	240cc	90cc			Yes	
3.15	240cc		Coughed	Few drops		
4.45		90cc			Yes	
6.10			Coughing	Soaked Underwear		
6.35		60cc			Yes	
7.00			Getting out of bath	Emptied bladder		
7.30	240cc					
9.00		120cc			Yes	
9.10	240cc					
10.00		210cc			Yes	
10.30		180cc			Yes	
11.05		60cc				
TOTAL	1680cc	1560cc				

Figure 7.2 Urinary diary showing input and output for each day. Timing, amount of leakage, whether it was associated with urgency or warning, and what activity precipitated it can be recorded.

They are aware of hesitancy, difficulty in voiding, poor stream, having to stand to void, and incomplete emptying, but these symptoms are uncommon. Acute retention, which is the most serious symptom, needs to be defined. It is usually painful, and catheterization is required for its relief, but it is important to note that the volume removed should be at least 50% of the functional bladder capacity. (Catheterization is sometimes carried out mistakenly in the belief that retention is present, and amounts much less than this are removed.) The prevalence of these symptoms in the general population is unknown. The prevalence of symptoms of confirmed voiding disorders in new attenders at a urodynamic unit is 12%; however, a further 2% of patients attending had asymptomatic voiding difficulties (Stanton et al., 1983). No one symptom seemed to accord more accurately with the clinical situation, but "poor stream" was the most common. Hesitancy is an uncommon symptom, but its postpartum prevalence in a group of healthy women without previous urological abnormality is between 8% and 10% (Stanton, Kerr-Wilson, and Harris, 1980).

Neurological history

The frequent occurrence of bladder disturbances associated with neurological disease makes it imperative that a neurological history and examination be completed. Evidence of general neurological disease should be sought and questions directed toward motor and sensory abnormalities, particularly those affecting sacral roots S2 to S4. The common neurological diseases that may appear are multiple sclerosis, peripheral neuropathy associated with diabetes mellitus, cerebrovascular accident, parkinsonism, and autonomic dysreflexia (with symptoms of sweating, palpitations, and headaches). It is important to question the patient about visual changes (blurred or double vision), back pain, disturbance of balance, and alteration in bowel control.

Gynecological history

Because of the close embryological, anatomical, and physiological relationships between the urological and genital tracts, lesions of either may affect both.

The urothelium is estrogen sensitive and dependent. Changes in functional urethral length but not pressure have been correlated with E_2 levels (Van Geelen et al., 1981). However, Hilton (1981),

studying patients who had urological symptoms, found significantly higher maximum urethral closure pressure in the early luteal phase than at any other time in the menstrual cycle. Smith (1972) has demonstrated the symptomatic and cytological changes associated with postmenopausal estrogen deficiency and the benefits of estrogen therapy. Thus the relationship of the menstrual cycle and menopause to urethral function is important.

The association of genital prolapse with stress incontinence is established. About 40% of patients with urethral sphincter incompetence will have significant anterior vaginal wall descent (Cardozo and Stanton, 1980).

The relationship between urological symptoms and gynecological surgery is important. Occasional repair of uncomplicated prolapse may cause postoperative urethral sphincter incompetence, believed to result from operative interference and postoperative scarring of the urethral sphincter mechanism. In a pre- and postoperative study of anterior colporrhaphy and vaginal hysterectomy for prolapse with or without stress incontinence, we could find no evidence of increase in symptoms of urgency and frequency postoperatively (Stanton et al., 1982). Jequier (1976) studied patients' symptoms before and after total abdominal hysterectomy and found no overall increase in urological symptoms. The colposuspension operation for urethral sphincter incompetence can lead to initial postoperative dyspareunia and also to symptoms and signs of enterocele. Usually, urgency and frequency are decreased following colposuspension, but sometimes symptoms arise de novo, with or without detrusor instability.

Ovarian and uterine enlargement may cause symptoms of frequency, and sometimes, if impaction occurs, urinary retention can result. Endometriosis involving the bladder can lead to frequency, urgency, and cyclical hematuria. Frequency and urgency may also be associated with pelvic inflammatory disease. Oral contraception (either combined estrogen and progestogen or progestogen only) is not found to cause specific urological symptoms.

Medical history

Any condition increasing abdominal pressure, for example, constipation or chronic cough, may induce stress incontinence caused by urethral sphincter incompetence by altering the pressure gradient between bladder and proximal urethra. Cardiac and renal failure will produce frequency, and diabetes mellitus and insipidus should be considered when polydipsia and polyuria or frequency appear.

Psychiatric history taking is discussed in detail in Chapter 30. For elderly patients who might be suffering from dementia, a dementia score to determine the awareness and degree of understanding and cooperation is helpful in their assessment (Chapter 28). The patient's appearance and behavior at the interview, mood state (for example, sad or elated), form and content of "talk," level of consciousness (where appropriate), and intelligence and orientation are important. Various self-administered psychiatric questionnaires are available for patient assessment; however, these are usually research tools and not widely used in routine clinical practice. Examples include the Wakefield Self-Assessment of Depression Inventory (WDI) to detect depression, Middlesex Hospital Questionnaire (MHQ) to detect neuroticism, and the Minnesota Multiphasic Personality Inventory (MMPI) to detect personality change. Referral to a psychiatric colleague is advisable if psychiatric disease is suspected.

Drug history

The current drug regime is important. Drugs taken directly for gynecological or urological symptoms and drugs taken for other conditions that might indirectly affect the lower urinary tract should be noted. It is relevant to confirm that the patient is taking her drugs at the correct time; a common cause for nocturia is late administration of diuretic therapy.

Past history

The obstetrical history should include parity, method of delivery, and weight of the largest infant (which can indicate late onset diabetes mellitus if over 4.5 kg). Details of the length of labor are often incorrectly recalled by the patient and are not helpful.

All past major surgery should be recorded. Pelvic surgery is of particular importance, especially when the bladder or urethra was involved; full operative and postoperative data are required, and any resultant side effects and complications should be detailed. Often a patient with a current voiding disorder has had a troublesome past surgical history requiring recurrent catheterization and a prolonged spontaneous voiding time. Surgery involving the vertebral column, for example, laminectomy, should be included because of potential damage to the nerve supply to the bladder, urethra, and pelvic floor.

Urinary tract infection and its treatment should be inquired about, and the frequency of episodes over the past 2 years and whether or not a positive bacterial culture was obtained before treatment should be recorded.

A history of past enuresis may indicate the likelihood of ongoing detrusor instability. Retention of urine, its antecedent causes such as surgery or childbirth, and its subsequent treatment should be inquired about. Finally, a note should be made of drug allergy and of any drug treatment for lower urinary tract disorders and the outcome.

EXAMINATION

Before commencing, it is important to place the patient at ease by reassuring her that no embarrassment should be felt if she loses urine during the course of the examination. The attitude and demeanor of the patient and any obvious personality or mental disorders should be noted. The height and weight of the patient is recorded and a simple "score" made of her mobility (for example, walks unaided, requires a walking stick, or is restricted to a wheelchair). After a general examination is completed, the remaining examination is divided into neurological and gynecological parts.

Neurological examination

A simplified neurological examination should be performed to screen all patients. Referral to a neurologist is advised if the neurological history and examination are abnormal. (Decision to refer is exercised if upper or lower motor neuron lesions are detected on cystometry alone.) The pupils are tested for pupillary reflex and nystagmus. Limbs are tested for tone, power, reflex, and sensation. Particular attention is paid to sensation over the sacral root dermatomes S2 to S4 (Figure 7.3). The back is examined for lesions such as spina bifida (overt or occult [Figure 7.4]) and prolapsed intervertebral disk or spondylosis. A Romberg test is used to confirm that balance is normal. A rectal examination is carried out to check anal sphincter tone.

Special neurological tests to confirm an intact sacral reflex include stroking the skin lateral to the anus to elicit contraction of the external anal

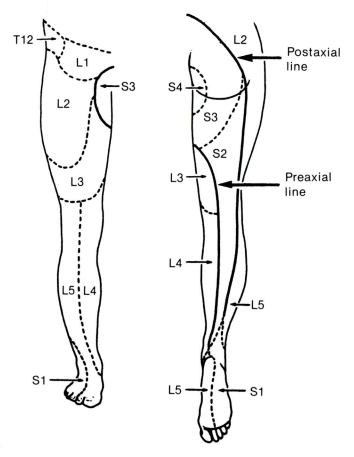

Figure 7.3 Cutaneous distribution of sacral nerve roots S2 to S4. (From Last, R.J. 1977. Anatomy regional and applied. ed. 5. Edinburgh. Churchill Livingstone.)

sphincter and tapping and squeezing the clitoris, which will produce a contraction of the ischio- and bulbocavernosus muscles (the bulbocavernosus reflex), which can also be elicited by pulling on a suprapubic or Foley catheter.

Gynecological examination

As part of the abdominal examination, renal enlargement or a palpable bladder should be detected; the latter may be difficult in the obese patient, but a bimanual examination may enable ballottement of the bladder by the vaginal hand; a crude estimate can be made of the residual urine. The external appearance of the vulva should be noted to detect congenital abnormalities such as epispadias (Figure 7.5) or an opening of an ectopic ureter, which may be difficult to detect. Vulval excoriation will give some indication of the severity of incontinence. The presence of stress incontinence may be detected equally in the supine or erect position but

is more noticeable when the patient has a comfortably full bladder (Robinson and Stanton, 1981). ''Wetness'' within or around the vagina needs differentiation between healthy vaginal discharge (which is clear or opalescent and without symptoms) and pathological vaginal discharge (which is white or yellow and associated with symptoms of discomfort and the presence of vaginitis). After drying the vagina with a swab, the physician should observe the patient for a while with a speculum in place and ask her to cough. Provided urine has not leaked from the external urethral meatus, any fresh appearance of urine suggests a fistula.

The presence of atrophic genital change should be noted and the capacity and mobility of the vagina determined; these may have been compromised by previous pelvic surgery and certainly affect the choice of subsequent incontinence surgery. The vagina should normally accommodate two fingers, which should be able to be separated and moved

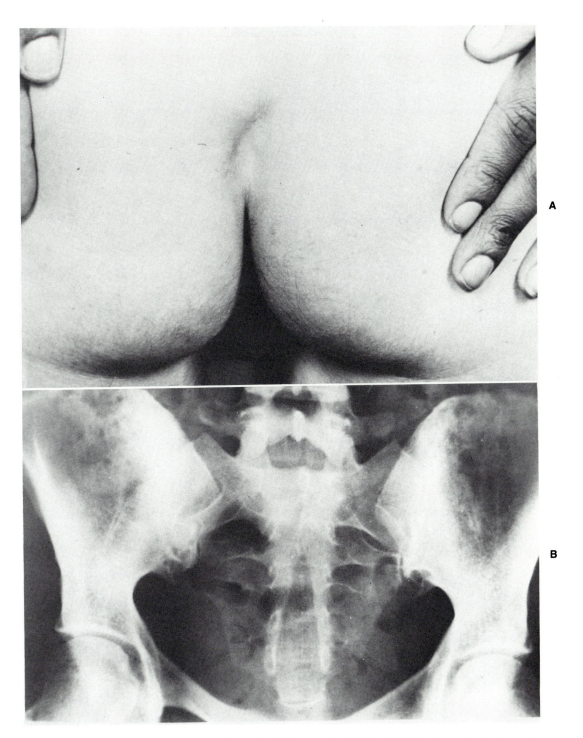

Figure 7.4 A, Sacral hollow found overlying spina bifida occulta of S2 to S4. **B,** Radiograph showing spina bifida occulta of S2 to S4.

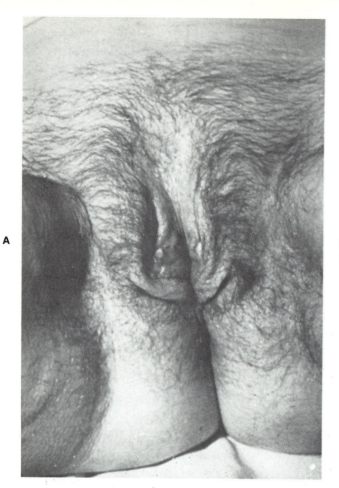

A

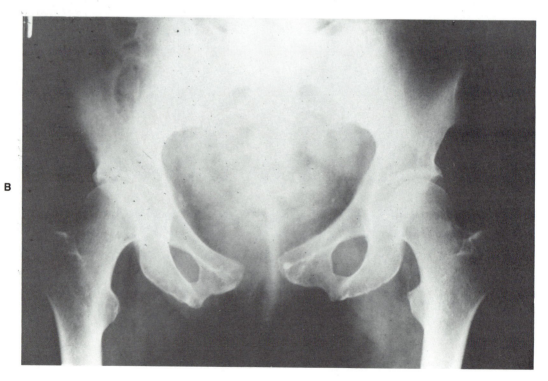

Figure 7.5 A, Female epispadias, showing separation of clitoris.

Fig. 7.5, cont'd. B, Underlying symphysial separation.

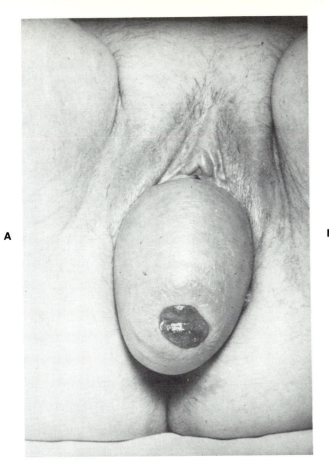

A

Figure 7.6 A, Procidentia with cervical erosion.

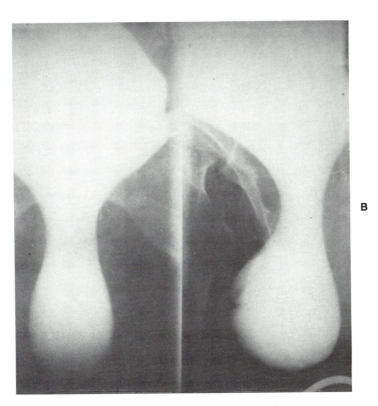

B

Figure 7.6, cont'd. B, Lateral and anteroposterior radiographs showing bladder descent associated with procidentia.

anteroposteriorly. If a colposuspension is to be performed, the fingers should be able to elevate the lateral vaginal fornices to the ipsilateral ileopectineal ligament. The urethra is examined for discharge, inflammation, rigidity, or fixation. An anterior vaginal wall mass may be either a urethral diverticulum or a paraurethral or vaginal cyst. A bimanual examination will confirm the presence of normal or abnormal pelvic organs and detect any bladder enlargement caused by residual urine or neoplasm. Genital prolapse, comprising descent of the anterior and posterior vaginal wall and uterus, may be detected on coughing and straining with the use of a Sims or similar speculum (Chapter 26). Some clinical grading of prolapse is helpful: I divide anterior wall descent into cystocele and cystourethrocele; a urethrocele on its own is rare. Descent may be slight (within the vagina) or marked (descent to or beyond the introitus). Uterine descent is graded as first degree—descent within the vagina; second degree—descent to the introitus; and third degree or procidentia—descent beyond the introitus, taking with it the bladder and terminal portions of the ureters (Figure 7.6). Posterior vaginal wall prolapse comprises enterocele (pouch of Douglas descent containing small bowel, usually) and rectocele, and these are graded similarly to anterior wall prolapse.

The examination is concluded by a rectal examination to exclude a rectal or anal pathological condition and in particular fecal impaction. The integrity of the pelvic floor and anal sphincter innervation is confirmed by asking the patient to squeeze on the examining finger.

REFERENCES

Bates, C.P., Loose, H., and Stanton, S.L. 1973. Objective study of incontinence after repair operations. Surg. Gynecol. Obstet. **136**:17-22.

Bungay, G.T., Vessey, M.P., and McPherson, C.K. 1980. Study of symptoms in middle life with special reference to the menopause. Br. Med. J. **281**:181-183.

Cardozo, L., and Stanton, S.L. 1980. Genuine stress incontinence and detrusor instability: a review of 200 patients. Br. J. Obstet. Gynaecol. **87**:184-190.

Cardozo, L., Stanton, S.L., and Bennett, A.E. 1978. Design of a urodynamic questionnaire. Br. J. Urol. **50**:269-274.

Farrar, D., et al. 1975. A urodynamic analysis of micturition symptoms in the female. Surg. Gynecol. Obstet. **141**:875-881.

Hilton, P. 1981. Urethral pressure measurement by microtransducers: observations on methodology, the pathophysiology of genuine stress incontinence and the effects of its treatment in the female. M.D. thesis. University of Newcastle-upon-Tyne.

Hodgkinson, C.P. 1963. Urinary stress incontiencne in the female: a programme of preoperative investigations. Clin. Obstet. Gynaecol. **6**:154-177.

Jarvis, G.J., et al. 1980. An assessment of urodynamic examination in the incontinent woman. Br. J. Obstet. Gynaecol. **87**:893-896.

Jequier, A. 1976. Urinary symptoms and total hysterectomy. Br. J. Urol. **48**:437-441.

Robertson, J. 1974. Ambulatory gynecologic urology. Clin. Obstet. Gynecol. **17**:255-275.

Robinson, H., and Stanton, S.L. 1981. Detection of urinary incontinence. Br. J. Obstet. Gynaecol. **88**:59-61.

Smith, P. 1972. Age changes in the female urethra. Br. J. Urol. **44**:667-676.

Stanton, S.L., Kerr-Wilson, R., and Harris, V.G. 1980. Incidence of urological symptoms in normal pregnancy. Br. J. Obstet. Gynaecol. **87**:897-900.

Stanton, S.L., Williams, J.E., and Ritchie, D. 1976. The colposuspension operation for urinary incontinence. Br. J. Obstet. Gynaecol. **83**:890-895.

Stanton, S.L., et al. 1983. Clinical and urodynamic effects of anterior colporrhaphy and vaginal hysterectomy for prolapse with and without incontinence. Br. J. Obstet. Gynaecol. **89**:459-463.

Susset, J., et al. 1976. Urodynamic assessment of stress incontinence and its therapeutic implications. Surg. Gynecol. Obstet. **142**:343-352.

Van Geelen, J.M., et al. 1981. Urodynamic studies in the normal menstrual cycle: the relationships between hormonal changes during the menstrual cycle and the urethral pressure profile. Am. J. Obstet. Gynecol. **141**(4):384-392.

Warrell, D. 1965. Investigation and treatment of incontinence of urine in the female who has had a prolapse repair operation. Br. J. Urol. **37**:233-239.

chapter 8

Cystometry

B.L.R.A. COOLSAET

Cystometry is a technique by which the pressure-volume relationship of the urinary bladder is measured. The aims of cystometry are as follows:

1. To find out the causes of dysfunction of the urinary bladder
2. To evaluate the possible role of the bladder in patients with symptoms of lower urinary tract dysfunction, such as incontinence or frequency
3. To evaluate the consequences of known or suspected pathological processes on the bladder, such as intravesical obstruction or neurogenic lesions
4. To evaluate the functional state of the bladder, for instance, after long-term isolation
5. To perform pharmacological and other testing procedures in the treatment of pathological processes and to evaluate objectively therapeutic results
6. To investigate the possible role of the urinary bladder with regard to supravesical urinary tract dysfunctions

Basically the bladder has a twofold function: to store various volumes of urine at a nearly constant pressure, the collection phase, and to expel urine under voluntary control, the evacuation phase. During clinical cystometry, bladder properties related to both phases will be evaluated.

TECHNIQUE

The technique varies considerably from one center to another. Under physiological conditions the kidneys excrete urine at a rate of about 0.5 ml/min. Pressure measurement with these physiological filling rates might appear to be the only reliable technique, since cystometry is performed under the same circumstances from which the complaints originate. However, even when the filling rate is physiological the pressure measurement itself, by whatever technique might be used, disturbs the physiological environment of the patient in such a way that no cystometry is really physiological. The question also arises as to whether the investigation has to be physiological, since provocative tests are common and valuable in medical practice. The means of provocation will be determined by the

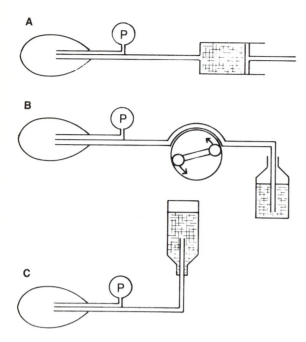

Figure 8.1 Infusion technique. **A,** Infusion pump. **B,** Roller pump. **C,** Drip set.

parameters for which the investigation is looking.

More rapid filling of the bladder can be obtained after fluid load and a diuretic agent. This method's only advantage is that the fluid medium is at body temperature and not irritating; its disadvantage is that no quantitative relationship between intraluminal volume and pressure is obtained, since the volume changes are variable and unknown.

Therefore it is advisable to use an infusion technique by which a nonirritating fluid at body temperature can be infused at constant and well-known infusion rates. Both the infusion pump (Figure 8.1, *A*) and the roller pump (Figure 8.1, *B*) are suitable for this purpose. Normal diuresis (0.5 to 1 ml/min) had to be added to this filling rate. The use of a gravity feed intravenous set (Figure 8.1, *C*) might be less expensive and relatively safe but has the disadvantage that the infusion rate is dependent on the difference between the pressure in the drip set and the back pressure in the bladder lumen. For routine clinical use, however, the intravenous set technique is sufficient to obtain most of the parameters for which the clinician is looking.

The use of gas (CO_2) had no fundamental advantages. It is irritating to bladder mucosa and compressible and has major disadvantages in combined urodynamic investigation (Gleason, Bottacini, and Reilly, 1977). Its use therefore will not

be discussed here, although it might have a place in rapid routine cystometry to detect whether or not high-pressure unstable contractions are present. The filling rates will be discussed later, since their selection is determined by the parameters needed and the basic bladder properties.

The intravesical pressure is determined by the active and passive properties of the bladder, the intraabdominal pressure, and the gravitational pressure of the fluid, which seldom exceeds 5 cm H_2O. The pressure in the bladder lumen is usually measured either by an external pressure transducer (Figure 8.2, *A*), which is connected to the bladder via a liquid-filled catheter, or by an internal pressure transducer (microtip pressure transducer Figure 8.2, *B*), which measures pressures in the bladder lumen directly.

Since the intravesical pressure is the pressure in the bladder lumen as compared to atmospheric pressure measured at the same external level as the bladder, the external pressure transducer should be located at the bladder level, which is about the upper edge of the symphysis pubis. The major advantages of the microtip pressure transducer are that errors resulting from volume displacement in the connecting tubes are avoided, the size of the catheters can be reduced to a minimum, and multiple pressure transducers can be fitted in one catheter so that simultaneous measurement of intravesical and urethral pressures can be registered. These catheters, however, are expensive, fragile, and sensitive to temperature changes. Most of them are rigid, which might cause artifacts in measuring urethral pressure. For routine clinical use the external pressure transducers are very sufficient when one adheres to some simple rules, such as the position of the transducer, regular calibration of the transducer, and the size (approximately 5 French) and length (approximately 75 cm) of the connecting tubes, which have to be manufactured of flexible but indistensible material.

Highly suitable double-lumen catheters are available so that there is no further need to use a single-channel catheter through which the bladder is filled and the pressure is measured, which leads to unnecessary artifacts. The intravesical pressure is influenced by intraabdominal forces. These forces are not uniformly distributed, which makes the exact measurement of their impact on intravesical pressure rather difficult. However, for clinical purposes the pressure recording of a space surrounding the bladder is sufficient. This is measured

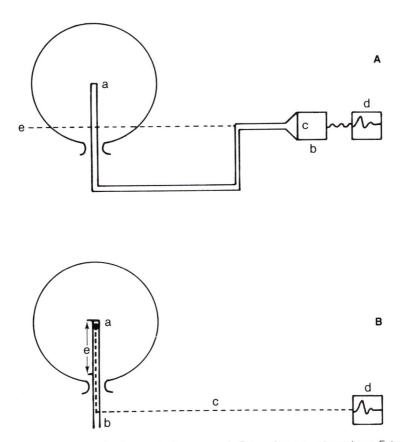

Figure 8.2 Technique for measuring intravesical pressure. **A,** *External pressure transducer.* External pressure transducer, *b,* is connected to bladder via liquid-filled catheter, *a.* Intravesical pressure is pressure in bladder lumen as compared to atmospheric pressure at same level as bladder. Therefore external pressure transducer should be located at bladder level, *e.* Catheter, *a,* is connected to external pressure transducer, *b,* via dome, *c.* Pressure measurement is not influenced by level of *a* in bladder lumen. *d,* Recorder. **B,** *Microtip pressure transducer.* Microtip pressure transducer, *a,* is located in bladder and connected via wire, *c,* to recorder. Pressure is measured with reference to atmospheric pressure via internal connection from pressure sensor to atmospheric pressure, *b.* Measured pressure depends on location of microtip pressure transducer in bladder, *e.*

in practice in the retropubic prevesical space (Nijman and Sjöberg, 1981) or in the rectum by using a simple standard Nélaton catheter. Since the rectum does not contain fluid, it might be advisable to fit a partially filled balloon around the tip of the catheter. The catheter is connected by means of a similar fluid-filled connecting tube to an external transducer at the same level as the one connected to the bladder lumen. More complicated catheters with intrarectal balloons to fixate the catheter are unnecessary and might even be disturbing in provoking anal-detrusor reflexes.

The reliability of the abdominal pressure measurement is tested by asking the patient to cough and strain, which must result quantitatively in the same pressure rises in the bladder lumen and in the prevesical or intrarectal space. The disadvantage of the intrarectal recording is that intrinsic rectal contractions might occur and could induce artifacts when both pressures are subtracted. The detrusor pressure is defined as the intravesical pressure diminished by the intraabdominal pressure. It might seem practical to subtract the abdominal pressure from the intravesical pressure electronically and to record the detrusor pressure only. Separate recordings are absolutely necessary because intrarectal pressures might contain artifacts.

Cystometry can be performed with the patient supine, sitting, or standing. Although less comfortable for the patient, standing cystometry must be included in the urodynamic investigation, since the correlation between symptoms and urodynamic

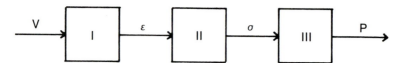

Figure 8.3 Block scheme. Volume signal, *V*, causes relative elongation of wall, (ε) through geometry of bladder, *I*. Elongation of wall results in stress, σ (force per unit area), determined by wall properties, *II*. Stress is measured in bladder lumen as pressure, *P*, again determined by geometry of bladder, *III*.

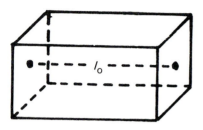

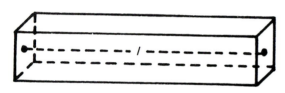

Figure 8.4 l_o indicates unstretched length of bladder wall, and *l*, length to which detrusor is stretched. Strain is defined as relative change of length: $\frac{l - l_o}{l_o}$.

findings is much better (Mayo, 1978). Jumping and walking on the spot might also be included.

The results of mobile cystometry (Frohneberg et al., 1981) are still preliminary but promising. Intravesical and abdominal pressures are transmitted by a telemetric system the patient carries while walking around, climbing steps, and so forth.

ORIGIN OF DETRUSOR PRESSURE

The detrusor pressure measured in the bladder lumen only partly represents the forces in the bladder wall. Indeed (Figure 8.3) a volume signal (V) causes a relative elongation of the wall (ε) through the geometry of the bladder. This elongation of the wall results in stress (σ) of the wall, and this stress is measured in the bladder lumen as pressure, again influenced by the geometry of the bladder.

Volume-strain relationship

Strain (ε) is defined as the relative change of the length. In a formula this means:

$$\epsilon = \frac{l - l_o}{l_o} \qquad (1)$$

where l_o indicates the unstretched length and *l* the length to which the detrusor is stretched (Figure 8.4). Since l_o and *l* cannot be measured directly, they must be calculated from the volume introduced (V) and the volume to which the bladder can be filled without stretching the wall (V_o), as follows:

$$\epsilon = \left(\frac{V}{V_o}\right)^{1/3} - 1 \qquad (2)$$

Strain-stress relationship

The relationship between strain and stress of the bladder wall can be described in terms of viscoelasticity (Coolsaet et al., 1973; van Mastrigt, Coolsaet, and van Duyl, 1978). In elastic material the stress depends on the *size* of deformation. This can be expressed in the following formula:

$$\sigma = f_1(\epsilon) \qquad (3)$$

where σ denotes stress, that is, the force per unit area in Newtons per square meter.

In viscous material the stress depends on the *rate* of deformation. This behavior can be represented by the following formula:

$$\sigma = f_2(\dot{\epsilon}) \qquad (4)$$

where $\dot{\epsilon}$ represents the rate of the relative changes in length.

Viscoelasticity is a combination of both length (size) and rate. It means that the force in the bladder wall will depend on both the length to which the bladder wall is strained (length dependency) and the rate at which the strain is applied (rate dependency). When a strip of the bladder wall is strained very slowly (Figure 8.5, *A*), only a slight increase of the stress will be generated, depending on the elastic, length-dependent properties. On the contrary, when the same strip is strained very fast to the same length, the stress will increase to a higher level, and when kept at that constant length, the stress will decrease to the level reached by slow

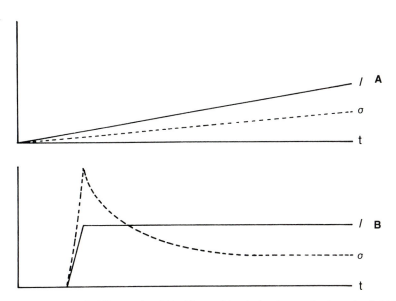

Figure 8.5 Rate dependency. **A,** When strip of bladder wall is strained very slowly, only slight increase of stress, σ, will be generated. **B,** When same strip is strained rapidly onto same strain level, stress will increase quickly. When kept at that constant length, stress decreases to level reached by slow straining.

straining (Figure 8.5, B). This rate dependency, which means that the stress depends on how fast the detrusor wall is strained, and the time dependency, which means that when the tissue is strained fast and maintained at constant length a decrease of the stress occurs that depends on time, are characteristics of viscoelastic behavior. Thus the relationship between strain (elongation of the wall) and stress (force in the wall) is determined by these viscoelastic properties. From experiments on bladder wall strips (Coolsaet et al., 1975a; Coolsaet, 1977) it turned out that this behavior can be mathematically described by three exponential functions and a constant:

$$\sigma = A \cdot e^{-\alpha t} + B \cdot e^{-\beta t} + C \cdot e^{-\gamma t} + K \quad \textbf{(5)}$$

The coefficients (A, B, C, K) represent the elastic, length-dependent properties, while the decay constants (α, β, γ) represent the time-dependent properties. The constant K represents the stress in the wall when no more time-dependent phenomena are involved. It denotes the static length dependency of stress in the wall.

This mathematical model can be visualized by a mechanical model (Figure 8.6) consisting of one Maxwell element (one spring and one dashpot) for each exponential function. The spring represents the elastic properties, the dashpot the viscous properties. The constant K is represented by the parallel elastic element E_o.

An additional characteristic of bladder wall tissue is that the unstretched length of the tissue increases after stretching, which means that the tissue becomes longer (increase of l_o). Therefore a plastic element (P_l) must be added in series. The plastic elongation caused by the stretch probably is reset in vivo by some metabolic processes.

Stress-pressure relationship

Stress in the bladder wall is measured as pressure in the bladder lumen influenced by the geometry of the bladder. The modified Laplace formula indicates this relationship:

$$\sigma = \frac{PR}{2d} \quad \textbf{(6)}$$

where P indicates pressure, R the radius of the bladder, and d the thickness of the bladder wall. The Laplace relation is derived from the principle that in a thin-walled sphere (Figure 8.7) the forces that push the two halves out of each other ($\pi R^2 P$) equal the forces that keep the walls in the circumference together ($2\pi RT$):

$$\pi R^2 P = 2\pi RT \quad \textbf{(7)}$$

$$T = \frac{PR}{2} \quad \textbf{(8)}$$

Since T stands for tension per unit length and one needs the force per unit area, the formula is adapted to the bladder wall according to formula 6. From

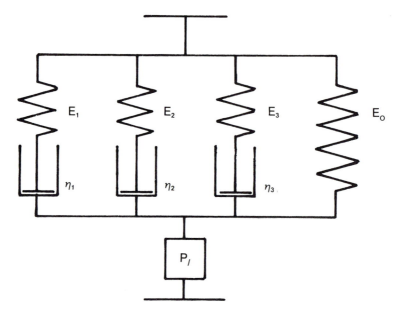

Figure 8.6 Mechanical model of bladder wall. Springs represent elastic properties (E_1, E_2, E_3, E_o), dashpots represent viscous properties (η_1, η_2, η_3). Force that remains when no more time-dependent phenomena are involved is represented by parallel spring, E_o. Plastic element in series, P_l, must be added, since unstretched length of bladder tissue increases after stretching.

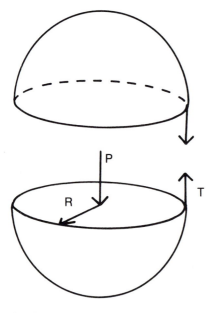

Figure 8.7 Representation of Laplace's formula. Halves of sphere are forced apart by force ($P \cdot \pi R^2$) and held together by force ($T \cdot 2\pi R$).

formula 6 it can be understood that an increase of the stress in the wall can result in a constant pressure in the bladder lumen, since the radius (R) increases with increasing volume.

To analyze the viscoelastic properties, the bladder must be filled quickly (10 ml/sec) until a peak pressure of about 40 cm H_2O is reached (Figure 8.8), after which a pressure decrease is seen with no further change in volume (stepwise cystometry—Coolsaet et al., 1973; Coolsaet, 1977). This pressure decrease curve can be analyzed using the mathematical model (formula 5). From these exponential functions the elastic parameters (coefficients) and viscoelastic parameters (decay constants) can be calculated using different fitting methods:

1. Graphic method (Kondo, Susset, and Lefaivre, 1972)
2. Electronic simulation (van Duyl et al., 1978)
3. Numerical procedures (van Mastrigt, 1977)

NEARLY FLAT SLOPE OF CYSTOMETROGRAM DURING COLLECTION PHASE

The nearly constant pressure during slow filling of the bladder has been ascribed to inhibition reflex mechanisms and more recently to viscoelastic prop-

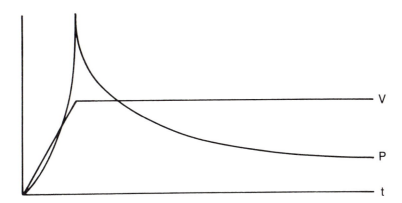

Figure 8.8 Stepwise cystometry. Bladder is filled very rapidly (10 ml/sec) until pressure peak of about 40 cm H₂O is reached. Then pressure decrease is seen with no further change in volume. This pressure decrease curve can be analyzed by using mathematical model. V, Volume of bladder; P, bladder pressure; t, time.

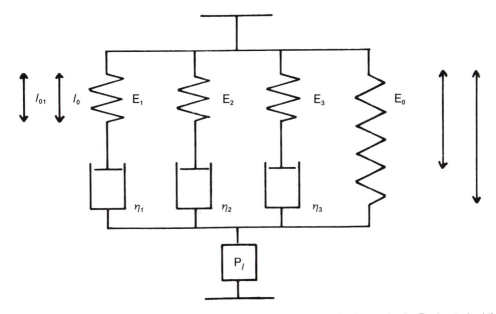

Figure 8.9 Representation of mechanical model after it had been stretched very slowly. Dashpots had time to follow elongation, so that springs, E_1, E_2, E_3, are not elongated, $l_{o1} = l_o$, and no force is produced in three Maxwell elements. Force in model will thus only be determined by elastic element in parallel, E_o, which is elongated indeed.

erties and the geometry of the bladder. Let us first consider what is happening in the bladder wall.

According to our mechanical model (Figure 8.6) one can easily understand that when the model is stretched very slowly, only the force of the parallel elastic element (E_o) will be measured (Figure 8.9) because the Maxwell elements produce no force, since the dashpots have time to follow the elongation, so that the springs, which generate force, will not be elongated. The force in the model and the stress in the bladder wall will thus only be determined by E_o. Experiments have shown that with increasing strain, the stress in the wall increases, as illustrated in Figure 8.10. This increasing stress is measured as pressure influenced by the geometry of the bladder. This pressure shows an S-shaped curve (Figure 8.11). Hence, no active adaptation mechanisms are necessary to explain the flat slope of the cystometrogram. Classical cystometry provides only information on this static elas-

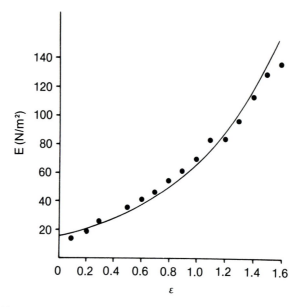

Figure 8.10 Relationship between stress in wall (represented by elastic modulus in ordinate) and strain level (represented by ε in abscissa). Stress in wall increases with increasing strain.

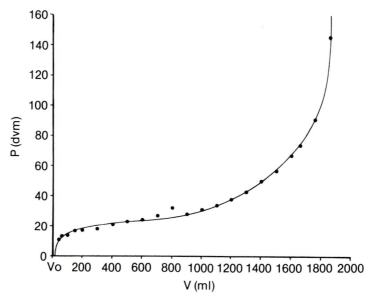

Figure 8.11 Pressure that results from increasing stress (Figure 8.10) shows S-shaped curve because of geometry of bladder.

tic element and its volume dependence.

To obtain this *static cystometrogram*, when no time-dependent mechanisms are involved, the bladder must be filled very slowly, in the range of about 3 ml/min, which is nearly the physiological rate. In practice, however, this method is too time consuming. Therefore we have to look for a method whereby filling rates are used with time-dependent mechanisms within an acceptable range of error. It turns out that filling rates up to 50 ml/min do not alter the shape of the cystometrogram in most cases.

When filling rates higher than the ones necessary to obtain a static cystometrogram are used, rate-dependent mechanisms are involved. The cystometrogram can nevertheless be performed slowly enough so that no time-dependent behavior can be observed. This is called a *pseudostatic cystometrogram*. A simple test can be performed to determine whether one cystometrogram is comparable to another (Coolsaet, 1980a). When the infusion is stopped during filling and no pressure decay is observed (Figure 8.12, *A*), the filling rate is within an acceptable range and the cystometrogram thus obtained is comparable to others that fulfill the same condition. When, on the contrary, the filling rate is too high, a pressure decay will be observed after stopping the infusion (Figure 8.12, *B*). In the

past this phenomenon has often been interpreted as an involuntary contraction of the detrusor.

The following lists the standardization of infusion rates as proposed by the International Continence Society (1976):

1. Slow filling cystometry: <10 ml/min
2. Medium filling cystometry: 10 to 100 ml/min
3. Rapid filling cystometry: >100 ml/min

These are valuable as a first approximation but rather arbitrary, since the division is not based on fundamental properties.

ENTEROCEPTION AND TEMPERATURE SENSITIVITY

Enteroceptive bladder innervation can be tested by using a cold solution at the beginning of the investigation. Normal individuals are sensitive to the temperature change. This temperature test is only used when a sensory neuropathic dysfunction is suspected. Routinely the bladder is filled from the start with a solution at body temperature.

ENTEROCEPTION AND BLADDER CAPACITY

During filling the first sensation is noticed as well as the volume at which a strong desire to void is perceived. The latter is generally accepted as the maximum bladder capacity. This strong desire

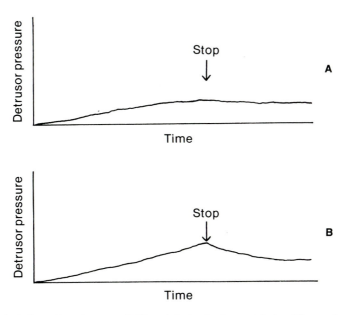

Figure 8.12 Pseudostatic cystometrogram. **A,** When infusion is stopped during filling and no pressure decay is observed, filling rate is within acceptable range and cystometrogram thus obtained is comparable to others that fulfill same condition. **B,** When, on the contrary, filling rate is too high, pressure decay will be observed because of time-dependent phenomena involved. Slope of this cystometrogram is not comparable to others.

probably is provoked by stress receptors in the wall and not directly related to the pressure in the lumen. The value of the capacity differs from one investigation to another and is, among other factors, dependent on the rate of filling, which determines the stress in the wall. The bladder also shows plasticity, which means that the wall becomes longer after stretching. The capacity might therefore increase when repeated cystometries are performed. Results of pharmacological testing in which bladder capacity is used as a parameter therefore have to be considered carefully.

DETRUSOR ACTIVITY

Besides having passive viscoelastic properties, the detrusor muscle also has the ability to contract (Figure 8.13), both slowly (tonic contraction), which results in an increase of tone, and more quickly (phasic contraction), which may be observed during the filling phase as spontaneous or provoked detrusor contractions and during evacuation as micturition contraction.

Tone

The term *tone* has been used and misused in the past, which has resulted in much confusion in the literature. A shift of the micturition contraction to the left or to the right has been defined, respectively, as "hypertonicity" or "hypotonicity", although shifting is only related to the onset of the micturition contraction and bladder capacity.

Tone is defined as "a long continued state of stress in the muscle maintained by activity of the contractile elements" (Landowne and Stacy, 1957). Difficulties arise in defining tone in numerical terms, since the pressure originates, among other factors, in both active and passive properties,

the latter causing rate dependency among other effects. So the steepness of the cystometrogram also depends on the relative changes of length per unit of time. When a small-capacity bladder is filled with the same infusion rate as a large-capacity one, the relative changes of length will be greater in the smaller bladder, which will result in a steeper increase of the pressure. Therefore the terms *hypotonic bladder* and *hypertonic bladder* should only be used when it can be proved that the pressure characteristics are related to active muscular mechanisms, which is rather difficult at this stage of knowledge.

Unstable contractions

On many cystometrograms waves of active detrusor contraction resulting in pressure rises ranging from a few centimeters of water to 70 to 80 cm H_2O are observed. On a rather arbitrary basis these pressure increases are defined as unstable contractions when they are at least 15 cm H_2O (International Continence Society, 1976). Pressure increases below this level are left to the interpretation of the investigator. These contractions are defined as provoked when they are induced by provocative maneuvers such as coughing, changing position, rapid filling, or catheter movement. They are spontaneous when they occur in the absence of these provocations, which supposes that routine urodynamic investigations, including the use of catheters, needles, and so forth, are not provocative.

The incidence of these unstable contractions shows a wide spread in the literature, ranging from 10% to 60%. This spread is the result of differences in the technique of cystometry, the provocative tests, the position of the patient, and the interpre-

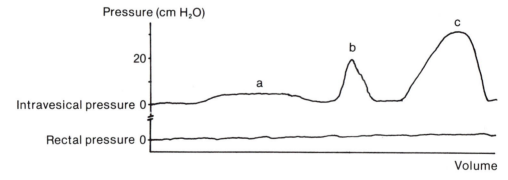

Figure 8.13 Cystometrogram including intravesical pressure and rectal pressure. During collection phase, slow tonic contractions, *a,* and faster phasic contractions, *b,* of detrusor muscle can be observed. During evacuation phase, phasic contraction, *c,* originates micturition.

tation of the data. Further sources of different interpretation arise from the fact that for some, an unstable contraction might not be suppressed by the patient, while for others, it is simply an involuntary contraction.

Further fundamental research is needed to better understand these contractions. It has been shown in animals that the bladder wall is continuously contracting in some parts, while it is relaxing in others (Coolsaet, van Duyl, and Blok, 1981). This continuous activity has been demonstrated in vitro on bladder wall strips (Van Duyl, 1980). In these preparations it has been clearly shown that the force in the wall depends on the width of the contracting area. Also, the magnitude of the spontaneous contractions increases with increasing stretch. When this normal spontaneous detrusor activity is ac-

cepted, one comes to the conclusion that every bladder is unstable, that is, spontaneously active. The height of the pressure waves observed during the filling phase of the bladder depends on the propagation and synchronization of the spontaneous contracting areas.

Based on these principles the appearance of the unstable contractions can be better understood: increasing pressure waves with increasing volume (Figure 8.14, *A*), subthreshold unstable contractions (<15 cm H_2O) (Figure 8.14, *B*), high-pressure unstable contractions (Figure 8.14, *C*), and synchronization of contracting areas, leading to micturition contraction (Figure 8.14, *D*). Special attention must be drawn to subthreshold unstable contractions that cause leakage (Figure 8.15, *A*). In the presence of a low urethral closure pressure,

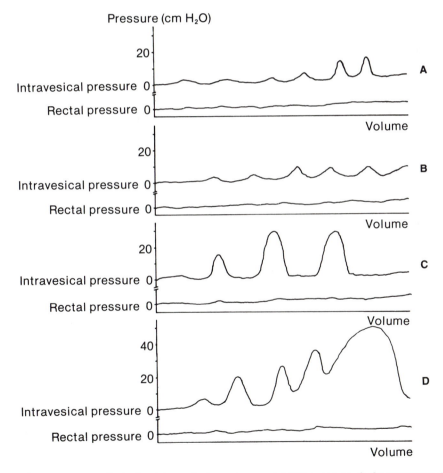

Figure 8.14 Cystometrogram including intravesical pressure and rectal pressure. **A,** Spontaneous detrusor contractions resulting in low pressure waves at low intravesical volume. Pressure waves increase (>15 cm H_2O) with increasing volume. **B,** Subthreshold unstable contractions (<15 cm H_2O) appearing during collection phase. **C,** High-pressure unstable contractions (>15 cm H_2O). **D,** High-pressure unstable contractions with increasing baseline, leading to micturition contraction.

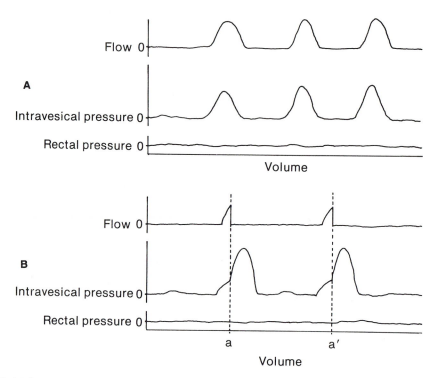

Figure 8.15 Subthreshold unstable contractions. **A,** Subthreshold unstable contractions (<15 cm H$_2$O) that cause leakage. Since urethra opens and flow starts, no further increase of detrusor pressure is observed. **B,** When during flow the bladder neck is suddenly occluded, a,a', isometric value of pressure caused by subthreshold unstable contraction is obtained. This isometric pressure is often above threshold (>15 cm H$_2$O).

urine may leak at low detrusor pressures. Once the value of the urethral resistance is reached, flow starts and no further increase of the detrusor pressure is observed. However, if during leakage the bladder neck is suddenly occluded by the balloon of the stop-flow catheter,* the isometric value of the unstable contraction is obtained, which often provides a higher level (>15 cm H$_2$O) of unstable contractions (Figure 8.15, *B*).

Standardization of terminology becomes more difficult when incontinence occurs during filling cystometry. Genuine *stress incontinence* is defined (International Continence Society, 1976) as the involuntary loss of urine from the urethra when the intravesical pressure exceeds the maximum urethral pressure but in the absence of detrusor activity. *Urge incontinence* is the involuntary loss of urine caused by unstable detrusor contractions. These definitions, however, can lead to misdiagnosis and erroneous treatment. Some practical situations might illustrate the complexity of the problem. The use of the urethral closure pressure

*Stop-flow Urodynamic catheter, Porgès.

enables better understanding of different possibilities (Figure 8.16). Incontinence provoked by cough may be the result of either an insufficient rapid pressure increase (Figure 8.16, *A*) in the urethra (passive, active, or a combination of both) or a low urethral closure pressure (Figure 8.16, *B*).

Provoked unstable contractions (Figure 8.16, *C* to *E*) or provoked subthreshold unstable contractions (Figure 8.16, *F* and *G*) may or may not cause leakage, depending on the urethral closure pressure. Unstable detrusor contractions (Figure 8.16, *H* and *I*) or subthreshold unstable contractions (Figure 8.16, *J* and *K*) may or may not cause leakage, depending on urethral closure pressure. All these possibilities and relations make clear-cut definitions rather difficult.

A major problem in the management of incontinence is the presence of unstable contractions. In contradistinction to previous opinions, unstable contractions associated with stress may or may not disappear after colposuspension (Meyhoff et al., 1980). Whether or not the remaining contractions will cause leakage will depend on the in-

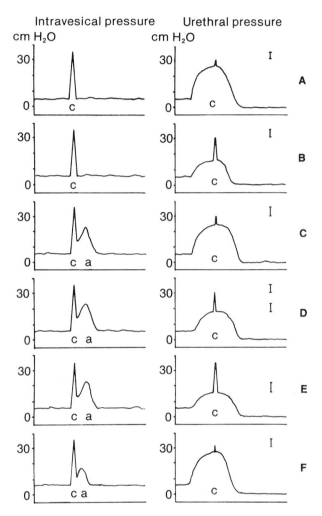

Figure 8.16 Schematic representation of different causes for incontinence related to intravesical pressure and urethral pressure. **A,** Incontinence caused by insufficient rapid pressure increase in urethra during stress. *c,* Cough. **B,** Incontinence resulting from low urethral closure pressure. Rapid pressure increase during stress is sufficient. **C,** Provoked unstable contraction, *a.* Incontinence is the result of insufficient rapid pressure increase during stress. Provoked unstable contraction does not cause leakage because of sufficient urethral closure pressure. **D,** Incontinence caused by both insufficient rapid pressure increase and provoked unstable contraction that causes higher pressure than urethral closure pressure. **E,** Incontinence resulting from provoked unstable contraction, since rapid pressure increase is sufficiently high. **F,** Incontinence caused by insufficient rapid pressure increase. Provoked subthreshold unstable contraction does not cause leakage because of higher urethral closure pressure. *Continued.*

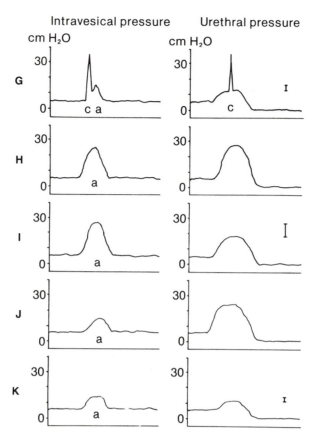

Figure 8.16, cont'd. G, Incontinence as a result of provoked subthreshold unstable contraction. Rapid pressure increase is sufficient but urethral closure pressure is low. **H,** High-pressure unstable detrusor contraction does not cause leakage because of higher urethral closure pressure. **I,** High-pressure unstable detrusor contraction causes incontinence because of low urethral closure pressure. **J,** Subthreshold unstable detrusor contraction does not cause incontinence because of sufficient urethral closure pressure. **K,** Subthreshold unstable detrusor contraction causes incontinence because of insufficient urethral closure pressure.

creased urethral closure pressure. Whether or not they will cause urge incontinence remains difficult to predict.

The major clinical problem consists of selecting those patients whose instability will be cured by colposuspension. We therefore introduced the *bladder neck elevation test* (Coolsaet, Blok, and van Venrooij, 1981). When unstable contractions are registered during standing cystometry, the bladder neck is elevated by the Bonney maneuver. The anterior vaginal wall and bladder neck are gently brought retropubically, simulating colposuspension (Figure 8.17). In some groups of patients the contractions will disappear during the test, reappearing after stopping the test (Fig. 8.18, *A*). In others the pressure waves will be less and postponed to a larger volume (Figure 8.18, *B*), while in still others they do not change. Based on the result of this test, colposuspension may or may not be indicated.

Detrusor contractility during voiding

When the patient has a strong desire to void after the command to pass urine, the detrusor contracts actively and the detrusor pressure rises to about 20 to 40 cm H_2O. From the moment the urethra opens and flow starts, the detrusor pressure is maintained during flow until the bladder is completely empty (Figure 8.19). This normal voiding pattern, however, is not seen in every patient. Some patients do not void during the urodynamic investigation. This might be because of psychogenic inhibition and an impaired micturition reflex. However, when the patient is left alone in a quiet atmosphere, micturition generally occurs.

In some patients, micturition is induced by an increase in abdominal pressure (Figure 8.20, *A*), and in some, voiding only occurs after the Valsalva maneuver (Figure 8.20, *B*). In these cases one could conclude that the detrusor is not contracting.

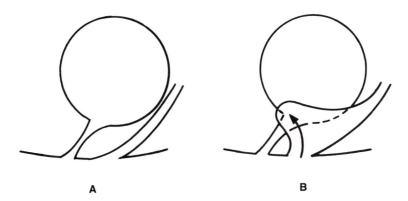

Figure 8.17 Bladder neck elevation test. Anterior vaginal wall and bladder neck are gently pushed up retropubically. **A,** At rest; **B,** on elevation.

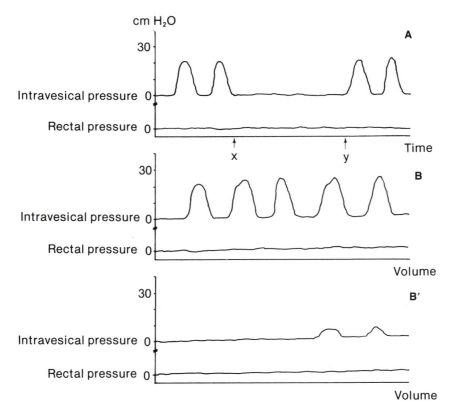

Figure 8.18 Bladder neck elevation test. **A,** In group of patients, unstable detrusor contractions disappear during test, $x \rightarrow y$ and reappear after stopping test. **B,** In other patients, unstable detrusor contractions remain unchanged. **B′,** In still other patients, contractions will be lower and postponed to larger volumes.

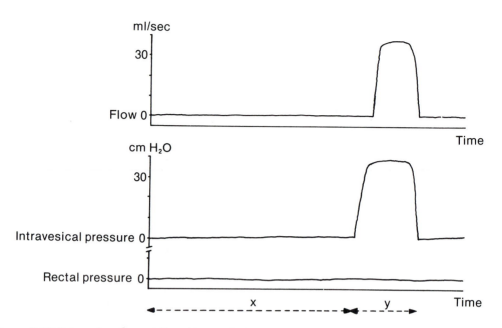

Figure 8.19 Schematic representation of intravesical pressure and rectal pressure during collection phase, *x,* and evacuation phase, *y.*

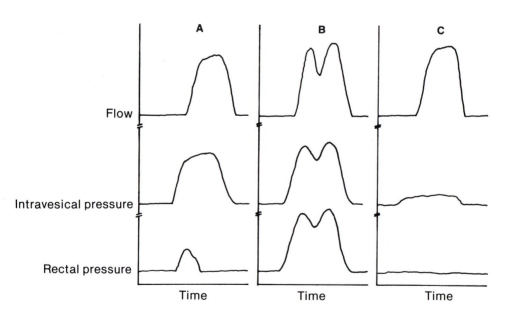

Figure 8.20 Different types of micturition. **A,** Micturition is induced by increased abdominal pressure. **B,** Micturition only occurs by increased abdominal pressure. **C,** Micturition characterized by normal flow but very low detrusor voiding pressure.

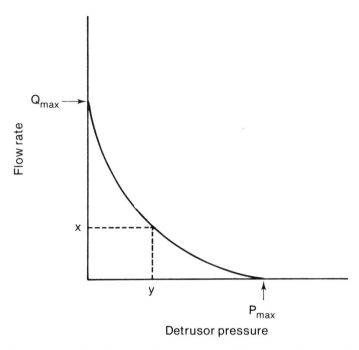

Figure 8.21 Bladder output relation. Detrusor with given contractility at given bladder volume can generate, for instance, high pressure at low flow rate or low pressure at high flow rate. P_{max}, Highest detrusor pressure that can be generated at zero flow rate. Q_{max}, Highest flow rate that can potentially be generated at zero pressure.

However, when cystometry is repeated, many patients will show a normal micturition pattern without increased abdominal pressure. It is therefore very useful to perform cystometry repeatedly during the same urodynamic session.

Some patients have a normal flow during voiding but only a very small voiding pressure (Figure 8.20, *C*). The question arises whether detrusor contractility can be determined by measuring the detrusor pressure during voiding. A straight measurement of detrusor pressure by itself is certainly not an adequate measure of detrusor contractility, because the detrusor pressure during voiding depends on the rate of urine flow out of the bladder. The detrusor with a given contractility at a given bladder volume can generate, for instance, a high pressure at a low flow rate or a low pressure at a high flow rate (Figure 8.21).

The relationship between detrusor pressure and flow rate has been described by Griffiths (1977) as the "bladder output relation," Thus certainly both detrusor pressure and flow rate must be considered. For example, a detrusor producing a normal pressure and a good flow rate has normal contractility, whereas if the pressure is normal but the flow rate is low (for a given bladder volume), then the contractility is poor.

To quantify contractility it is helpful to consider two parameters:
1. The highest detrusor pressure that can be generated at zero flow rate (P_{max})
2. The highest flow rate that can potentially be generated at zero pressure (Q_{max})

The first of these, the maximal detrusor pressure (P_{max}), can be obtained by shutting off the urethra suddenly during micturition (Gjertsen, 1961; Griffiths, 1977; Coolsaet, 1980b). Note that it may depend, in principle, on the bladder volume (Griffiths et al., 1979). It is important to notice that the detrusor is not always contracting with the same force. This might depend on the degree of stimulation, the width of the contracting area, and the condition of the detrusor before the contraction.

Stop-flow test. In practice the shutting off of the urethra can be realized in different ways:

1. The patient is asked to stop flow during voiding, which usually result in a rapid increase of the detrusor pressure (Figure 8.22). The P_{max} thus obtained should represent the isometric detrusor pressure (Gjertsen, 1961; Griffiths, 1977). Some difficulties arise in using this method:
   a. Some individuals cannot stop flow suddenly; this results in a lower $P_{max\ 1}$, which does not represent the real isometric pressure.

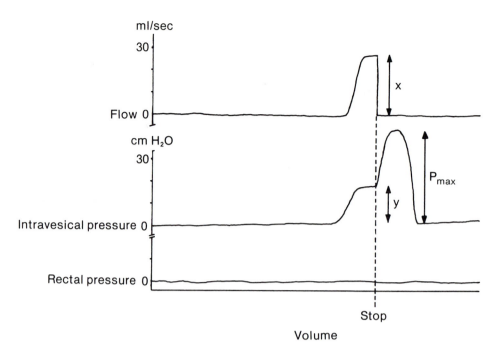

Figure 8.22 Stop-flow test. When during micturition characterized by flow, x, and voiding pressure, y, flow is suddenly interrupted, pressure usually increases rapidly to maximum pressure, P_{max}.

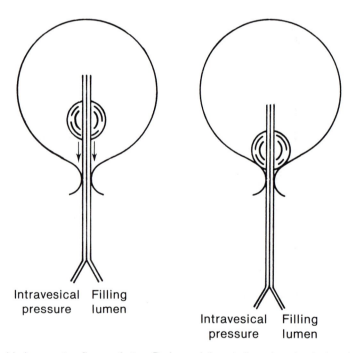

Figure 8.23 Double-lumen stop-flow catheter. During voiding, balloon is retracted suddenly to occlude bladder neck.

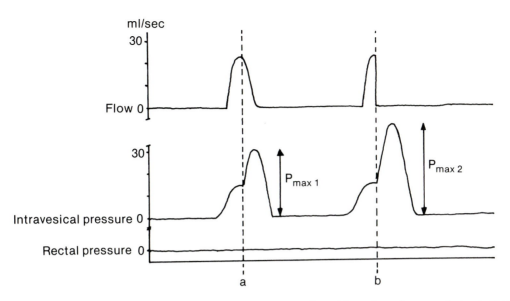

Figure 8.24 Maximum pressure obtained by voluntary interruption of flow, $P_{max\ 1}$, is generally lower than maximum pressure obtained by sudden occlusion of bladder neck using stop-flow catheter, $P_{max\ 2}$.

b. Some individuals do not show any pressure rise when the urethra is shut off suddenly.

2. An alternative (Coolsaet, 1981) is the use of the double-lumen stop-flow catheter. The catheter contains one channel for infusion, one channel for pressure measurement, and a balloon that lies in the bladder lumen during filling cystometry. During voiding the balloon is retracted suddenly to occlude the bladder neck (Figure 8.23); the $P_{max\ 2}$ thus obtained (Figure 8.24) is generally higher than the one obtained by the first method.

3. The maximum pressure is the pressure that should be obtained when the urethra does not open at the onset of micturition. We therefore introduced another method of using the same stop-flow catheter. The balloon is gently retracted when the command to void is given. The detrusor contraction, which normally stabilizes when the urethra opens, will continue to rise to its maximal value (Figure 8.25). When maximal detrusor pressure is reached, flow may be allowed in two ways:

   a. The catheter is relaxed so that the bladder neck becomes free and flow can start. During the following voiding the balloon can be retracted once or several times to obtain the P_{max} at different volumes.

   b. The catheter remains in place but its lumen is opened to allow flow through the lumen of the catheter. The lumen might be occluded several times during voiding to obtain the P_{max} related to volume.

Force-velocity relation. The most characteristic parameters of contracting muscle are its maximum velocity of contraction at zero force (V_{max}) and the maximum force it can generate in isometric conditions (F_{max}) (Hill, 1938; Griffiths, 1977; Griffiths et al., 1979; van Mastrigt and Griffiths, 1979; van Duyl, Coolsaet, and van Mastrigt, 1978; van Mastrigt, 1980). This force-velocity relation can be obtained by two methods: one based on the "bladder output relationship" and one on the isometric contraction at the beginning of micturition.

Bladder output relationship. The bladder output relationship is a hyperbolic function with known curvature (Figure 8.21). Usually the relationship can be obtained from measurements of two points on the curve. These two points are known from the stop-flow test:

   1. The flow rate (a) and detrusor pressure (b) just before the moment of interruption of the flow
   2. The P_{max} at zero flow rate, which is obtained by sudden interruption of the flow

The relationship between detrusor pressure and flow rate can be converted by a simple geometrical transformation to a relation between the active force (F) in the detrusor muscle and the velocity of shortening (v). The transformations are as follows:

$$v = Q/2R^2 \qquad \textbf{(9)}$$

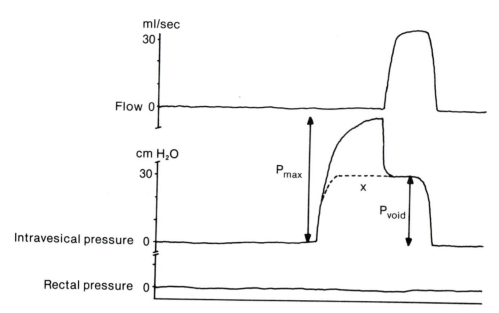

Figure 8.25 Maximum pressure is obtained by occluding bladder neck onset of micturition, P_{max}. Since no flow can occur, maximum pressure will be higher than voiding pressure, x.

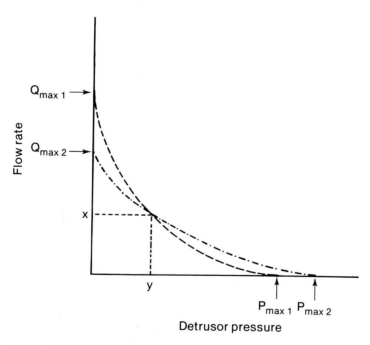

Figure 8.26 Since maximum velocity of contraction is derived from Q_{max} value, which is obtained by extrapolation, it might be erroneously concluded that in patients who do not stop flow suddenly, $P_{max\,1}$, maximum velocity of contraction is higher than it really is. Indeed, when bladder neck is suddenly occluded, $P_{max\,2}$ generally is higher, which will result in a lower Q_{max}, $Q_{max\,2}$, and a lower velocity of contraction.

where v is the velocity of contraction, Q is the flow rate, and R is the radius, and:

$$F = \pi R^2 P \qquad \textbf{(10)}$$

where F is the force, R is the radius of the bladder (assumed spherical), and P is the pressure.

Since the curvature of the function that describes the relationship between P_{max} and Q is known, the maximum velocity of contraction (v_{max}), which is a rather theoretical parameter, can be obtained by extrapolation. Since this parameter is obtained by extrapolation, it depends on the obtained P_{max} value. A lower P_{max}, since it is generally obtained by voluntary interruption of the flow, will result in a higher Q_{max} value (Figure 8.26). This might lead to the erroneous conclusion that patients who cannot interrupt flow suddenly have an increased velocity of contraction.

Isometric contraction. Another method of obtaining this force-velocity relation is based on the isometric contraction that occurs at the beginning of micturition, before the onset of flow (Figure 8.27). When micturition starts, the detrusor muscle contracts isometrically until the urethra opens and flow starts. This isometric pressure rise is recorded and analyzed by a computer using Hill's model (1938) (Figure 8.28) for behavior of contracting muscle. During the isometric contraction the total

length of the muscle remains constant. Shortening of the contractile element results in an elongation of the series elastic element, thus developing force. The relationship between length and force of the series elastic element has been determined in experimental situations. So the changes of length can be determined from the changes of force. The rate of change of this length is equal to the velocity of shortening. The force-velocity data are fitted with a hyperbolic curve, which again yields the two parameters: the maximum contraction velocity (v_{max}) and the maximum force (F_{max}). These two parameters represent, respectively, the ability of the detrusor to generate pressure (P_{max} or F_{max}), and its ability to contract fast and generate flow (Q_{max} or v_{max}), that is respectively, the *strength* and the *speed* of the detrusor muscle.

PHARMACOLOGICAL TESTING

It is possible to perform pharmacological testing during cystometry. One of the major problems to be solved is whether or not the detrusor is arreflexic. Therefore the bethanechol supersensitivity test has been widely used. The test is based on the denervation law, which indicates that denervated organs are more sensitive for some chemicals, for instance, neurotransmitter. In denervated bladders the detrusor pressure should rise more than 15 cm

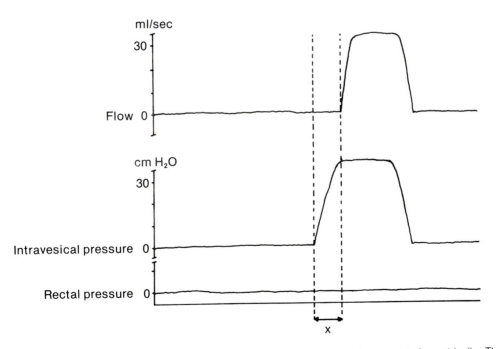

Figure 8.27 At onset of micturition, before urethra opens, detrusor muscle contracts isometrically. This isometric pressure rise can be recorded and analyzed by computer to obtain force-velocity relationship.

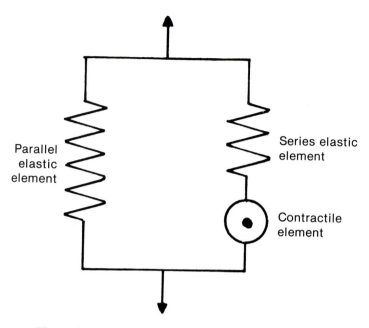

Figure 8.28 Hill's model for behavior of contracting muscle.

H_2O after subcutaneous injection of 2.5 mg betha-nechol chloride. However, since the test provides about 25% false-negative and about 50% false positive results, cystometry even combined with pharmacological testing is still unable to indicate or exclude denervation.

REFERENCES

Coolsaet, B.L.R.A. 1977. Stepwise cystometry: a new method to investigate properties of the urinary bladder. Thesis. Rotterdam University.

Coolsaet, B.L.R.A. 1980a. The pseudostatic cystometrogram: a simple method to test whether cystometrograms are comparable. Proceedings of the European Urological Association meeting. Athens.

Coolsaet, B.L.R.A. 1980b. Stop-test: une détermination qualitative de la contractilité du détrusor chez les patients qui souffrent d'une incontinence d'effort. J. Urol. **86:**187-191.

Coolsaet, B.L.R.A. 1981. The stop-flow test and its implications in bladder function. Proceedings of the seventy-sixth American Urological Association meeting. Boston.

Coolsaet, B.L.R.A., Blok, C., and van Venrooij, G.E.P.M. 1981. Bladder neck elevation test. Proceedings of the Urodynamics Society meeting. Boston.

Coolsaet, B.L.R.A., van Duyl, W.A., and Blok, C. 1981. Spontaneous detrusor activity. Proceedings of the Urodynamics Society meeting. Boston.

Coolsaet, B.L.R.A., et al. 1973. Stepwise cystometry of urinary bladder. Urology **2:**255-257.

Coolsaet, B.L.R.A., et al. 1975a. Viscoelastic properties of bladder wall strips. Invest. Urol. **12:**351-356.

Coolsaet, B.L.R.A., et al. 1975b. Viscoelastic properties of the bladder wall. Urol. Int. **30:**16-26.

Coolsaet, B.L.R.A., et al. 1976. Viscoelastic properties of bladder wall strips at constant elongation. Invest. Urol. **13:**435-440.

Frohneberg, D., et al. 1981. Telemetric urodynamic investigations in patients with infravesical obstruction. Paper presented at the seventy-sixth meeting of the American Urological Association meeting. Boston.

Gjertsen, K.T. 1961. Paradoxical incontinence in prostatic patients: a cystometrical and clinical study. Norwegian Monographs on Medical Science. Oslo. Norwegian Universities Press.

Gleason, D.M., Bottacini, M.R., and Reilly, R.J. 1977. Comparison of cystometrograms and urethral profiles with gas and water media. Urology **9:**155-160.

Griffiths, D.J. 1977. Urodynamic assessment of bladder function. Br. J. Urol. **49:**29-36.

Griffiths, D.J., et al. 1979. Active mechanical properties of the smooth muscle of the urinary bladder. Med. Biol. Eng. Comput. **17:**281-290.

Hill, A.V. 1938. The heat of shortening and the dynamic constants of muscle. Proc. R. Soc. Lond. **126:**136-195.

International Continence Society. 1976. First report. Br. J. Urol. **48:**39.

Kondo, A., Susset, J.G., and Lefaivre, J. 1972. Visco-elastic properties of bladder. I. Mechanical model and its mathematical analysis. Invest. Urol. **10:**154-163.

Landowne, M., and Stacy, R.W. 1957. Glossary of terms: 'tissue elasticity.' In Remington, J.W., editor. papers arising from a conference held at Dartmouth College, Hanover, NH., Sept. 1-3, 1955. Washington. American Physiological Society. pp. 191-201.

Mayo, M.E. 1978. Detrusor hyperreflexia: the effect of posture and pelvic floor activity. J. Urol. **119:**635-638.

Meyhoff, H.H., et al. 1980. Incontinence surgery in females with motor urge incontinence. Proceedings of the International Continence Society-Urodynamics Society meeting. Los Angeles.

Nijman, C.R., and Sjöberg, G. 1981. Direct transmural measurement of the detrusor pressure. Invest. Urol. **18**:392.

van Duyl, W.A. 1980. Determination and interpretation of micromotion in urinary bladder smooth muscle: viscomotion model. Proceedings of the twentieth International Conference on Biological engineering. London.

van Duyl, W.A., Coolsaet, B.L.R.A., and van Mastrigt, R. 1978. A new clinical parameter for the assessment of the contracility of the urinary bladder. Urol. Int. **33**:31.

van Duyl, W.A., et al. 1978. An electronic device for quick analysis of exponential decay curves. Urol. Int. **33**:50.

van Mastrigt, R. 1977. A system approach to the passive properties of the urinary bladder in the collection phase. Thesis. Rotterdam University.

van Mastrigt, R. 1980. The on-line determination of the maximal contraction velocity of the urinary bladder from an isometric contraction. Proceedings of the International Continence Society-Urodynamics Society meeting. Los Angeles.

van Mastrigt, R., and Griffiths, D.J. 1979. Contractility of the urinary bladder. Urol. Int. **34**:410.

van Mastrigt, R., Coolsaet, B.L.R.A., and van Duyl, W.A. 1978. Passive properties in the collection phase. Med. Biol. Eng. Comput. **16**:471-482.

chapter 9

Radiology

STUART L. STANTON

Investigation of disorders of micturition includes the lower and upper urinary tracts and the spinal cord, which is intimately involved here. Careful selection of the radiological studies is necessary because of the hazard of cumulative irradiation and the invasive nature of some of the investigations (Table 9-1).

PLAIN ABDOMINAL AND PELVIC RADIOGRAPHS

A plain abdominal or pelvic radiograph may be taken to investigate a visible abnormality or as a control film during an intravenous urogram. The following conditions may cause incontinence or are related to its treatment.

Epispadias (see Figure 7.5) and bladder exstrophy are obvious congenital anomalies. The wide separation of the pubic bones in exstrophy (Figure 9.1) is a characteristic radiological feature. Traumatic separation of the symphysis pubis (see Figure 16.3) and opening of the pelvic ring are found following automobile accidents in which injury to the pelvis is often associated with other injuries to the bony pelvis and its soft-tissue contents. There may be no obvious injury to the lower urinary tract at the time. Less marked symphysial separation may also be found following symphysiotomy for cephalopelvic disproportion in labor.

The likelihood of past syphilitic infection may be deduced from heavy metal deposits (for example, bismuth) in the buttocks as shown in Figure 9.2. This particular patient had chronic retention and overflow, a variable sensory deficit, and absence of lower limb reflexes. An intravenous urogram showed hydronephrosis and a large amount of residual urine. Urinary retention (Figure 16.6) may be found during investigation of a lower abdominal mass and has to be distinguished from ascites or an ovarian cyst. The "fluid level" shown

TABLE 9.1 Irradiation dosages to the ovaries following radiological procedures	
Radiological procedures	**Dosage (mGy)**
Plain pelvic anteroposterior radio-graph	0.8
Anteroposterior and lateral views of lumbosacral spine	2.0
Lumbar myelogram	2.0
Intravenous urogram	2.6
Micturition cystography	8.4
Videocystourethrography	2.7
Urethrogram	5.7

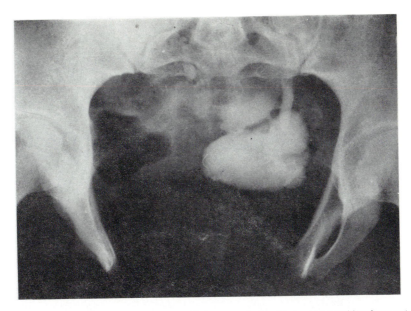

Figure 9.1 Pelvis in bladder exstrophy showing widely separated pubic bones resulting from outward rotation of pubis and innominate bones. There is contrast in reconstructed bladder.

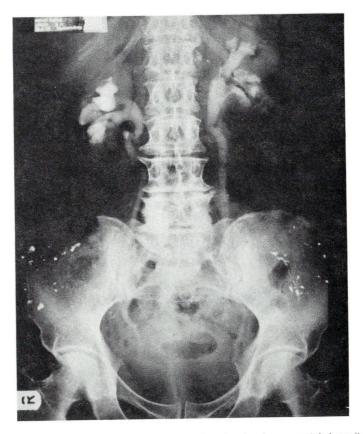

Figure 9.2 Radiograph during intravenous urogram series showing heavy metal deposits in buttocks and bilateral hydronephrosis.

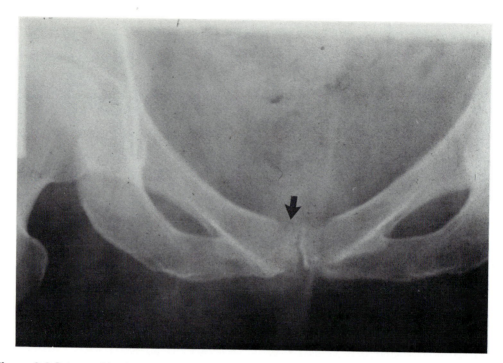

Figure 9.3 Osteomyelitis of pubis resulting from osteitis pubis following Marshall-Marchetti-Krantz procedure. Arrow shows area of osteomyelitis.

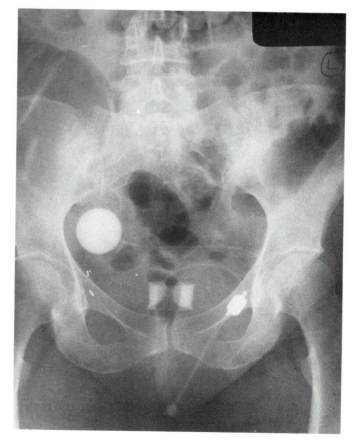

Figure 9.4 Activated artificial urinary sphincter (AMS 792) showing reservoir, cuff, and pump filled with contrast.

here is due to a urinary tract infection by gas-producing organisms.

Osteitis pubis is a known complication of the Marshall-Marchetti-Krantz procedure (see Chapter 16), and in the case illustrated in Figure 9.3 osteomyelitis had developed in both pubic rami and required curettage.

The artifical urinary sphincter (see Chapter 16) is shown in the activated mode, with the cuff, reservoir, and pump containing 12.5% Hypaque, which is the normal hydraulic fluid (Figure 9.4). The role of the radiograph is to confirm that fluid is present within all components; this may be in doubt if the incontinence recurs following implantation.

VERTEBRAL COLUMN RADIOGRAPHS

Vertebral column radiographs include plain lateral and anteroposterior radiographs, myelograms, and spinal angiograms. The following outline indicates the conditions that may be investigated:

Disorders involving the spinal cord that cause disturbance of micturition

I. Congenital
   A. Sacral agenesis
   B. Spina bifida occulta
   C. Diastomatomyelia
   D. Myelomeningocele
II. Trauma
III. Tumor
   A. Intramedullary
   B. Extramedullary
IV. Inflammatory
   A. Extradural abscess
   B. Spinal arachnoiditis
V. Spinal lumbar canal (stenosis)
VI. Prolapsed intervertebral disk
VII. Spondylolisthesis

Sacral agenesis (Figure 9.5) will produce urinary symptoms only if three or more sacral segments are absent. Spina bifida occulta (see Figure 7.4), which is found in up to 50% of the population without any clinical significance, will produce symptoms and signs if the cord is tethered by an abnormally thick filum terminale. If the cord is bifurcated by a spur or bone or cartilage growing from the back of the vertebral body, as in diastomatomyelia (Figure 9.6), symptoms and signs of neuropathic bladder will occur as the child grows: upward movement of the conus medullaris produces traction on nerve roots from the bony spur or tethered filum.

Myelomeningocele is most common in the lumbar region and is an important cause of neuropathic disorders in childhood. The radiograph will indicate the level and extent of the lesion (Figure 9.7);

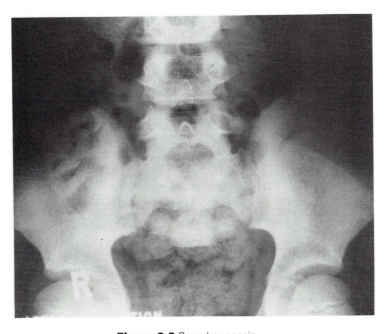

Figure 9.5 Sacral agenesis.

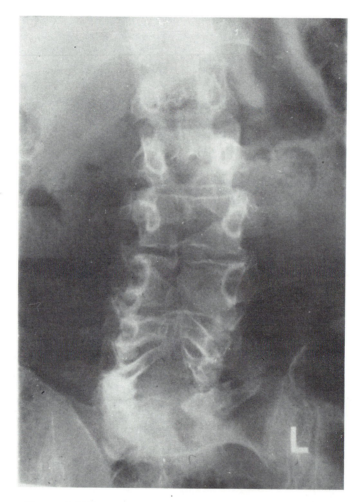

Figure 9.6 Diastomatomyelia involving lower lumbar vertebrae.

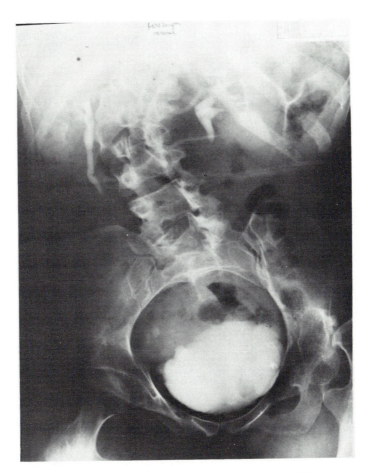

Figure 9.7 Radiograph during intravenous urogram series showing spina bifida involving L4 and L5, with lumbar scoliosis and congenital dislocation of left hip.

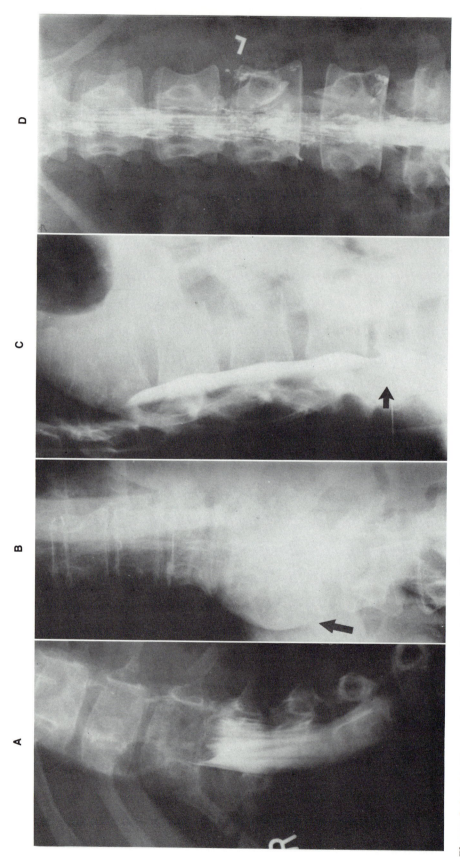

Figure 9.8 A, Myelogram showing complete obstruction at T12 to L1 by astrocytoma of spinal cord. **B,** Anteroposterior view of thoracolumbar spine showing showing paravertebral tissue abscess. Arrow shows lateral border of abscess. **C,** Lateral myelogram showing destruction of intravertebral disk space at T11 and T12 and collapse of T11 and T12 with cord compression *(arrow)*. **D,** Anteroposterior view of lumbar spine showing chronic adhesive arachnoiditis. Contrast has "brush-painted" appearance. (**A** courtesy of Mr. Michael Torrens; **B, C,** and **D** courtesy of Dr. James Ambrose.)

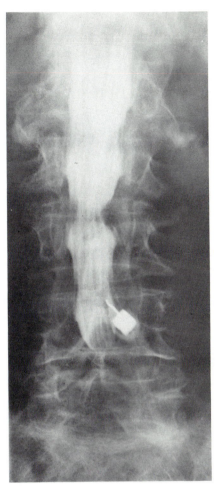

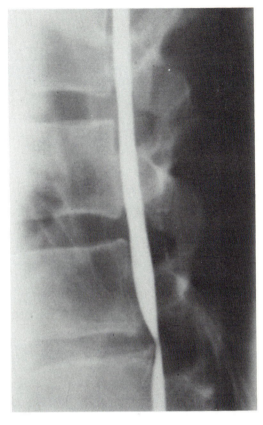

Figure 9.9 Anteroposterior view of lumbar radiculogram showing stenosis at L4 and L5 effectively causing complete obstruction. (Courtesy of Dr. James Ambrose.)

Figure 9.10 Prolapsed intravertebral disk with compression of spinal cord.

the same radiograph may demonstrate abnormalities of the pelvic bones, particularly the hip joints.

Trauma to the spinal cord, intra- or extramedullary tumors, and extradural abscess will produce disturbance of micturition, the precise form depending on the level and extent of the lesion. Spinal arachnoiditis (usually caused by Myodil) causes obstructive symptoms and frequency; incontinence is uncommon. The radiological appearances of these lesions are shown in Figure 9.8. Lumbar spinal stenosis, which is a combination of degeneration of the intervertebral disk and osteoarthritic change producing osteophytes along the posterior margins of the vertebral bodies and degenerative changes around the posterior intervertebral joints, leads to compression of the spinal cord and nerve roots

(principally L4, L5, and S1). Neurogenic claudication affecting the legs and urinary retention are common symptoms; radiological changes (Figure 9.9) include narrowing of the lumbar canal, shortening of the pedicles, and anteroposterior flattening of the exit foramina of the nerve roots. Myelography will show narrowing and multiple waistlike anterolateral and posterolateral indentations on the thecal sac.

Prolapsed intervertebral disk is most common at the L4-5 space and at the L5 and S1 levels and causes compression of the corresponding lateral roots (Figure 9.10). Central compression may cause a cauda equina syndrome.

Spondylolisthesis (Figure 9.11) commonly of L5 slipping on S1 will cause mainly frequency.

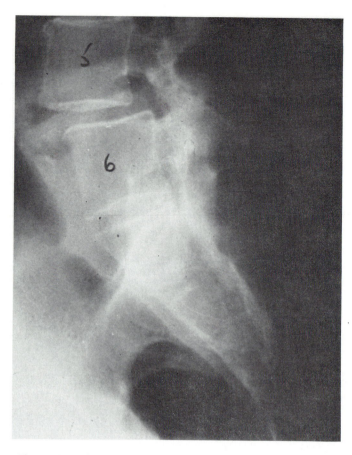

Figure 9.11 Spondylolisthesis, with slipping forward of L5 on L6.

INTRAVENOUS UROGRAPHY AND RETROGRADE UROGRAPHY

The indications for intravenous urography in this context are:

1. Continuous incontinence with an otherwise normal voiding pattern
2. Diurnal incontinence
3. Recurrent urinary tract infection
4. Obstructive uropathy
5. Neuropathic bladder
6. Persistent "vaginal" discharge

Here the main indication for a retrograde urogram is to identify a ureterovaginal fistula.

The following conditions may be detected by intravenous urography: An ectopic ureter (Figure 9.12) is bilateral in 5% to 25% of cases and is more common in the female than in the male. The ectopic opening may be detected by urethrocystoscopy or careful vaginal examination. Only if the ectopic ureter opens distal to the bladder neck or in the vagina will incontinence occur. Recurrent urinary tract infection may be a presenting feature.

A ureterocele (Figure 9.13) is a cystic dilatation of the terminal ureter within the bladder or urethra. An "ectopic" ureterocele is located distal to the trigone and may project into the urethra; 10% are bilateral. In the neonate a ureterocele can be seen as a urinary tract infection and failure to thrive; urinary retention can occur if the ectopic ureterocele prolapses through the bladder neck. Incontinence may result if the ureterocele interferes with the competence of the urethral sphincter mechanism.

Hydronephrosis and hydroureter may be a sequel to outflow obstruction and vesicoureteric reflux. These are an index of deterioration in renal function and are therefore important to detect (Figure 9.14).

A ureterovaginal fistula may be demonstrated by an intravenous urogram (Figure 9.15) or retrograde ureterography (Figure 9.16). Third-degree uterine prolapse (procidentia) may lead to residual urine, recurrent urinary tract infection, and rarely compression of the ureters leading to hydronephrosis (Figure 9.16). An intravenous urogram will

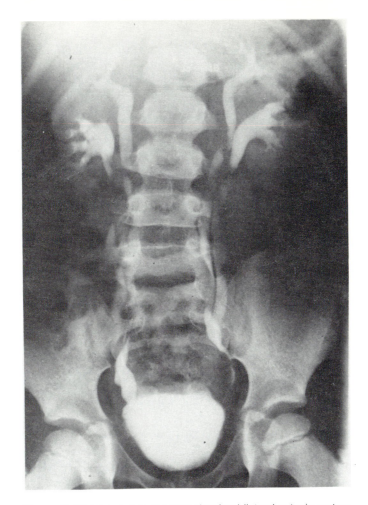

Figure 9.12 Intravenous urogram showing bilateral ectopic ureters.

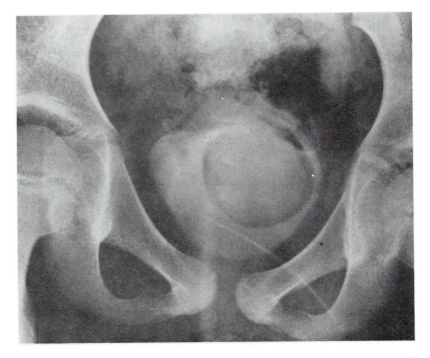

Figure 9.13 Intravenous urogram showing left orthotopic ureterocele. (Courtesy of Drs. C. Kasby and K. Parsons.)

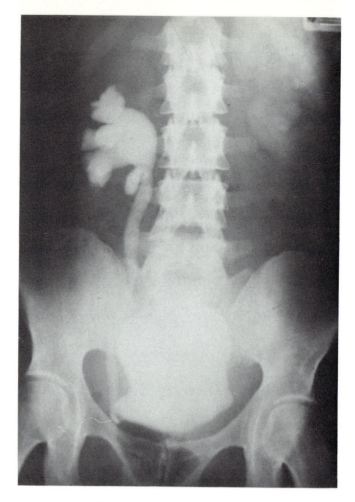

Figure 9.14 Intravenous urogram showing right hydronephrosis and hydroureter. Left kidney is nonfunctioning.

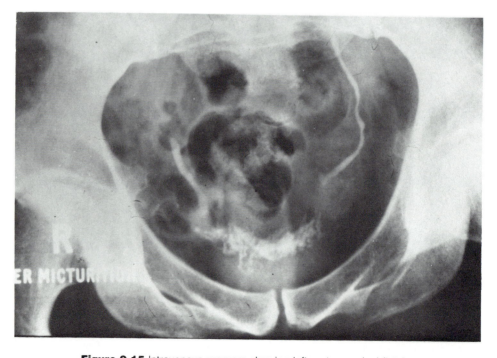

Figure 9.15 Intravenous urogram showing left ureterovaginal fistula.

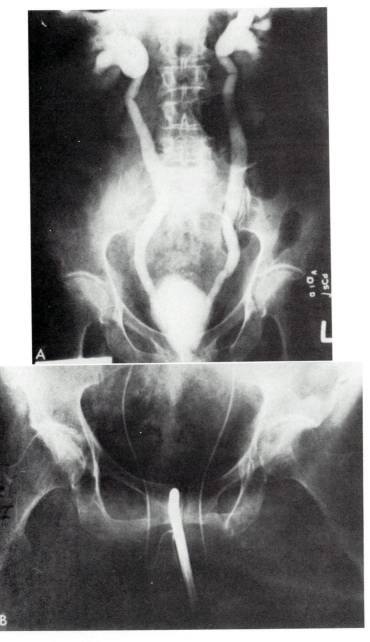

Figure 9.16 Intravenous urogram showing bilateral hydronephrosis and hydroureter resulting from compression of ureter as result of procidentia. Lower radiograph is retrograde pyelogram showing extent of ureteric descent. (Courtesy of Drs. Herbert Buchsbaum and Joseph Schmidt.)

demonstrate the involvement of the upper urinary tract and the degree to which the ureters may be displaced—a sometimes unrecognized hazard at vaginal hysterectomy and anterior repair in these cases.

BLADDER

Radiological investigation of female bladder function has undergone many changes since cystography was first used at the beginning of the century; advances in radiological technology and evolution of concepts of lower urinary tract function have led to increasingly complex but informative procedures. Early cystography consisted of anteroposterior views using a manual cassette changer. Fluoroscopy was used in the 1920s, and oblique and lateral views were taken. However, the unacceptably high radiation dose was a limiting factor. Chain cystography was introduced in the late 1930s, and lateral views began to be used extensively in the 1950s. The development of image intensification allowed longer screening using a much smaller current than previously. The image could now be filmed, and a permanent and dynamic record of the act of micturition could be obtained.

The static cystogram lateral views were studied extensively by Jeffcoate and Roberts (1952) and led to their theories on the posterior urethrovesical angle, which were to stand unchallenged for 20 years. However, a change in emphasis away from morphological toward physiological measurements and the pioneer work by Enhorning (1961) with urethral and bladder pressure measurements led to the development of a combination of cineradiographic screening of the bladder during micturition, with simultaneous bladder and urethral pressure measurements by Enhorning, Miller, and Hinman in 1964. Bates, Whiteside, and Turner-Warwick (1970) refined this, and the technique was gradually adopted as a practical method of investigation in many urological centers. Use of videocystourethrography, which allowed instant replay and rerecording if necessary, made the procedure even more versatile.

The techniques for bladder imaging may be classified as shown in the outline below:

I. Static radiograph
   A. Erect
      1. Oblique
      2. Lateral
      3. Anteroposterior
   B. Sitting
      1. Lateral
II. Micturition cystography
III. Videocystourethrography

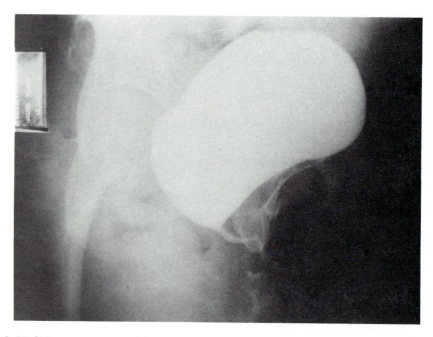

Figure 9.17 Oblique erect nonstraining radiograph showing bladder neck open and contrast in proximal urethra.

Static radiographs may be plain, use a metallic bead chain, use contrast media of differing densities, and outline the vagina or rectum. They may be taken at rest, on straining, squeezing, or during voiding.

Static radiograph

This is the most common technique of radiological investigation of the bladder. It may be taken in a variety of views as described previously. A sitting position is of course more natural for a woman patient but requires greater irradiation to penetrate the superimposed femora to visualize the bladder neck. The lateral erect position will demonstrate the relationship of the bladder, bladder neck, and urethra to the symphysis. Oblique views are less informative, but they can be obtained with a lower dose of radiation. Anteroposterior views are less popular and only show changes in descent of the bladder and because of superimposition; it is not possible to define the position of the bladder neck separate from the base of the bladder. This is seen more readily on lateral or oblique views. An oblique erect nonstraining radiograph is shown in Figure 9.17; the bladder neck is open and contrast is in the proximal urethra. Without simultaneous bladder and abdominal pressure recordings, it is difficult to differentiate between (1) an uninhibited detrusor contraction, (2) leakage of contrast in response to coughing caused by urethral sphincter incompetence, (3) voluntary voiding, and (4) a bladder neck held open by fibrosis with incomplete milk-back. Measurement of the posterior urethrovesical angle (in a lateral view) has no significant diagnostic application nowadays.

More use can be made of static radiographs by taking serial radiographs at rest and on straining, squeezing, and voiding, after the technique of Olesen and Walter (1977) (Figure 9.18). In addition, the vagina may be outlined with 15 ml of ordinary barium contrast. This gives further information about the supports of the bladder base and urethra and pelvic floor function. The technique relies, however, on an experienced radiologist detecting the precise time at which these individual actions occur and being certain that exposure is made at the time of maximum effort.

Further information on the relationship of other soft tissues in the pelvis was obtained by Béthoux and Bory (1962), who instilled contrast into the rectum (colpocystogram) and took lateral still radiographs at rest, during straining, and on contraction of the pelvic floor.

To outline the urethra and determine its anatomical relationship to the bladder and symphysis, a metallic bead chain may be introduced into the urethra and bladder together with contrast media. Radiographs taken at rest and during straining may indicate downward movement and backward rotation of the bladder and displacement of the urethrovesical junction to the lowermost bladder level (Hodgkinson, 1958) (Figure 9.19).

Studies by Hertogs (1983) indicate the usefulness of this technique in detecting the relationship of the proximal urethra to the symphysis pubis in patients after failed and successful incontinence procedures (Figure 9.20).

Use of contrast media of differing densities provides further visualization of the bladder neck and urethra. When 12% sodium iodide and iodized oil (Lipiodol) are introduced into the bladder, the iodized oil settles to the base of the bladder and outlines the bladder neck (Figure 9.21).

In summary, the advantage of the static radiograph is simplicity and a low radiation dose. The disadvantages include the low yield of information, difficulty in recording a dynamic activity on still radiographs and an inability to diagnose detrusor instability.

Micturition cystography

Micturition cystography consists of radiological screening of the bladder in the standing or sitting position. The images are either recorded as static radiographs on 35 mm film or as a continuous procedure on cine film. The latter is preferable because micturition is a dynamic process and should be recorded as such. Micturition cystography may be used to demonstrate vesicoureteric reflux (Figure 9.22), vesicovaginal fistula (Figure 9.23), bladder diverticulum (Figure 9.24), and urethral diverticulum (Figure 9.25). Incontinence may be demonstrated, but detrusor instability cannot be accurately diagnosed unless there are synchronous bladder and abdominal pressure measurements. Urethral sphincter incompetence may be diagnosed, but difficulty may arise in those patients in whom detrusor instability and urethral sphincter incompetence coexist. Similarly, little can be inferred from the presence of an open bladder neck unless pressure recordings are taken simultaneously.

A large bladder with a large postmicturition residual as a result of lower motor neuron disease is shown in Figure 9.26. Marked descent of the blad-

Text continued on p. 101.

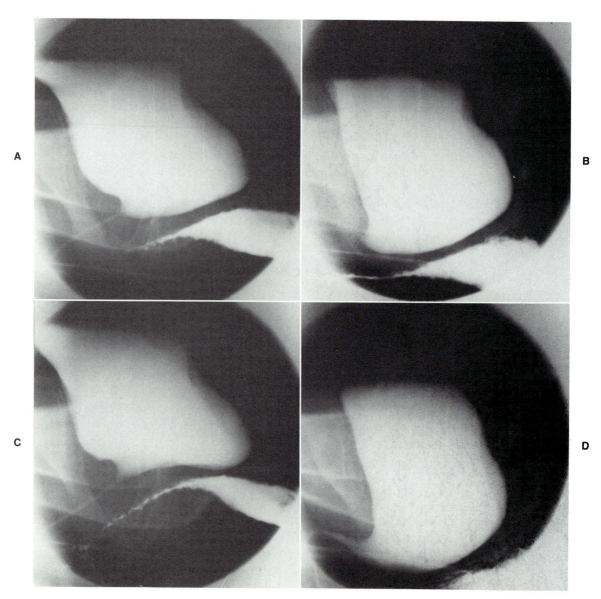

Figure 9.18 Colpocystourethrography (lateral voiding cystourethrography with barium contrast in vagina). **A,** Bladder at rest showing some descent. **B,** Coughing, with further descent of bladder. **C,** Tightening of pelvic floor showing repositioning of bladder to its normal configuration. **D,** Voiding, with typical posterior descent and "teapot deformity." (Courtesy of Dr. Klud Olesen.)

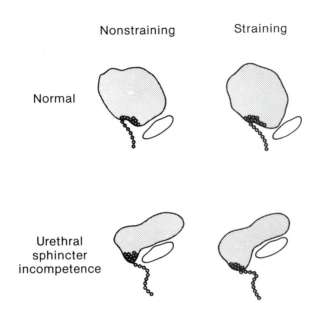

Normal Nonstraining Straining

Urethral sphincter incompetence

Figure 9.19 Drawings from lateral radiograph of bladder and symphysis with bladder base and urethra outlined by metallic bead chain. There is greater descent of bladder neck at rest and on straining in patient with urethral sphincter incompetence. (Courtesy of Dr. C. Paul Hodgkinson.)

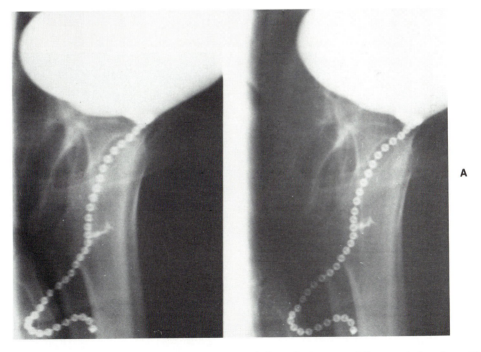

A

Figure 9.20 A, Lateral radiograph of metallic bead chain in patient successfully operated on for urethral sphincter incompetence. *Left,* During straining; *right,* at rest. Note elevated position of bladder neck and alignment of bladder neck and proximal urethra to posterosuperior aspect of symphysis pubis.

Continued.

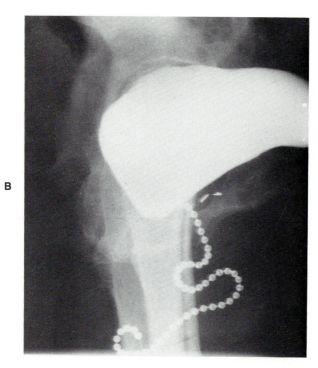

Figure 9.20, cont'd. B, Recurrent urethral sphincter incompetence with failure of elevation of bladder neck and lack of alignment of bladder neck and proximal urethra to symphysis pubis. (Courtesy of Mr. Keith Hertogs.)

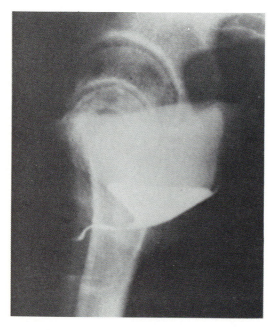

Figure 9.21 Erect lateral radiograph outlining bladder and urethra by using opaque media of different specific gravities. (Courtesy of Drs. J. Edward Morgan and Grant Farrow.)

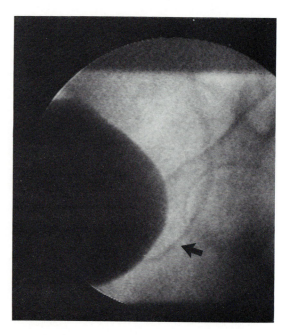

Figure 9.22 Micturition cystogram showing left vesicoureteric reflux.

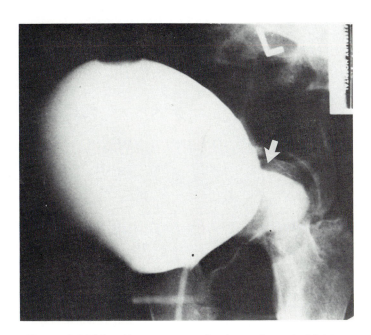

Figure 9.23 Micturition cystogram showing vesicovaginal fistula.

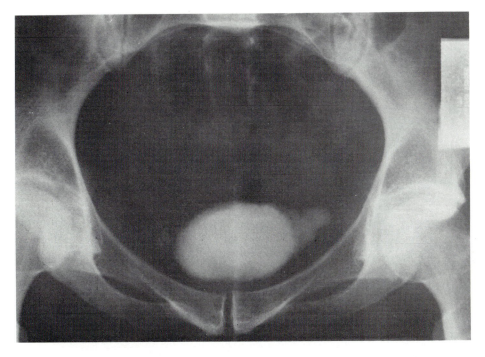

Figure 9.24 Micturition cystogram showing bladder diverticulum on left.

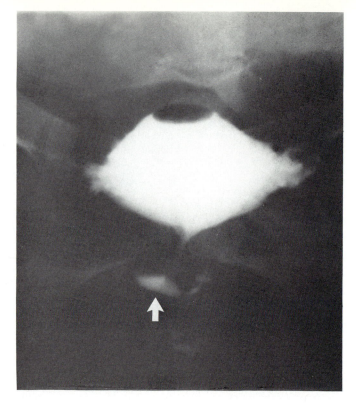

Figure 9.25 Micturition cystogram showing urethral diverticulum *(arrow)*.

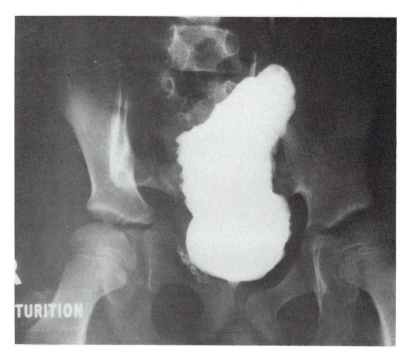

Figure 9.26 Micturition cystogram showing large bladder containing large postmicturition residual as result lower motor neuron disease.

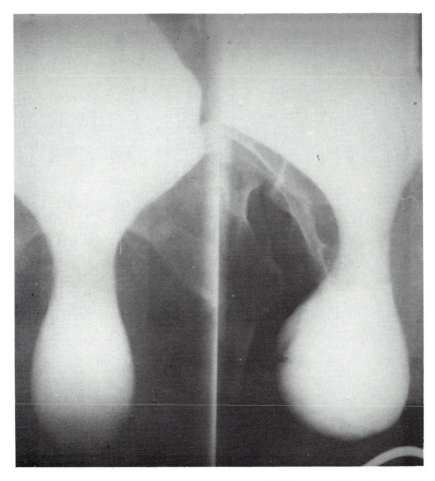

Figure 9.27 Micturition cystogram showing marked cystocele. *Left,* Anteroposterior view, *Right,* Lateral view.

der with residual urine associated with third-degree uterine descent and descent of the anterior vaginal wall is illustrated in Figure 9.27.

Videocystourethrography

The technique of synchronous radiological screening of the bladder and measurement of bladder and abdominal pressure and urine flow rate recorded with sound on videotape is known as videocystourethrography (Figure 9.28).

In addition to those indications for micturition cystography, the following are specific indications for videocystourethrography:

1. Failed incontinence surgery
2. Complex symptomatology associated with incontinence
3. Suspect detrusor instability
4. Voiding difficulty

With a patient lying supine on a tilting radiological table, sterile urethral catheterization is performed with a No. 12 Fr catheter (to measure the residual urine and fill the bladder) and a soft 1 mm external diameter fluid-filled catheter (to measure bladder pressure (Figure 9.29). A 2 mm external diameter fluid-filled catheter (with its end protected by a fingerstall) is inserted just into the rectum, to record the rectal pressure (equivalent to the abdominal pressure). Both catheters are connected to pressure transducers; electronic subtraction of the rectal pressure from the intravesical pressure gives the detrusor pressure. The bladder is filled with contrast media at a rate of 100 ml/min (a neuropathic bladder is filled more slowly, between 2 and 5 ml/min), which is recorded using a weighing transducer. First sensation and full capacity are noted. The patient coughs several times during fill-

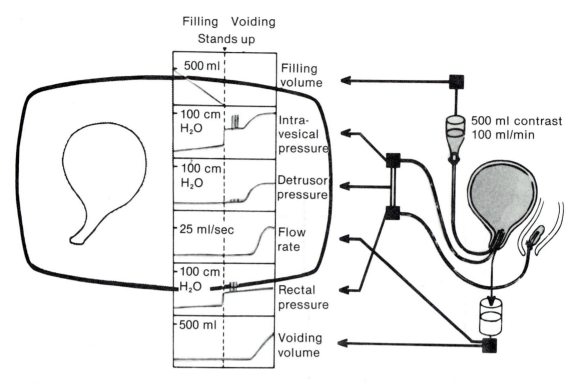

Figure 9.28 Videocystourethrography schema. Simultaneous recording of bladder and rectal pressure changes during supine cystometry combined with display of bladder filling volume is shown on left side of polygraph trace. On voiding, bladder and rectal pressures with voiding rate and volume are recorded on right of trace. Television cameras select three parameters (intravesical pressure, detrusor pressure, and voiding rate) that are added to radiographic image of bladder (extreme left of diagram) and recorded with sound commentary on videotape.

ing (to confirm that the pressures are being satisfactorily recorded and subtracted and to act as a provocative stimulus for detrusor instability). The filling catheter is then removed and the patient positioned erect and radiologically screened in the erect oblique or in the sitting position. She is asked to cough, and leakage and bladder neck and bladder base descent are noted. She is then asked to void and interrupt her stream. The peak urine flow rate and volume voided are recorded on a uroflowmeter, simultaneous with measurement of the detrusor pressure (maximum voiding pressure). The ability to milk-back contrast from the proximal urethra into the bladder is noted. She completes voiding and is rescreened to detect any residual contrast media. When erect, approximately 20% of women have difficulty voiding, which may be overcome by moving the patient with pressure lines in situ to an adjacent side room where the patient can void in privacy, seated on a flowmeter. All data are recorded on a six-channel recorder. During the voiding phase, a television camera is positioned

above the recording chart. Three channels (intravesical and detrusor pressures and peak flow rate) are selected and with the aid of a mixing device, a fused image of the bladder and urethra and pressures and flow data are created. This is displayed on a television monitor and the combined picture, together with sound commentary, is recorded on videotape for instant and later replay (Figure 9.30).

Provocative tests for detrusor instability include rapid bladder filling, coughing during filling, passive posture change, and coughing and filling in the erect position. The total screening time is less than 1 minute, and using an image intensifier, the radiation dose to the ovaries is approximately 700 mrad/min. Each examination takes about 20 minutes; six patients can easily be screened in one session.

The following features are found in a normal female bladder:

Residual urine less than 50 ml

First sensation at 150 to 200 ml

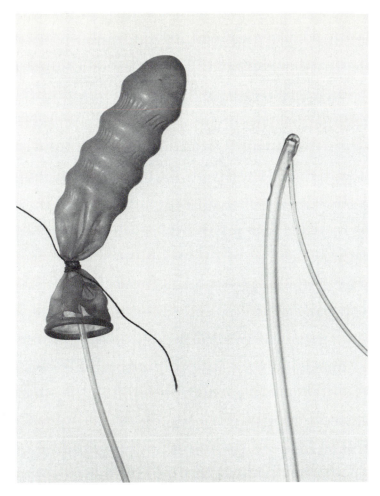

Figure 9.29 Catheters used for videocystourethrography. *Left,* Rectal catheter protected by fingerstall. *Right,* No. 12 Fr gauge filling catheter with 1 mm external diameter intravesical pressure–measuring catheter slotted into its side.

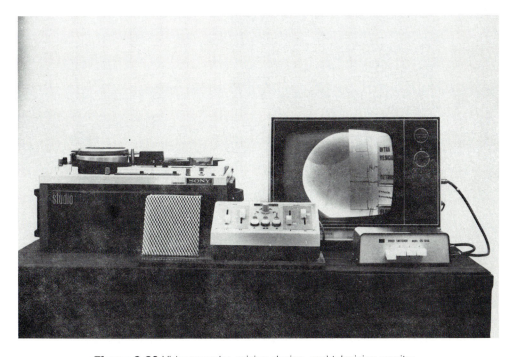

Figure 9.30 Videorecorder, mixing device, and television monitor.

Strong desire to void at 400 to 500 ml

Detrusor pressure rise on filling, standing, and coughing below 15 cm of water

No loss of contrast and only slight descent of the bladder neck and bladder base on coughing

A rise of detrusor pressure on voiding not greater than 70 cm of water with a peak flow rate greater than 15 ml/sec for a volume voiding of at least 150 ml

Ability to cease voiding on command with milk-back of contrast from the midurethra to the bladder (During this time, the isometric contraction pressure gradually falls as the bladder neck closes)

No vesicoureteric reflux

A series of still frames from a normal video-cystourethrogram is shown in Figure 9.31. The importance of videocystourethrography is illustrated

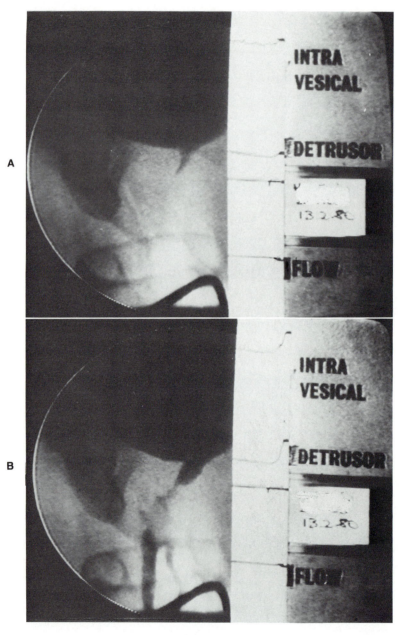

Figure 9.31 Series of still frames from videocystourethrogram showing normal micturition with voluntary interruption. **A,** Bladder neck opening and contrast visible in proximal urethra. Detrusor pressure begins to rise. **B,** Contrast outlining all of urethra and beginning to enter flowmeter. Detrusor pressure is 25 cm of water.

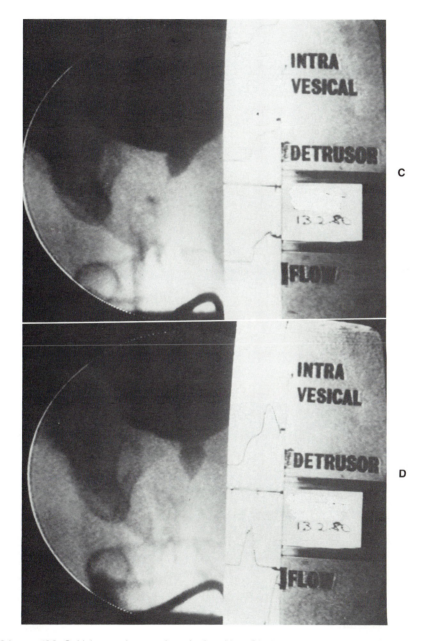

Figure 9.31, cont'd. C, Voluntary interruption of micturition. Bladder neck is open, but extrinsic sphincter is contracted. Detrusor pressure rises at start of isometric contraction phase. Flow rate is 15 ml/sec. **D,** Isometric contraction phase almost finished and detrusor pressure has fallen to prestop level. Bladder neck is still kept open by detrusor contraction. Flow rate is zero. *Continued.*

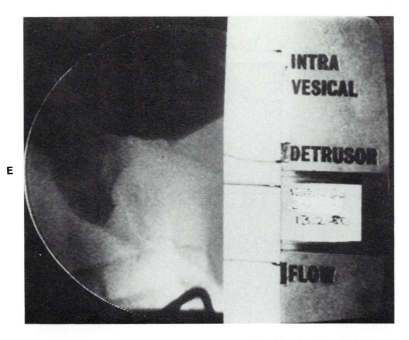

Figure 9.31, cont'd. E, Detrusor pressure has fallen to premicturition level, and bladder neck has closed. Flow rate is zero.

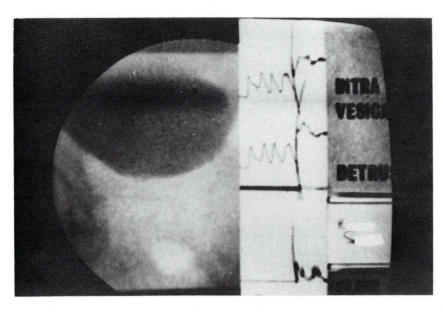

Figure 9.32 Videocystourethrogram image showing uninhibited detrusor contractions during filling with detrusor pressure rise of 20 cm of water on standing.

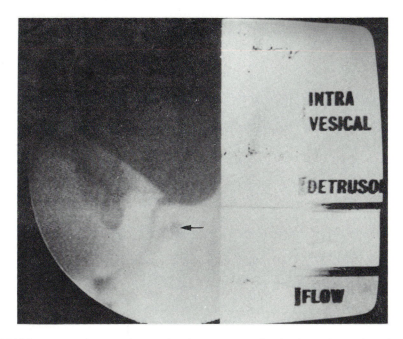

Figure 9.33 Videocystourethrogram image showing contrast collecting in vagina during micturition, owing to altered vaginal anatomy following abdominoperineal resection.

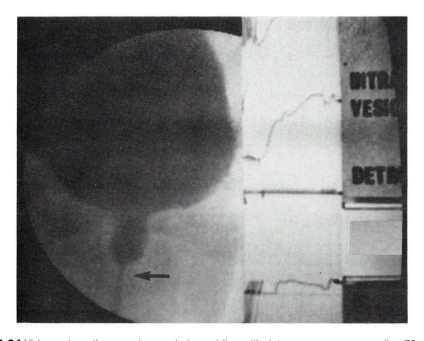

Figure 9.34 Videocystourethrogram image during voiding with detrusor pressure exceeding 70 cm of water and flow rate of 8 ml/sec. There is narrowing of distal urethra as result of external urethral sphincter spasm or distal urethral stenosis.

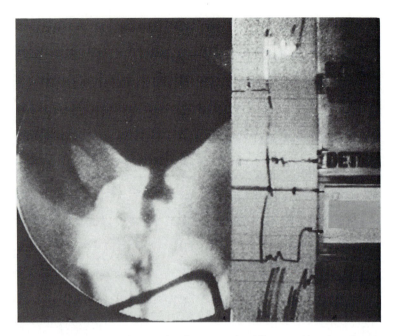

Figure 9.35 Videocystourethrogram image showing normal voiding resulting from increase in abdominal pressure with pelvic floor relaxation but without any rise in detrusor pressure. Urethral diverticulum is present.

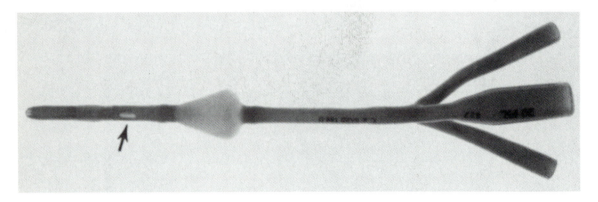

Figure 9.36 Tratner triple-lumen catheter for urethrography. There are two balloons. On inflation they are positioned respectively at internal and external urethral meatuses. Contrast is injected by third lumen to outline urethra.

in the following cases of incontinence. Figure 16.7 demonstrates incontinence caused by urethral sphincter incompetence; the bladder neck is open, and leakage is seen with a cough sequence in progress. There is no evidence of uninhibited detrusor contraction. Uninhibited detrusor activity is demonstrated in Figures 9.32 and 17.5. An unusual case of incontinence is seen in Figure 9.33 where postmicturition dribbling occurs as a result of vaginal reflux following an abdominoperineal resection.

Voiding difficulties may be identified by a lower motor neuron trace showing delayed first sensation, a large capacity bladder, and a minimal detrusor pressure rise. External urethral sphincter spasm or distal urethral stenosis (Figure 9.34) may be present. Figure 9.35 shows how normal voiding may occur without a detrusor contraction, owing to a rise in abdominal pressure and relaxation of the pelvic floor. A urethral diverticulum is shown.

URETHROGRAM

Selective radiography of the urethra is used to detect a urethral diverticulum that may otherwise be diagnosed on videocystourethrography or ure-throscopy. A Tratner or Davies catheter is used (Figure 9.36), which has three channels, two to fill the distal and proximal balloons that are positioned respectively at the internal and external ure-thral meatus, and the remaining channel to allow contrast to escape into the urethra to demonstrate the diverticulum. This catheter can also be used to demonstrate a urethrovaginal fistula.

REFERENCES

Bates, C.P., Whiteside, C.G., and Turner-Warwick, R. 1970. Synchronous cine/pressure/flow/cystourethrography with special reference to stress and urge incontinence. Br. J. Urol. **42:**714-723.

Béthoux, A., and Bory, S. 1962. Les mecanismes statiques visceraux pelviens chez la femme: a la lumiere de l'exploration fonctionelle du dispositif en position debout. Ann. Chir. **16:**887-916.

Enhorning, G. 1961. Simultaneous recording of intravesical and intra-urethral pressure. Acta. Clin. Scand. Suppl. **276:** 1-68.

Enhorning, G., Miller, A.E., and Hinman, F., Jr. 1964. Urethral closure studies with cine roentgenography and simultaneous bladder-urethra pressure recording. Surg. Gynecol. Obstet. **118:**507-516.

Hertogs, K. 1983. Personal communication.

Hodgkinson, C.P., Doub, H., and Keely, W. 1958. Urethrocystograms: metallic bead technique. Clin. Obstet. Gynecol. **1:**668-677.

Jeffcoate, N., and Roberts, H. 1952. Stress incontinence. Br. J. Obstet. Gynaecol. **59:**685-720.

Olesen, K., and Walter, S. 1977. Colpocystourethrography: a radiological method combined with pressure-flow measurements. Dan. Med. Bull. **24:**96-100.

Urethral pressure measurement

PAUL HILTON

From the definition of incontinence given in Appendix II, it may be presumed that the state of continence is the retention of urine in the bladder between voluntary episodes of micturition. It is evident that continence is dependent on "the powers of urethral resistance exceeding the forces of urinary expulsion." This concept was, however, first expressed by Barnes in 1940 and first demonstrated by simultaneous intravesical and urethral pressure measurement by Enhorning as recently as 1961. To maintain continence, it is vital that the urethral lumen seal completely. Zinner, Ritter, and Sterling (1976) have described three major elements of urethral function necessary to achieve this hermetic property: urethral inner wall softness, inner urethral compression, and urethral outer wall tension. Although any elastic tube can be closed if sufficient compression is applied, the efficiency of its closure is dramatically increased if its lining possesses the property of plasticity, or the capacity to mold into a watertight seal. This has been demonstrated in crude physical models (Zinner, Sterling, and Ritter, 1979), although demonstration in human subjects is still awaited. The property of urethral softness, or plasticity, is only effective in producing continence if the urethral lining is under compression. Although greater plasticity of a given urethral lining reduces the degree of compression required, compression is nevertheless a vital component of the continence mechanism. Compression is itself a consequence of the mural tension that results from the passive and active characteristics of the components of the urethral wall and periurethral tissues. It is therefore the sum of behavioral characteristics of all of these structures at any instant in time that determines continence or micturition.

NATURE OF URETHRAL PRESSURE

Pressure measurement within the urethra is different from pressure measurement of many other biological tubes. In blood vessels, for instance, in which the lumen is filled with fluid in constant flow, the pressure in the liquid is in equilibrium with the forces exerted by the walls. This latter function is itself a compound of the active and passive tensions generated by the wall, by surrounding structures, and by transmission from adjacent body cavities. In the urethra, however, the intraluminal pressure is seldom measured when fluid is present, that is, during micturition; nor is it measured when the urethra is completely empty, since all methods of measurement require the presence of a measuring instrument within the lumen. The significance of error induced by the instrument is determined by the distensibility of the urethra, that is, by the extent to which urethral pressure rises as the urethra is distended (Abrams, Martin, and Griffiths, 1978). If the urethra were a rigid tube, very great changes in pressure would occur with small changes in cross-sectional area; a single pressure measurement at an arbitrarily imposed diameter would therefore be meaningless. In a highly distensible tube, however, pressure changes very little over a wide-range, cross-sectional area; a single pressure measurement is much more representative of the physical characteristics of the tube (Griffiths, 1980). This appears much more appropriate to the normal urethra, and although the measured pressure depends on catheter size, this dependence is slight in the region of maximum pressure (Plevnik, 1976).

The most obvious feature of the urethral pressure profile in women is the symmetry around the point of maximum pressure in the urethra. Although the morphological contributors to this characteristic of the profile are difficult to determine, from a hydrodynamic point of view this region may be accurately termed an *elastic constriction* (Griffiths, 1969). It is the region that would show the minimum cross-sectional area, or maximum flow rate,

if the urethra were perfused at constant pressure. It is therefore the region that determines the resistance relation of the urethra as a whole and controls the flow rate for a given bladder pressure. In the context of continence one might also expect this region to be of major importance in maintaining urethral closure. The concept of urethral pressure measurement as a means of defining the mechanical properties of the urethra would thus appear valid, at least in the proximal parts of the urethra, up to the region of maximum resting pressure.

URETHRAL PRESSURE MEASUREMENT AT REST AND ON STRESS

The development of reliable methods for measuring urethral pressure over the last 20 years has led to several reports seeking to relate impairment of urethral closure with the development of genuine stress incontinence. Enhorning (1961) demonstrated that maximum urethral closure pressure fell with increasing age and was lower in stress-incontinent women than in continent women. Toews (1967) confirmed these findings and in addition noted that severity of symptoms was inversely correlated with urethral pressure. Henriksson, Andersson, and Ulmsten (1979) were unable to define any lower limit of urethral closure pressure that definitely predisposed an individual to stress incontinence, and a number of other workers have emphasized the overlap of urethral closure perameters between normal and stress-incontinent groups. Others have considered that the distinction between these groups is better made by examining the urethral pressure profile under provocation. Glen and Rowan (1973) showed that in continent women the urethral closure pressure tended to increase with increasing bladder volume, whereas in stress-incontinent patients a fall in the profile was often noted. Similar changes have been found in response to postural change; that is, in normal women the closure pressure increases on assuming the erect posture, whereas in those with genuine stress incontinence there was either no change or a fall (Henriksson, Ulmsten, and Andersson, 1977a, b).

More recent studies have concentrated on the importance of the effect of transmission of intraabdominal pressure rises to the urethra (Figure 10.1). Barnes (1940) introduced the concept of the proximal urethra being an abdominal organ, subjected to intraabdominal pressure variations in a fashion similar to the bladder. Confirmation of this concept was obtained by Enhorning (1961) by simultaneous

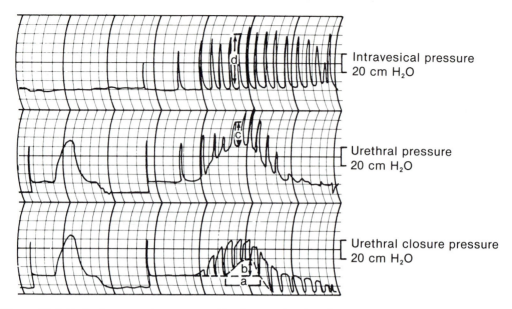

Figure 10.1 Urethral pressure trace on coughing in normal patient. Pressure transmission ratios calculated from formula $c/d \times 100$, where c is increment of urethral pressure and d is simultaneous increment of bladder pressure. *a*, Functional length of urethra during stress. *b*, Maximum closure pressure on stress. $c/d \times 100$, Pressure transmission ratio.

bladder and urethral pressure measurements at rest and on stress. The use of stress profiles in the assessment of urethral function has subsequently been shown to be of considerable value (Henriksson and Ulmsten, 1978; Eberhard and Lienhard, 1979; Hilton and Stanton, 1981). Lindstrom and Ulmsten (1978) suggest that a measuring system should have a rise time approximately three times faster than that of the physiological events being recorded. The rise times involved in a cough sequence may be between 50 and 200 msec. Thus to be applicable in these situations the measuring system should ideally be capable of a rise time of around 20 msec or have a frequency response of at least 25 Hz.

TECHNIQUES OF URETHRAL PRESSURE MEASUREMENT

Over the last 50 years several different techniques have been introduced for the assessment of urethral function. While the majority purport to measure intraluminal urethral pressure either as a static measurement or a continuous profile, attempts have also been made to determine the distribution of mural tension along the urethra. Various aspects of each technique are described here, including their development and use in clinical practice.

Retrograde sphincterometry

Retrograde sphincterometry was first described by Bonney (1923), reporting the work of Rivett. Several workers employed the technique in the 1940s and 1950s. Later, when most centers had long since abandoned the method as unreliable, Robertson (1974) reintroduced it, using carbon dioxide.

The technique of retrograde sphincterometry is a method for determining the total resistance of the urethra to the retrograde instillation of fluid. A urethral catheter connected to a manometer tube is introduced just within the external urethral meatus. The manometer level is then raised until the pressure head is just sufficient to overcome the urethral resistance and allow fluid to pass into the bladder. With carbon dioxide sphincterometry, the pressure is recorded within the gas source. There seems to be little reason to assume that the urethral resistance to retrograde instillation of fluid bears any relationship to its ability to contain urine in an antegrade fashion. Although carbon dioxide sphincterometry remains in use in a number of centers in the United States, it is generally held that inconsistencies in results, exacerbated by the compressibility of the gas and the high flow rates required, are such that the procedure has little clinical value (Tanagho, 1979).

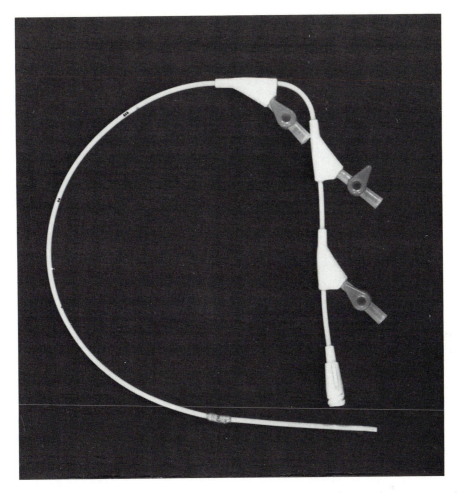

Figure 10.2 No. 7 French four-lumen membrane catheter. Three channels record pressures and fourth permits bladder filling.

Balloon or membrane catheters

The technique of pressure measurement using a balloon catheter was first applied to the urethra by Simons (1936). The technique as currently applied uses as small as a No. 7 French catheter with two or more lumina (Figure 10.2). The distal end of the catheter is usually open to allow recording of the intravesical pressure. In some reports an infusing channel also opens distally (Tanagho, 1979). Between 5 and 8 cm proximally, one or more membranes or cylindrical balloons are mounted over side holes in the catheter. Each pressure-measuring lumen is connected to its own transducer and then to an amplifier and recorder. Before use, the space beneath the membranes is filled with fluid to a pressure marginally greater than atmospheric pressure. The catheter is then introduced into the urethra so that all channels lie initially within the blad-

der. After flushing the open-ended intravesical pressure channel, all channels are zeroed to the same level, and the catheter is then withdrawn either incrementally or continuously at a slow, steady rate down the urethra so that the profile is obtained. This system perceives mural contributions from the whole urethral circumference and thus records a true hydrostatic pressure. The system has a rise time of around 40 msec (Enhorning, 1961) and therefore theoretically is not able to give an accurate indication of urethral response to physiological stresses. Despite this, several workers have attempted to use the technique for stress profiles. The membrane usually has a significant length (on the order of 5 to 10 mm) in comparison with urethral length, and a smoothing effect is therefor introduced into the profile. The main disadvantages of this method, however, are difficulties in construction of the catheters and in calibration of the equipment. In particular, freeing the membranes of air bubbles is often troublesome (Harrison, 1976; Jonas and Klotter, 1978).

Force gauges

Shelley and Warrell (1965) described the use of a force gauge in the urethra. The aim of this device was not to record the intraluminal pressure to record but the total forces closing the urethra. The system had the disadvantage of measuring over a length of 12 mm and therefore had an averaging effect. Although it provides useful information regarding urethral mechanics, this technique has not yet found any clinical application.

Fluid perfusion system

The fluid perfusion method of pressure measurement was first reported by Toews (1967), although it only came into popular use after the description of Brown and Wickham (1969). The Brown and Wickham system involved recording the pressure at the side hole of a catheter that was constantly perfused with an intravenous saline solution. Several minor defects in this system have been modified by subsequent workers. Harrison and Constable (1970) introduced a motor-driven syringe pump, allowing more accurate control of the infusion rates. With the addition of a catheter position transducer and an XY plotter, they could superimpose serial profiles for comparative purposes. Others have obviated the need for this by using mechanical or electrical catheter withdrawal devices: Glen and Rowan (1973) developed a two-channel system, with which continuous urethral closure pressure profiles could be obtained; Ghoneim et al. (1975) suggested that inaccuracies caused by axial rotation could be overcome by using a multiholed catheter. While water and saline solutions have been the most commonly used fluids in the United Kingdom, carbon dioxide has been advocated by Raz and Kaufman (1977) and is commonly employed in the United States.

The method most commonly used involves a one- or two-channel No. 7 Fr urethral catheter. A centrally placed lumen terminates at the catheter tip in an end or side hole for recording intravesical pressure, and the second lumen terminates in one or more circumferentially arranged side holes approximately 5 cm proximally. Both lumina are connected with Portex extension tubes to standard Statham blood pressure transducers. The connections

are made through three-way taps so that the system can be flushed to exclude air bubbles. The urethral lumen is linked through a Y junction, the third limb being linked to a syringe driver and infused at a fixed rate of 2 ml/min. With the bladder filled to a known volume, the catheter is passed through the urethra so that both lumina open into the bladder. It is then connected to a catheter withdrawal device. The whole system is flushed with saline to exclude air bubbles, and the infusion is begun. This system has been shown capable of recording a maximum pressure gradient of between 34 (Abrams, et al., 1978) and 50 (Hilton and Stanton, 1981b) cm H_2O/sec. This limits the use of the fluid perfusion system to the resting situation, and the rate of catheter withdrawal must be calculated accordingly.

Fluid bridge test. Brown and Sutherst (1978) described a procedure developed from the fluid perfusion method of urethral pressure measurement for use under stress situations and for the identification of incompetence of the bladder neck. The apparatus used for the test is the same as that used for the standard fluid perfusion closure pressure profile. When a resting profile has been performed, the catheter is reintroduced so that both lumina open into the bladder. Withdrawal is then begun again until the urethral side hole is 0.5 cm from the bladder neck. The fluid infusion is then discontinued. This has the effect of impairing the frequency response of the system to an extreme degree, and response is only restored if fluid continuity between the side hole and the bladder is made. This continuity is called a "fluid bridge." Thus if a patient is asked to cough with the catheter so located, when a fluid bridge is created, the bladder and urethral pressure traces will coincide at some point in the sequence (Figure 10.3, A). If the bladder neck remains competent, the cough spike will not be transmitted to the urethral sensor (Figure 10.3, B).

Although this is a useful addition to the standard resting urethral closure pressure profile, the relationship between bladder neck incompetence and the diagnosis of genuine stress incontinence is unproven. Sutherst and Brown (1980), comparing the fluid bridge test with other urodynamic investigations, showed a 28% false-positive rate with their technique. Hilton (1981) also found evidence of bladder neck incompetence in 25% of women entirely free of urinary symptoms. The demonstration of a fluid bridge cannot therefore be said to relate

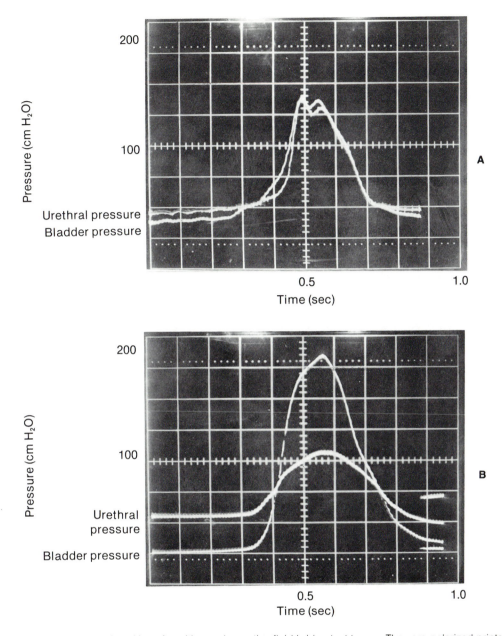

Figure 10.3 Examples of position of positive and negative fluid bridge test traces. They are polarized prints of superimposed urethral and bladder pressure recordings displayed on cathode-ray tube. **A,** Positive test. Urethra opens as far as measuring point, and fluid bridge is established; urethra and bladder pressure recordings are identical. **B,** Negative test. Urethra remains dry at measuring point, and no fluid bridge is established. (Courtesy of Mr. John Sutherst, Royal Liverpool Hospital).

closely to a diagnosis of genuine stress incontinence.

Microtransducers

The measurement of intraurethral pressure with a receptor placed directly within the urethra was introduced by Karlson (1953). The technique was not used further, however, until the receptor was miniaturized by Millar and Baker (1973). Since that time, it has been used extensively for urethral pressure profile measurements and for simultaneous urethrocystometry.

The method has been criticized because of the high cost and fragility of the instruments. If used carefully, however, these catheters have a considerable working life; Asmussen (1981) has used the same catheter for over 6 years, performing several thousand investigations without significant breakdown.

The advantages of the microtransducer system are several. The small size of the pressure-sensitive area means that there is little smoothing effect, and an accurate profile is achieved. The repeatability and reproducibility of profiles are significantly better than those obtained by other techniques (Hilton and Stanton, 1981b). The fine caliber of catheters available limits errors caused by urethral distension. Since the method involves no fluid infusion or connection tubing, it is very easy to perform and has improved patient acceptability. The most significant advantage of this measuring system over previous methods, however, lies in its high-frequency response. Since the pressure sensor lies within the lumen concerned, frequency response has been calculated at over 2000 Hz (Asmussen, Lindstrom, and Ulmsten, 1975). This means it has more than adequate capacity to record any physiological event, in particular the pressure changes involved in the voiding cycle, rapid cough sequences, and pelvic floor contraction.

The technique employed is similar to that just described for a fluid perfusion system. With a known volume in the bladder, the dual-sensor catheter (Figure 10.4) is passed through the urethra so that both transducers lie in the bladder. It is then secured to an electronic withdrawal device (Figure 10.5) and connected to a polygraph recorder. In the examples shown later in this chapter, profiles at rest were made with a catheter withdrawal rate of 15 cm/min, and profiles during coughing were made at a withdrawal speed of 5 cm/min. The chart paper speed is a standard 2.5 mm/sec. When the patient is comfortable and relaxed, three resting profiles are performed to ensure consistency of results. The catheter is then returned so that both transducers lie in the bladder, and the patient is asked to give a series of coughs with maximum effort while the catheter is withdrawn down the urethra again. At the reduced withdrawal rate, the patient can comfortably cough every 2 to 3 seconds, which corresponds approximately to every 2 mm of urethral length. After the profiles are completed, the proximal sensor of the catheter is relocated at the region of maximum resting pressure. After resting pressure over a period of 20 to 30 seconds is

recorded, the patient is asked to give one or two single coughs and then a rapid series of coughs to assess the response of this particular region to repeated stresses.

Micromanometers

A new and entirely different type of micromanometer transducer was described by Hok (1976). This instrument is perhaps more accurately called a micromanometer, and its sensitivity depends on the variation in conductance between two electrodes bathed to a variable depth in saline solution. The first report of the use of this technique for urethral pressure measurement came from Forman et al. (1979), and there are as yet no other reports of its value in clinical practice.

The frequency response of this instrument is less than that of a standard microtransducer, although it is perfectly adequate for use in resting and stress urethral profiles at around 240 Hz. It is less expensive to construct and rather more robust and flexible than other transducers, and by virtue of its small size, multiple elements may be combined into fine-caliber catheters so that real-time sequences may be visualized. The development of this technique is very much in its infancy, and it will be some time before it replaces the standard microtransducer system.

INDICATIONS

There has been much concern in recent years as to whether the urethral pressure profile has any place at all in the practice of clinical urodynamics. Indeed, the International Continence Society, at their tenth annual meeting in 1980, saw fit to debate this very issue. Its conclusion was, however, favorable toward the use of the procedure in the investigation of female urinary incontinence (International Continence Society, 1980). There are, of course, several other clinical and research situations in which it might be considered to have a place.

Clinical

Clinical applications of the urethral pressure profile include:
1. Female urinary incontinence
2. Female voiding difficulties
3. Prostatic obstruction in the male
4. Urethral stricture in the male
5. Incontinence after prostatectomy

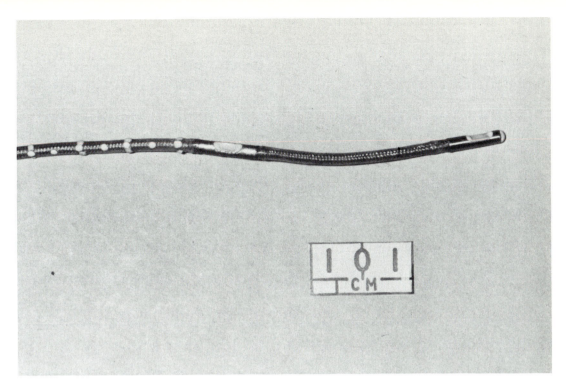

Figure 10.4 Dual-sensor microtransducer catheter. (Gaeltec Ltd., Isle of Skye, Scotland.)

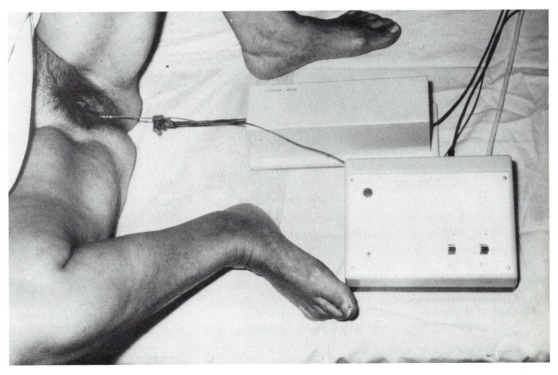

Figure 10.5 Technique of urethral pressure profile measurement using microtransducer catheter and electronic withdrawal device.

Research

Research applications of the urethral pressure profile include:

1. Assessment of incontinence surgery
2. Assessment of operative procedures on the outflow tract, including prostatectomy, urethrotomy, urethroplasty, and implantable prosthesis
3. Assessment of drug therapy on the urethra
4. Assessment of physiotherapy or electrical therapy
5. Investigation of the mechanism of continence

CLINICAL EXAMPLES

The results of resting and stress profiles in several clinical situations are described here. The traces illustrated were obtained by a microtransducer technique. The procedure employed has been described in detail elsewhere (Hilton, 1981).

Symptom-free women

The profile parameters of a group of 20 symptom-free women (mean age 46 years) are listed in Table 10.1 (Hilton, 1981).

These results compare closely with previously published results (Abrams, 1979), although it should be noted that there is considerable variation between patients and considerable overlap between symptomatic and symptom-free groups (Figure 10.6). Much more characteristic of the symptom-free state is the appearance of the cough profile, an example of which is shown in Figure 10.7. Most of the urethral length considered functional at rest remains functional on stress, and the closure pressure is maintained; indeed, often at a point just distal to the resting profile peak, an accentuation in closure pressure on stress may be seen, perhaps resulting from a reflex pelvic floor contraction.

Genuine stress incontinence

Several studies have demonstrated that the maximum closure pressure at rest is lower in stress-incontinent women than in symptom-free groups. Hilton and Stanton (1980) have shown that the more severe the stress incontinence, the lower the maximum urethral closure pressure. However, whether a specific value for this parameter may be defined, below which an individual is definitely predisposed to stress incontinence and above which this symptom is unlikely (as suggested by Bunne and Obrink [1978]), is open to doubt. It seems likely that a defect in the mechanism of transmission of intraabdominal pressure rises to the urethra is a more important etiological factor in most cases of genuine stress incontinence. Several other features of urethral function, and in particular urethral response to stress, have been identified that may be responsible for the failure of stress incontinence in some individuals (Hilton, 1981). Figure 10.8 illustrates resting and stress profiles from a patient with genuine stress incontinence, which results from a low resting closure pressure and impaired pressure transmission. Figure 10.9 also shows profiles from a patient with genuine stress inconti-

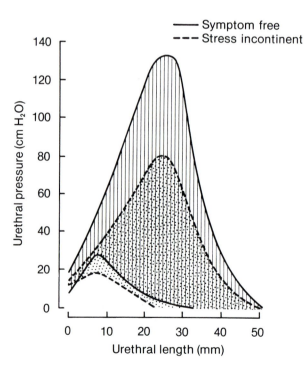

Figure 10.6 Resting urethral closure pressure profiles in stress incontinent and symptom-free women. Profiles are constructed from mean ± 2 standard deviations for conventional profile parameters.

TABLE 10.1 Profile parameters of 20 symptom-free women

Parameter	Mean	(SD)
Total profile length (mm)	41.6	(4.6)
Functional profile length (mm)	31.3	(5.5)
Length to peak pressure (mm)	16.6	(4.6)
Maximum urethral pressure (cm H_2O)	80.8	(26.4)
Maximum urethral closure pressure (cm H_2O)	68.2	(28.9)

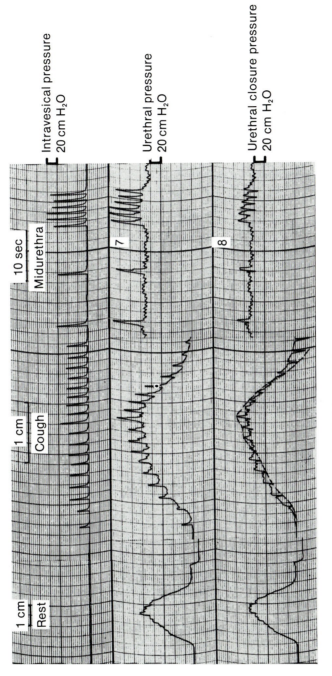

Figure 10.7 Resting and cough profiles in symptom-free woman.

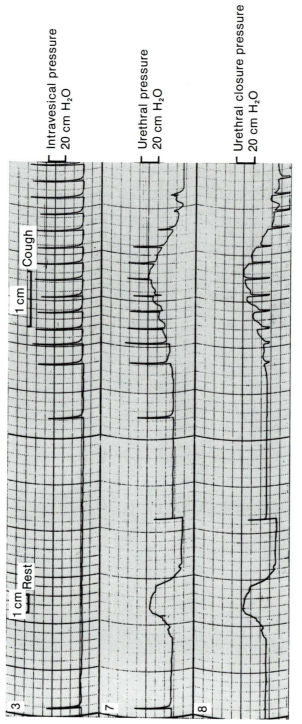

Figure 10.8 Resting and cough profiles in woman with genuine stress incontinence.

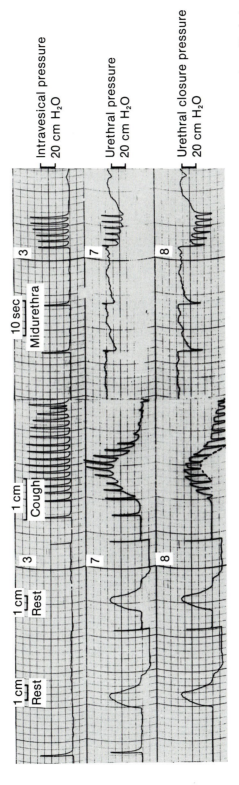

Figure 10.9 Resting and cough profiles in woman with genuine stress incontinence. Positive closure pressure is maintained during the cough profile (---), but after rapid sequence of coughs (right), maximum urethral closure pressure shows sustained relaxation.

nence. Here the resting pressure is slightly higher, and the transmission of intraabdominal pressure, as calculated on the stress profiles, is rather better than in the previous case. The latter part of the pressure trace, however, shows that in response to one or several coughs, the urethral closure pressure shows a sustained relaxation. The nature of this effect is as yet unknown, although it certainly accounts for the frequently recognized clinical finding of a patient who fails to demonstrate stress incontinence when giving a single cough but does so when giving a rapidly repeated series of coughs.

Detrusor instability

Detrusor instability is considered in Chapter 17. By virtue of the definitions given there, it can be seen that this is a diagnosis made only on the basis of continuous filling cystometry. Few studies have looked at urethral profilometry in this condition, although it is generally held to be associated with a normal or high resting closure pressure and a normal urethral response to filling, postural change, and stress (Tanagho, 1979). By means of continuous monitoring of both urethral and bladder pressure, urethrocystometry, several patterns of urethral function may be identified that suggest that even in so-called idiopathic detrusor instability, the prime defect may lie centrally.

Most patients labeled on the basis of simple filling cystometry as having idiopathic detrusor instability show normal resting urethral closure pressure profiles (Figure 10.10). During continuous urethrocystometry, however, it is seen that each uninhibited detrusor contraction is preceded by a reduction in urethral pressure. While several authors have used the term *urethral instability* to describe this situation, it is perhaps better considered as ''an unstable micturition pattern.''

Urethral instability

Unstable urethra is a term used to describe the situation in which negative urethral closure pressure results from an involuntary fall in intraurethral pressure in the absence of detrusor activity (Bates et al., 1979; see also Appendix II). In this condition, conventional urethral pressure profile measurements may again be entirely normal as may filling cystometry. The abnormality is only identified by continuous urethrocystometry, during which spontaneous, cough-provoked, or filling-provoked urethral relaxation may be demonstrated (Figure 10.11).

Effects of surgery

Several studies have attempted to examine the effect of surgery on urethral pressure. However, only the more recent studies involving profiles obtained on stress have identified any significant effects from successful incontinence operations. It has now been shown that while there are no significant changes in functional length or maximum urethral closure pressure at rest following the pubococcygeal vaginal repair (Obrink, et al., 1978), the Marshall-Marchetti-Krantz procedure (Henriksson and Ulmsten, 1978), the Stamey endoscopic bladder neck suspension (Constantinou, Faysal, and Govan, 1980), and the Burch colposuspension and alloplastic sling (Hilton and Stanton, 1981c) lead to an enhancement of the transmission of intraabdominal pressure rises to the urethra. This in turn led to an improved maximum closure pressure and functional length on stress (Figure 10.12).

Just which aspects of the procedures account for the enhanced pressure transmission is uncertain. It has been suggested that it simply reflects an eversion of the bladder neck and proximal urethra into an intraabdominal position (Enhorning, 1976). Results of the Burch colposuspension and Stamey procedures, however, have shown even greater transmission values than could be achieved by this mechanism. It has been postulated that this effect may result from improved efficiency of the pelvic floor reflex aiding urethral closure on stress. However, I believe a purely mechanical explanation resulting from the relocation of the urethra in a retropubic position is more likely (Hilton, 1981).

Following unsuccessful incontinence surgery, these changes in pressure transmission are not observed (Hilton and Stanton, 1981c); indeed, a reduction in resting urethral closure pressure is often noted (Hilton, 1981).

At present it is not possible to determine the most appropriate form of incontinence surgery for an individual patient based on the characteristics of the resting and stress urethral pressure profiles. While it seems likely that the lower the resting maximum closure pressure is the less likely a successful surgical outcome is, no value for this parameter can be determined below which a cure is unlikely or above which incontinence is assured.

Effects of drugs

Many attempts have been made in the past to define urethral physiology in terms of the changes

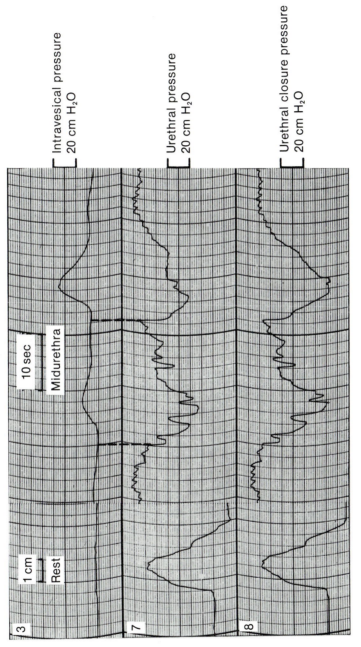

Figure 10.10 Resting urethral pressure profile *(left)* and continuous urethrocystometry *(right)* in patient with idiopathic detrusor instability.

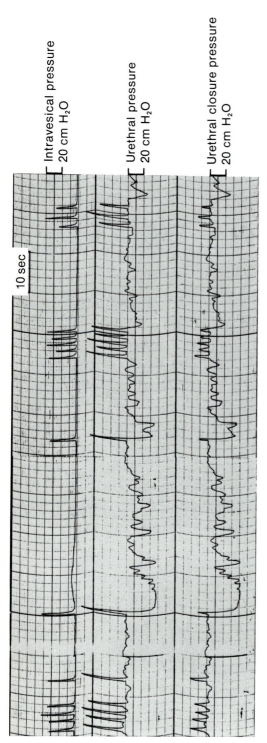

Figure 10.11 Continuous urethrocystometry in patient with cough-provoked urethral instability.

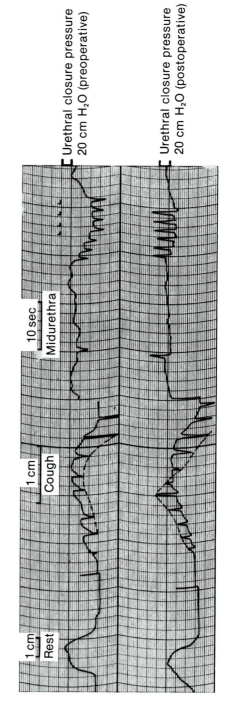

Figure 10.12 Resting and stress urethral closure pressure profiles obtained before *(top)* and after *(bottom)* successful Burch colposuspension.

induced in the urethral pressure profile by the administration of drugs. However, results have rarely been consistent between studies. The two groups of drugs that have caused the most controversy in recent years have been estrogens (considered in detail Chapter 27) and adrenergic stimulant drugs. Ek et al. (1978) reported a significant increase in the maximum urethral pressure and maximum urethral closure pressure following an adminsitration of the α-adrenergic stimulant norephedrine. Obrink and Bunne (1978), however, examining multiple parameters of the urethral pressure profile at rest and on stress, found no significant changes with this drug. Montague and Stewart (1979) noted a 20% increase in the maximum urethral pressure of stress-incontinent women following the use of phenylpropanolamine (Propadrine). Jonas (1977) found a 30% increase in maximum urethral pressure but a simultaneous 35% increase in bladder pressure following the use of midodrine; he found similar results in both continent and stress-incontinent women. Hilton (1981), again examining parameters of profiles both at rest and on stress, found no significant changes following the use of phenylpropanolamine. Obviously, differences in measuring techniques and the degree of blindness and control in these various studies contribute to disparities in results. It would appear, however, that at present, urethral pressure measurement has little to offer in the prediction of the therapeutic efficacy of drugs in abnormalities of urethral function.

CONCLUSION

The validity of urethral pressure measurement as a means of defining the physical properties of the organ is beyond doubt; however, the value of the investigation in clinical practice is questioned by many. Certainly, the standard urethral pressure profile as recorded by fluid perfusion or membrane catheter techniques has little to offer the practicing gynecologist or urologist. However, the assessment of the urethral response to stress by means of microtransducer techniques is a more useful tool and one for which several clinical and research applications have been defined and illustrated.

REFERENCES

Abrams, P.H. 1979. Perfusion urethral profilometry. Urol. Clin. North Am. **6**(1):103-109.

Abrams, P.H., Martin, S., and Griffiths, D.J. 1978. The measurement and interpretation of urethral pressures obtained by the method of Brown and Wickham. Br. J. Urol. **50**:33-38.

Asmussen, M. 1975. Urethrocystometry in women. Lund, Sweden. Studentlitteratur.

Asmussen, M. 1981. Personal communication.

Asmussen, M., Lindstrom, K., and Ulmsten, U. 1975. A catheter-manometer calibrator: a new clinical instrument. Biol. Med. Eng. **10**:175-180.

Barnes, A.C. 1940. The method of evaluating the stress of urinary incontinence. Am. J. Obstet. Gynecol. **40**:381-390.

Bates, P., et al. 1979. The fourth report on the standardisation of terminology of the lower urinary tract function. Glasgow International Continence Society.

Bonney, V. 1923. On diurnal incontinence of urine in women. J. Obstet. & Gynecol. Br. Emp. **30**:358-365.

Brown, M., and Sutherst, J. 1978. Detection of fluid entry into the proximal urethra during coughing. Proceedings of the eighth International Continence Society meeting. Manchester, England.

Brown, M., and Wickham, J.E.A. 1969. The urethral pressure profile. Br. J. Urol. **41**:211-217.

Bunne, G., and Obrink, A. 1978. Urethral closure pressure with stress: a comparison between stress incontinent and continent women. Urol. Res. **6**:127-134.

Constantinou, C.E., Faysal, M.H., and Govan, D.E. 1980. The impact of bladder neck suspension on the mode of distribution of abdominal pressure along the female urethra. Proceedings of the tenth International Continence Society meeting. Los Angeles.

Eberhard, J., and Leinhard, P. 1979. Stress incontinence in women: the evaluation and interpretation of intra-urethral pressure profiles obtained by microtransducers. Geburtshilfe Frauenheilkd. **39**:195-208.

Ek, A., Andersson, K.E., and Ulmsten, U. 1978. The effects of norephedrine and bethanechol on the human urethral closure pressure profile. Scand. J. Urol. Nephrol. **12**:97-104.

Enhorning, G.E. 1961. Simultaneous recording of the intravesical and intraurethral pressure. Acta Chir. Scand. [Suppl.] **276**:1-68.

Enhorning, G.E. 1976. A concept of urinary continence. Urol. Int. **31**:3-5.

Forman, A., et al. 1979. A new transducer (micromanometer) for intra-luminal pressure recordings. J. Med. Eng. Technol. **3**:295-298.

Ghoneim, M.A., et al. 1975. Urethral pressure profile: standardization of technique and study of reproducibility. Urology **5**:632-637.

Glen, E.S., and Rowan, D. 1973. Continuous flow cystometry and urethral pressure profile measurement with monitored intra-vesical pressure: a diagnostic and prognostic investigation. Urol. Res. **1**:97-100.

Griffiths, D.J. 1969. Urethral elasticity and micturition hydrodynamics in females. Med. Biol. Eng. **7**:201-215.

Griffiths, D.J. 1980: Urodynamics. Bristol. Adam Hilger.

Harrison, N.W. 1976. Urethral pressure profile. Urol. Res. **4**:95-100.

Harrison, N.W., and Consable, A.R. 1970. Urethral pressure measurement: a modified technique. Br. J. Urol. **42**:229-233.

Henriksson, L., Andersson, K.E., and Ulmsten, U. 1979. The urethral pressure profiles in continent and stress incontinent women. Scand. J. Urol. Nephrol. **13**:5-10.

Henriksson, L., and Ulmsten, U. 1978. A urodynamic evaluation of the effects of abdominal urethrocystopexy and vaginal sling urethroplasty in women with stress incontinence. Am. J. Obstet. Gynecol. **113**:78-82.

Henriksson, L., Ulmsten, U., and Andersson, K.E. 1977a. The effects of changes in posture on the urethral closure pressure in healthy women. Scand. J. Urol. Nephrol. **11:**201-206.

Henriksson, L., Ulmsten, U., and Andersson, K.E. 1977b. The effects of changes in posture on the urethral closure pressure in stress incontinent women. Scand. J. Urol. Nephrol. **11:**207-210.

Hilton, P. 1981. Urethral pressure measurement by microtransducer: observations on methodology, the pathophysiology of genuine stress incontinence, and the effects of its treatment in the female. M.D. thesis. Newcastle-upon-Tyne, England.

Hilton, P., and Stanton, S.L. 1980. Urethral pressure measurement by microtransducer. Paper presented at the Gynaecologic Urology Society Meeting. New Orleans.

Hilton, P., and Stanton, S.L. 1981a. Urethral measurement by microtransducer: a comparison of stress profiles obtained on coughing and straining. Proceedings of the International Continence Society eleventh annual meeting. Lund, Sweden.

Hilton, P., and Stanton, S.L. 1981b. Urethral pressure measurement by microtransducer: an analysis of variance and an analysis of rotational variations. Proceedings of the International Continence Society eleventh annual meeting. Lund, Sweden.

Hilton, P., and Stanton, S.L. 1981c. The urodynamic effects of successful and failed incontinence surgery. Paper presented at the International Urogynecologists Association meeting. Stockholm, Sweden.

Hok, B. 1976. New microtransducer for physiological pressure recordings. Med. Biol. Eng. **13:**279-284.

Jonas, D. 1977. Treatment of female stress incontinence with midodrine: preliminary report. J. Urol. **118:**980-982.

Jonas, U., and Klotter, J.H. 1978. Study of three urethral pressure recording devices: theoretical considerations. Urol. Res. **6:**119-125.

Karlson, S. 1953. Experimental studies on the functioning of the female urinary bladder and urethra. Acta Obstet. Gynecol. Scand. **32:**285-307.

Lindstrom, K., and Ulmsten, U. 1978. Some methodological aspects on the measurement of intra-luminal pressures in the female urogenital tract in vivo. Acta Obstet. Gynecol. Scand. **57:**63-68.

Millar, H.D., and Baker, L.E. 1973. Stable ultraminiature catheter tip pressure transducer. Med. Biol. Eng. **11:**86-89.

Montague, D.K., and Stewart, B.H. 1979. Urethral pressure profiles before and after Ornade administration in patients with stress urinary incontinence. J. Urol. **122:**198-199.

Obrink, A., and Bunne, G. 1978. The effects of alpha adrenergic stimulants in stress incontinence. Scand. J. Urol. Nephrol. **12:**205-208.

Obrink, A., et al. 1978. Urethral pressure profile before, during and after pubococcygeal repair for stress incontinence. Acta Obstet. Gynecol. Scand. **57:**49-61.

Plevnik, S. 1976. Model of the proximal urethra: measurement of the urethral stress profile. Urol. Int. **31:**23-32.

Raz, S., and Kaufman, J.J. 1977. Carbon dioxide urethral pressure profile in female incontinence. J. Urol. **117:**765-769.

Robertson, J.R. 1974. Gas cystometrogram urethral pressure profile. Obstet. Gynecol. **44:**72-76.

Shelley, T., and Warrell, D.W. 1965. Measurement of intravesical and intraurethral pressure in normal women and in women suffering from incontinence of urine. Br. J. Obstet. Gynaecol. **72:**926-929.

Simons, I. 1936. Studies on bladder function: the sphincterometer. J. Urol. **35:**96-102.

Sutherst, J.R., and Brown, M.C. 1980. Detection of urethral incompetence in women using the fluid bridge test. Br. J. Urol. **52:**138-142.

Tanagho, E.A. 1979. Membrane and microtransducer catheters: their effectiveness for profilometry in the lower urinary tract. Urol. Clin. North Am. **6**(1):118-119.

Toews, H. 1967. Intra-urethral and intra-vesical pressures in normal and stress incontinent women. Obstet. Gynecol. **29:**613-624.

Zinner, N.R., Ritter, R.C., and Sterling, A.M. 1976. The mechanism of micturition. In Williams, D.I., and Chisholm, G.D., editors. Scientific foundations of urology. London. William Heinemann, Ltd.

Zinner, N.R., Sterling, A., and Ritter, R.C. 1979. Role of inner urethral softness in urethral continence. Proceedings of the ninth International Continence Society meeting. Rome, Italy.

chapter 11

Uroflowmetry

PAUL ABRAMS

HISTORICAL INTRODUCTION

The importance of urine flow rates was realized half a century ago (Ballenger, Elder, and Mc-Donald, 1932). Drake (1948) made the first accurate measurements of urine flow. He used a spring balance; a pen that wrote on a kymograph was attached to one end, and a receptacle for the voided urine was attached to the other end. By rotating the kymograph drawn at a known speed, Drake obtained a trace of voided urine volume against time. He calculated the maximum urine flow rate by a measurement of the steepest part of the volume-time curve. It is evident from his description that the apparatus was relatively crude and difficult to use. Furthermore, urine flow rates had to be calculated from volume-time data. Drake's flowmeter was never produced commercially. Kaufman (1957) commercially produced a modification of Drake's flowmeter that was more refined but similarly made no direct recording of flow rate.

The advent of electronics in medical instrumentation allowed the mass production of accurate and reliable recording devices. Von Garrelts (1956) designed the first of the electronic urine flowmeters, which consisted of a tall urine-collecting cylinder with a pressure transducer in the base. The pressure transducer measured the pressure exerted by an increasing column of urine as the patient voided. Since a direct relationship existed between the volume voided and the pressure recorded, von Garrelts was able to produce a direct recording of urine flow rate by electronic differentiation with time.

DEFINITIONS OF URINE FLOW RATE MEASUREMENTS

In any field of scientific measurement it is important that all workers use standardized terminol-

Findings

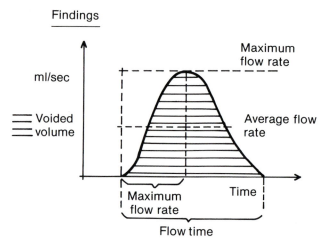

Figure 11.1 Diagrammatic urine flow curve with measured parameters.

ogy. Urine flow rates are measured in milliliters per second (ml/sec^{-1}). Figure 11.1 denotes the definitions for urine flow rate measurements as suggested by the Standardisation Committee of the International Continence Society (1977):

Flow rate is the volume expelled from the baldder per second.

Maximum flow rate is the maximum measured rate of the flow rate.

Flow time is the time over which measurable flow occurs. Flow time is easily measured if flow is continuous, unless there is a lengthy terminal dribble that may be noted but not included in the flow time. If urine flow is intermittent, the time intervals between flow episodes are not included.

Volume voided is the total volume expelled through the urethra.

Average flow is the volume voided divided by the flow time. The volume voided may be calculated from the area beneath the flow time curve.

METHODS OF URINE FLOW RATE MEASUREMENT

There are many potential methods of urine flow measurement varying from electromagnetic techniques through audiometric methods to an ultrasonic device. However, the most common method has been that of Drake (1948) modified by von Garrelts and Strandell (1972)—the measurement of urine weight.

In addition, flowmeters have been produced that use the principles of air displacement, water displacement, resistance to gas flow, photoelectricity, capacitance, and a revolving disk.

Flowmeters employing the principles of weight

transduction, a rotating disk, and a capacitance transducer are the best known and the most completely tested and validated of the flowmeters available.

The weight transducer type of flowmeter (Figure 11.2, *A*) weighs the voided urine and by differentiation with time produces an "on-line" recording of urine flow rate:

$$\left(FR = \frac{dV}{dt} \right)$$

where dV is the change in volume of urine over change in time, dt.

The rotating disk flowmeter (Figure 11.2, *B*) depends on a servomotor maintaining the rotation of the disk at a constant speed. Urine hits the disk, and the extra power required to maintain the speed is electronically converted into a measurement of flow rate.

The capacitance flowmeter is the simplest of the three flowmeters. This flowmeter consists of a funnel leading urine into a collecting vessel. The transducer is in the form of a dipstick made of plastic and coated with metal, which dips into the vessel containing the voided urine (Figure 11.2, *C*).

All three types of flowmeter perform accurately and efficiently. The capacitance (dipstick) flowmeter is the least expensive to buy and has the advantage of no moving parts, which means mechanical breakdowns are eliminated.

CLINICAL MEASUREMENT OF URINE FLOW RATE

The environment for patient flow rate recording is of considerable importance. Female patients are

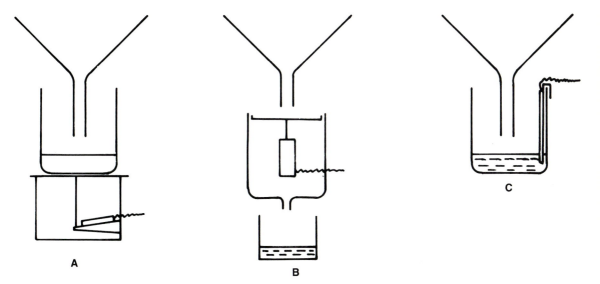

Figure 11.2 Urine flowmeters. **A,** Weight transducer. **B,** Rotating disk. **C,** Capacitance (dipstick).

used to voiding in circumstances of almost complete privacy. It is essential in the clinical situation that every effort is made to make the patient feel comfortable and relaxed. If these refinements are ignored, a higher proportion of patients will fail to void in a representative way. When videostudies are combined with pressure-flow recordings in the radiology department, up to 30% of women may fail to void.

Having established a satisfactory environment for urine flow study measurement, the clinician should ensure that the patient voids a satisfactory volume of urine. It is recommended that in the week before the flow study, the patient completes a frequency-volume chart (urinary diary). On this chart the patient enters the volumes of fluid drunk and the volumes of urine voided. In this way the clinican can estimate the patient's average voided volume. It is desirable that the measured urine flow rate should be for a volume within the patient's normal range (average, 200 to 550 ml). If either a much smaller or much larger volume is voided, the flow rate may be misleading. Urine volumes of less than 100 ml are passed at a slow flow by most patients irrespective of their individual lower urinary tract properties. Urine volumes above the patient's normal range may lead to a low urine flow rate as a result of reduced detrusor contraction from the bladder being overstretched. Ideally, the patient should be asked to remain for 2 to 3 hours and repeat her urine flow rates on several occasions.

FACTORS INFLUENCING URINE FLOW RATE

Urine flow depends on the relationship between the bladder and the urethra during voiding. The situation during voiding is the antithesis of the situation required for continence. Continence depends on intraurethral pressure being higher than intravesical pressure. For voiding to occur intravesical pressure must exceed intraurethral pressure.

Enhorning (1961) and later Asmussen and Ulmsten (1976) showed clearly that before any rise in intravesical pressure, a fall in intraurethral pressure occurred. This suggests that the urethra actively relaxes during voiding rather than being passively "blown open" by the detrusor contraction. Soon after the urethra has relaxed and pelvic floor descent has occurred, the detrusor contracts. The detrusor normally contrives to contract until the bladder is empty, producing a continuous flow curve. Changes in intraabdominal pressure also influence urine flow. Some women appear to void entirely by increasing intraabdominal pressure, that is, by contraction of the diaphragm and the anterior abdominal wall muscles.

It follows from this discussion that the urine flow may differ from normal as a result of abnormalities of the urethra or the detrusor.

Urethral factors

Anatomical factors. The urethra may be abnormally narrow, or the urethra may not be straight.

The narrowest part of the urethra, as shown by videostudies of voiding, is usually the midzone. However, the urethra may become narrowed and the most common site is at the external meatus associated with estrogen deficiency in the postmenopausal woman. Bladder neck obstruction in the female is excessively rare (Turner-Warwick et al., 1973). The female urethra is usually straight, and deviation from this state is most common in anterior vaginal wall prolapse. Vaginal repair of the prolapse may produce no significant alteration in flow rate, irrespective of whether or not stress incontinence is present (Stanton et al., 1981). However, correction of anterior vaginal wall prolapse by a colposuspension does lead to deterioration in flow rate (Stanton and Cardozo, 1979).

Pathological factors. Unusual congenital conditions such as urethral duplication, urethral diverticulum, or urethral cysts may obstruct voiding. Infective lesions as in urethritis or infected paraurethral cysts may lead to voiding difficulties. Posttraumatic strictures and urethral neoplasms will have a similar effect. Intravaginal abnormalities, such as prolapse or foreign bodies, may also obstruct micturition.

Functional factors. Abnormal urethral behavior during voiding may lead to alteration in the urine flow rate recording. Urethral closure may be due to contraction of the intraurethral striated muscle or to contraction of the pelvic floor. In the neurologically abnormal patient contraction of the intraurethral striated muscle with or without the pelvic floor is known as detrusor sphincter dyssynergia. In the nervous and anxious but neurologically normal patient the urethra may be closed by pelvic floor contraction, and this may be termed detrusor pelvic floor dyssynergia.

Detrusor factors

Contractility. It is well known that when neurological disease occurs, bladder behavior may be altered. However, in patients with no neurological disease poor detrusor contractility may be responsible for a slow flow rate. Such patients may have urinary tract infections or urinary retention. These patients have normal urethral function as judged by pressure profilometry or radiology. Their reduced flow rates are secondary to a weak and poorly sustained detrusor contraction. A proportion of this clinical group go on to demonstrate classical neurological disease such as multiple sclerosis.

Innervation. Normal detrusor behavior depends on normal innervation. Bladder contractions are preserved if the sacral reflex arc is intact even when the upper motor neurons are damaged. However, if the sacral reflex arc is damaged, bladder contractions are generally absent. The only form of contractile activity possible when the lower motor neuron is damaged is locally mediated—the "autonomous" bladder. The urine flow rates produced by the abnormally innervated bladder are usually reduced and interrupted.

Pathological factors. Although little specific literature on the subject exists, it is evident that gross disease of the detrusor will result in abnormal urine flow rates. The fibrosis resulting from irradiation tuberculosis, cystitis, or interstitial cystitis is likely to impair detrusor contractility.

URINE FLOW PATTERNS
Normal

The normal flow trace shows a symmetrical peak with maximum flow rate achieved within 5 seconds of the beginning of voiding (Figure 11.3). Normal urine flow rate values change little with age in female patients. For a series of 137 normal women (aged 20 to 49) that were urologically asymptomatic the average flow rate was 23.6 ml/sec for an average voided volume of 413 ml. The average flow rate of the second series of 50 women (aged 50 to 69) was 24.4 ml/sec for a voided volume of 425 ml (Shepherd, 1979). Data given by other authors are similar: Walter et al. (1979) give a median figure of 25.3 ml/sec (range 14.6 to 30.6) for 11 normal middle-aged women. Drach, Ignatoff, and Layton (1979), for a patient group of 121 with an average age of 33 years, quote an average figure for maximum urine flow rate of 26 ml/sec (± 14, being 1 standard deviation from the average). Therefore it is reasonable to use 15 ml/sec for volumes in excess of 200 ml as the lower limit of normal for maximum urine flow rates in female patients.

Abnormal—continuous flow

Reduced. Maximum urine flow rates of less than 15 ml/sec for voided volumes greater than 200 ml may be regarded as abnormally reduced (Figure 11.4). Maximum flow for reduced rates tends to be achieved within 10 seconds, and the flow then slowly reduces until voiding stops. A reduced flow rate may be due either to a urethral obstruction or to a poor detrusor contraction. It is necessary to perform full pressure flow studies to demonstrate the cause of a reduced urine flow rate.

Reduced and fluctuating. A reduced and fluc-

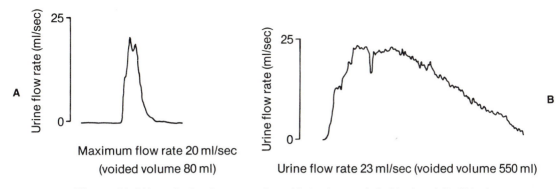

Maximum flow rate 20 ml/sec
(voided volume 80 ml)

Urine flow rate 23 ml/sec (voided volume 550 ml)

Figure 11.3 Normal urine flow traces for voided volumes of, **A,** 80 ml and, **B,** 550 ml.

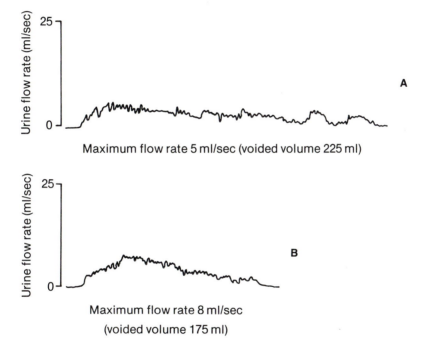

Maximum flow rate 5 ml/sec (voided volume 225 ml)

Maximum flow rate 8 ml/sec
(voided volume 175 ml)

Figure 11.4 Reduced urine flow trace caused by, **A,** detrusor underactivity (maximum detrusor pressure 20 cm H_2O) and **B,** outflow obstruction (meatal stenosis, maximum detrusor pressure 54 cm H_2O).

tuating flow pattern (Figure 11.5) is usually associated with an incompletely sustained detrusor contraction as may be seen in patients with multiple sclerosis. As well as being incompletely sustained, the maximum detrusor pressure is usually below normal; hence the reduced flow.

Abnormal—interrupted flow

Voluntary sphincter contraction. In the anxious, nervous patient the distal urethral sphincteric mechanism may close. Flow rate may decrease or stop (Figure 11.6). Characteristically, the rate of change of flow rate is rapid, indicating sphincter closure. As was seen in Figure 11.5, when flow

rate changes are due to changes in the desturor activity, the rate of change is slow.

Detrusor sphincter dyssynergia. Detrusor sphincter dyssynergia is an involuntary phenomenon in which the expected coordination of detrusor contraction and urethral relaxation is lost. Despite an effective detrusor contraction, the urethral mechanism remains closed for longer periods of time (up to several minutes). Detrusor sphincter dyssynergia may result in a large residual urine together with upper tract dilatation and renal failure and is often associated with repeated infection. Detrusor sphincter dyssynergia only occurs in neurologically abnormal patients, most classically in

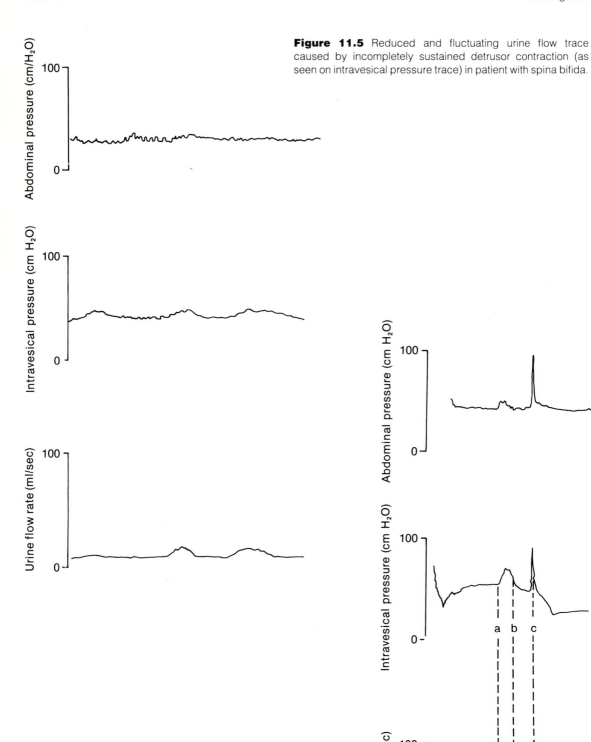

Figure 11.5 Reduced and fluctuating urine flow trace caused by incompletely sustained detrusor contraction (as seen on intravesical pressure trace) in patient with spina bifida.

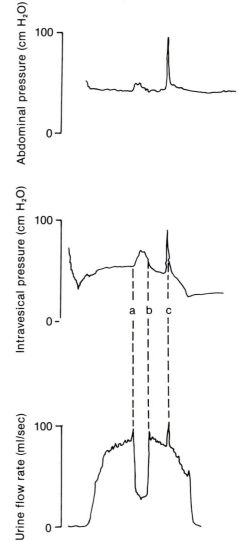

Figure 11.6 Interrupted urine flow trace caused by voluntary sphincter contraction in anxious patient. At point *a* sphincter closes with increase in intravesical pressure and decrease in flow rate. Converse occurs at point *b*. At point *c* patient raises her intraabdominal pressure, and as sphincter is open flow rate increases.

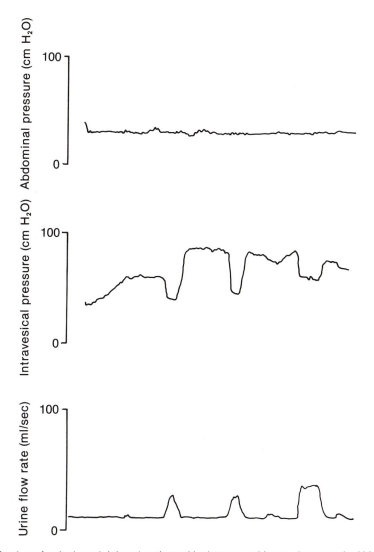

Figure 11.7 Tracing of spinal cord–injured patient with detrusor sphincter dyssynergia. Urine flow trace is interrupted and flow only occurs when sphincter relaxes at which time intravesical pressure falls.

high spinal cord trauma. The flow rate produced by detrusor sphincter dyssynergia is usually reduced and always interrupted (Figure 11.7).

The flow patterns that have been described are secondary to pathophysiological problems. The patient may modify her flow tract by straining, using abdominal wall and diaphragmatic muscles. Before a flow rate measurement, the patient should be asked whether or not she usually strains to void. If she does usually strain, she should be asked whether she can void without straining. If she has to strain to void, it is likely that detrusor activity is reduced or absent. If the patient claims not to void by straining, she should be asked to void in a relaxed manner and without straining. Straining

produces changes in flow rate of moderate speed and usually the flow remains continuous (Figure 11.8). However, straining may be used by any patient with any coexisting lower urinary tract problem.

INDICATIONS FOR UROFLOWMETRY

Flow rates should only be regarded as a screening test. Flow studies in female patients are less useful than in male patients. This is because in the male patient a high proportion of lower urinary tract problems are related to outflow obstruction. In the female the incidence of outflow obstruction is low, whereas the incidence of incontinence and associated abnormalities of bladder behavior is high.

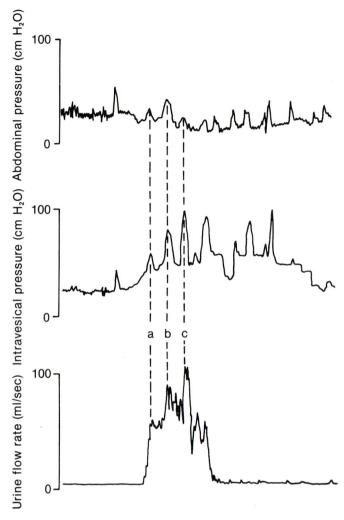

Figure 11.8 Irregular urine flow trace of patient with normal lower urinary tract who is straining while voiding. At points *a*, *b*, and *c*, patient strains with consequent increase in abdominal pressure and intravesical pressure, and on each occasion urine flow rate rises.

However, the demonstration of an abnormal flow trace is an indication for further urodynamic investigation, that is, inflow cystometry and pressure-flow studies, with or without simultaneous videocystourethrography.

Urine flow studies are useful screening tests for all patients with lower urinary tract problems. These problems fall into the following broad groups.

Urinary tract infection

Lower urinary tract infections are common in female patients. However, in most instances the underlying cause remains obscure although urine flow studies do demonstrate the occasional patient with obstruction who will benefit from urethral dilatation.

Symptoms suggestive of outflow obstruction

Whereas the symptoms of slow stream, hesitancy, the feeling of incomplete emptying, and the need to strain to void are common in male patients, they are infrequently encountered in women patients. Only 3.9% of women referred for urodynamic studies prove to have an obstruction. If urine flow rates prove to be normal in this group, further investigation is unnecessary, however if flow rates are low, pressure-flow studies are indicated.

Symptoms suggestive of bladder overactivity

Flow studies are only a preliminary to cystometry that is often necessary to define the urodynamic abnormality responsible for the symptom complex of frequency, nocturia, urgency, and urge incontinence.

Genuine stress incontinence

Flow studies alone are a useful prognostic indication as to the success of surgery for genuine stress incontinence. Assuming genuine stress incontinence has been demonstrated, a normal flow rate reassures the surgeon that voiding difficulties are unlikely to follow an operation to cure stress incontinence. However, if flow rates are reduced, this may be indicative of relative detrusor weakness. Since effective surgery usually results in an increase in urethral resistance in this group of patients, incomplete emptying or even persistent failure to void may follow surgery (Stanton et al., 1978). Therefore urine flow studies with or without pressure-flow studies are to be recommended before surgery.

Neuropathic lower urinary tract dysfunction

Voiding problems in patients with neuropathic lower urinary tract dysfunction consist of three main types. Patients may experience incontinence as a result of bladder instability. The main problem may be failure to empty the bladder because of a poorly sustained detrusor contraction. Detrusor sphincter dyssynergia may prevent an effective detrusor contraction from emptying the bladder with the consequent possible complications of recurrent infections and renal failure. Urine flow studies may suggest the origin of the problems experienced by this group of patients, although video-pressure-flow studies are desirable in almost every case.

Radical pelvic surgery

Detection of voiding difficulty before radical pelvic surgery is an indication to ensure adequate bladder drainage until spontaneous voiding occurs; this in itself may be considerably delayed if there is damage to the nerve supply of the bladder in the course of surgery.

REFERENCES

Asmussen, M., and Ulmsten, U. 1976. Simultaneous urethrocystometry with a new technique. Scand. J. Urol. Nephrol. **10**:7-11.

Ballenger, E.G., Elder, O.F., and McDonald, H.P. 1932. Voiding distance decrease as important early symptom of prostatic obstruction. South. Med. J. **25**:863.

Drach, G.W., Ignatoff, J., and Layton, T., 1979. Peak urinary flow rate: observations in female subjects and comparison to male subjects. J. Urol. **122**:215-219.

Drake, W.M., 1948. The uroflowmeter: an aid to the study of the lower urinary tract. J. Urol. **59**:650-658.

Enhorning, G. 1961. Simultaneous recording of intravesical and intraurethral pressure. Acta Chir. Scand. [Suppl.] **276**:1-68.

International Continence Society. 1977. Second report on the standardisation of terminology of lower urinary tract function. Br. J. Urol. **49**:207-210.

Kaufman, J. 1957. A new recording uroflowmeter: a simple automatic device for measuring voiding velocity. J. Urol. **78**:97.

Shepherd, A.M. 1979. The effects of gynaecological surgery on bladder function. M.D. thesis. University of Bristol.

Stanton, S.L., Hilton, P., Norton, C., and Cardozo, L. 1982. Clinical and urodynamic effects of anterior colporrhaphy and vaginal hysterectomy for prolapse, with and without incontinence. Br. J. Obstet. Gynaecol. **89**:459-463.

Stanton, S.L., et al. 1978. Clinical and urodynamic features of failed incontinence surgery in the female. Obstet. Gynaecol. **51**:515-520.

Turner-Warwick, R., et al. 1973. A urodynamic view of the clinical problems associated with bladder neck dysfunction and its treatment by endoscopic incision and trans-trigonal posterior prostatectomy. Br. J. Urol. **45**:44-59.

von Garrelts, B. 1956. Analysis of micturition: a new method of recording the voiding of the bladder. Acta Chir. Scand. **112**:326.

von Garrelts, B., and Strandell, P. 1972. Continuous recording of urinary flowrate. Scand. J. Urol. Nephrol. **6**:224-227.

Walter, S., et al. 1979. Bladder function in urologically normal middle aged females. Scand. J. Urol. Nephrol. **13**:249-258.

chapter 12

Cystourethroscopy

PETER H.L. WORTH

Cystourethroscopy is essentially an examination to establish if disease is present in the bladder or urethra. It is not the investigation to decide whether a bladder neck is obstructed or incompetent; this can only be satisfactorily established by urodynamic testing. It may, however, be of help in deciding how to operate on a patient with incontinence.

PREPARATION

Cystoscopy in the female can be carried out quite easily without an anesthetic, and whether local anesthesia is put into the urethra makes little difference. Apart from observation of the inside of the bladder, usually no additional procedures are carried out except for gentle urethral dilatation. Occasionally a patient tolerates diathermy, provided that it is not on the trigone. If a general anesthetic is going to be used for cystoscopy, one should have additional equipment available to carry out definitive procedures when indicated. It is bad practice to carry out a cystoscopy as a single procedure under anesthesia without being prepared to proceed to biopsy or diathermy. (Any specialist carrying out a cystoscopy should have had proper training in its use and at least be able to biopsy the bladder.)

Cystoscopic equipment has improved in the last 10 years, and, together with solid rod lens systems designed by Professor Harold Hopkins and solid state diathermy machines, endoscopic surgery has been able to progress considerably. There is little to choose from among the various cystoscopes on the market, and everyone has his or her personal preferences (Figure 12.1). It is better to keep to one make because systems are not interchangeable, and it is important to have a good basic set consisting of a cystoscope, resectoscope, catheterizing bridge, and 70-degree and 30-degree telescopes. For examination of the urethra a 0-degree telescope is preferable but not essential. In addition to this endoscopic equipment, some means of dilating the urethra is needed. An Otis urethrotome is ideal, but other types of dilators such as Cany Ryall, Wyndham Powell, or Hegars will do. In gynecological practice there is no need to use anything but water to irrigate the bladder.

TECHNIQUE

Before the cystoscope is passed, the external urethral meatus should be inspected to exclude any local pathological condition, such as a urethral caruncle or urethral mucosal prolapse. The urethra is

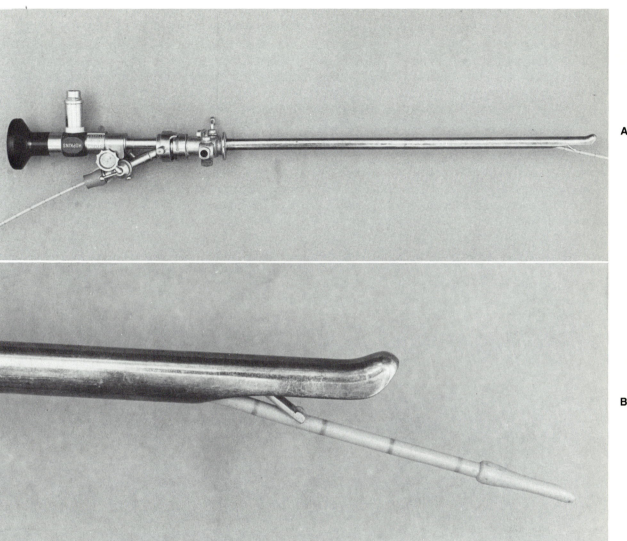

Figure 12.1 A, Standard cystoscope with catheterizing bridge and Hopkins telescope. **B,** Close-up shows bulb catheter that is used for ascending ureterograms.

a difficult area to examine in women, and it is probably best inspected on withdrawal of the cystoscope rather than on entry as in men.

The instrument having been passed, residual urine can be measured. It is not necessarily a very accurate assessment, because there is no guarantee that the individual has recently made an effort to empty the bladder. If the bladder is found to be full of clot when it is first inspected, it is important to wash out the clot with an Ellik evacuator; this may take quite a long time, but useful information cannot be gained as long as clot remains in the bladder. While using the 70-degree telescope, the first thing to do is to orient oneself, identify the trigone and the interureteric bar (not always easy in the female), and find the ureteric orifices. Then look for the air bubble, which is always to be found in the dome of the bladder and is a useful reference point because, when changing from a 70-degree to a 30-degree telescope and taking a biopsy, it may be difficult to reorient oneself. Examine the lateral walls of the bladder in turn, and look very carefully between the air bubble and the bladder neck. If the bladder is already too full, this may be out of sight, but suprapubic pressure should bring it into view.

Try not to overdistend the bladder, and be careful when emptying the bladder because in certain conditions it may cause the bladder to bleed and make reexamination very difficult. It is important to note how much fluid has gone into the bladder from the filling bag so that the capacity can be roughly assessed. Accurate measurement by emptying the bladder into a jug is not usually necessary, unless it is thought that the capacity is abnormally low. At this stage the bladder neck and urethra should be examined, preferably with a 30-degree or 0-degree telescope. If a catheterizing cystoscope is used, leakage will occur because of the shape of the beak, and therefore a standard cystoscope or urethroscope should be used when the urethra has to be specifically inspected. The appearance of the bladder neck does not correlate with function, and it is dangerous to draw conclusions from the endoscopic appearance. The degree of laxity may signify incompetence. The opening of a urethral diverticulum is often difficult to identify unless one knows from previous radiology where it is to be found.

GENERAL POINTS
Trabeculation

Trabeculation (Figure 12.2) is readily recognized, but interpretation of what it means is very difficult. In women it is not usually associated with obstruction and does not signify a high pressure system, and so a bladder neck resection is not indicated and should never be undertaken, unless there is urodynamic evidence of obstruction. When trabeculation becomes marked, sacculation may form between the trabeculae, and eventually a diverticulum may be formed. When a diverticulum is present, attempts should be made to look inside it (not always easy) because it may be harboring disease, for example, a carcinoma or a stone. It is also important to locate the opening of the diverticulum in relation to the ureteric orifices.

Cystitis

Cystoscopy should be avoided in the presence of active cystitis because it is potentially dangerous

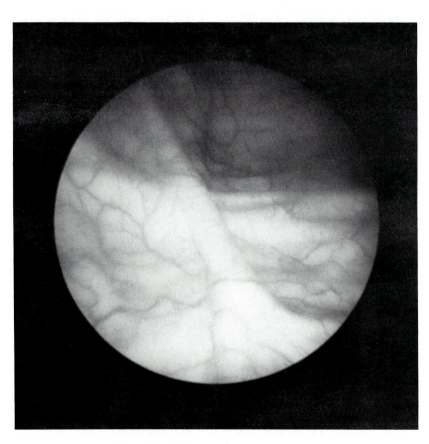

Figure 12.2 Marked bladder trabeculation.

and may cause bacteremia or septicemia. If cystoscopy is undertaken quite soon after acute cystitis has been treated, the mucosa is reddened and tends to bleed on decompression.

In recurrent bouts of cystitis or urethrotrigonitis the bladder may be normal, but there may be marked squamous change on the trigone. Whether this should be treated by diathermy, resection, urethral dilatation, sphincterotomy, or by no action at all is debatable.

Chronic cystitis is a collection of conditions not usually associated with bacterial infection but producing recurrent bouts of frequency and a great deal of suprapubic pain. In tuberculosis discrete red areas may be visible in the bladder, and the ureteric orifices may be rigid and open. In interstitial cystitis linear splits, which bleed on decompression, may be visible in the dome of the bladder. More often there is a generalized vascularity in the dome, and very often the capacity is reduced. In any of these conditions a biopsy should be taken. A biopsy forceps passed through a cystoscope or resectoscope makes obtaining a biopsy of the bladder wall very easy, and it is safely away from the base of the bladder even in the relatively thin bladder of the female. Biopsies of the trigone are best obtained by using a resectoscope loop because the mechanism of the biopsy forceps using the 30-degree telescope does not allow biopsies to be taken close to the bladder neck.

Recurrent pyelonephritis with reflux

When ureteric reflux is present in the prepubertal child, it is important to assess the position of the ureters. Often the trigone is abnormally wide, with the ureteric orifices laterally placed. In addition, the configuration of the orifice may give some guide to the possibility of the reflux ceasing—a big open ureter laterally placed is unlikely to become competent, whereas a normally appearing ureter in the correct place may improve.

Duplications

Completely duplicated ureters usually open quite close together in the bladder either side by side or on the ureteric ridge a short distance apart; the lower ureteric orifice always drains the upper part of the kidney. An ectopic ureter may open near the bladder neck but may open also in the urethra or vagina or in the perineum and be very difficult to

detect even if the patient has been given a dye, because the function of the upper part of the kidney may be so poor.

Ureterocele

A ureterocele is caused by a bag of mucosa at the lower end of the ureter and may be associated with obstruction of varying degrees. A ureterocele may be single and orthotopic or part of a duplex system and either orthotopic or ectopic. They have a very characteristic appearance and may be flattened when the pressure in the bladder rises and may even prolapse back up the ureter. In a young child a ureterocele may occasionally be so big that it is seen as a mass at the urethral orifice, having prolapsed out of the bladder (see Fig. 22-20).

Fistulae

Large vesicovaginal fistulae are no problem to diagnose, but when they are small, diagnosis may be difficult. Outpatient methylene blue testing may have already established that a vesicovaginal fistula rather than a ureterovaginal fistula is present. This test involves placing three swabs in the vagina and then filling the bladder through a catheter (better placed before the swabs are inserted) with water and methylene blue. Pressure should be applied to the bladder with the catheter clamped. This may cause some leakage into the superficial swab; but if the middle swab is clean and the dye is present on the deepest swab, a vesicovaginal fistula must be present. If the swab is damp but not discolored, the presence of a ureterovaginal fistula is a possibility. Sometimes it is easier to find the fistula by filling the bladder; then, with a speculum in the vagina, water may be seen to be spurting out of the fistula. A small probe or ureteric catheter can then be passed through the hole, and the opening in the bladder can be recognized. It is important to note the relationship of the fistula to the ureteric orifices and trigone. A vesicocolic fistula is rarely a hole big enough to see but is often indicated by the presence of a red patch on the left lateral wall of the bladder a fair distance from the ureteric orifices. It is unlikely to occur in a woman who has not had a hysterectomy.

In a patient with nonfunction of a kidney apparent on an intravenous urogram, the possibility of an absent kidney may be raised. At cystoscopy a hemitrigone will be seen. If a ureteric orifice is present, ascending ureterography should be per-

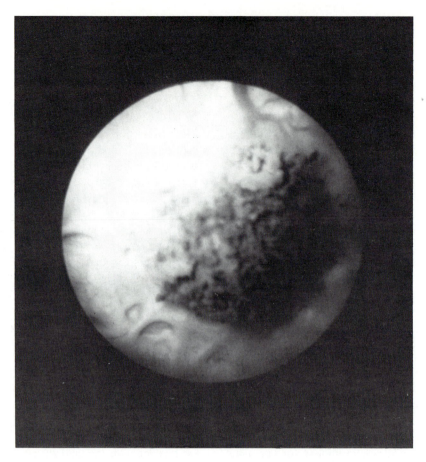

Figure 12.3 Typical papillary tumor with some adherent blood clot. Visible bladder wall shows trabeculation and sacculation.

formed. A special Chevasseau catheter (Figure 12.1), which has a conical end, is placed in the ureteric orifice, and, while contrast is injected, screening is undertaken to see where the contrast goes and whether there is any obstruction. It is bad practice to put too much contrast into an obstructed system because it may cause chemical irritation and worsen the clinical condition. It is rarely necessary to perform a retrograde pyelogram when the catheter is passed up to the renal pelvis, since this sort of information should be obtained by a good intravenous urogram.

Bladder cancer

The majority of bladder cancers are discrete papillary tumors with an orange color more often than not found on the base of the bladder or above and lateral to the ureteric orifices. Biopsy resection with the resectoscope loop effectively cures the lesion. It is important to be certain that the lesion is single

rather than multiple, and it is necessary to inspect the mucosa around the tumor very carefully; if it is abnormal, it should be biopsied (Figure 12.3).

Solid tumors may be extensive and should have generous biopsies taken, preferably with the resectoscope loop. Tumor in the bladder may be a result of cervical cancer and may occasionally be related to rectal cancer. They look different, they tend to be relatively flat and have an irregular surface, and the mucosa may be essentially intact.

The important examination at the time of cystoscopy in the case of bladder cancer is the bimanual examination to assess staging of the tumor. If there is a mass present, it is important to know whether it is mobile and whether it extends through the bladder wall. This information, together with a histological report, helps to decide how to manage the patient.

chapter 13

Special investigations

STUART L. STANTON

There are a variety of investigations; some are well established and others lie between research and current urodynamic practice. Their common link is that they are not in routine use but are reserved for resistant clinical problems whose answers have not been provided by existing conventional studies.

QUANTIFYING URINARY LOSS

Failure to demonstrate urine loss either on clinical examination or when the patient strains or coughs at full bladder capacity during cystometry or videocystourethrography can be overcome using a simple noninvasive test designed by James et al. (1971), which uses a Urilos diaper or pad. It consists of a disposable pad containing aluminium strip electrodes and dry electrolyte and is worn in proximity to the vulva. It is connected to a Urilos monitor that can be worn on the shoulder; this in turn is linked by cable or telemetering to a recorder situated at a distance (Figure 13.1). The patient attends with a comfortably full bladder, and during 45 minutes she is given a fluid load to drink and encouraged to carry out maneuvers normally likely to precipitate incontinence during her daily activity, for example, coughing, walking, jogging, and washing. Any urinary leakage onto the pad causes a change in electrical capacitance that is detected by the monitor and recorded. The pad has an approximate capacity of 100 ml of urine (Stanton and Ritchie, 1977). The original hope that this would provide accurate quantification of urinary loss has not been realized, and a more absorbent plastic-backed pad is preferred. This is nonelectronic and is worn for a period of up to 2 hours, during which time the patient takes a standardized fluid intake and exercise schedule. One or more pads are used; they are weighed at the end to give the urine loss (Sutherst, Brown, and Shawer, 1981).

The other application of Urilos is in the ambulant and nonambulant elderly or disabled patient, who may be unaware of urine loss and of the need to have the clothing changed when it occurs.

BETHANECHOL TEST

Lapides et al. (1962) suggested that decentralization of the detrusor could be detected and distinguished from other causes of a noncontractile detrusor by the subcutaneous administration of 2.5 mg bethanechol chloride during a cystometric examination. This was based on Canon's law of denervation, whereby there is supersensitivity of "denervated" (decentralized) smooth muscle to its natural neurotransmitter, acetylcholine.

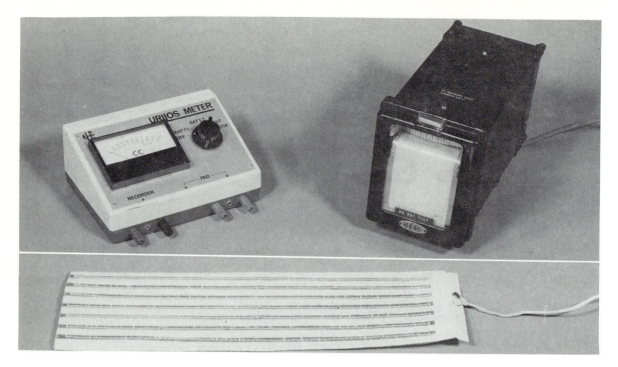

Figure 13.1 Urilos electronic nappy (diaper) with meter and recorder.

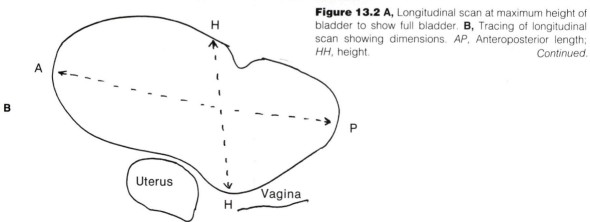

A

B

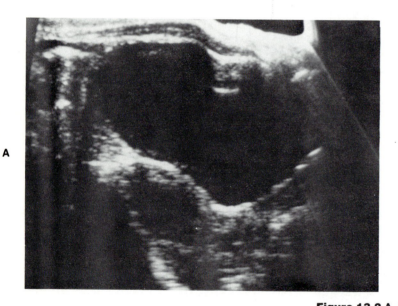

Figure 13.2 A, Longitudinal scan at maximum height of bladder to show full bladder. **B,** Tracing of longitudinal scan showing dimensions. *AP,* Anteroposterior length; *HH,* height. *Continued.*

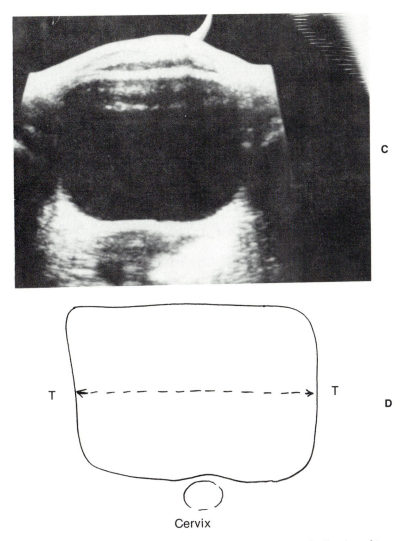

Cervix

Figure 13.2, cont'd. C, Transverse scan at maximum height of bladder. **D,** Tracing of transverse scan showing dimensions. *TT,* Transverse width. (Courtesy of Dr. R.H. Patel.)

Cystometry is performed, and the bladder pressure is noted at a volume of 100 ml. Thirty minutes after a subcutaneous administration of 2.5 mg bethanechol, the cystometrogram is repeated at the same filling rate. An increase in pressure of more than 15 cm of water is indicative of "denervation."

Many clinicians find that this test is not specific and does not in fact distinguish decentralization from other causes of neuropathy (Blaivas, 1979). Tests therefore should be interpreted cautiously and not relied on as a single confirmatory investigation.

ULTRASOUND

Residual urine can be estimated on bimanual palpation, but this is not accurate, catheterization is an invasive procedure accompanied by a potential risk of urinary tract infection. Ultrasound assessment is not invasive and is reasonably accurate. Using a static B scanner, the product of the greatest superoinferior and anteroposterior measurements in the saggital plane and the greatest transverse measurement in the transverse plane is calculated, but as the bladder is not a cube a correction factor has to be applied (Figure 13.2). Using a value of 0.7, a standard error of 21% was achieved (Poston, Joseph, and Riddle, 1983).

More detailed information on bladder and urethral morphology can be obtained using a transrectal real-time linear scanner in combination with conventional urodynamic studies (Nishizawa et al.,

1982). The technique gives information on bladder and urethral movement during filling, coughing, voiding, and voluntary interruption of the urinary stream, together with any associated movement of the vagina and pelvic floor.

ELECTROMYOGRAPHY

Electromyography is the study of bioelectrical potentials generated by smooth and striated muscle. A motor unit consists of an individual motor nerve cell and the muscle fibers it activates; the potential it generates during voluntary contraction is known as a motor unit action potential. Normally each motor unit action potential is biphasic, triphasic, or quadriphasic. Polyphasic potentials are sometimes found in normal muscle, but usually their presence indicates an incomplete lower motor neuron lesion. At rest, normal skeletal muscle is electrically quiescent or silent. As the muscle contracts, an increasing number of motor units are recruited and fire off, producing multiple action potentials.

In an early complete motor neuron lesion, spontaneous action potentials may be seen that are either single or polyphasic (fibrillation) potentials. Later, as the muscle atrophies, there is disappearance of the spontaneous potential. If the lower motor neuron lesion is incomplete, the amount of activity is proportional to the extent of the injury. There may be spontaneous activity at rest, and individual action potentials are increased in amplitude and duration, with an increased number of polyphasic potentials. In an upper neuron motor lesion, there is loss of voluntary control. Individual motor unit potentials are normal, and motor unit activity is normal or increased.

Studies on the electromyographic activity of the smooth and skeletal muscles of the lower urinary tract have shown variable degrees of clinical usefulness. Despite several attempts to record and evaluate detrusor electromyograms (Boyce, 1952; Franksson and Peterson, 1953; Stanton, Hill, and Williams, 1973; Doyle, Hill, and Stanton, 1975), there has been a disappointing correlation between the recording and clinical function. Craggs and Stephenson (1976) believe that much of the discrepancy was due to a physicochemical source, including tissue and fluid movement and some skeletal electromyogram interference. More recently, Takaiwa et al. (1982) have used carbon fiber surface electrodes mounted on a urethral catheter and claim recording superior to the conventional metal electrodes as a result of lessened interference from mechanical movement of the bladder wall.

A variety of methods have been used to record "urethral sphincter activity," depending on which muscles are studied. The external anal sphincter is the most frequently used on the basis that its action is similar to the urethral sphincter because its innervation by sacral spinal segments S2 to S4 is similar. However, several clinicians (Blaivas, Labib, Bauer, and Retik, 1977; Vereecken, de Meirsman, and Puers, 1981; Koyanagi, Ankado, Takamatsu, and Tsuji, 1982) have demonstrated that the levator ani, external anal urethral sphincter, and external striated urethral sphincter (rhabdosphincter) can all contract and relax independently of each other (Figure 13.3). Therefore it may be unreliable to monitor the anal sphincter as an indicator of urethral sphincter activity. The periurethral muscles (levator ani, transverse perinei) can be monitored easily, but the rhabdosphincter muscle is more inaccessible and doubt must exist sometimes about the validity of its recordings.

The most common mode of recording external anal sphincter activity is with an anal plug electrode, which can be modified to include a catheter for simultaneous recording of the intraabdominal (rectal) pressure (Figure 13.4). A ground electrode is needed, which is conveniently taped to the thigh. This is a noninvasive and painless procedure and therefore particularly suitable for children. However, surface electrodes do not permit assessment of individual motor unit potentials. More accurate recordings can be obtained by using concentric needle electrodes, which consist of an inner and outer recording electrode. This can be inserted through unanesthetized skin into either the external anal sphincter or the periurethral muscles; the latter are located 5 mm lateral to the external urethral meatus and approximately 1.5 to 2 cm deep and parallel to the urethra (Stanton, Hill, and Williams, 1973). The presence of striated muscle electromyographic activity with a good signal-to-noise ratio is confirmed using a portable electromyograph, with the electrode adjusted if necessary. The signal can be recorded at gains of 50 to 100 μV/cm deflection, with a low frequency time constant of 0.03 seconds and an upper cutoff frequency of 70 Hz.

An alternative method of recording urethral sphincter activity is to use a urethral catheter that can record urethral or vesical pressure with two ring electrodes mounted on it (Figure 13.5). It has all the disadvantages of a surface electrode and in addition is quite likely to produce artifacts. Finally, it is uncertain from which muscle groups the recordings are made—striated rhabdosphincter, peri-

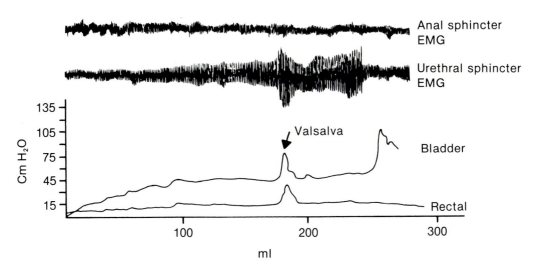

Figure 13.3 Synchronous cystometry and electromyographic investigation. Discrepancy between anal sphincter and urethral sphincter electromyogram is notable.

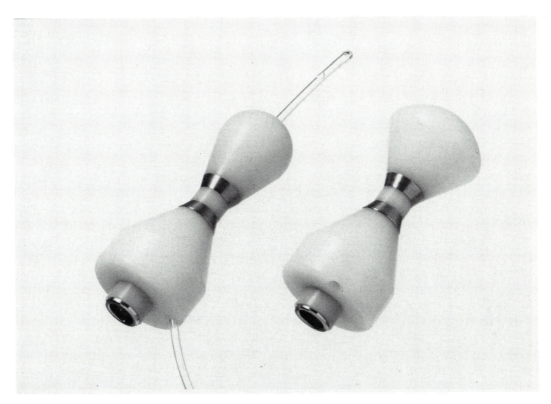

Figure 13.4 Anal plug electrodes. *Left,* Plug electrode with 1 to 2 mm external diameter polyethylene catheter for measurement of rectal (abdominal) pressure during investigation. (DISA, Copenhagen.)

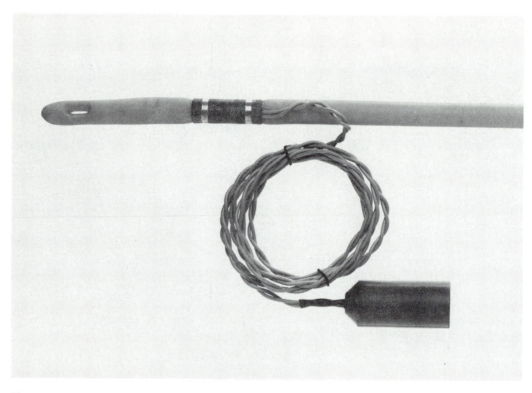

Figure 13.5 No. 10 to 14 Fr gauge urethral ring catheter with two platinum ring electrodes situated just below balloon. Electrodes are separated by 1 cm.

urethral muscle, or smooth urethral muscle. It is more useful as a stimulating electrode for the production of sacral-evoked responses.

Greater accuracy can be achieved by using single-fiber electromyography. A needle electrode with a very small recording surface (diameter 25 μm) detects extracellular activity from a single muscle fiber at minimum voluntary activity. When a motor nerve is partially damaged, the remaining axons sprout to reinnervate those muscle fibers that have been denervated. Each of the remaining axons supply a greater number of muscle fibers. A quantitative estimate can be made with the number of muscle fibers of a single motor unit within the area of the recording electrode, which is called the motor neuron fiber density. This is increased in neuropathy and myopathy and may be an index of reinnervation following denervation (Anderson, 1983).

SACRAL-EVOKED RESPONSES

The sacral-evoked response technique assesses the integrity of the sacral reflex arc by measuring the conduction time or latency period between a stimulus to a peripheral nerve and an evoked neurological response such as a muscle contraction or a cerebral cortical potential.

Sacral-evoked responses allow distinction to be made between neuropathic, myopathic, and functional bladder disorders and will effectively localize neurological lesions of the conus medullaris or corda equina. It is a more sensitive indicator of denervation and neuropathy than single-fiber electromyography.

Square-wave stimuli (1 Hz at 0.05 to 1 msec) are delivered to the skin over the dorsal nerve of the clitoris or via a urethral electrode to the urethral or bladder mucosa. A concentric electromyograph needle is placed into a convenient recording site, for example, anal sphincter or levator ani muscle. A ground electrode is placed on the thigh. An electromyographic amplifier with an oscilloscope and signal averager are required to monitor the sacral-evoked response.

The normal and abnormal responses are shown in Figure 13.6. The sensory threshold occurs at

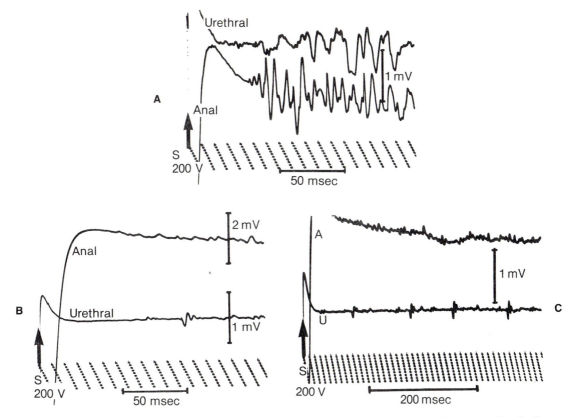

Figure 13.6 A, Evoked response in periurethral muscle (urethral) and external anal sphincter (anal) after perianal stimulation in normal continent woman. Normal latency of 50 msec is seen in anal sphincter and 52 msec in periurethral muscle. **B,** Evoked response in periurethral muscle and external anal sphincter after perianal stimulation in woman with urethral sphincter incompetence. Weak response with latency of 60 msec is seen in anal sphincter and single motor unit is seen in periurethral muscle after latency of 110 msec. **C,** Evoked response from same subject at slower speed showing response in anal sphincter for greater than 400 msec and sporadic activity in periurethral muscle for 300 msec. (Courtesy of Mr. Robert S. Anderson.)

about 25 V, but a strength of 50 to 60 V, may be required, which can be uncomfortable (Abrams, Feneley, and Torrens, 1983). The response has an early component and a late component. The latency period of the former can be used as a measure of response time and may represent a neural potential, whereas the second component may represent a muscle potential. Alternatively, both components may represent the involvement of separate afferent pathways through the spinal cord that vary in the number of synapses (Krane and Siroky, 1980).

CEREBRAL-EVOKED RESPONSES

The development of computer averaging techniques has allowed recording of low-level stimulus-related signals from the background electroencephalograph. Gerstenberg, Hald, and Meyhoff (1981) have described the technique of urethral stimulation via a urethral ring electrode using a square wave impulse of 0.2 msec duration, with a rate of 2 Hz. Current amplitude was just above the urethral preception threshold. The cortical response was detected on the sensory cortex in the midline. The short latency period of 65 msec and amplitude of 4 μV suggests the response may be related to proprioceptive pelvic floor afferents rather than represent bladder sensation.

URETHRAL SENSITIVITY

Urethral sensation as an index of function has been investigated by Powell and Feneley (1980) in a variety of bladder conditions, including bladder hypersensitivity (frequency and urgency with a normal cystometrogram apart from reduced capacity), neuropathy, detrusor instability, chronic retention, outflow obstruction, and "stress incontinence." A

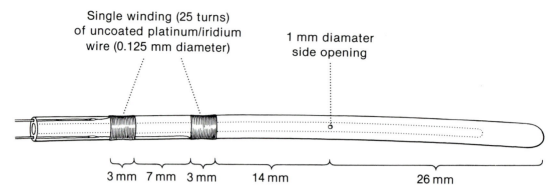

Single winding (25 turns)
of uncoated platinum/iridium
wire (0.125 mm diameter)

1 mm diamater
side opening

3 mm 7 mm 3 mm   14 mm   26 mm

Figure 13.7 Urethral sensitivity catheter. Modified No. 12 Fr triple-lumen Rossier catheter. Equal volume of normal saline and K-Y Jelly is used as lubricant for catheter. Stimulus parameters are 0.3 msec pulses, 20 Hz, and 0 to 20 mA. Catheter is positioned using fluid bridge technique to ensure that electrodes are in same position for each test. (Courtesy of Mr. K. Murray.)

No. 10 Fr urethral catheter with two platinum electrodes separated by 1 cm and situated 1.5 cm below the balloon was used. The catheter was inserted into the bladder, the balloon was just inflated and then withdrawn so that it fitted snugly at the level of the bladder neck, and the electrodes were then sited in the posterior urethra. Square wave impulses at the rate of 20/sec at an increased intensity of constant current were applied until the patient experienced the sensation of tingling. It was found that urethral hyposensitivity (requiring a high current to stimulate the sensation) was more common among patients with neuropathy and in the few patients with recurrent urinary tract infection, while urethral hypersensitiviry was found commonly in the group with hypersensitive bladders, those with chronic urinary retention, and in a small number of patients with stress incontinence. Patients with detrusor instability exhibited a wide range of response.

Murray (1982) used a modified No. 12 Fr Rossier catheter (Figure 13.7) to study urethral sensitivity in relation to change in bladder capacity in a variety of patients. He also investigated the relationship of sensitivity in cases of neuropathic bladder and urethral syndrome and the role of endogenous opiates in bladder function before and after administration of potentiating and antagonizing drugs.

URETHRAL SOFTNESS

The concept of softness of the inner urethral wall as a major contribution to continence control was originally described by Zinner, Ritter, and Sterling (1976). They hypothesized that the soft urothelial lining (which is partly estrogen sensitive and atro-

phies when estrogen is deficient) alters in response to surgery and at the time of the menopause and that this is conducive to decreasing hermetic closure and incontinence.

In 1981 Plevnik and Vrtacnik described the use of a No. 10 Fr Plexiglas transducer catheter that could measure the deformation of the inner urethral wall and could quantify its softness. The principle was the measurement of electrical impedance of tissue introduced between two electrodes in the catheter. Later, a No. 15 Fr catheter (Figure 13.8) was used that allowed urethral pressure (using the perfusion technique of Brown and Wickham [1969]) to be recorded. This catheter has a measuring aperture in which there are two calibration electrodes and two measuring electrodes for detecting deformation of the internal urethral wall. The catheter is introduced into the urethra and the measuring aperture placed at the desired site. Pressure exerted by the urethral wall at the site of the measuring aperture is registered using the perfusion technique (Figure 13.9). The perfusion channel is then disconnected and the tissue allowed to be introduced into the aperture. The depth of tissue introduction (that is, the deformation) was measured as a change in electrical impedence between the measuring electrodes situated along the aperture. The change in electrode area in contact with the tissue is proportional to the depth of the introduced tissue, and the softness of the inner urethral wall can be expressed in the form of a constant, representing pressure/deformation ratio.

TELEMETRY

Most urodynamic techniques are carried out as tests in isolation from the normal day-to-day ac-

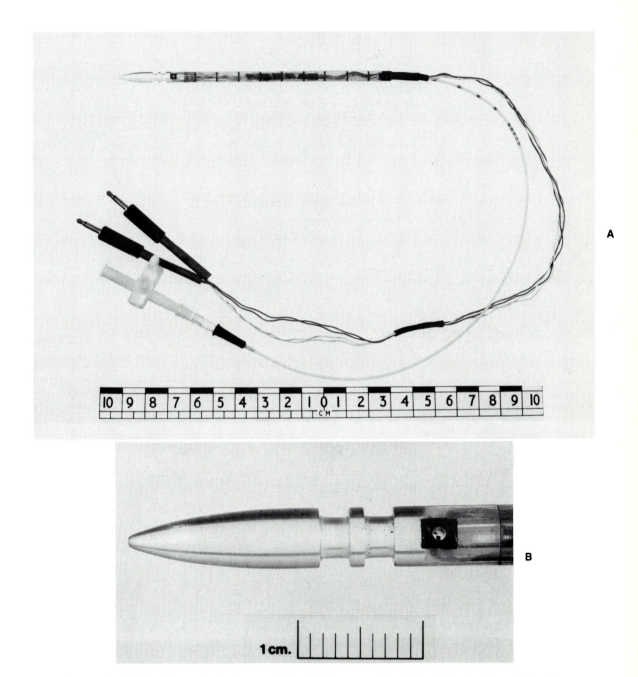

Figure 13.8 A, Plevnik's urethral softness catheter. **B,** Close-up of front of catheter showing retaining rings and measuring aperture.

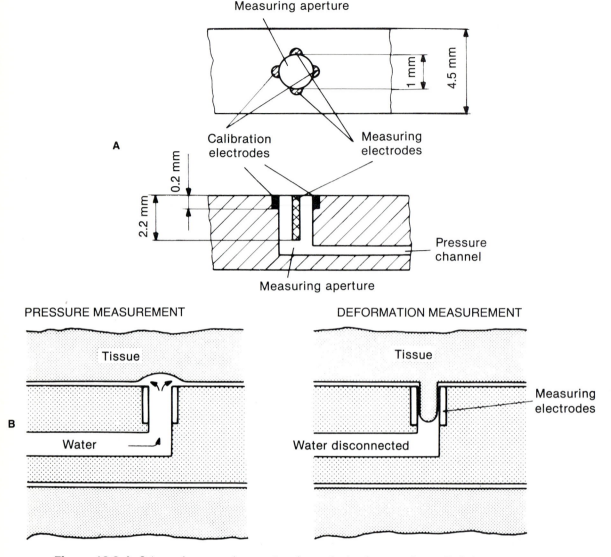

Figure 13.9 A, Schema for measuring aperture for urethral softness catheter. **B,** Schema for measuring pressure *(left)* and deformation *(right)* of inner urethral wall. Urethral wall softness is inversely related to pressure needed to introduce tissue to known depth in cylindrical side aperture of catheter. Introduction of tissue to 0.5 mm depth will be noted by detecting amount of current flowing through electrode in wall of aperture at corresponding depth.

tivity of the patient, and it is not surprising when discrepancies are encountered between clinical symptoms and urodynamic findings.

To overcome this, various clinicians have carried out ambulatory monitoring of patients, either coupling the patient by an electric cable (which still poses an artificial limit) or using radiotelemetry to link with a recording device. Warrell, Watson, and Shelley (1963) described the use of a pressure-sensitive "radio pill" that could be introduced into the bladder and would transmit intravesical pres-

sure (Figure 13.10). It measured 15 mm by 9 mm and a fine thread was attached to one end to allow retrieval. It was able to transmit information up to 30 cm. The disadvantages included occasional discomfort on insertion, it had a limited life, it cost over $450, and finally it measured total bladder pressure and a similar pill would have to be inserted into the rectum to obtain the abdominal pressure and allow calculation of the detrusor pressure.

Attempts to measure bladder and urethral pressure during ambulation by using fluid-filled lines

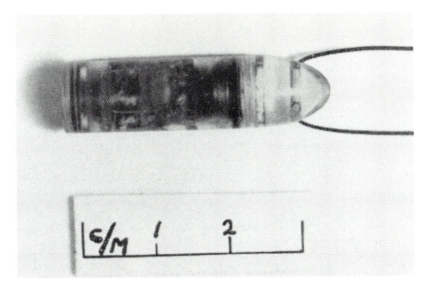

Figure 13.10 "Radio pill" that is inserted into bladder and retrieved by means of nylon thread at one end.

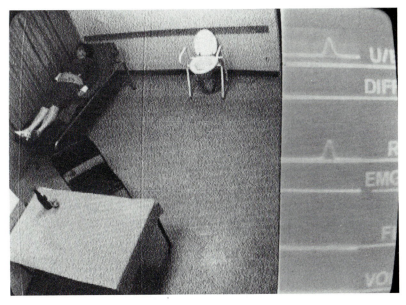

Figure 13.11 Patient recumbent while telemetric urodynamic investigations are in progress. On right are urodynamic parameters. (From Thuroff, J., et al. In Zinner, N., and Sterling, A. 1981. Female incontinence. New York. Alan R. Liss, Inc.)

are bedevilled by inaccuracies as a result of movement of liquid within the catheters. To overcome this James (1979) has used air-filled balloon catheters to measure urethral and bladder pressure. The catheter is linked to a transducer attached to the patient's thigh, which is in turn linked to a recording device. While the bladder pressure can be reliably measured, it is difficult to maintain the urethral balloon at precisely the same place within the urethra while the patient moves around.

Comprehensive telemetering was obtained by Thuroff et al. (1981), who carried out urodynamic recordings and observed the patient under closed-circuit television in a special investigation room where the patient could exercise, void, and rest undisturbed. Bladder filling was obtained using an oral fluid load and a diuretic, and all data were recorded on video for future replay (Figure 13.11).

This is a complicated, time-consuming, and expensive maneuver and probably only indicated for those patients in whom detection of urine leakage, detrusor instability, or a voiding disorder of likely psychogenic origin have already defied conventional assessment, or for the purposes of research into diurnal and nocturnal rhythms of the lower urinary tract.

REFERENCES

Abrams, P., Feneley, R., and Torrens, M. 1983. Urodynamics. Heidelberg. Springer-Verlag.

Anderson, R. 1984. A neurogenic element to urinary genuine stress incontinence. Br. J. Obstet. Gynaecol. **91**:31-45.

Blaivas, J.G. 1979. A critical appraisal of specific diagnostic techniques. In Krane, R., and Siroky, M., editors: Clinical neurourology. Boston. Little, Brown & Co.

Blaivas, J.G., Labib, K., Bauer, S., and Retik, A. 1977. A new approach to electromyography of the external urethral sphincter. J. Urol. **117**:773-777.

Boyce, W. 1952. Bladder electromyography: a new approach to the diagnosis of urinary bladder dysfunction. J. Urol. **67**:650-668.

Brown, M., and Wickham, J. 1969. Urethral pressure profiles. Br. J. Urol. **41**:211-217.

Craggs, M., and Stephenson, J. 1976. The real bladder electromyogram. Br. J. Urol. **48**:443-451.

Doyle, P., Hill, D., and Stanton, S.L. 1975. Electromyography of the detrusor muscle. J. Urol. **114**:208-212.

Franksson, C., and Peterson, I. 1953. Electromyographic recording from the normal human urinary bladder, internal urethral sphincter and ureter. Acta. Physiol. Scand. Suppl. **106**:105-156.

Gerstenberg, T., Hald, T., and Meyhoff, H. 1981. Urinary cerebral evoked potentials mediated through urethral sensory nerves: a preliminary report. In Zinner, N., and Sterling, A., editors. Female incontinence. New York. Alan R. Liss, Inc.

James, D. 1979. Continuous monitoring. Urol. Clin. North Am. **6**:125-135.

James, E., Flack, F., Caldwell, K., and Martin, M. 1971. Continuous measurement of urine loss and frequency in incontinent patients. Br. J. Urol. **43**:233-237.

Koyanagi, T., Ankado, K., Takamatsu, T., and Tsuji, I. 1982. Experience with electromyography of the external sphincter and spinal cord injury patients. J. Urol. **127**:272-278.

Krane, R., and Siroky, M. 1980. Studies on sacral-evoked potentials. J. Urol. **124**:872-876.

Lapides, J., Friend, C.R., Ajemian, E., and Reus, W. 1962. Denervation supersensitivity as a test for neurogenic bladder. Surg. Gynecol. Obstet. **114**:241-244.

Murray, K. 1982. Urethral sensitivity: an integral component of the storage phase of the micturition cycle. Neurourol. Urodynamics **1**:193-197.

Nishizawa, O., Takada, H., Morita, T., Satoh, S., and Tsuchida, S. 1982. Combined ultrasonotomagraphic and urodynamic monitoring. Proceedings of twelfth annual meeting of the International Continence Society. Leiden.

Plevnik, S., and Vrtacnik, P. 1981. How to measure inner urethral wall softness. In Zinner, N., and Sterling, A., editors. Female incontinence. New York. Alan R. Liss, Inc.

Poston, G., Joseph, A., and Riddle, P. 1983. The accuracy of ultrasound and the measurement of changes in bladder volume. Br. J. Urol. **55**:361-363.

Powell, P., and Feneley, R.C. 1980. The role of urethral sensation in clinical urology. Br. J. Urol. **52**:539-541.

Stanton, S.L., Hill, D., and Williams, J.P. 1973. Electromyography of the detrusor muscle. Br. J. Urol. **45**:289-298.

Stanton, S.L., and Ritchie, D. 1977. Urilos: practical detection of urine loss. Am. J. Obstet. Gynecol. **124**:461-463.

Sutherst, J., Brown, M., and Shawer, M. 1981. Assessing the severity of urinary incontinence by weighing perineal pads. Lancet **1**:1128-1130.

Takaiwa, M., Date, T., Fukaya, Y., Shiraiwa, Y., Katahira, K., and Tsukahara, S. 1982. Clinical electromyogram of detrusor bladder using carbon fibre electrode. Proceedings of twelfth annual meeting of the International Continence Society. Leiden.

Thuroff, J., Jonas, U., Petri, E., and Frohneberg, D. 1981. Telemetric urodynamic investigation in female incontinence. In Zinner, N., and Sterling, A., editors. Female incontinence. New York. Alan R. Liss, Inc.

Vereecken, R., de Meirsman, J., and Puers, B. 1981. Sphincter electromyography in female incontinence. In Schulman, C., editor: Advances in diagnostic urology. Heidelberg. Springer-Verlag.

Warrell, D.W., Watson, B., and Shelley, T. 1963. Intravesical pressure measurement in women during movement using a radio-pill and an air-probe. Br. J. Obstet. Gynaecol. **70**:959-967.

Zinner, N., Ritter, R., and Sterling, A. 1976. The mechanism of micturition. In Williams, D.I., and Chisholm, G., editors. Scientific foundation of urology. London. William Heinemann Medical Books, Ltd.

chapter 14

Physical aspects of urodynamic investigations

DEREK JOHN GRIFFITHS

In this chapter I examine, from a physical (that is, mechanical) point of view, some of the urodynamic measurements that are commonly made in gynecological urology. Some artifacts are pointed out, and, where possible, "best" methods are recommended.

FILLING CYSTOMETRY
Gas or water

The choice of medium—gas or water—is bound up with the choice of system—one channel or two (Figure 14.1). In a two-channel system the bladder pressure is measured directly, whereas in a one-channel system the measured pressure differs from the bladder pressure because of the extra pressure needed to drive the infusion through the resistance of the catheter. With water the catheter resistance is relatively higher, so that with a one-channel sys-

tem under steady conditions the measured pressure can be noticeably higher than the pressure in the bladder, unless the infusion rate is limited to relatively low values. Thus with water a two-channel system is usual.

With gas the catheter resistance is much lower, so that a much faster rate of infusion can be used before this error in the pressure measurement becomes significant under steady conditions. Thus a one-channel system is usually used for gas cystometry.

When the bladder pressure changes significantly during filling, as during a contraction, the dead volume of the pump and tubing may become important (Figure 14.1). Its effect depends on whether gas or water is used.

With water, when the bladder contracts, the amount of fluid in the dead volume does not change

153

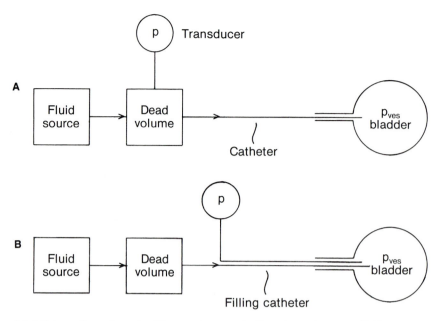

Figure 14.1 Schematic systems for filling cystometry. **A,** One-channel system. **B,** Two-channel system. In two-channel system pressure transducer may be either external or catheter mounted.

significantly, so that the volume in the bladder remains essentially constant; furthermore, the measured volume delivered by the pump is equal to the volume infused into the bladder.

With gas the situation is different because of its compressibility. If the dead volume is relatively large, then, when the bladder pressure rises, a considerable quantity of gas is forced out of the bladder and backwards through the catheter into the dead volume, until the pressure there becomes approximately equal to the bladder pressure. Thus the bladder contraction is not isovolumic, and the volume in the bladder differs from the volume apparently delivered by the pump. When the bladder relaxes, the gas flows back through the catheter into the bladder. The dead volume should therefore be made small in comparison with the smallest bladder volume of interest (for example, 20 ml) and should be specified by the manufacturer. However, even if the dead volume is negligible, the volume of the bladder falls by some 10% for a pressure rise of 100 cm H_2O as its gaseous contents are compressed. Thus the bladder contraction is not isovolumic, and the volume in the bladder is not equal to that delivered by the pump, although the error is not very large.

A further disadvantage of one-channel gas cystometry is that the dead volume, together with the resistance of the catheter, leads to a smoothed-out version of the pressure changes in the bladder. This can make it difficult to distinguish detrusor contractions from abdominal straining, since on the gas cystometrogram they appear equally smooth, and of course an abdominal pressure measurement is not normally made.

Other disadvantages are undetected gas leakage, which can make the calculated bladder volume even more unreliable (Gleason and Reilly, 1979), and the fact that the gas cannot be used for a subsequent flow study. One advantage is the easy registration of an intraurethral EMG signal during bladder filling and (quasi)voiding. Nevertheless, gas cystometry as normally practiced can only be considered as a quick and convenient screening examination; water cystometry with a two-channel system is technically clearly superior.

With water one may choose either an external or a catheter-tip transducer. An external transducer is sensitive to artifacts caused by movement of the water-filled tube that connects it to the bladder. It must be positioned at the level of the bladder, that is, the level of the upper edge of the symphysis pubis, (International Continence Society, 1979); this can be a nuisance if the patient moves during the procedure. It has the advantages that the zero reading usually does not drift during the measure-

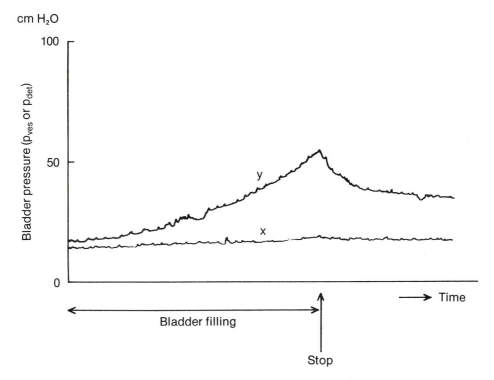

Figure 14.2 Bladder pressure as measured during filling cystometry. *x*, Small pressure rise, little pressure relaxation when filling is stopped; *y*, large pressure rise (low-compliance bladder), significant pressure relaxation after filling stops.

ment* and that suspected drift can immediately be checked by opening the transducer to the atmospheric pressure.

A catheter-tip transducer moves with the patient and is not sensitive to movement artifacts. However, it can begin to drift after being inserted into a warm, urine-filled bladder, and this drift cannot be checked until after the measurement is completed.

External and catheter-tip transducers respond differently to vertical movement of the catheter tip within the bladder (Griffiths, 1980), but the difference is unlikely to exceed 10 cm H_2O, which is not significantly greater than the other uncertainties in the measurements. Thus with care both types of transducers can give satisfactory results.

Rate of filling

The faster the bladder is filled, the higher the pressures that are measured during the filling. If fast filling is interrupted, the bladder pressure "re-

laxes" back toward a lower value, corresponding to very slow filling (Van Mastrigt and Griffiths, 1981). With a "medium" rate of filling (10 to 100 ml/min) (International Continence Society, 1979), two situations typically arise (Figure 14.2). The pressure remains low (<10 cm H_2O rise) throughout filling (apart from obvious detrusor contractions). In this case the potential for relaxation is obviously limited, and the measured pressures are similar to those that would have been measured at a much slower filling rate. (2) The pressure rises more steeply during filling (by >20 cm H_2O); that is, the bladder has a low compliance. In this case there is more room for relaxation, and in my own experience it can nearly always be observed. One can look at this in two ways: (a) the filling rate is too fast, so that artificially high pressures are being generated, or (b) the steep rise is abnormal, an important sign of a pathological condition. Taking this second view, one would like to distinguish a passive (viscoelastic) from an active (hypertonic) cause of the pressure rise. Unfortunately, the relaxation appears to be very similar in both cases.

---

*This is not so if the transducer dome is provided with a membrane to ensure sterility. Domes with membranes are therefore not recommended.

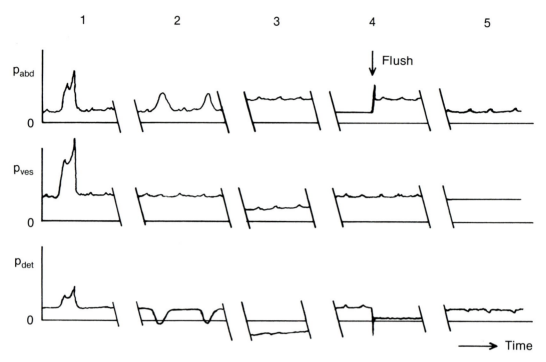

Figure 14.3 Examples of malfunctioning or artifacts in pressure measurements. *1*, Straining unequally transmitted to bladder (P_{ves}) and rectum (P_{abd}); *2*, phasic contractions of rectum; *3*, abdominal pressure too high (that is, significant rectal tone); *4*, rectal catheter not functioning (respiration not registered) until flushed through; *5*, bladder catheter not functioning.

ABDOMINAL PRESSURE

During filling cystometry and pressure-flow studies of micturition the measurement of abdominal (usually rectal) pressure helps to distinguish detrusor contractions from abdominal pressure variations. Usually it is subtracted from the intravesical pressure to form the detrusor pressure (International Continence Society, 1979). Although valuable, this procedure is liable to artifacts.

No general abdominal pressure may exist; the pressure exerted on the rectum may differ from that exerted on the bladder (Figure 14.3).

The rectum may have its own tone. Regular contractions are easily recognized because they are not present in the intravesical pressure (Figure 14.3), but a significant steady tone is difficult to distinguish, since it results only in an unusually low or negative detrusor pressure (Figure 14.3).

To measure a real (fluid) pressure in the rectum, a few drops of water must be introduced and maintained by flushing the measuring catheter whenever necessary. It appears to make little difference whether the end of the catheter is enclosed in a loosely fitting, noninflated balloon. The working of the catheter should be continually checked by observing whether all variations in abdominal pressure (for example, respiration) are subtracted from the detrusor pressure (Figure 14.3, *D*). Display of all three pressure traces (intravesical, abdominal, and detrusor pressure) helps to check catheter functioning and to identify artifacts.

The transducers for intravesical and rectal pressure should in principle be at the same level. This is sometimes difficult to arrange with catheter-tip transducers, but other errors are likely to be larger.

URETHRAL PRESSURE

The pressure measured with a catheter in a closed urethra is different in character from a "real" fluid pressure, and this gives rise to difficulties in interpretation. The mere use of the term *urethral pressure* implies some assumptions that may or may not be valid for a particular urethra.

What is meant by urethral pressure

Imagine an open urethra, filled with fluid, and concentrate on one point along its length (Figure 14.4). If the pressure of the fluid rises, the urethra is forced further open, and vice versa; thus there

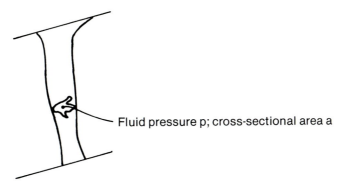

Figure 14.4 Fluid-filled urethra with noncircular lumen. When fluid pressure is *p*, lumen cross-sectional area is *a*, at point shown.

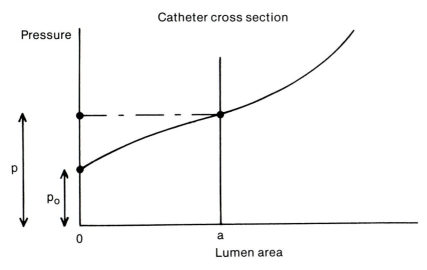

Figure 14.5 Possible relation between fluid pressure and lumen area at point shown in Figure 14.4. p_o, Fluid pressure needed to open lumen at this point; *p*, pressure that would be measured by catheter of cross-sectional area, *a*, ignoring any difference between natural form of urethral lumen (Figure 14.4) and that of catheter. Here *p* is significantly greater than p_o because this urethra is not particularly highly distensible.

is a relation between the fluid pressure and the lumen area (Figure 14.5). If the fluid pressure is reduced, the lumen eventually closes (at the point in question) when the pressure is p_o. If the pressure of the fluid nearby were gradually raised from a low value, the lumen would begin to open when it reached p_o. Thus p_o is the pressure at which leakage can occur past the given point, and it is therefore the urethral pressure that we are interested in when assessing incontinence. Notice that p_o is an ordinary fluid pressure and so cannot vary, for example, with the rotation of a measuring catheter.

In practice, however, p_o cannot be directly measured. Instead, a catheter of finite cross-sectional area, *a*, is inserted in the urethra, and measures the pressure, *p*, when the lumen area is *a* (Figure 14.5). Obviously, $p > p_o$. However, if we make the assumptions that the urethra is highly distensible and that it seals well when it closes, then p_o does not vary much with *A* (Figure 14.6); thus p is not much larger than p_o, and the measurement is a good approximation of the desired urethral pressure.

Since the catheter cross section is round, the measured pressure may in principle differ from that in Figure 14.5, where the lumen has its natural shape. Furthermore, because of this distortion a transducer on one side of the catheter may give different readings as it is rotated in the urethra, even though the desired urethral pressure, p_o, does not itself depend on orientation. Provided that the assumption of high distensibility is valid, however,

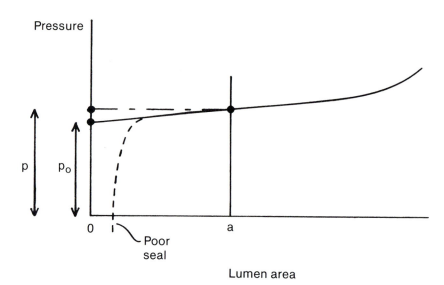

Figure 14.6 Possible relation between fluid pressure and lumen area for highly distensible urethra. *Full curve*, Urethra seals well and *p* is approximately equal to p_o. *Broken curve*, If seal is poor, lumen may remain open even at zero (atmospheric) pressure, so that p_o does not even exist at ordinary pressures.

these effects should be small. The rotational variations sometimes observed probably result from a different type of distortion, as discussed later.

If the assumption of high distensibility is not valid, any catheter will significantly overestimate the urethral pressure p_o; if the urethra does not seal properly, p_o may not even exist within the normal range of pressures, and leakage can then always occur past the point in question, whatever the pressure reading given by a urethral catheter (Figure 14.6).

Maximum urethral closure pressure

The difference between the bladder pressure and the pressure measured by a catheter in the urethra is called the urethral closure pressure. It is often supposed that the maximum value of the closure pressure is a measure of the capacity of the urethra to resist leakage. Clearly this may be so if the assumptions of high distensibility and a good seal are valid at the point of maximum pressure, but, if they are not valid, the maximum urethral closure pressure may grossly overestimate the capacity to resist leakage. In practice, this means that a high maximum urethral closure pressure is an important factor in the capacity to resist leakage but cannot by itself guarantee it.

Which method of measurement

If the assumptions of high distensibility and a good seal are valid, all the methods of measuring

urethral pressure should give similar results (although with their own peculiarities, which are discussed later). If the assumptions are not valid, the methods may give different results, but none of them gives a reliable assessment of the capacity to resist leakage. No method can be called "best," although all have some value.

In addition to these physical points, one must realize that under the conditions in which leakage is likely, functional changes in the urethral pressure are also probable (such as relaxation or tightening of the periurethral muscles, and "transmission" of abdominal pressure changes). A static urethra pressure profile gives little or no information about these changes. A stress profile (with coughing or straining) is better in principle but demands a measuring system with a high speed of response to pressure changes.

Membrane/balloon catheter

Advantages. The advantages of membrane/balloon catheter measurements are of a real fluid pressure, no rotational effects, and high speed of response to pressure changes.

Disadvantages. The disadvantages of membrane/balloon catheter measurement are that it tends to be big. The large cross section can exaggerate the difference between measured p and p_o; length can smooth out fine features in pressure profile.

Catheter-tip transducer

Advantages. The advantages of catheter-tip

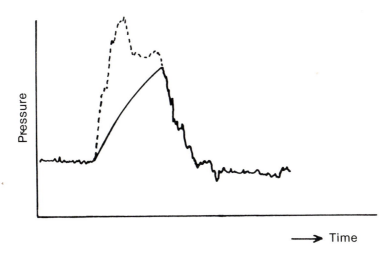

Figure 14.7 Distortion of urethral pressure peak, which can occur with poorly designed perfusion system. *Broken curve,* True course of pressure. *Solid curve,* measured pressure, showing typical "sawtooth" distortion.

transducer measurements are its smallness and high speed of response.

Disadvantages. The disadvantages of catheter-tip transducer measurements are that they are not a direct measurement of a real fluid pressure and are therefore subject to artifacts: for example, recessed transducer reads too low a pressure (Hilton and Stanton, 1981b), sometimes shows rotational effects (Hilton and Stanton, 1981a, see also later), and is somewhat fragile.

Perfusion (Brown-Wickham) method, with water as perfusion fluid

Advantages. The advantages of the perfusion method are that it can be made reasonably small, is a direct measure of the pressure needed to cause leakage (except in the presence of a catheter), and is a simple and robust apparatus.

Disadvantages. The disadvantages of the perfusion method are that its slowness in responding to rising pressure can cause distortion (Figure 14.7) (Griffiths, 1980; Brown, Sutherst, and Shawer, 1980). This distortion can be overcome by careful design, provided that water, not gas, is used as the perfusion fluid. This method sometimes shows rotational effects, depending on catheter stiffness (see later) and number of perfusion sideholes; the reading depends somewhat on perfusion rate, but this can be turned to advantage, since it allows the assumption of high distensibility to be checked. For normal use 2 to 4 ml/min is suitable.

Rotational artifacts. The rotational effects

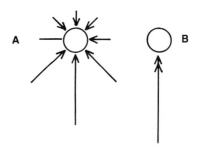

Figure 14.8 When catheter with side-mounted transducer or single perfusion sidehole is rotated in urethra, it may register greater pressure in one orientation than in others. **A,** Scheme of distribution of forces exerted by urethral wall on catheter in this situation. **B,** Results of these forces, that is, net sideways force exerted by urethral wall on catheter at point in question. ("Sideways" here means perpendicular to axis of catheter and urethra.)

sometimes observed with the catheter-tip and perfusion methods involve a higher measured pressure when the transducer or sidehole(s) is oriented in one particular direction (Hilton and Stanton, 1981a). Thus under these circumstances the urethra exerts a strong sideways force on the catheter (Figure 14.8). The most likely explanation is that a stiff catheter has been inserted in a curved urethra. The resulting bending automatically generates sideways forces (Figure 14.9). This artifact can be reduced by using a more flexible catheter, but it appears in any case to be less pronounced in the female urethra than in the more severely curved male urethra.

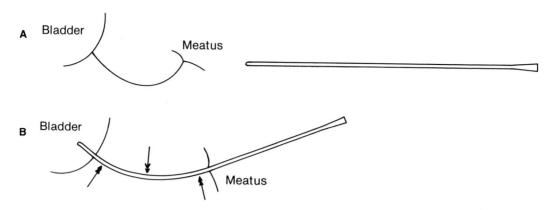

Figure 14.9 A, Curved urethra and straight catheter. **B,** When catheter is inserted into urethra, both assume an intermediate curvature. Arrows show schematically the distribution of net sideways forces that urethra must exert on catheter to bend it to this curvature.

UROFLOWMETRY

The weakest link in most commonly used flow-meters is the collecting funnel. It delays and distorts the flow pattern; changes in stream direction and angle appear as dips and peaks in the flow curve (as artifacts) (Scott, 1973; Rollema, 1981). Careful design—for instance, ribs to prevent swirling and a wide, short outlet—can reduce but not eliminate these artifacts. Isolated peaks in an otherwise smooth flow curve should be regarded with suspicion as possible artifacts.

Once the fluid has been collected, the flow rate can be measured in many different ways, each with its own peculiarities.

1. Rotating disk (DISA) has its advantages: direct measurement of the flow rate itself; quickness of response to changes, subject to limitations of the funnel; and insensitivity to mechanical disturbance (such as knocks). It has disadvantages as well: reading of volume depends on density of liquid (contrast or water), so initial calibration may be necessary; and the motor unit must be kept dry.

The other common methods all measure the quantity of liquid voided and derive the flow rate by electrical differentiation with respect to time.

2. Measurement of weight is simple (no funnel necessary) and fast in response; however, the reading depends on the liquid density, and it is extremely sensitive to knocks, since the collecting vessel tends to wobble on the weight transducer.

3. Measurement of liquid level in a vessel of known cross section (various methods) tends to be sensitive to knocks and to be slower in response to changes because level disturbances caused by

the inflow must be damped out. In some designs the damping is insufficient, and level oscillations can be seen as artifacts in the flow curves. Some methods follow:

Measurement of pressure at the bottom of the vessel: cheap and robust, but reading depends on liquid density.

Measurement of electrical capacitance between liquid and a dipstick immersed in it: cheap and robust; reading is relatively insensitive to properties of voided fluid.

Measurement of time for ultrasound pulse to travel to surface and back: robust and can be installed as a normal looking (flushing) toilet; reading depends only slightly on liquid density.

PRESSURE-FLOW MICTURITION STUDIES
Urethral resistance

In women real anatomical urethral obstruction is rare, although it can occur (Griffiths and Scholtmeijer, 1981). A poor flow is usually caused by an insufficient detrusor contraction and/or by functional urethral obstruction (insufficient relaxation). Such functional abnormalities may be either neurogenic or psychogenic. Characteristically they are rather variable, resulting in a complicated, changing pattern of pressure and flow.

Pressure at maximum flow. Often the maximum flow rate occurs when the urethra is at its most relaxed. The corresponding detrusor pressure is then a measure of the minimum urethral resistance attained in that micturition. (The delay and distortion of the flow measurement should be taken into account.) This pressure at maximum flow is useful if anatomical obstruction is a possibility, since one can then say that the "anatomical" part of the urethral resistance is certainly not greater than this. An abnormally low detrusor pressure at maximum flow may sometimes be of interest, but one must remember that a normal value is already low, and that an error in the abdominal pressure (and therefore the detrusor pressure) of 10 cm H_2O is likely.

In normal and functionally obstructed urethras a calculated resistance factor has little meaning. A graphic method of expressing the urethral resistance is to be preferred in general (International Continence Society, 1979).

Maximum micturition pressure. If functional effects are present, the maximum detrusor pressure developed during micturition may be important in itself. Because of the way in which the detrusor responds to urethral changes, the highest pressure is often attained when the urethra is least relaxed, that is, most nearly shut off. The pressure is then close to the isometric detrusor pressure and gives more information about detrusor function than about urethral resistance (see later).

Effect of a urethral catheter

In the majority of girls (and, *a fortiori*, in women) a No. 8 Fr urethral catheter has very little mechanical effect on the urethral resistance (Griffiths and Scholtmeijer, 1981). In a minority, those with distal urethra or meatus calibrating at about No. 20 Fr or less, it can cause significant obstruction. In true obstructive stenosis (caliber No. 16 Fr or less) it exaggerates the degree of anatomical obstruction.

More commonly the presence of a urethral catheter (together with the other circumstances surrounding a urodynamic examination) has an inhibiting effect on micturition—that is, causes some functional obstruction and/or detrusor contraction.

Bladder contractility: the stop test. In many patients, if voiding is suddenly interrupted by sphincter action, the detrusor pressure rapidly rises to a higher value. This behavior reflects a fundamental myogenic property of the contracting detrusor—a trade-off between the pressure generated and the flow delivered. The detrusor pressure attained on stopping, the isometric detrusor pressure, ought to be a more reliable measure of the detrusor

contraction than the pressure during voiding, which depends also on the flow rate and therefore on the urethral resistance (Griffiths, 1979).

In the routine clinical use of this "stop test" there are difficulties: (1) The detrusor contraction may be partially inhibited when the urethra is shut off, or the flow may be interrupted by inhibiting the detrusor instead of by shutting the sphincter. (2) The patient may be unable on command to interrupt the flow completely. Both (1) and (2) lead to too low an isometric pressure. Although a high isometric pressure may imply a good contraction, a low value may be untrustworthy. A partial solution may be suddenly to block the urethra with a balloon (Coolsaet, private communication).

Other methods of assessing the detrusor contraction, based on the maximum flow rate and the corresponding detrusor pressure (Abrams and Griffiths, 1979) or on the rate of rise of the detrusor pressure at the beginning of a contraction (Van Mastrigt and Griffiths, 1981), have not been much used in the clinic area.

All these methods suffer from the disadvantage that they assess only the detrusor contraction at that moment and not the contractility itself, that is, the ability to contract. Thus, although a good contraction, maintained until the bladder is empty, implies good contractility, a weak or absent contraction does not necessarily imply poor contractility.

There are also practical difficulties. When micturition is near normal, the tests may indeed be applicable, although probably unnecessary. However, in abnormal micturition, in which detrusor contractility is in doubt, they are often difficult to apply. A typical problem is the woman who micturates with much straining but little or no rise in detrusor pressure, giving rise to a poor flow and perhaps residual urine. The question is, will she void satisfactorily if, after an operation, the urethral resistance is raised? A stop test is hardly possible because both an extra interruption in the flow and a small rise in detrusor pressure would be masked by irregular changes and artifacts caused by straining. One can, however, say that since the maximum flow rate and the detrusor pressure at maximum flow (and throughout micturition) are low, the detrusor contraction is poor in this micturition. Nevertheless, the possibility of an improvement after the operation cannot be ruled out because the potential contractility has not been assessed.

DESIRABLE DEVELOPMENTS

There are two problems for which I would like to see solutions.

1. Urethral capacity to resist leakage. The urethral pressure profile (with or without "stress") is useful but insufficient. Measurement of urethral softness (as a measure of its sealing ability) is one possibility (Plevnik et al., 1981), but a direct measurement of the capacity to resist real leakage, with no catheter in the urethra is really required.

2. Bladder contraction/contractility. At least two difficult situations arise. (a) Steep pressure rise (low compliance) during filling cystometry—is it active or passive? For this a reliable detrusor EMG would be helpful. (b) The woman who micturates apparently only by straining. Is the detrusor contracting or not? If not or only poorly contracting, is it capable of contracting adequately under other circumstances? Again, a detrusor EMG might be helpful.

That such problems still exist at such a basic level after so many years of urodynamics should make us realize that urodynamic measurements do not automatically provide exact answers to clinical questions. A liberal dose of experience is necessary, first, to recognize and discard artifacts, and, second, to interpret the remaining measurements and apply them in the clinical situation. This is likely to remain true however sophisticated the measurements themselves may become in the future.

REFERENCES

Abrams, P.H., and Griffiths, D.J. 1979. The assessment of prostatic obstruction from urodynamic measurements and from residual urine. Br. J. Urol. **51**:129-134.

Brown, M.C., Sutherst, J.R., and Shawer, M. 1980. A standard specification for the speed of response of urethral pressure measuring apparatus. Clin. Phys. Physiol. Meas. **6**:85-87.

Coolsaet, B.L.R.A. Private communication.

Gleason, D., and Reilly, R. 1979. Gas cystometry. In Clinical urodynamics. Urol. Clin. North Am. **6**:85-87.

Griffiths, D.J. 1979. Uses and limitations of mechanical analogies in urodynamics. In Clinical urodynamics. Urol. Clin. North Am. **6**:143-148.

Griffiths, D.J. 1980. Urodynamics: The mechanics and hydrodynamics of the lower urinary tract. Bristol, U.K. Adam Hilger Ltd.

Griffiths, D.J., and Scholtmeijer, R.J. 1981. Precise determination of the obstructive effect of meatal stenosis in little girls. Proceedings of eleventh annual meeting of International Continence Society, Lund, Sweden.

Hilton, P., and Stanton, S.L. 1981a. Urethral pressure measurement by microtransducer. II. An analysis of rotational variation. Proceedings of eleventh annual meeting of International Continence Society. Lund. Sweden.

Hilton, P., and Stanton, S.L. 1981b. Urethral pressure measurement by microtransducer. IV. The effect of transducer design on the urethral profile. Proceedings of eleventh annual meeting of International Continence Society. Lund, Sweden.

International Continence Society. 1979. First, second, and third reports on the standardisation of terminology of lower urinary tract function. U. Urol. **121**:551-554.

Plevnik, S., et al. 1981. Urethral softness distribution in the female urethra. Proceedings of eleventh annual meeting of International Continence Society. Lund. Sweden.

Rollema, H.J. 1981. Uroflowmetry in males. Thesis. State University of Groningen. Netherlands. pp. 40-42.

Scott, F.B. 1973. Correlation of flow rate profile with diseases of the urethra in man. In Lutzeyer, W., and Melchior, H., editors. Urodynamics. New York. Springer-Verlag New York, Inc.

van Mastrigt, R., and Griffiths, D.J. 1981. First results of contractility measurements on children using isometric contractions. Proceedings of the eleventh annual meeting of International Continence Society. Lund, Sweden.

part THREE

PATHOPHYSIOLOGY: CLINICAL CONDITIONS

chapter 15

Classification of incontinence

STUART L. STANTON

DEFINITION

Incontinence is defined according to the International Continence Society* as "a condition in which involuntary loss of urine is a social and hygienic problem and is objectively demonstrable."

Involuntary aspects

Incontinence is considered to be involuntary; for two categories of patients it needs further explanation. In children the diagnosis of incontinence can be made before the age of 3 (when most children are continent) if the child is wet between voids. After this age it should not be too difficult to confirm the parent's observation that the child is incontinent. The physically fit but mentally frail or demented patient, who has lost her social consciousness or appreciation of the need to be continent (Chapter 30) can be diagnosed as incontinent.

*The International Continence Society was formed in 1971 to promote the scientific study of lower urinary tract function in men and women. It draws members from many disciplines including urology, gynecology, neurosurgery, gerontology, physics, biomedical engineering, anatomy, physiology, pharmacology, nursing, and physiotherapy. There is an annual meeting with published proceedings.

Social problem

There is no more distressing lesion than urinary incontinence—a constant dribbling of the repulsive urine soaking the clothes which cling wet and cold to the thighs making the patient offensive to herself and her family and ostracising her from society.

Howard A. Kelly, 1928

It is important to realize that in an otherwise fit patient incontinence is a social problem leading to ostracism and isolation, since the patient becomes rejected by friends and relatives and may be forced to enter an institution for care. The patient may need institutional care by virtue of mental or physical frailty yet be barred because of incontinence.

Hygienic problems

Wet as a ditch, day in day out. She got through fifteen pairs of knickers a day, not to mention all her bed linen.

Lara in Akenfield by Roland Blythe

That incontinence is a hygiene problem of some magnitude is readily understood. It is believed to occupy about 25% of nursing time in hospitals. No smell is more upsetting to visitors and relatives than a urinous odor pervading the environment of a room or ward.

TERMINOLOGY

The terminology of the subject of incontinence is confusing because each authority has developed a separate language for it. In 1973 the International Continence Society, in its wisdom, decided to establish a Standardisation Committee to overcome the multiplicity of terms and attempt to produce internationally acceptable working definitions and names. In a large measure it has succeeded, and so far four reports have been produced. The first report (1976) dealt with terminology of lower urinary tract function; the second (1977) and third (1980) reports dealt with procedures relating to evaluation of micturition, flow, rate, pressure measurement, and symbols. The fourth report (1981) dealt with terminology related to neuromuscular dysfunction of the lower urinary tract (see Appendix II).

In 1928 Sir Eardley Holland coined the term *stress incontinence,* which meant loss of urine during physical effort. This came to be understood as the name of a disorder that gives rise to this symptom and sign.

As the pathophysiology of urinary incontinence became more clearly understood, it was apparent that the term *stress incontinence* was ambiguous because it could apply to a symptom, a sign, and a diagnosis. Indeed, the symptom and sign of stress incontinence can be found in most types of incontinence. The International Continence Society sought to clarify this situation by adopting the following terminology: The symptom "stress incontinence" indicates the patient's statement of involuntary loss of urine when exercising physically. The sign "stress incontinence" denotes the observation of involuntary loss of urine from the urethra immediately on an increase in abdominal pressure.

In 1976 the International Continence Society adopted the term *genuine stress incontinence* to mean "involuntary loss of urine when the intravesical pressure exceeds the maximum urethral pressure but in the absence of a detrusor contraction" (Appendix II). This condition has a number of synonyms, such as the following:

Urethral sphincter incompetence
Stress urinary incontinence
Anatomical stress incontinence
Pressure equalization incontinence

I prefer the term *urethral sphincter incompetence* because "genuine stress incontinence" is too similar to "stress incontinence," and it adds nothing to our understanding of the condition. Urethral

sphincter incompetence implies that the sphincter mechanism is no longer able to withstand the rise of detrusor pressure, resulting in incontinence.

Similarly the condition or term *detrusor instability,* originally proposed by Bates et al. in 1970, described a condition well known before that called *dyssynergic detrusor dysfunction* by Hodgkinson, Ayers, and Drukker in 1963. The other terms used are:

Dyssynergic detrusor dysfunction
Urge incontinence
Uninhibited bladder
Unstable bladder/detrusor instability

In 1979 the International Continence Society (Appendix II) defined an unstable detrusor as one

. . . shown objectively to contract spontaneously or on provocation, during the filling phase while the patient is attempting to inhibit micturition. An unstable detrusor may be asymptomatic and its presence does not necessarily imply a neurological disorder: when an objectively defined neurological disorder exists, the term "detrusor hyperreflexia" should be used.

CLASSIFICATION

The causes of incontinence may be divided into urethral and extraurethral conditions (Figure 15.1); this is not entirely satisfactory, since congenital conditions appear in both. However, it has the merit of emphasizing that fistulae are an important cause of incontinence and that an ectopic ureter can remain as an undetected cause of incontinence even through to adulthood.

Urethral conditions

Urethral sphincter incompetence. The most common form of incontinence is urethral sphincter incompetence; it is present from the teens onward.

Detrusor instability. The cause of detrusor instability is still imprecise but may be divided into neuropathic, or hyperreflexic—found from birth onwards—and nonneuropathic, or idiopathic—thought to have a psychosomatic cause among other causes and found from the teens onward. In some patients with detrusor instability the sphincter mechanism is competent at a normal bladder pressure. When the detrusor pressure rises, the sphincter begins to open and lose its competence; the patient's symptoms are predominantly urge incontinence with some stress incontinence. In other patients the sphincter mechanism is incompetent at a normal bladder pressure, and this is aggravated by any subsequent pressure rise. These patients com-

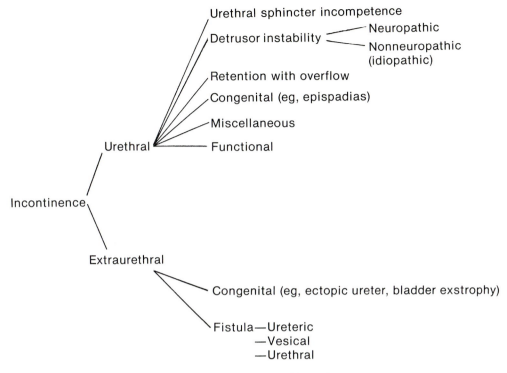

Figure 15.1 Classification of incontinence.

plain of stress incontinence and urge incontinence with or without a rise in detrusor pressure. It is important to distinguish between the two groups because the former may respond to conservative management alone, whereas the latter may require conventional bladder neck surgery in addition to any conservative therapy.

Urinary retention with overflow. Urinary retention with overflow may be acute or chronic. The acute form is usually painful. There may be an obvious antecedent cause such as an impacted pelvic mass or an acute genital infection, for example, herpes vulvitis. Chronic retention, on the other hand, is often painless and insidious and is frequently undetected, so that errors in diagnosis are often made. It is more common in the elderly and is often a result of a neuropathy such as the peripheral neuropathy of diabetes mellitus or cerebrovascular artherosclerosis.

Congenital disorders. Congenital disorders such as epispadias should be detected during childhood, but occasionally they are not diagnosed until later. An etopic ureter can be a notoriously difficult condition to diagnose and may not be present until after childhood.

Miscellaneous. Other causes may include ure-

thral diverticulum, urinary tract infection (temporary, and more common in the elderly), and drugs (such as α-blocking agents) (see Chapter 35).

Incontinence caused by functional disorder. Incontinence caused by a functional disorder is rare and is discussed in Chapter 30. Before this diagnosis is made, the patient has to be fully investigated, since this diagnosis is made when all other causes have been excluded. Any symptom may be simulated, but frequently incontinence is complained of and is said to occur continuously or at any time and without apparent cause. Findings from a clinical examination and investigation may be normal; however, as mentioned earlier, the symptoms and cystometric findings characteristic of nonneuropathic detrusor instability may be found (which may have a psychosomatic cause).

Extraurethral conditions

Extraurethral disorders are distinguished from urethral disorders by the symptom of continuous incontinence.

The extraurethral congenital disorders are ectopic ureter and bladder exstrophy (see Chapter 22); frequently these have been attended to in childhood by a pediatric urologist. Urinary fistulae in the western world are largely iatrogenic, the majority of them occurring after abdominal surgery for benign conditions (see Chapter 20). Great skill and patience are required sometimes to detect the fistula, especially if it is quite small. Common to all iatrogenic fistulae is the history of an antecedent abdominopelvic operation, followed at a variable time by incontinence.

REFERENCES

Bates, C.P., Whiteside, C., and Turner Warwick, R. 1970. Synchronous cine stroke pressure stroke flow stroke cystourethrography with special reference to stress and urge incontinence. Br. J. Urol. **42:**714-723.

Hodgkinson, C.P., Ayers, M.A., and Drukker, B.H. 1963. Dyssynergic detrusor dysfunction in the apparently normal female. Am. J. Obstet. Gynecol. **87:**717-730.

chapter 16

Urethral sphincter incompetence

STUART L. STANTON

Incontinence resulting from urethral sphincter incompetence may be defined as involuntary urethral loss of urine when the intravesical pressure exceeds the maximum urethral pressure in the absence of detrusor activity (Bates et al., 1976). Functioning of the sphincter is complex, and maintenance of a higher pressure in the urethra than in the bladder depends on intact innervation and on the following factors: urethral smooth muscle, external sphincter (striated muscle), blood vessel turgor within the urethral muscle, elastin and collagen within the urethral wall, and urethral epithelium. The important contributory adjacent structures—are the periurethral striated muscle (levator ani), the perineal muscles, and the bony pelvis. The bladder neck is supported by the posterior pubourethral ligaments, the pubocervical fascia, the levator ani, and the pelvic floor muscles. Increases in intraabdominal and detrusor pressures impair urinary control.

TERMINOLOGY

Increases in knowledge concerning the anatomy and physiology of the lower urinary tract have led to changes in terminology. The term *stress incontinence* was first proposed by Sir Eardley Holland in 1928. This is now considered unsatisfactory as a diagnostic term because the signs and symptoms of stress incontinence can occur in many different types of incontinence. Instead the term *genuine stress incontinence* was proposed by the International Continence Society in 1974 (Bates et al., 1976). Alternative terms include *anatomical stress incontinence* and *pressure equalization incontinence*. I prefer *urethral sphincter incompetence,* since this is germane to the subject and suggests the likely pathogenesis.

ETIOLOGY

The following are possible causes of urethral sphincter incompetence. Sometimes more than one may be responsible.

Congenital anatomical defect

Weakness. Studies indicating the prevalence of stress incontinence in young nulliparous women (Nemir and Middleton, 1954; Wolin, 1969; Thom-

as et al., 1980) show that 5% to 15% regularly have troublesome stress incontinence. In the absence of an obvious anatomical abnormality, this probably results from a fundamental anatomical weakness, associated partly with the evolutionary change from the horizontal to the vertical position. When a woman is on her hands and knees, the bladder and urethra are located at a relatively high position in relation to the short vertical axis of the abdominal cavity, where gravity has little additional influence on the intraabdominal pressure. The urethra exits from the posterior wall of the bladder, passing over the symphysis pubis (Figure 16.1, *A*). By contrast, in the vertical position the urethra leaves the bladder at a point of combined intraabdominal pressure and maximum gravity force, without the buttressing support of the symphysis (Figure 16.1, *B*). These anatomical relationships are deleterious to urinary control (Hodgkinson, 1970).

Abnormality. Epispadias (see Chapter 22) is the main congenital urinary system abnormality and should be easily identifiable in the neonatal period. It is characterized by continuous or daytime incontinence. Rarely the condition may escape detection until adulthood (Figure 16.2, *A*). The urethra and bladder neck are imperfectly formed because of faulty migration and midline fusion of the mesoderm, resulting in a widened bladder neck, a

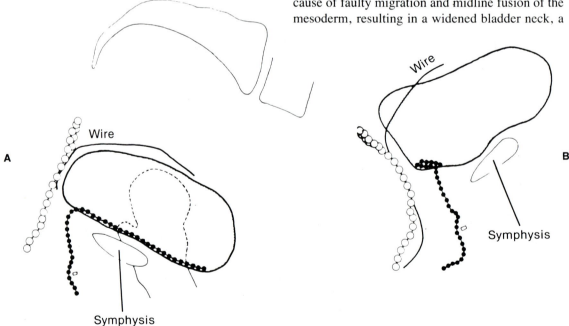

Figure 16.1 A, Chain urethrocystogram with patient in nonstraining, lateral, "all fours" position, showing urethra exiting from high position in bladder and supported by symphysis. **B,** Patient erect, showing bladder neck junction at lowest level of bladder and without symphysial support. (From Hodgkinson, C.P. 1970. Am. J. Obstet. Gynecol. **108:**1141-1168.)

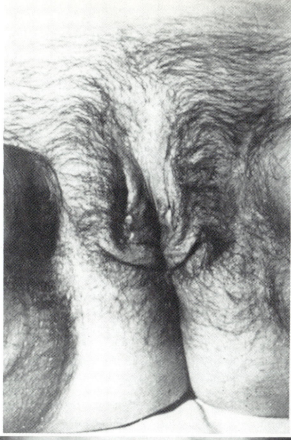

A

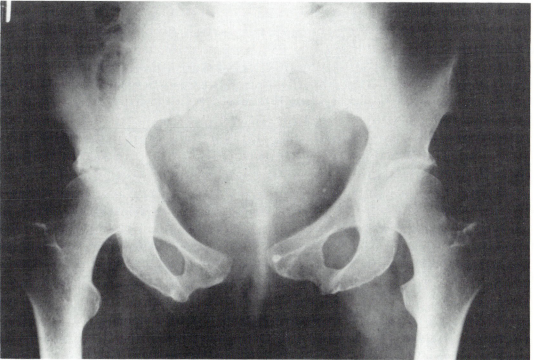

B

Figure 16.2 A, Epispadias. Clitoris is separated into two distinct bodies, and there is flattening of pubic region and loss of pubic hair in midline. **B,** Underlying separation of symphysis pubis accompanies epispadias.

short urethra with defective smooth and striated musculature, and underlying separation of the symphysis pubis (Figure 16.2, *B*).

Acquired anatomical defect

An anatomical defect may result from trauma (for example, anteroposterior compression of the bony pelvis during a traffic accident) or occasionally from symphysiotomy. The symphysis separates, and there is damage to the underlying soft tissue supports of the bladder neck, particularly the posterior pubourethral ligaments (Figure 16.3). This results in a downward displacement of the bladder neck (Stanton, Cardozo, and Riddle, 1981).

Parity

Childbearing is considered to be an important factor in the causation of pelvic floor weakness. Thomas et al. (1980) have shown that the prevalence of incontinence is higher among multiparous women than among nulliparous women. No data are available concerning the role of duration of the second stage of labor, weight of the infant or mode of delivery in causing pelvic floor weakness. It is speculative to suggest that in recent years the decrease in parity and shortening of the second stage may lead to a decrease in the incidence of urethral sphincter incompetence.

Menopause

The incidence of incontinence rises linearly with age (see Chapter 27). Estrogen deprivation produces atrophy of muscle and ligaments and a decrease in urethral closure pressure and in the hermetic closure of the urethra, which is effected by the urothelium.

Past surgery

Operations around the bladder neck to correct prolapse or urethral sphincter incompetence may produce recurrent incontinence. The precise reasons are unknown but may include interference with or damage to the urethra and sphincter mechanism at the time of surgery (leading to a decrease in urethral resistance or closure pressure), postsurgical fibrosis affecting the urethra and paraurethral tissue, fixation of the urethra to the back of the symphysis with loss of elasticity, and failure to elevate the bladder neck or production of its descent.

PATHOPHYSIOLOGY

The mechanism of continence and the causes of incontinence are reviewed in Chapter 3. The factors relevant to the development of incontinence as a result of urethral sphincter incompetence are the maximum urethral pressure at rest, the intrinsic variability in urethral pressure and the sustained response to stress of this pressure, the intraabdominal pressure, and the pressure transmission ratio, which depends on bladder neck elevation. Hilton (1981) uses the term *margin to continence* to describe the interrelationship of these factors and their roles in determining continence (Figure 16.4).

Maximum urethral closure pressure at rest

The maximum urethral closure pressure at rest may be lower in incontinent women and varies according to the degree of severity of incontinence. It falls as age increases but is not affected by parity. Recurrent unsuccessful surgery often leads to a low urethral pressure.

Variability and response to stress

Urethral pressure has an intrinsic variability in both continent and incontinent women. In women predisposed to incontinence, it may be one of several factors responsible for this disorder and for determining its severity. Similarly, the lack of a sustained urethral pressure response to acute rises in intraabdominal pressure may precipitate incontinence and determine its severity (Hilton 1981).

Intraabdominal pressure

Variations in the extent and dissipation of intraabdominal pressure rise affect the detrusor and urethral pressures. Incontinence is more likely to develop in an obese woman with a chronic cough than in her thin, healthy counterpart. The intravesical pressure rise in response to coughing is higher in women with urethral sphincter incompetence than in continent women (Hilton 1981).

Pressure transmission ratio

The pressure transmission ratio in continent women is greater than 100% in the proximal three fourths of the functional urethral length, whereas incontinent women have a linear decrease in transmission from bladder neck to external meatus, with values below 100%. Maintenance of a ratio in excess of 100% is due to a high urethral closure

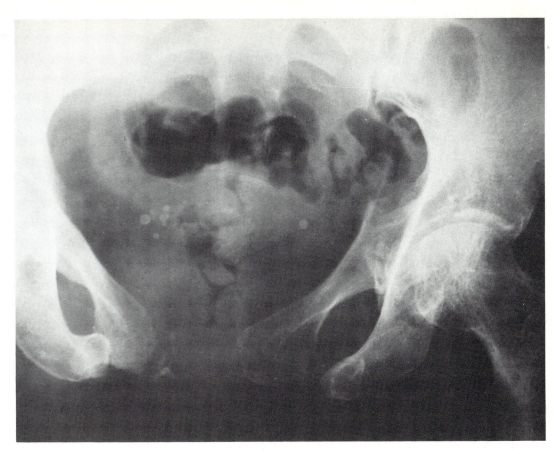

Figure 16.3 Traumatic diastasis of symphysis and fractures of internal pelvic ring. (From Stanton, S.L., Cardozo, L., and Riddle, P.R. 1981. Br. J. Urol. **53:**453-454.)

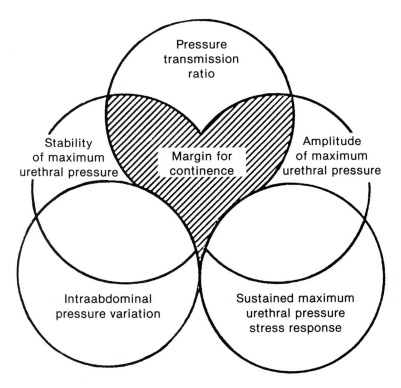

Figure 16.4 Diagram of interaction of morphological and functional factors and their role in determining continence. (Courtesy of P. Hilton.)

pressure at rest and to the position of the bladder neck within the abdominal zone of pressure (Enhörning, 1961), supported by the posterior pubourethral ligaments, the pubocervical fascia, and the pelvic floor musculature.

PRESENTATION
Symptoms

The history informs the clinician of the nature, severity, and duration of the complaint. The bladder is an unreliable indicator, however, and it may be quite misleading to diagnose the cause of incontinence on the basis of the clinical history alone (Bates, Loose, and Stanton, 1973; Jarvis et al., 1980). Nevertheless, the complaint of stress incontinence alone may reliably indicate urethral sphincter incompetence in more than 90% of patients.

Patients are usually multiparous, and the symptoms commonly appear in pregnancy, worsening after successive pregnancies (Francis, 1960; Stanton, Kerr-Wilson, and Harris, 1980). Patients often

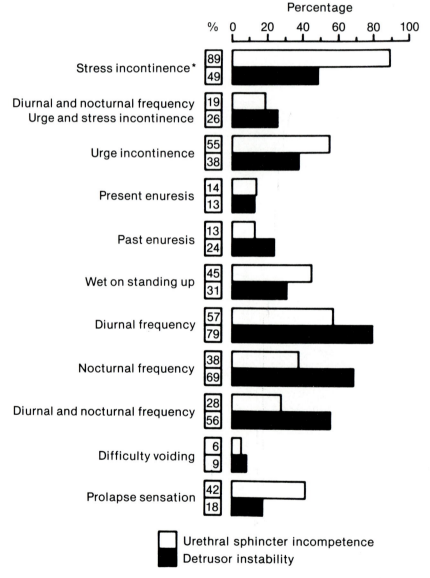

Figure 16.5 Incidence of symptoms associated with urethral sphincter incompetence and detrusor instability. *Stress incontinence is dominant; other symptoms include urgency, diurnal frequency, and nocturnal frequency. (From Cardozo, L., and Stanton, S.L. 1980. Br. J. Obstet. Gynaecol. **87:**184-190.)

seek advice and treatment in middle age. There may be a history of operations to correct stress incontinence. In a study of 100 patients with urethral sphincter incompetence and 100 patients with detrusor instability, 91% of the former group were multiparous. Their mean age at initial examination was 50 years, and their mean number of previous operations was 0.6. Stress incontinence was the most common symptom, followed by diurnal frequency, urge incontinence, and incontinence on standing (Figure 16.5) (Cardozo and Stanton, 1980). Stress incontinence may be greater in the week preceding the menstrual period. Ability to interrupt the urinary stream was equally present in both groups of patients, although more patients with detrusor instability seemed uncertain of their ability to interrupt the stream (Table 16.1).

Signs

Usually there are no special features on general or neurological examination. Epispadias is readily recognizable (Figure 16.2). Cardozo and Stanton (1980) have studied the incidence of genital prolapse on vaginal examination in 100 patients with urethral sphincter incompetence. Their findings are as follows:

Cystocele or cystourethrocele	42
2-degree vault or cervical descent	5
Rectocele	23
Enterocele	1

Genital prolapse has been confirmed by other clinicians to be present in approximately half of the patients with urinary sphincter incompetence.

INVESTIGATION

Although the diagnosis may be determined with over 90% accuracy on the basis of the history alone when stress incontinence is the sole presenting symptom, usually urinary sphincter incompetence has a polysymptomatic presentation. Because of the adverse effects of surgery on patients with either detrusor instability, voiding difficulties, complicated symptoms, or past bladder neck surgery, urodynamic investigations are usually performed.

Plain radiographs

A plain radiograph can detect symphysial diastasis of either congenital (Figure 16.2, B) or traumatic (Figure 16.5) cause or a full bladder resulting from chronic retention, which can masquerade as urethral sphincter incompetence, especially in the elderly (Figure 16.6).

Cystometry and videocystourethrography

The radiological diagnosis of urethral sphincter incompetence is based on demonstration of urine or contrast leakage simultaneous with physical effort (such as coughing or Valsalva's maneuver), in the absence of detrusor activity. After bladder filling with the patient supine, the patient is asked to stand and cough several times. Any urinary leakage is noted (Figure 16.7). Because small leakage may not be detected by radiological screening, the patient should always be asked if leakage has occurred. Other causes of urine loss, such as detrusor instability, urethral diverticulum, and urinary fistula, should be excluded during the radiological examination.

Urilos test

Failure to demonstrate urine loss by either physical examination or cystometry and videocystourethrography should be followed by a Urilos test. This is a simple, objective, and noninvasive method of demonstrating urine loss (Stanton and Ritchie, 1977). Quantitative estimation may be ob-

---

TABLE 16.1   Ability of patients with urethral sphincter incompetence or detrusor instability to interrupt their urinary stream

	Can interrupt	Cannot interrupt	Unsure
Urethral sphincter incompetence			
Interview	38	50	12
Videocystourethrography	85	15	—
Detrusor instability			
Interview	31	46	23
Videocystourethrography	82	18	—

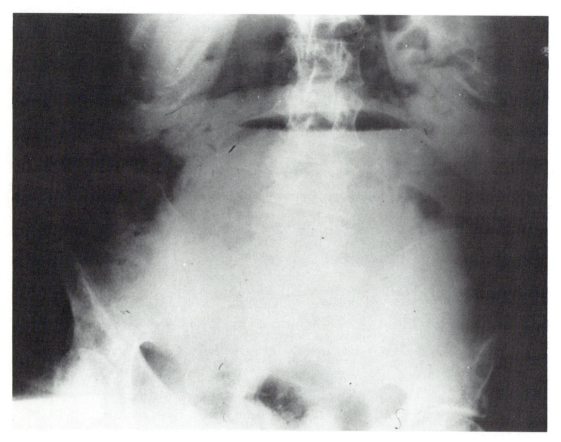

Figure 16.6 Chronic retention of urine, which can imitate urethral sphincter incompetence by causing stress incontinence.

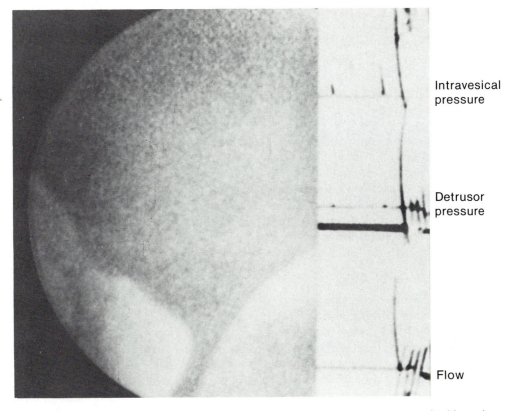

Intravesical
pressure

Detrusor
pressure

Flow

Figure 16.7 Videourethrocystographic image of stress incontinence resulting from urethral sphincter incompetence. There is absence of detrusor pressure rise except that briefly caused by cough impulse. Contrast outlines open bladder neck and urethra.

tained by perineal pad weighing (Sutherst, Brown, and Shawer, 1981). The patient's bladder should be comfortably full at the start of the test. She wears a diaper or sanitary napkin. If the exact moment of urine loss is critical, an electronic recording pad can be used instead. The patient exercises for 30 to 40 minutes, during which time she is encouraged to drink fluids, see running water, wash her hands, and carry out the activities that normally precipitate urine loss during the day. If no leakage is observed, it is unlikely that her incontinence is a significant problem, and treatment should be deferred and the patient reevaluated in 6 months.

Urethral pressure measurement

Hilton (see Chapter 10) has discussed the clinical role of urethral pressure measurement. The resting maximum urethral closure pressure value is of some help in predicting the outcome of surgery, with a lower value indicating a decreased chance of success. When gradual urethral relaxation in response to stress is present, continuous recording of urethral pressure for 20 seconds or more while the patient is performing some activity, such as coughing, will demonstrate urethral relaxation with a decrease in maximum urethral closure pressure (see Figure 10.9).

Uroflowmetry

The measurement of urine flow rate is a simple, noninvasive screening test for voiding difficulties (see Chapter 6). The prevalence of voiding difficulties in the healthy female population is unknown, but among patients in a urodynamics clinic it was found to be 16%, of whom 2% were asymptomatic (Stanton, Oszoy, and Hilton, 1983). Because suprapubic bladder neck surgery to correct incontinence may induce voiding difficulties, prior uroflowmetry should always be performed. If a voiding disorder is detected, it should be evaluated and the decision to proceed with bladder neck surgery should be reviewed. If surgery is decided on, the patient should be informed of a likely delay in resumption of voiding and the need for a prolonged period of catheter drainage.

The peak flow rate value, the shape of the curve,

the mean flow rate, the flow time, and the presence of abdominal straining should all be considered. Several flow rate tests carried out in comfort and privacy may be necessary. The volume voided should be greater than 150 ml for the result to be meaningful.

TREATMENT

Urethral sphincter incompetence may be treated conservatively or surgically or by a combination of both. There have been few authoritative studies of the prophylaxis of urinary incontinence. The roles of episiotomy, a shortened second stage of labor, decline in parity, postnatal exercises, and preemptive hormone replacement therapy have yet to be objectively evaluated.

Conservative treatment

Conservative treatment is indicated when (1) mild stress incontinence owing to urethral sphincter incompetence exists; (2) the patient is medically unfit for or declines surgery; (3) further childbearing is contemplated; and (4) the patient has both detrusor instability and urinary sphincter incompetence. (In the last situation, if a trial of reasonable conservative treatment fails, surgery may be tried.)

The methods available are discussed in the relevant chapters: drug therapy in Chapter 35, electrical therapy in Chapter 36, pads and mechanical methods in Chapter 40, and physiotherapy in Chapter 41. The advantages of conservative therapy include minimum side effects (which cease when treatment ceases) and the avoidance of hospitalization.

Surgical treatment

The aim of surgery is to elevate the bladder neck within the abdominal zone of pressure so that there is positive transmission of any rise in intraabdominal pressure to the proximal urethra (Figure 16.8). Some operations produce an increase in outlet resistance, which may be disadvantageous if it causes voiding difficulties. Such an increase can be beneficial for patients with a reduced urethral closure pressure if continence rather than retention results.

Although more than 100 operations exist to correct stress incontinence resulting from urinary sphincter incompetence, most have not been fully evaluated or have not stood the test of time. They may be subdivided into vaginal and suprapubic operations depending on the route of access. Green (1962) suggested a schema based on the magnitude of the posterior urethrovesical angle and the inclination of the urethral axis as shown by the lateral standing/straining urethrocystogram. Patients with minor anatomical defects (type I) would be candidates for vaginal surgery (such as anterior colporrhaphy), and patients with major defects (type II) would be candidates for suprapubic surgery (such as the Marshall-Marchetti-Krantz operation). Unfortunately, the concept of the posterior urethrovesical angle as an aid to continence is no longer credible, since some women with an excellent posterior urethrovesicular angle are incontinent and

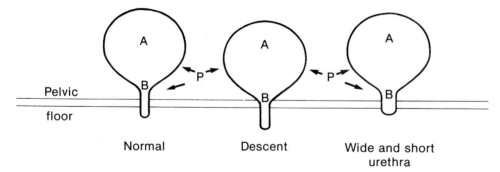

Figure 16.8 Effects of transmission of intraabdominal pressure. *Left,* Normally situated bladder neck above pelvic floor, with equal transmission of intraabdominal pressure to bladder and proximal urethra. This maintains positive pressure gradient between bladder and urethra and secures positive transmission to proximal urethra. *Center,* Bladder neck has descended to or beyond pelvic floor, so there is no transmission of intraabdominal pressure to proximal urethra, and positive pressure gradient is lost. *Right,* Bladder neck is elevated satisfactorily, but intraurethral pressure is equivalent to bladder pressure. Transmission of intraabdominal pressure to bladder and urethra is equal, but this will not raise urethral pressure above bladder pressure.

some women without this angle are dry. Green's excellent results are a tribute to his surgical expertise. The overall results of vaginal surgery are much less satisfactory (Table 16.2).

Hodgkinson (1970) has rightly stated that the first operation should be the most effective procedure, and other clinicians with a special interest in incontinence (Tanagho, 1976; Morgan and Farrow, 1977) support him, believing that the suprapubic approach leads to better and longer-lasting results than those provided by the vaginal operations. However, the anterior colporrhaphy, a vaginal operation, is quicker to perform, may cause less postoperative morbidity, and can correct genital prolapse at the same time.

Vaginal surgery

Anterior colporrhaphy. The anterior colporrhaphy has been in use for more than 100 years and is still perhaps the most commonly performed operation to correct urethral sphincter incompetence or genital prolapse.

With the patient in the lithotomy position, a vertical incision is made in the anterior vaginal wall, starting just below the external urethral meatus and extending down to the bladder base. The bladder and bladder neck are exposed, one or two Kelly bladder neck sutures are inserted, and the pubocervical fascia is coapted. Some clinicians place sutures in the tissue left on the bladder after reflecting the anterior vaginal wall flaps. I have found that this is usually only bladder muscle and that the plane of dissection has left the pubocervical fascia still attached to the vaginal flaps. The anterior vaginal wall is closed and any excess skin is excised.

The bladder is usually drained for 2 to 5 days. The main intraoperative complications, which are rare, are damaging the urethra during dissection and opening, but failing to identify, a urethral diverticulum. The main postoperative complications are recurrence of incontinence and a decreased mobility and capacity of the vagina as a result of paraurethral scarring. This renders subsequent surgery to correct incontinence more difficult to perform and more likely to fail. We found no increase in urgency, frequency, or voiding difficulties following this procedure (Stanton et al., 1982). The advantages of the colporrhaphy are its ability to correct coexistent cystourethrocele, the relative freedom from postoperative pain, and low morbidity.

Suprapubic surgery. Many suprapubic operations exist, and the appropriate choice is not easy to make. Figure 16.9 shows a schema to select the procedure, based partly on the degree of elevation of the bladder neck and partly on clinical assessment of the mobility of the vagina.

Nonsling procedures

MARSHALL-MARCHETTI-KRANTZ PROCEDURE. First described in 1949, the Marshall-Marchetti-Krantz operation has had widespread use and is frequently performed as a primary procedure. It does not correct coexistent cystourethrocele or increase outflow resistance on urethral pressure studies (Henriksson, 1977). Sjoberg (1981) found significant postoperative elevation of the urethral closure pressure but no change in peak flow rate or maximum voiding pressure during normal voiding. When voiding was accompanied by straining, the peak flow rate was reduced and the residual urine was increased.

In the original account, three No. 1 chromic catgut sutures were placed in the paraurethral tissues, taking a double bite to ensure a secure hold. A fourth suture was placed at the level of the bladder neck (Figure 16.10). The sutures were inserted into the periosteum of the pubis and also into the symphysial cartilage where feasible. When tied, the urethra and bladder neck were apposed to the symphysis and posterior aspect of the rectus muscles. Additional sutures were placed in the anterior wall of the bladder and the posterior aspect of the rectus muscle. Symmonds (1972) modified this by opening the bladder at the dome to facilitate dissection between the symphysis and the bladder and urethra and to inspect the internal urethral meatus. If the bladder neck was patent, the proximal urethra was opened and then plicated. In a greatly simplified version, Krantz (1980) suggested the use of

---

TABLE 16.2   Comparison of results of anterior colporrhaphy in the treatment of urethral sphincter incompetence

Investigators	Total cases	Failures (%)
Bailey (1954)	83	61.5
Jeffcoate (1967)	—	40
Low (1967)	74	54
Stanton and Cardozo (1979a)	25	64

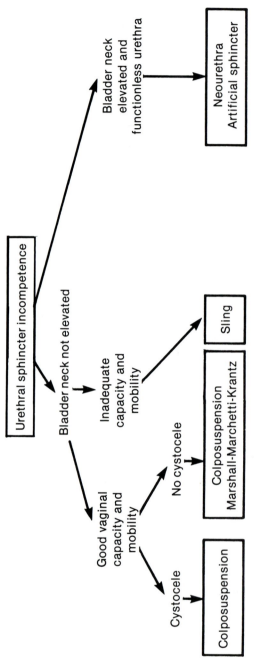

Figure 16.9 Schema for selection of suprapubic operation to correct urethral sphincter incompetence.

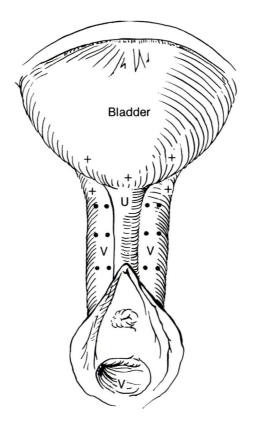

Figure 16.10 Position of sutures according to original description of Marshall-Marchetti-Krantz procedure.

just two sutures (Mersilene 2.0 braided), one on either side of the bladder neck and attached to the pubic periosteum (Figure 16.11).

The success rate of this operation as a primary procedure is about 95% (Green, 1978; Krantz, 1980). The most feared complication is osteitis pubis, which occurs in more than 5% of cases.

BURCH COLPOSUSPENSION. The Burch colposuspension involves suturing paravaginal fascia of the lateral vaginal fornices to the ipsilateral ileopectineal ligaments. In his original description, Burch noted that this procedure also corrects anterior vaginal wall prolapse. He did not state precisely the level of his sutures in the paravaginal fascia (Burch, 1961, 1968, 1978). There are several variations of this procedure. In the colpocystourethropexy of Tanagho (1976), two pairs of No. 1 Dexon sutures are inserted, the distal pair at the level of the midurethra and the proximal pair at the bladder neck. Both are attached to the ileopectineal ligament. Tanagho emphasized the need to place the sutures well lateral to the bladder neck and to avoid compressing the urethra against the symphysis pubis, which he maintained would compromise rather

than enhance the competence of the sphincter mechanism.

I use four pairs of No. 1 Dexon sutures to secure a more extensive elevation of the anterior vaginal wall (Figure 16.12) (Stanton and Cardozo, 1979; Hodgkinson and Stanton, 1980). The most distal (caudad) pair is inserted at the level of the bladder neck, and the second, third, and fourth are inserted more proximal (cephalad) alongside the bladder base. They are inserted into the ipsilateral iliopectineal ligament and tied, elevating the bladder neck and anterior vaginal wall (Figure 16.13). Any enterocele is corrected by a Moschowitz procedure. If uterine prolapse is present, this can be dealt with by carrying out an abdominal hysterectomy beforehand. Indeed, all forms of genital prolapse can be corrected abdominally with this technique, except a rectocele, which still requires a posterior repair. A Redivac drain is placed in the retropubic space, and a Bonanno suprapubic catheter drains the bladder. The Bonanno catheter is removed when the residual urine is less than 100 ml.

Intraoperative complications include ureter and

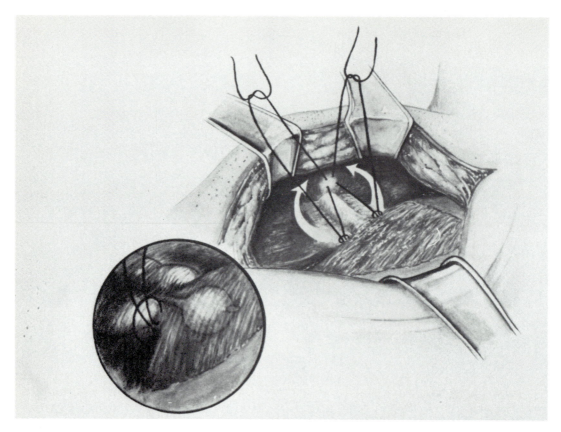

Figure 16.11 Marshall-Marchetti-Krantz procedure. Inset shows double bite of vaginal wall with 2.0 Mersilene suture. This is inserted into periosteum on posterior aspect of symphysis pubis. Suture is repeated on other side of bladder neck. (From Krantz, K. 1980. Marshall-Marchetti-Krantz procedure. In Stanton, S.L., and Tanagho, E.A., editors. Surgery of female incontinence. Heidelberg. Springer-Verlag.)

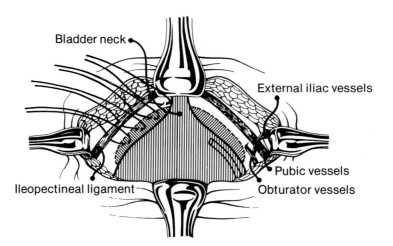

Figure 16.12 Modified colposuspension. Anatomy of retropubic dissection and placement of sutures between paravaginal fascia and ileopectineal ligaments. Oblique shading indicates where bladder has been dissected medially, off paravaginal fascia, to permit placement of sutures without injury to bladder and ureter.

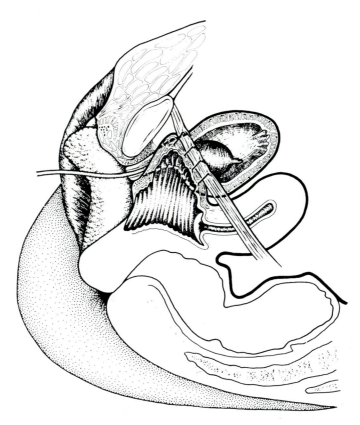

Figure 16.13 Modified colposuspension. Sagittal section showing elevation of bladder neck and anterior vaginal wall by approximation of paravaginal fascia to each ileopectineal ligament.

bladder trauma and venous hemorrhage. Postoperative complications include voiding difficulties, recurrence of incontinence, and detrusor instability (Cardozo, Stanton, and Williams, 1979).

Burch's results in performing colposuspension on 143 patients showed a subjective success rate of 93% (Burch, 1978). The follow-up monitoring in these cases ranged from less than 10 months to more than 5 years. Only 11 patients had an enterocele, an occurrence rate of 7.6%. Of our series of 440 patients operated on over 7 years, with preoperative and postoperative urodynamic assessment, 60 were available for follow-up evaluation 5 years after surgery. Objective assessment indicated an overall cure rate of 83% at 1 year and 72% at 5 years. Among patients without previous bladder neck surgery, the cure rate was 97% at 1 year and 79% at 5 years. With previous surgery, the cure rate after 1 year and 5 years was 71% and 65% respectively.

Sling procedures. Sling procedures are more complicated than nonsling procedures and are usually reserved for the treatment of recurrent stress incontinence. The bladder neck is elevated by passing a sling underneath it and attaching the sling to a higher point in the pelvis. Both organic and inorganic slings have been used.

ORGANIC SLINGS. The earliest description of an organic sling is that of Goebell (1910), who used the pyramidalis muscle as a sling. This was modified by Frangenheim (1914) who used the pyramidalis muscle attached to strips of overlying fascia. Stoeckel (1917) modified this even further by combining it with bladder neck plication, a procedure now known as the Goebell-Frangenheim-Stoeckel technique. The technique described by Aldridge in 1942 has remained a standard procedure. Through a vertical anterior vaginal wall incision, a plane of cleavage is created on either side of the urethra and bladder neck, upward and behind the symphysis pubica. The urethra and bladder neck are imbricated by mattress sutures. Through a Pfannensteil incision, two strips of rectus sheath fascia (6 cm and 1.5 cm) are prepared from either side of the midline, with the point of attachment at the midline. The strips are passed through each rectus mus-

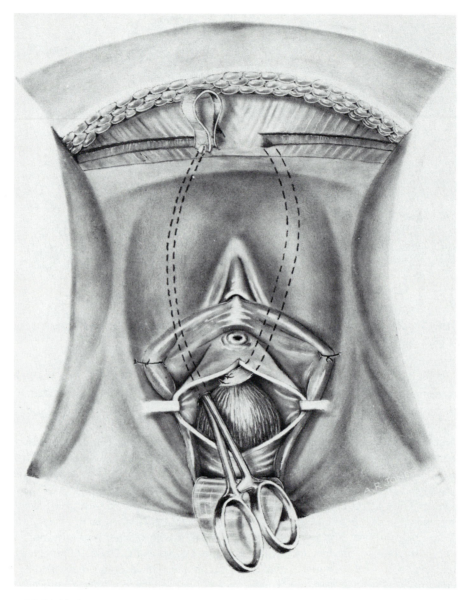

Figure 16.14 Aldridge sling procedure. Two strips of rectus sheath fascia are guided downward retropubically into vaginal incision and sutured together below bladder neck. (From Aldridge, A. 1942. Am. J. Obstet. Gynecol. **44:**398-411.)

cle, down alongside the bladder neck to the vaginal dissection, where they are united beneath the bladder neck with sufficient tension to elevate it slightly (Figure 16.14).

Studdiford (1944) modified this procedure by using a continuous fascial strip and reuniting this to the rectus fascia after passing it underneath the bladder neck. To avoid using vaginal incision (with the risk of carrying infection into the retropubic space), Millin and Read (1948) positioned a rectus sheath strip employing only a transverse suprapubic incision. The tunnel under the bladder neck was created by blind dissection, which has the obvious risk of urethral and bladder trauma. Other variations were described by Michon (1943), Delinotte (1956), and Narik and Palmrich (1962). The use of lyophilized dura was reported by Havlicek (1972). Heterologous tissues have included ox fascia and porcine skin.

The advantage of using organic tissue is the minimum adverse reaction in the host. The disadvantages include lack of consistent tensile strength and sometimes difficulty in obtaining suitable rectus sheath (or fascia lata substitute). These problems led to a trial of inorganic materials.

INORGANIC SLINGS. The inorganic slings have been made of nylon (Bracht, 1956) and polyethylene (Mersilene)(Moir, 1968), which are relatively inelastic. Polypropylene (Marlex) was used by Morgan (1970) and Morgan and Farrow (1977). Both Moir and Morgan favor a combined vaginal and suprapubic access and anchor a narrow sling (approximately 2 cm wide) to the bladder neck. Although this approach has the risk of vaginal contamination and infection, which is serious when using inorganic material, it minimizes the risk of trauma to the urethra and bladder, permits accurate positioning of the sling, and affords good hemostasis. Moir and Morgan agree that the tension should be just enough to elevate the bladder neck; the correct tension is difficult to estimate and to convey to other clinicians because of its subjective nature and the total absence of objective measurements.

The main disadvantage of all the inorganic materials mentioned so far is the fibrous reaction they cause around the urethra and bladder neck, despite being theoretically inert. Because of scar tissue, further surgery to release the sling (if causing voiding difficulties or retention) or to replace it if stress incontinence continues is technically difficult.

To overcome these disadvantages, Stanton and Brindley (1982) devised a Silastic sling by bonding 0.5 mm (0.02 inch) medical-grade Silastic to 0.17 mm (0.007 inch) Dacron-reinforced Silastic, with small tantalum markers at regular intervals for postoperative radiological screening (Figure 16.15). The sling measures 20×1 cm and can be shaped according to need. It can be extended approximately 1% and has a breaking force of 7.2 kg. Because it does not react with the surrounding tissues, it must be securely fixed to the ileopectineal ligaments with unabsorbable sutures such as polybutylate-coated polyester (Ethibond). Ten days after surgery the sling is freely mobile and can be easily tightened or loosened if necessary. Within 3 months a fibrous sheath forms around the sling. Although the sling is mobile within the sheath, it can easily be replaced. The sheath must be gently broken down to secure full mobility of the proximal urethra and bladder neck.

In 1973 Stamey described a modification of Pereyra's procedure (1959), in which the bladder neck is elevated by a nylon suture passed from the suprapubic region to the vagina under both direct and endoscopic vision. The anterior vaginal wall is incised to display the bladder neck. Bilateral suprapubic incisions are made, and a nylon suture is introduced on a special Stamey needle alongside the bladder neck to the vaginal incision. A 1 cm sleeve of 5 mm Dacron is inserted in the nylon loop, and the nylon is returned to the suprapubic region by a second insertion of the needle. This is repeated on the other side, leaving a threaded Dacron sleeve on either side of the bladder neck (Figure 16.16). The vaginal incision is closed, and the nylon sutures are tied to the rectus sheath, elevating the bladder neck. The suprapubic incisions are then closed. By endoscope viewing during the operation, the surgeon confirms that the sutures have not entered the bladder and are positioned correctly at the bladder neck. The advantages of this procedure are its simplicity and speed. The disadvantages are trauma by the needle to the bladder and urethra and risk of infection from endoscopy with an open vaginal wound and foreign body material in situ. Stamey (1980) reported a 91% rate of cure of incontinence, with minimum postoperative pain and infection.

MECHANISM OF ACTION. Henrikssen and Ulmsten (1978), using a twin microtip transducer catheter to evaluate the effects of sling procedures, found an increase in maximum urethral closure pressure during coughing and a positive closure pressure in

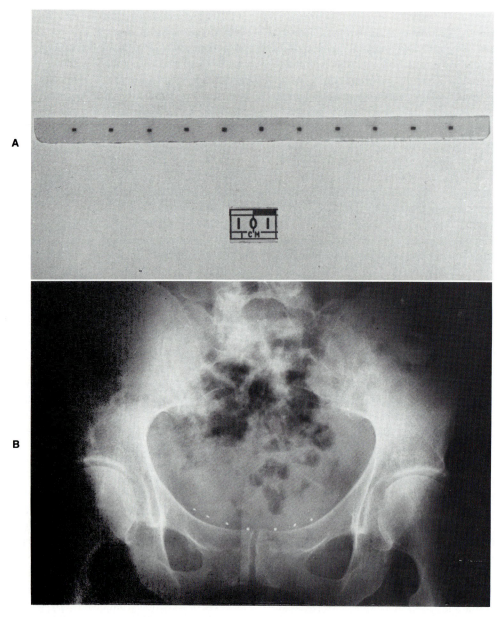

Figure 16.15 A, Sling measuring 20 cm × 1 cm made of medical grade Dacron-reinforced Silastic. **B,** Pelvic radiograph showing sling in situ attached to both ileopectineal ligaments. Tantalum markers are shown at 1 cm intervals. (**A** from Stanton, S.L., and Brindley, G. 1982. A Silastic sling for urinary incontinence. Proceedings of the twelfth annual meeting of the International Continence Society. Leiden.)

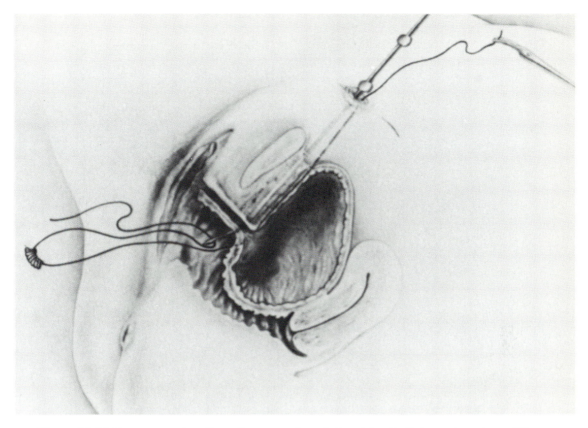

Figure 16.16 Stamey procedure. Second passage of needle 1 cm lateral to first, carrying nylon and Dacron sleeve. (From Stanton, S.L., and Tanagho, E.A., editors. Surgery of female incontinence. Heidelberg. Springer-Verlag.)

the proximal urethra. Hilton (1981), using a similar technique, found the functional length of the urethra and the maximum urethral closure pressure during coughing to be increased, with positive transmission in the proximal three fourths of the functional urethral length. The peak flow rate was significantly reduced, and the maximum voiding pressure was unchanged. Outlet obstruction was thought unlikely to be related to cure because some successful cases showed no postoperative reduction in flow rate and some failed cases showed a significant reduction.

RESULTS. Overall results are difficult to assess because few series have been validated by objective findings. In series employing organic slings, Jeffcoate (1956) and McLaren (1968) reported 86% and 87% cure rates, respectively; the rate in the latter series declined to 71% after 16 years. Beck et al. (1974), using fascia lata, achieved a 76% cure rate at 2 years by objective assessment.

In series using inorganic slings, Moir (1968) achieved an 83% cure or improvement rate, and

Morgan and Farrow (1977) showed a 93% cure rate. Both studies were subjective. Using the Morgan procedure, I found an objective improvement rate of 77% in a group of 31 women.

The main intraoperative complication is trauma to the bladder and urethra during dissection to free the bladder neck and bladder from scar tissue resulting from previous surgery. Postoperatively, the most troublesome problem is delayed voiding and later voiding difficulties. Beck (1978) states that this is so common that he has included catheterization in routine postoperative care. The average time for his patients to require catheterization has been 24 days. In our series of 31 patients with a Marlex sling, 7 to 46 days were required until spontaneous voiding without a suprapubic catheter, with an average of 17 days. Other postoperative complications include sling erosion into the urethra and exposure into the vagina, urinary tract infection if there is persistent residual urine, and occurrence of detrusor instability.

Zacharin operation. The Zacharin operation is

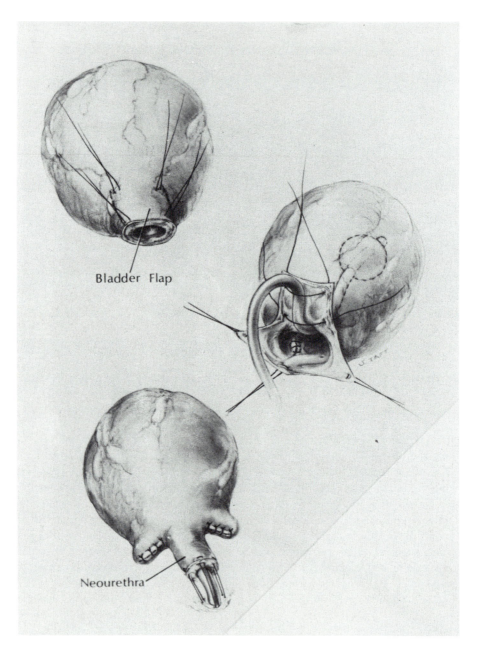

Figure 16.17 Neourethra. A 2.5 cm flap is raised from anterior bladder wall and formed into tube around catheter. Bladder neck is then reconstructed and either anastomosed to residual segment of urethra or brought out independently into vulva, just above vaginal opening. (From Tanagho, E.A. 1980. Neo-urethra: rationale, surgical techniques and indications. In Stanton, S.L., and Tanagho, E.A., editors. Surgery of female incontinence Heidelberg. Springer-Verlag.)

unusual in that is uses the posterior pubourethral ligaments to elevate the bladder neck (Zacharin and Gleadell, 1963). A synchronous combined technique through a Pfannenstiel incision and an inverted Y incision on the anterior vaginal wall exposes the posterior pubourethral ligaments. Rectus fascial strips are passed through each ligament at the point of its paraurethral attachment, and each is sutured to the paraurethral tissue. A 5-year subjective cure rate of 72% was achieved (Zacharin, 1977).

Neourethra. Construction of a new urethra was devised by Tanagho (1976) for use in congenital absence of the urethra and when the urethra is functionless because of scarring and fibrosis resulting from repeated bladder neck surgery for incontinence. Transection of the urethrovesical junction is followed by tubularization of a strip of anterior bladder wall. This is attached to the distal portion of the urethra to produce a new urethral outlet (Figure 16.17) (Tanagho, 1980). Construction of a urethra is a major procedure and is reserved for a small

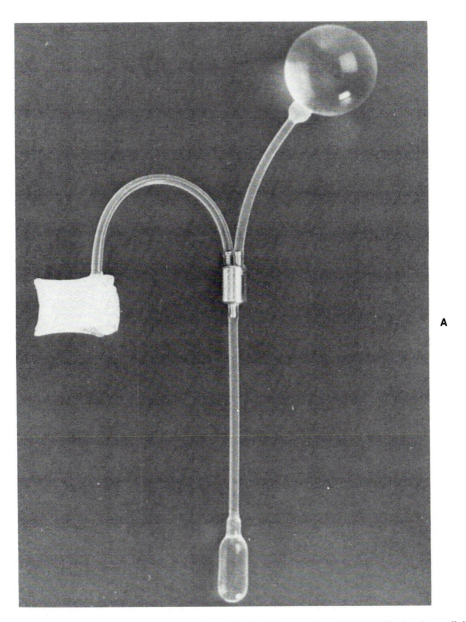

A

Figure 16.18 A, Artificial urinary sphincter (American Medical Systems, Inc., Model 792), showing cuff, fluid resistor, pressure-regulating balloon, and pump.   *Continued.*

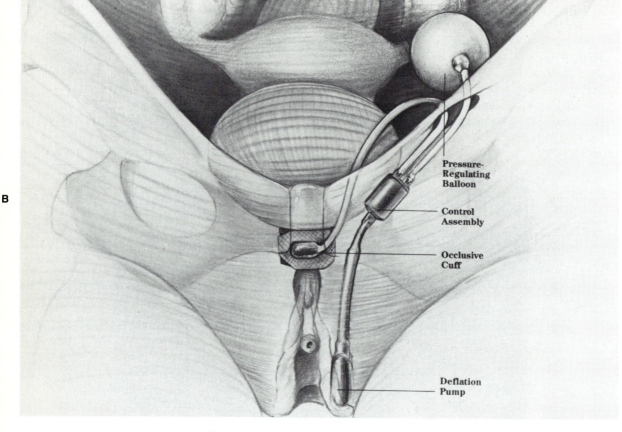

B

Pressure-Regulating Balloon

Control Assembly

Occlusive Cuff

Deflation Pump

Figure 16.18, cont'd. B, Sphincter in place.

group of patients who, as a result of recurrent surgery or epispadias, have no functional urethral resistance. To date, I have carried out this procedure in seven patients, five of whom have had an improvement in continence control.

Artificial sphincter. One of the boldest and most imaginative techniques of biomedical engineering has been the construction of a practical artificial urinary sphincter by Scott, Bradley, and Timm (1973). It may be used for adults and children of both sexes and is suitable for incontinence caused by urethral sphincter incompetence, epispadias, and low-pressure detrusor hyperreflexia. The currently available model (American Medical systems, Inc., Model 792) is made partly of medical-grade Silastic and consists of a pressure-regulating balloon (placed in the prevesical space), a fluid resistor (placed subcutaneously), a deflating pump (placed in the labium majus), and an inflatable cuff (inserted around the bladder neck) (Figure 16.18). It is available in several sizes according to the di-

ameter of the bladder neck. Complications include urethral and bladder neck erosion, mechanical failures, and infection. Erosion can be minimized by ensuring that the cuff pressure does not exceed 50 cm H_2O and by employing a delayed activation technique, especially when vascularization of the bladder neck is in doubt. The sphincter is implanted, but the circuit is not connected and the cuff is left in the deflate mode for 2 months. If no erosion has occurred, the circuit is then connected in a second, minor operation. Scott et al. (1981) achieved a 90% cure rate for postoperative stress incontinence in a group of 21 male and female patients.

Urinary diversion. Although the attainment of continence is not lifesaving, it is socially and hygienically desirable. Diversion should be considered for any women who has resistant incontinence and requests such a procedure, provided she is medically fit and aware of the need to be dry. Ileal loop ureterocolic anastomosis and continent vesicostomy are standard but major procedures, and careful patient selection is necessary. It is beneficial for the patient to meet a successfully treated patient before surgery to discuss day-to-day living with a diversion.

CONCLUSION

There are many factors in the causation of urethral sphincter incompetence, and each must be considered in the treatment of this disorder. Of the many treatment options, surgery usually offers the most effective long-term cure. There is a role for conservative therapy in the management of mild cases of incontinence, both as an interim measure and as an adjunct to surgery.

REFERENCES

Aldridge, A. 1942. Transplantation of fascia for relief of urinary stress incontinence. Am. J. Obstet. gynecol. **44**:398-411.

Bailey, K.V. 1954. A clinical investigation into uterine prolapse with stress incontinence: treatment by modified Manchester colporrhaphy. I. J. Obstet. Gynaecol. Br. Emp. **69**:291-301.

Bates, C.P., Loose, H., and Stanton, S.L. 1973. The objective study of incontinence after repair operation. Surg. Gynecol. Obstet. **136**:17-22.

Bates, P., et al. 1976. Standardisation of terminology of lower urinary tract function. Br. J. Urol. **48**:39-42.

Beck, R.P. 1978. The sling operation. In Buchsbaum, H.J., and Schmidt, J.D., editors. Gynecologic and obstetric urology. Philadelphia. W.B. Saunders Co.

Beck, R.P., et al. 1974. Recurrent urinary stress incontinence treated by the fascia lata sling procedure. Am. J. Obstet. Gynecol. **120**:613-621.

Bracht, E. 1956. Eine besondere Form der Zügelplastik. Geburtshilfe Frauenheilkd. **16**:782-790.

Burch, J. 1961. Urethrovaginal fixation to Cooper's ligament for correction of stress incontinence, cystocele and prolapse. Am. J. Obstet. gynecol. **81**:281-290.

Burch, J. 1968. Cooper's ligament urethrovesical suspension for stress incontinence. Am. J. Obstet. Gynecol. **100**:764-772.

Burch, J. 1978. Personal communication.

Cardozo, L., and Stanton, S.L. 1980. Genuine stress incontinence and detrusor instability: a review of 200 patients. Br. J. Obstet. Gynaecol. **87**:184-190.

Cardozo, L., Stanton, S.L., and Williams, J.E. 1979. Detrusor instability following surgery for genuine stress incontinence. Br. J. Urol. **51**:204-207.

Delinotte, P. 1956. Incontinence d'urine orthostatique chez la femme, suspension, simplifiée du col vésical par voie vaginale. Urologie **3**:327-354.

Enhörning, G. 1961. Simultaneous recording of the intravesical and intra-urethral pressures. Acta Chir. Scand. Suppl. **276**:1-68.

Francis, W.J. 1960. The onset of stress incontinence. J. Obstet. Gynaecol. Br. Emp. **67**:899-903.

Frangenheim, P. 1914. Zur operativen Behandlung der Inkontinenz der mannlichen Harnrohre. Verh. Dtsch. Ges. Chir. **43**:149-154.

Goebell, R. 1910. Zur operativen Beseitigung der Angeborenen Incontinentia Vesicae. Z. Gynäkol. Urol. **2**:187-191.

Green, T. 1962. Development of a plan for the diagnosis and treatment of urinary stress incontinence. Am. J. Obstet. Gynecol. **83**:632-648.

Green, T. 1978. Urinary stress incontinence: pathophysiology, diagnosis and classification. In Buchsbaum, H.J., and Schmidt, J.D., editors: urology. Philadelphia. W.B. Saunders Co.

Havlicek, S. 1972. Schlingenoperationen mit Lyoduraband bei rezidivierender Harninkontinenz der Frau. Geburtshilfe Frauenheilkd. **32**:757.

Henriksson, L. 1977. Studies on urinary stress incontinence in women. Thesis. Mälmo.

Henriksson, L., and Ulmsten, U. 1978. A urodynamic evaluation of the effects of abdominal urethrocystopexy and vaginal sling urethroplasty in women with stress incontinence. Am. J. Obstet. Gynecol. **131**:77-82.

Hilton, P. 1981. Urethral pressure measurement by microtransducer: observations on methodology, the pathophysiology of genuine stress incontinence and the effects of its treatment in the female. MD thesis. University of Newcastle-upon-Tyne.

Hodgkinson, C.P. 1970. Stress urinary incontinence. Am. J. Obstet. Gunecol. **108**:1141-1168.

Hodgkinson, C.P., and Stanton, S.L. 1980. Surgery of female incontinence. Heidelberg. Springer-Verlag.

Holland, E. 1928. Cited in Jeffcoate, T.N. 1967. Principles of gynaecology. ed. 3. London. Butterworth & Co.

Jarvis, G., et al. 1980. An assessment of urodynamic examination in incontinent women. Br. J. Obstet. Gynaecol. **87**:893-896.

Jeffcoate, T.N. 1956. The results of the Aldridge sling operation for stress incontinence. J. Obstet. gynaecol. Br. Emp. **63**:36-39.

Jeffcoate, T.N. 1957. Principles of gynaecology. ed. 3. London. Butterworth & Co.

Krantz, K. 1980. Marshall-Marchetti-Krantz procedure. In Stanton, S.L., and Tanagho, E.A., editors. Surgery of female incontinence. Heidelberg. Springer-Verlag.

Low, J. 1967. Management of anatomic urinary incontinence by vaginal repair. Am. J. Obstet. Gynecol. **97**:308-315.

Marshall, V., Marchetti, A., and Krantz, K. 1949. The correction of stress incontinence by simple vesico-urethral suspension. Surg. Gynecol. Obstet. **44**:509-518.

McLaren, H.C. 1968. Late results for sling operation. Br. J. Obstet. Gynecol. **75**:10-13.

Michon, L. 1943. Traitment de l'incontinence d'une de la femme par suspension aponévrotique du col vésical. Mem. Acad. Chir. **69**:121-126.

Millin, T., and Read, C. 1948. Stress incontinence of urine in the female. Postgrad. Med. J. **24**:51-56.

Moir, J.C. 1968. The gauze hammock operation. Br. J. Obstet. Gynaecol. **75**:1-9.

Morgan, J.E. 1970. A sling operation, using Marlex polypropylene mesh for treatment of recurrent stress incontinence. Am. J. Obstet. Gynecol. **106**:369-377.

Morgan, J.E., and Farrow, G.A. 1977. Recurrent stress urinary incontinence in the female. Br. J. Urol. **49**:37-42.

Narik, G., and Palmrich, A. 1962. A simplified sling operation suitable for routine use. Am. J. Obstet. Gynecol. **84**:400-405.

Nemir, A., and Middleton, R. 1954. Stress incontinence in nulliparous women, Am. J. Obstet. Gynecol. **68**:1166-1168.

Pereyra, A.J. 1959. A simplified procedure for the correction of stress incontinence in women. West. J. Surg. Obstet. Gynecol. **67**:223-226.

Scott, F.B., Bradley, W.E., and Timm, G.W. 1973. Treatment of urinary incontinence by implantable prosthetic sphincter. Urology **1**:252-259.

Scott, F.B., et al. 1981. Current results with the AMS artificial sphincter. Proceedings of eleventh annual meeting of the International Continence Society. Lund.

Sjoberg, B. 1981. Hydrodynamics of micturition in stress-incontinent women following surgical correction. Thesis. Stockholm.

Stamey, T. 1973. Endoscopic suspension of the vesical neck for urinary incontinence. Surg. Gynecol. Obstet. **136**: 547-554.

Stamey, T. 1980. Endoscopic suspension of the vesical neck. In Stanton, S.L., and Tanagho, E.A., editors. In Surgery of female incontinence. Heidelberg. Springer-Verlag.

Stanton, S.L., and Brindley, G. 1982. A Silastic sling for urinary incontinence. Proceedings of the twelfth annual meeting of the International Continence Society. Leiden.

Stanton, S.L., and Cardozo, L. 1979a. A comparison of vaginal and suprapubic surgery in the correction of incontinence due to urethral sphincter incompetence. Br. J. Urol. **51**:497-499.

Stanton, S.L., and Cardozo, L. 1979b. Results of colposuspension for incontinence and prolapse. Br. J. Obstet. Gynaecol. **86**:693-697.

Stanton, S.L., Cardozo, L., and Riddle, P.R. 1981. Urological complications of traumatic diastasis of the symphysis pubis in the female. Br. J. Urol. **53**:453-454.

Stanton, S.L., Kerr-Wilson, R., and Harris, V.G. 1980. Incidence of urological symptoms in normal pregnancy. Br. J. Obstet. Gynaecol. **87**:897-900.

Stanton, S.L., Ozsoy, C., and Hilton, P. 1983. Voiding difficulty in the female: prevalence, clinical and urodynamic review. Obstet. Gynecol. **61**:164-167.

Stanton, S.L., and Ritchie, D. 1977. Urilos: a practical method of detecting urine loss. Am. J. Obstet. Gynecol. **128**: 461-463.

Stanton, S.L., et al. 1982. Clinical and urodynamic effects of anterior colporrhaphy and vaginal hysterectomy for prolapse with and without incontinence. Br. J. Obstet. Gynaecol. **89**:459.

Stoeckel, W. 1917. Uber die verwendung der Musculi Pyramidalis bei der operativen Behandlung der Incontinentia urinae. Zentralbl. Gynaekol. **41**:11-19.

Studdiford, W.E. 1944. Transplantation of abdominal fascia for relief of urinary stress incontinence. Am. J. Obstet. Gynecol. **47**:764-775.

Sutherst, J., Brown, M., and Shawer, M. 1981. Assessing severity of urinary incontinence in women by weighing perineal pads. Lancet. **1**:1128-1130.

Symmonds, R.E. 1972. Suprapubic approach to anterior vaginal relaxation and urinary stress incontinence. Clin. Obstet. Gynecol. **15**:1107-1121.

Tanagho, E.A. 1976a. Colpocystourethropexy: the way we do it. J. Urol. **116**:751-753.

Tanagho, E.A. 1976b. Urethrosphincteric reconstruction for congenitally absent urethra. J. Urol. **116**:237-242.

Tanagho, E.A. 1980. Neo-urethra: rationale, surgical techniques and indications. In Stanton, S.L., and Tanagho, E.A. Surgery of female incontinence. Heidelberg. Springer-Verlag.

Thomas, T., et al. 1980. Prevalence of urinary incontinence. Br. Med. J. **281**:1243-1245.

Wolin, L. 1969. Stress incontinence in young, healthy, nulliparous female subjects. J. Urol. **101**:545-549.

Zacharin, R.F. 1977. Abdominoperineal urethral suspension. Obstet. Gynecol. **50**:1-8.

Zacharin, R.F., and Gleadell, L.W. 1963. Abdominoperineal urethral suspension. Am. J. Obstet. Gynecol. **86**:981-994.

chapter 17

Detrusor instability

LINDA CARDOZO

A hundred years ago when Mosso and Pellacani first described the use of cystometry, they showed that the introduction of additional fluid volumes into the bladder did not result in an increase in bladder pressure. Fifty years later raised bladder pressure was reported in association with certain neurological disorders (Rose, 1931; Langworthy, Kolb, and Dees, 1936), but it was not until 1963 that the clinical significance of increased detrusor activity was realized when Hodgkinson, Ayers, and Drukker demonstrated urinary incontinence as a result of uninhibited detrusor contractions in 64 women without neurological disability.

DEFINITION

The term *unstable bladder* was introduced by Bates, Whiteside, and Turner-Warwick (1970), who defined it as an "objectively measured loss of ability to inhibit detrusor contractions even when it is provoked to contract by filling, change of position, coughing, etc." It is therefore a cystometric finding and cannot be diagnosed clinically. Other terms are used to describe this condition including

dyssynergic detrusor dysfunction (Hodgkinson, Ayers, and Drukker, 1963), uninhibited detrusor dysfunction (Torrens and Griffiths, 1974), and hyperreflexic detrusor dysfunction (Bradley and Timm, 1976), but detrusor instability is the most widely used and acknowledged name; hyperreflexia is now used to describe an unstable bladder of neuropathic etiology (International Continence Society, 1980).

INCIDENCE

Detrusor instability is the second most common cause of urinary incontinence in women during their reproductive years, and among elderly women it is the most common cause. The reported incidence varies considerably, but about 20% of all patients investigated for voiding disorders (Cardozo, 1979) and somewhere between 30% and 50% of cases investigated for incontinence are found to have detrusor instability (Moolgaoker et al., 1972; Torrens and Griffiths, 1974). In a personal series of 800 patients seen for urodynamic investigation, 36.5% of those who were incontinent had detrusor instability. The incidence of detrusor instability following surgery for incontinence is even higher and has been assessed at about 70% (Bates, Whiteside, and Turner-Warwick, 1970; Arnold et al., 1973). This is partly due to failure to diagnose instability before surgery.

ETIOLOGY

Detrusor instability may be caused by an upper motor neuron lesion affecting the bladder, such as multiple sclerosis. In men it may be caused by outflow obstruction and has been shown to be reversed by relief of the obstruction (Turner-Warwick et al., 1973). In women outflow obstruction is rare, and opinion as to whether or not it can produce an unstable bladder is divided. In a study of 92 women an 18.5% incidence of detrusor instability was discovered following a colposuspension operation for genuine stress incontinence (Cardozo, Stanton, and Williams, 1979). This was not a temporary phenomenon and may have been caused by the extensive dissection around the bladder neck that this operation involves. Detrusor instability following surgery for genuine stress incontinence has also been described by Jarvis (1981).

In most cases the cause of detrusor instability remains unknown, and these patients are referred to as having "idiopathic," "primary," or "non-neuropathic" detrusor instability. It may be that this type of detrusor instability is a variant of normal rather than an abnormality, and it has been suggested that up to 10% of the population may have relatively asymptomatic unstable bladders (Turner-Warwick, 1978). In elderly asymptomatic men two small studies have shown that the incidence of detrusor instability is as high as 50% and that it increases with age (Abrams, 1977; Anderson et al., 1978); however, there is no comparable study in women. Recently more and more evidence has been pointing to a psychosomatic cause for "idiopathic" detrusor instability because of its variable nature and the way it responds to psychotherapy.

PRESENTATION

Detrusor instability usually is seen with a combination of symptoms of varying severity. Patients may complain of frequency (voiding more than seven times during the day), nocturia (voiding twice or more at night), urgency, urge incontinence, stress incontinence, and nocturnal enuresis. In a study by Cardozo and Stanton (1980) of 100 women with detrusor instability the most common symptoms were urgency (80%) and diurnal frequency (79%), but these are very common symptoms among patients with any form of incontinence. Nocturnal frequency was present in 69% and enuresis in 27% of the cases. Stress incontinence was the only presenting symptom in 5% of the cases.

Farrar et al. (1975) found that patients complaining solely of frequency, recurrent urinary tract infections, or stress incontinence rarely demonstrated detrusor instability; whereas symptoms of urge incontinence and nocturia were closely associated with an unstable bladder. Whiteside and Arnold (1975) found that 50% of patients with childhood enuresis and 75% of patients with current enuresis had unstable bladders.

Clinical examination is not helpful in detrusor instability, since there are no distinctive physical signs. Stress incontinence may be demonstrated, but this will not help with diagnosis. A higher incidence of detrusor instability has been found in patients complaining of prolapse together with incontinence than among those without prolapse, but the instability was not cured by repairing the prolapse (Arnold et al., 1973). In cases where detrusor instability is caused by an upper motor neuron lesion, other neurological stigmata may be demonstrable on clinical examination. It is therefore worth examining the cranial nerves and S2 to S4 outflow in cases of detrusor instability of sudden onset, strange symptomatology, or where there is a history of other neurological symptoms.

DIAGNOSIS

The diagnosis of detrusor instability is made by subtracted cystometry or videocystourethrography with pressure and flow studies when detrusor contractions or a detrusor pressure rise greater than 15 cm H_2O occurs during bladder filling or on the provocative tests of coughing, passive posture change, catheter withdrawal, or coughing when standing erect (Turner-Warwick, 1975). Simple cystometry, which measures only the intravesical pressure, may be inconclusive in cases of detrusor instability, since increases in pressure may reflect changes in intraabdominal pressure rather than abnormal detrusor activity.

Usually a sense of urgency is associated with detrusor contractions, and if the intravesical pressure exceeds the urethral pressure during a detrusor contraction, the symptom of urge incontinence will be experienced. However, a few patients are unaware of their detrusor contractions and complain of stress incontinence that is the result of a detrusor contraction produced by coughing or some similar activity (Bates, Loose, and Stanton, 1973). Patients who complain of frequency of micturition do not always have a small bladder capacity; they sometimes allow large volumes of fluid to be introduced into their bladders at cystometry. This may reflect their drinking habits and cause polyuria, in which case a fluid balance chart is helpful in diagnosis.

Enuretic patients with detrusor instability often have no other symptoms and rarely leak on cystometry despite very high detrusor pressures. While awake they are able to remain continent because of the voluntary element of control, but this is lost when they are asleep, allowing the intravesical pressure to exceed the urethral pressure causing incontinence. Turner-Warwick and Whiteside (1976) feel that the reason that the patient does not wake to void is nonurological.

The cystometric pattern in detrusor instability may take three forms (Cardozo, Stanton, and Williams, 1979). Most commonly there are systolic detrusor contractions during bladder filling—type A (Figure 17.1), or the detrusor pressure may rise when the patient stands up—type B (Figure 17.2), or there may be a steep detrusor pressure rise during bladder filling—type C (Figure 17.3). The latter

shows noncompliance of the detrusor. This is not always considered to represent detrusor instability, but since the symptoms are the same as is the response to treatment, I feel it warrants inclusion as detrusor instability. It is possible that the shape of the cystometrogram alters with the duration of detrusor instability, but there is no published data on this aspect. A typical cystometrogram trace detrusor instability is shown in Figure 17.4, *A*. An example of noncompliant detrusor instability is shown in Figure 17.4, *B*.

Many patients with unstable bladders have coarse trabeculation that may be a finding at cystoscopy or may be noted when the bladder is radiologically screened during videocystourethrography or micturition cystography. Figure 17.5 shows typical coarse trabeculation in a patient with long-standing detrusor instability.

TREATMENT

Since the recognition of "urge incontinence" as a separate condition, many different forms of treatment have been tried with varying degrees of success. Conventional bladder neck surgery, as performed in genuine stress incontinence, gives poor results in detrusor instability unless there is concomitant urethral sphincter weakness, in which case stress incontinence may be improved but the symptoms of urgency, urge incontinence, and frequency of micturition are likely to remain unaltered

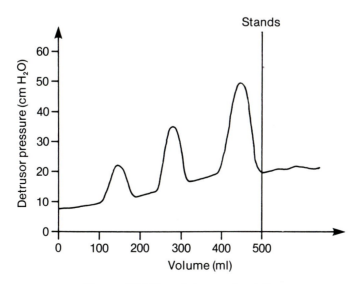

Figure 17.1 Type A detrusor instability.

Pressure rise on standing > 15 cm H₂O
without detrusor contractions

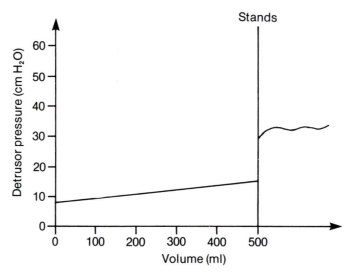

Figure 17.2 Type B detrusor instability

Pressure rise during filling > 15 cm H₂O without
detrusor contractions or pressure rise on standing

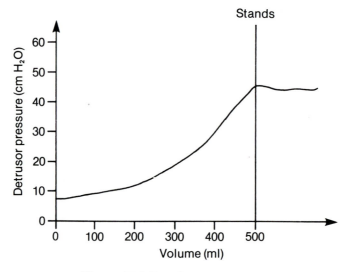

Figure 17.3 Type C detrusor instability.

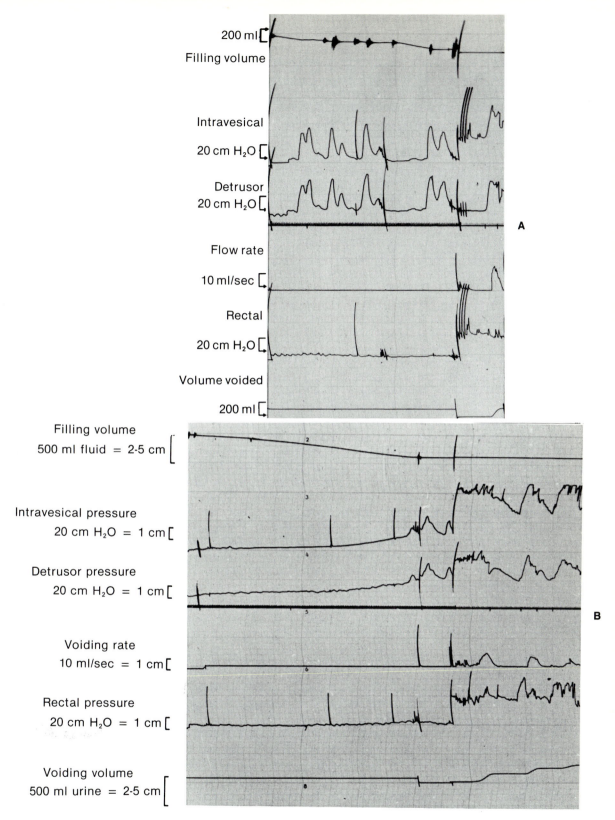

Figure 17.4 A, Cystometrogram trace from patient with detrusor instability showing detrusor contractions to 50 cm H_2O; only approximately 100 ml of fluid has filled the bladder. There is no detrusor pressure rise when standing or coughing. **B,** Cystometrogram trace from patient with noncompliant detrusor instability. Note gradual detrusor pressure rise during bladder filling followed by uninhibited detrusor contractions at end of bladder filling and further rise in detrusor pressure when patient passively stood up.

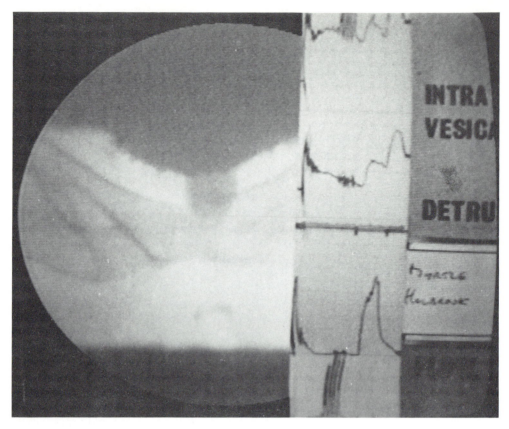

Figure 17.5 Videorecording of patient with severe detrusor instability. She has been asked to inhibit voiding. Note high rise in detrusor pressure after she has tried to stop voiding and inability to milkback urine from proximal urethra into bladder. There is marked coarse trabeculation.

(Stanton et al., 1978). This underlines the importance of an accurate diagnosis in all cases of urinary incontinence before treatment is undertaken, especially in patients who complain of multiple symptoms or in whom previous incontinence surgery has failed.

Vaginal denervation

The earliest surgical treatment reported for ''urge incontinence'' was bilateral resection of the inferior hypogastric plexus through the vagina. Ingelman-Sundberg (1959) treated 34 women by this method after first assessing the likely outcome by performing unilateral and then bilateral nerve blocks of the inferior hypogastric plexus. If this abolished abnormal detrusor activity on the cystometrogram and there was less than 150 ml residual urine, denervation was performed. Out of 34 patients 30 (88%) were initially cured or improved, but later symptoms recurred in 5 (15%) patients. This was thought to be due to the regrowth of

nerves. Although this operation does not have the high cure rates once hoped for and despite its complications (loss of bladder sensation and high residual urine), it has recently been used for patients with severe detrusor instability in whom drugs have failed (Warrell, 1977; Hodgkinson and Drukker, 1977). Ingelman-Sundberg (1978) now performs partial denervation on patients with urgency of micturition in association with reduced bladder capacity as well as those with detrusor instability.

Cystocystoplasty

In severe cases of detrusor instability cystocystoplasty has been performed. The bladder is denervated by supratrigonal transection with division of all inferior lateral communications, including the inferior vesical vessels, so that the bladder is attached only by the peritoneum and superior vesical vessels. The supratrigonal bladder is then resutured to the bladder base. Good subjective results have been reported (Turner-Warwick and Handley-Asken, 1966; Essenhigh and Yeates, 1973). However if too much of the bladder is resected, it will lose its sensation, and if not enough is cut, it will continue to contract uninhibitedly. Cecocystoplasty has also been tried, but the results are not good in cases of detrusor instability (Pengelly et al., 1981).

Sacral neurectomy

Selective sacral neurectomy has only been used in a small number of patients. Its likelihood of success can be assessed by preoperative bilateral selective nerve root blocks of S2 to S4. Uninhibited detrusor contractions are most commonly abolished by blocking S3 (Torrens, 1974). Torrens and Griffiths (1974) performed sacral neurectomy on nine patients and reported two who were cured, five who improved, and two who remained the same. The only side effect reported was large residual urine. Sacral neurectomy has not been widely used, but Clarke, Forster, and Thomas (1979) reported on nine patients, seven of whom were improved although six regressed later. They concluded that selective sacral neurectomy was a valuable procedure in a highly selected group of patients with neuropathic bladder dysfunction.

Cystodistension

Cystodistension was introduced as a method of treatment for carcinoma of the bladder (Helmstein, 1966). It was first used in the management of detrusor instability in Oxford from where the best results have been reported. Ramsden et al. (1976) reported on its use in 51 patients: 16 patients were cured, 25 improved, and 10 failed. Of the 13 redistensions following relapse, only 2 were cured and 6 were improved. Long-term results of the Oxford cystodistensions (Higson et al., 1978) showed that the beneficial effects of treatment lasted for about a year in 50% of patients treated. A more recent study has shown that although some patients obtained symptomatic relief, there were no objective conversions from unstable to stable cystometrograms (Pengelly et al., 1978). Since cystodistension is attended by a 5% risk of bladder rupture (Higson, Smith, and Whelan, 1978), it is possible that the side effects outweigh the usefulness. The technique used by Pengelly et al. (1978) was identical to that used in Oxford and the method of patient selection was the same, so it is interesting that the results were so different. This suggests that successful treatment of detrusor instability may be partially dependent on the personality and enthu-

siasm of the operator rather than the actual method of treatment.

Drug therapy

Drugs are currently the most popular type of treatment for detrusor instability. Many different preparations have been tried with variable results. At best, the drugs used currently produce temporary symptomatic relief, but when treatment is stopped, the symptoms recur. This may, however, be all that is required, since for many patients detrusor instability is a disorder characterized by spontaneous exacerbations and remissions. Therefore occasional courses of tablets prescribed when symptoms are most severe may relieve the problem until the condition improves. Although most of the drugs prescribed are not without side effects, this type of treatment is basically safe and is definitely economical in terms of time and cost, since treatment can be given on an outpatient basis.

Many different types of drugs have been tried, including ganglion blockers, anticholinergic preparations, musculotropic agents, β-adrenergic stimulants, prostaglandin synthetase inhibitors, and calcium antagonists (Table 17.1).

Traditionally emepronium bromide (Cetiprin), a ganglion blocker, and flavoxate hydrochloride (Urispas), a musculotropic agent, have been the two most widely used preparations. Stanton (1973) compared their efficacy in a double-blind trial and found that they both produced symptomatic relief, but only flavoxate hydrochloride was statistically significant. In a more recent study (Cardozo and Stanton, 1980a) neither drug given in standard therapeutic doses produced symptomatic relief in more than 30% of patients. Flavoxate hydrochloride has not been shown to produce objective improvement when administered parenterally, whereas emepronium bromide does effectively abolish detrusor contractions when given intramuscularly (Cardozo and Stanton, 1979). However, emepronium bromide is poorly absorbed when given orally (Ritch et al., 1977), and doses large enough to affect the bladder sometimes produce severe side effects of dry mouth, blurred vision, and impaired voiding.

Propantheline (Pro-Banthine) is a parasympathetic depressant that has a cholinergic blocking action at both ganglionic and end-organ receptors. It has potent antimuscarinic activity and is particularly effective in reducing urinary frequency. The dosage is 15 mg t.d.s. orally, which should be

TABLE 17.1 Drugs reducing detrusor activity

Type of drug	Example of drug	Dosage
Ganglionic blocker	Emepronium bromide	200 mg q.d.s.
Postganglionic blocker	Propantheline	15-30 mg t.d.s.
Anticholinergic agent	Oxybutynin chloride	5 mg t.d.s.
	Imipramine	25-20 mg t.d.s.
Musculotrophic agent	Flavoxate hydrochloride	200 mg q.d.s.
β-Adrenergic stimulant	Orciprenaline sulfate	20 mg q.d.s.
Prostaglandin synthetase inhibitor	Flurbiprofen	50-100 mg t.d.s.
Calcium antagonist	Terodiline	25 mg b.d.
Polysynaptic inhibitor	γ-Aminobutyric acid	5-20 mg t.d.s.

increased until side effects occur such as dry mouth or blurred vision; the dosage may then be reduced if necessary.

Imipramine, a tricyclic antidepressant, has long been used for children suffering from nocturnal enuresis. Although its exact mode of action is uncertain, it does produce parasympatholytic activity and acts centrally as an antidepressant. About 50% of adult patients with detrusor instability found that imipramine produced some symptomatic relief (Cardozo and Stanton, 1980a). It is particularly helpful in the management of nocturia and incontinence during coitus or at orgasm.

Prostaglandins are released during nervous stimulation of the bladder and have been shown to increase detrusor activity (Abrams and Feneley, 1976). Two prostaglandin synthetase inhibitors—indomethacin and flurbiprofen—have been tried in the treatment of detrusor instability. Both produced symptomatic improvement in frequency of micturition and flurbiprofen showed an increase in bladder volume at first detrusor contraction but side effects, particularly gastrointestinal, were common (Cardozo and Stanton, 1980b; Cardozo et al., 1980).

Calcium antagonists have been studied, and in a double-blind crossover trial on 12 patients terodiline (Bicor) (12.5 mg b.d.) was found to produce subjective and objective improvement in 11 patients without any reported side effects (Ekman et al., 1980). The same drug has been shown to abolish carbachol-induced contractions in an in vitro study on isolated human bladder preparations (Rud et al., 1980). So far calcium antagonists have only been used on a small number of patients, but if the initial findings are confirmed, these drugs should prove useful, especially in the management of patients with neuropathic detrusor instability.

Bladder retraining

Jeffcoate and Francis (1966) first described "bladder discipline" as a method of treatment for urgency incontinence. They admitted their 246 patients to the hospital, performed urethral dilatation, prescribed anticholinergic drugs, and instructed them to void by the clock and not according to desire, increasing the time intervals between voiding over a period of 2 to 3 weeks. After 1 year, 67% of their patients were cured and 22% were improved using this type of treatment. They pointed out the need to distinguish between stress and urge incontinence before treatment.

In 1970 Frewen suggested that idiopathic urge incontinence might be psychosomatic in origin. He found that the onset of symptoms usually dated back to a "trigger factor" that could be discovered by taking a careful history. Using bladder drill with supportive psychotherapy, Frewen (1972) achieved an 80% cure rate. His work was criticized because of its lack of objective evidence of detrusor instability before treatment and urodynamic changes produced by bladder drill. In 1978 he published a study in which cystometry was performed before and after treatment and demonstrated a cure or marked improvement in 82.5% of the patients studied (Frewen 1978). This method of treatment required up to 10 days in the hospital, and patients also received anticholinergic drugs during their hospital stay. However, Jarvis and Millar (1980) carried out a controlled trial of bladder drill in 30

TABLE 17.2   Results of biofeedback treatment for detrusor instability

	No. of patients	
	Subjective	**Objective**
Cured	11 (37%)	12 (40%)
Improved	13 (43%)	6 (20%)
Failed	6 (20%)	12 (40%)

patients with idiopathic detrusor instability and achieved a 90% cure rate with a mean hospital stay of 6 days without the use of drugs. Jarvis has also performed a randomized trial comparing bladder drill to a combination of drugs commonly used in the treatment of detrusor instability, and bladder drill proved to be a far more effective treatment (Jarvis, 1981b).

Biofeedback has also been tried as a method of treatment for idiopathic detrusor instability. This is a form of reeducation in which the patient receives information about a normally unconscious body process in the form of an auditory, visual, or tactile signal. The objective effects of biofeedback can be recorded on a polygraph trace, but subjective changes may be difficult to separate from the placebo effect.

In the original study (Cardozo et al., 1978a) biofeedback was performed during four to eight 1-hour sessions during which the patient's detrusor pressure was measured cystometrically and converted into auditory and visual signals from which the patient could appreciate changes in her detrusor pressure. The efficacy of biofeedback was assessed both subjectively, by means of a urinary diary that the patient completed each week, and objectively by cystometry. Thirty women between 16 and 65 years of age (mean, 41 years) suffering from idiopathic detrusor instability were treated in two centers (Cardozo et al., 1978b). They were given an average of 5.4 sessions of treatment. The outcome of treatment is shown in Table 17.2.

The six patients who failed to improve both subjectively and objectively all had severe detrusor instability with detrusor contractions greater than 60 cm H_2O and cystometric capacities of less than 200 ml; they found it impossible to inhibit abnormal detrusor activity, and one of them was later found to have multiple sclerosis. Biofeedback helps by giving the patient a better understanding of the mechanism of bladder function and of her particular bladder abnormality, but it is time consuming and requires each patient to be reasonably intelligent and highly motivated. The overall improvement rate of 80% is the same as that which Frewen achieved with bladder drill, and biofeedback does not require hospital admission, although skilled personnel are required to perform the training.

All forms of bladder retraining are advantageous, because no patient is ever made worse and there are no unpleasant side effects. It is becoming increasingly apparent that mild to moderate idiopathic detrusor instability in most patients can be satisfactorily treated by reeducation of the bladder. However the problem that now remains is how to manage patients with neuropathic detrusor instability or severe idiopathic detrusor instability that does not respond to retraining. For some of these patients urinary diversion may be helpful and should always be considered as an alternative to long-term catheterization, which is often unsatisfactory in patients with an unstable bladder. This is because there may be uninhibited detrusor contractions even when the bladder is relatively empty, causing leakage of urine around the catheter.

For any incontinent patient the most degrading aspect is often the odor and staining of clothes, which can often be helped by good advise regarding incontinence pads and garments. Other general help should include advice regarding drinking habits. Patients who suffer from nocturia should be advised not to drink late in the day, and all patients with detrusor instability should make sure they do not drink excessive quantities.

CONCLUSION

Detrusor instability is a common condition affecting people of all age groups and characterized by multiple symptoms. It is not life-threatening but may cause much embarrassment and a very restricted life-style. In most cases the cause remains a mystery, although we now know that there is a psychosomatic element in idiopathic detrusor instability and that exactly similar clinical and urodynamic manifestations may be due to a neurological lesion. Our lack of understanding of the underlying pathological condition is reflected in the numerous methods of treatment that are currently used, none of which is wholly satisfactory. Conventional bladder neck surgery is not helpful in detrusor instability, which emphasizes the need for an accurate diagnosis before treatment in all cases of incontinence. Denervation procedures and urinary diversion are reserved for severe disease. Bladder retraining seems to be the best treatment for idiopathic detrusor instability, but that still leaves the difficult problem of patients with detrusor instability resulting from a neurological lesion who are at present given ineffective drug therapy.

REFERENCES

Abrams, P.H. 1977. The investigation of bladder outflow obstruction in the male. M.D. thesis. Bristol.

Abrams, P.H., and Feneley, R.C.L. 1976. The action of prostaglandins on the smooth muscle of the human urinary tract, in vitro. Br. J. Urol. **48:**909-915.

Anderson, J.T., et al. 1978. Bladder function in healthy elderly males. Scand. J. Urol. Nephrol. **12:**123-127.

Arnold, E.P., et al. 1973. Urodynamics of female incontinence: factors influencing the results of surgery. Am. J. Obstet. Gynecol. **117:**805-813.

Bates, C.P., Loose, H., and Stanton, S.L. 1973. The objective study of incontinence after repair operations. Surg. Gynecol. Obstet. **136:**17-22.

Bates, C.P., Whiteside, C.G., and Turner-Warwick, R.T. 1970. Synchronous cine/pressure/flow cystourethrography with special reference to stress and urge incontinence. Br. J. Urol. **42:**714-723.

Bradley, W.E., and Timm, G.W. 1976. Cystometry. IV. Interpretation. Urology **2:**231-235.

Cardozo, L.D. 1979. The investigation and treatment of detrusor instability in women. M.D. thesis. Liverpool.

Cardozo, L.D., and Stanton, S.L. 1979. An objective comparison of the effects of parenterally administered drugs in patients suffering from detrusor instability. J. Urol. **122:**58-59.

Cardozo, L.D., and Stanton, S.L. 1980a. Genuine stress incontinence and detrusor instability: a review of 200 cases. Br. J. Obstet. Gynaecol. **87:**184-190.

Cardozo, L.D., and Stanton, S.L. 1980b. A comparison between bromocriptine and indomethacin in the treatment of detrusor instability. J. Urol. **123:**399-401.

Cardozo, L.D., Stanton, S.L., and Williams, J.E. 1979. Detrusor instability following surgery for genuine stress incontinence. Br. J. Urol. **51:**204-207.

Cardozo, L.D., et al. 1978a. Biofeedback in the treatment of detrusor instability. Br. J. Urol. **50:**250-254.

Cardozo, L.D., et al. 1978b. Idiopathic bladder instability treated by biofeedback. Br. J. Urol. **50:**521-523.

Cardozo, L.D., et al. 1980. Evaluation of flurbiprofen in detrusor instability. Br. Med. J. **280:**281-282.

Clarke, S.J., Forster, D.M., and Thomas, D.G. 1979. Selective sacral neurectomy in the management of urinary incontinence due to detrusor instability. Br. J. Urol. **51:**510-514.

Ekman, G., et al. 1980. A double blind crossover study of the effects of terodiline in women with unstable bladder. Acta Pharmacol. Toxicol. **46:**39-43.

Essenhigh, D.W., and Yeates, W.K. 1973. Transection of the bladder with particular reference to enuresis. Br. J. Urol. **45:**299-305.

Farrar, D.J., et al. 1975. A urodynamic analysis of micturition symptoms in the female. Surg. Gynecol. Obstet. **141:**875-881.

Frewen, W.K. 1970. Urge and stress incontinence: fact and fiction. Br. J. Obstet. Gynaecol. **77:**932-934.

Frewen, W.K. 1972. Urgency incontinence: review of 100 cases. Br. J. Obstet. Gynaecol. **79:**77-79.

Frewen, W.K. 1978. An objective assessment of the unstable bladder of psychosomatic origin. Br. J. Urol. **50:**246-249.

Helmstein, K. 1966. Hydrostatic pressure therapy: a new approach to the treatment of carcinoma of the bladder. Opusc. Med. **9:**328-333.

Higson, R.H., Smith, J.C., and Whelan, P. 1978. Bladder rupture: an acceptable complication of distention therapy? Br. J. Urol. **50:**529-534.

Higson, R.H., et al. 1978. An analysis of first time prolonged bladder distension in 65 patients with idiopathic detrusor instability. Proceedings of eighth International Continence Society meeting, Manchester.

Hodgkinson, C.P., Ayers, M.A., and Drukker, B.H. 1963. Dyssynergic detrusor dysfunction in the apparently normal female. Am. J. Obstet. Gynecol. **87:**717-730.

Hodgkinson, C.P., and Drukker, B.H. 1977. Infravesical nerve resection for detrusor dyssynergia (the Ingleman-Sundberg operation). Acta Obstet. Gynecol. Scand. **56:**401-408.

Ingelman-Sundberg, A. 1959. Partial denervation of the bladder. Acta Obstet. Gynecol. Scand. **38:**487-502.

Ingleman-Sundberg, A. 1978. Partial bladder denervation for detrusor dyssynergia. Clin. Obstet. Gynecol. **21:**797-805.

International Continence Society. 1980. Fourth report on the standardization of terminology of lower urinary tract function. Int. J. Urol. **53:**333-335.

Jarvis, G.J. 1981a. Detrusor muscle instability: a complication of surgery? Am. J. Obstet. Gynecol. **139:**219.

Jarvis, G.J. 1981b. A controlled trial of bladder drill and drug therapy in the management of detrusor instability. Br. J. Urol. **53:**565-566.

Jarvis, G.T., and Millar, D.R. 1980. Controlled trial of bladder drill for detrusor instability. Br. Med. J. **281:**1322-1323.

Jeffcoate, T.N.A., and Francis, W.J.A. 1966. Urgency incontinence in the female. Am. J. Obstet. Gynecol. **94:**604-618.

Langworthy, D.R., Kolb, L.G., and Dees, J.E. 1936. Behaviour of the human bladder freed from cerebral control. J. Urol. **36:**577-597.

Moolgaoker, A.S., et al. 1972. The diagnosis and management of urinary incontinence in the female. Br. J. Obstet. Gynaecol. **79:**481-497.

Pengelly, A.W., et al. 1978. Results of prolonged bladder distension as treatment for detrusor instability. Br. J. Urol. **50:**243-245.

Pengelly, A.W., et al. 1981. Results of caecocystoplasty. Proceedings of the annual meeting of the British Association of Urological Surgeons, London.

Ramsden, P.D., et al. 1976. Distension therapy for the unstable bladder: later results including an assessment of repeat distensions. J. Urol. **48:**623-629.

Ritch, A.E.S., et al. 1977. A second look at emepronium bromide in urinary incontinence. Lancet **1:**504-506.

Rose, D.K. 1931. Clinical application of bladder physiology. J. Urol. **26:**91-105.

Rud, T., et al. 1980. Terodiline inhibition of human bladder contraction: effects in vitro and in women with unstable bladders. Acta Pharmacol. Toxicol. **46:**31-38.

Stanton, S.L. 1973. A comparison of emepronium bromide and flavoxate hydrochloride in the treatment of urinary incontinence. J. Urol. **110:**529-532.

Stanton, S.L., et al. 1978. Clinical and urodynamic features of failed incontinence surgery in the female. Obstet. Gynecol. **51:**515-520.

Torrens, M.J. 1974. The control of the hyperactive bladder by selective sacral neurectomy. M.D. thesis. Bristol.

Torrens, M.J., and Griffiths, H.B. 1974. The control of the uninhibited bladder by selective sacral neurectomy. Br. J. Urol. **46:**639-644.

Turner-Warwick, R.T. 1975. Some clinical aspects of detrusor dysfunction. J. Urol. **113:**539-544.

Turner-Warwick, R.T. 1978. Communication to the Eighth International Continence Society Meeting, Manchester.

Turner-Warwick, R.T., and Handley-Asken. 1967. The functional results of partial, subtotal and total cystoplasty with special reference to ureterocaecocystoplasty, selective sphincterotomy and cystocystoplasty. Br. J. Urol. **39:**3-12.

Turner-Warwick, R.T., and Whiteside, C.G. 1976. A urodynamic view of clinical urology. In Hendry, W.F. Recent advances in urology. London. Churchill Livingstone.

Turner-Warwick, R.T., et al. 1973. A urodynamic view of the clinical problems associated with bladder neck dysfunction and its treatment by endoscopic incision and trans-trigonal posterior prostatectomy. Br. J. Urol. **45:**44-59.

Warrell, D.W. 1977. Vaginal denervation of the bladder nerve supply. Urol. Int. **32:**114-116.

Whiteside, C.G., and Arnold, E.P. 1975. Persistent primary enuresis: a urodynamic assessment. Br. Med. J. **1:**364-367.

chapter 18

Neuropathic bladder

ROBERT J. KRANE and MIKE B. SIROKY

Neuropathic bladder is defined as urinary retention or incontinence as a result of detrusor or urethral dysfunction caused by a neurological lesion. This definition therefore excludes voiding disorders or bladder dysfunction resulting from psychogenic disturbances, structural abnormalities, and local causes such as carcinoma, inflammation, or radiation. Functionally the lower urinary tract is best considered a single unit composed of the detrusor muscle, the smooth muscle of the proximal urethra, and the periurethral striated muscle (external urethral sphincter). To enhance our understanding of how neurological diseases affect the function of this unit, a brief introduction to neuroanatomical and neurophysiological aspects of the lower urinary tract is appropriate (see also Chapter 2).

NEUROANATOMY

Motor innervation. The parasympathetic nerves supplying the detrusor muscle arise from the sacral spinal cord, segments S2 to S4. This portion of the spinal cord, also called the conus medullaris, is situated approximately at the junction of the T12 and L1 vertebral bodies. These nerves course along the rectum where they are known as the pelvic nerves and join the hypogastric nerve to form the perivesical plexus at the base of the bladder. These are preganglionic fibers that synapse with postganglionic fibers within the bladder wall.

The sympathetic nervous system also contributes to bladder innervation, originating in the spinal cord at segments T11 and L2. These preganglionic fibers travel through the sympathetic paravertebral ganglia and follow the course of the great vessels into the pelvis. The majority of these sympathetic preganglionic fibers synapse in the inferior mesenteric and hypogastric plexuses and terminate as postganglionic fibers in the bladder, particularly in the trigone. The hypogastric or presacral nerves are synonymous with the sympathetic nerve supply of the bladder.

Embryologically, the bladder can be separated into the trigone (mesoderm) and the detrusor muscle (endoderm). Neuroanatomically, however, the trigone and the detrusor muscle beneath it are indistinguishable in their patterns of autonomic innervation. Therefore for clinical purposes it is more appropriate to divide the bladder into base (trigone and underlying detrusor) and body (detrusor of bladder dome) (Raezer et al., 1973).

Although few histochemical studies of cholinergic innervation have been performed in humans, it seems clear that acetylcholinesterase (ACHE)-positive nerves are abundant in all parts of the bladder musculature in both sexes (Ek et al., 1977). In addition, a dense cholinergic innervation of the smooth muscle of the bladder neck and proximal urethra occurs in the female (Gosling, Dixon, and

Lendon, 1977). Adrenergic innervation is particularly dense in the bladder base and far less profuse in the bladder body. In all areas of the bladder the density of adrenergic innervation is less than that of the cholinergic nerves. The smooth muscle of the proximal urethra has a rich adrenergic innervation similar to that at the bladder base. However, in human studies contradictory results have been reported by various investigators regarding the density of adrenergic innervation of the trigone and proximal urethra.

Afferent innervation. At present no available specific histochemical technique can positively identify visceral afferent nerve terminals in normal tissue. It is clear, however, that afferent axons travel by way of both the pelvic and the hypogastric nerves from the bladder. Pelvic nerve afferents appear to have a greater density in the muscle layers and the submucosa and are evenly distributed to all areas of the bladder. In contrast, hypogastric

nerve afferents are more dense in the submucosa and more prominent in the bladder base than in the body. Of some importance is the fact that the afferent impulses related to relex contractions of the bladder travel in the pelvic nerves (DeGroat, 1975) and are initiated by stretch receptors in the detrusor (Iggo, 1955). On the other hand, pain and temperature impulses from the trigone travel by way of the hypogastric nerve.

Innervation of periurethral striated sphincter. Most of the striated muscles of the pelvic floor are innervated by branches of the pudendal nerve. However, it is not clear whether the periurethral striated muscle receives its entire innervation by this pathway. Gosling, Dixon, and Lendon have proposed that this muscle is innervated by somatic nerve fibers traveling with the pelvic autonomic nerves. (Chapter 1 provides further information.)

CENTRAL NERVOUS CONTROL OF MICTURITION

It has long been accepted that the conus medullaris contains a segmental micturition reflex center (Figure 18.1) facilitated and inhibited by higher centers. Thus the sacral center is considered capable of coordinating a well-sustained detrusor contraction with both striated and smooth muscle sphincter relaxation (Tanagho, 1981). However, clinical experience with spinal cord transection has failed to conform to this scheme (Siroky and Krane,

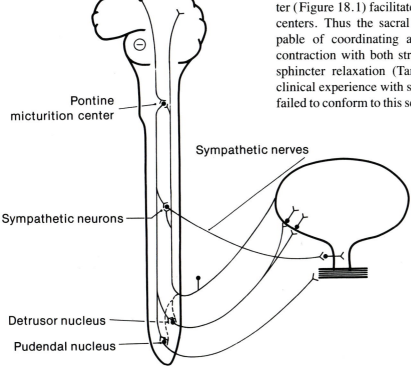

Figure 18.1 Schematic representation of long route reflex between lower urinary tract and pontine micturition center. Net effect on pontine micturition center by higher centers is inhibitory. At time of micturition vesical afferents ascend to pons and cerebrum, which results in voluntary release of cerebral inhibition and therefore allows micturition reflex to occur. Coordination of bladder contraction and sphincteric relaxation occurs at pontine level, although volitional (cerebral) relaxation also occurs in normal individual. (From Krane, R.J., and Siroky, M.B., editors. 1979. Clinical neuro-urology. Boston. Little, Brown & Co.)

1981). Suprasacral spinal injury (especially when complete) results in an isolated spinal cord that is capable of producing only poorly sustained detrusor contractions and, in most cases, uncoordinated sphincters (vesicosphincter dyssynergia)(Figure 18.2). In contrast, intracerebral lesions (cerebrovascular accident) may result in loss of voluntary (cerebral) control but do not disrupt vesicosphincter coordination (Figure 18.3). Thus the ''sacral reflex center,'' when removed from higher control, is not capable of controlling micturition in humans except in a rudimentary manner.

Barrington (1914) first emphasized the existence and importance of a pontine micturitional center. More recently the micturition reflex has been shown to have the characteristic latency of a long route reflex rather than a segmental one (DeGroat, 1975). In other words, the production of a bladder contraction by vesical distension is mediated through the spinal cord to the pontine micturition center rather than solely being a segmental reflex centered in the sacral cord.

The suprapontine central nervous system centers as a whole have a net inhibitory effect on micturition. Certain areas such as the posterior hypothalamus facilitate the micturition reflex. However, in the intact individual the net effect of the suprapontine centers is inhibitory. The concept of a pontine micturition center has practical clinical consequences. For example, in cases of complete suprasacral spinal cord transection the resultant interaction between the bladder and isolated cord differs significantly from the normal. Not only does the detrusor muscle lack inhibition by suprapontine centers, but it also appears to lack facilitation from the pontine micturition center and thus cannot sustain its contraction. As mentioned previously, the interaction of the bladder with the striated urethral sphincter is also affected. Normally, vesical contraction is associated with relaxation of the striated pelvic floor, which occurs before a bladder contraction. In cases of suprasacral cord transection, the bladder-sphincter coordination is greatly impaired, whereas in cases of suprapontine lesions, bladder sphincter coordination almost always remains normal. Thus it appears that coordination between the striated pelvic floor and detrusor muscle may take place in the area of the

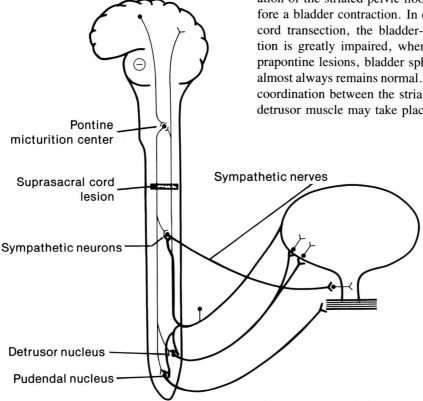

Pontine micturition center

Suprasacral cord lesion

Sympathetic nerves

Sympathetic neurons

Detrusor nucleus

Pudendal nucleus

Figure 18.2 Schematic representation of suprasacral cord lesion. Complete lesion through suprasacral cord will interrupt normal pathways between lower urinary tract and pontine micturitional center. With complete lesions this may result in loss of coordination between bladder and sphincters, producing syndrome of vesicosphincter dyssynergia. (From Krane, R.J., and Siroky, M.B., editors. 1979. Clinical neuro-urology. Boston. Little, Brown & Co.)

pons. Obviously there are exceptions to the dictum that complete transection of the suprasacral cord will lead to a dyssynergic state between the bladder and striated urethral sphincter, but these are rare. Furthermore, our experience has indicated the converse: that true vesicosphincter dyssynergia occurs only in cases of suprasacral cord lesions.

Neurological lesions above the pontine micturition center (for example, Parkinson's disease, cerebrovascular accident, brain tumor, and dementia) result in loss of inhibition of the pontine micturition reflex and therefore vesical hyperreflexia. However, the coordination between the bladder and the striated sphincter is preserved. Obviously, in certain poorly localized diseases of the central nervous system such as multiple sclerosis, wherein infrapontine and suprapontine plaques often coexist, a spectrum of abnormalities is related to the coordination of the bladder and sphincter (Goldstein et al., 1982).

NEUROUROLOGICAL EXAMINATION

History and physical examination. The patient with known or suspected neuropathic bladder should be assessed in a careful, systematic manner by using the history and physical and specialized urodynamic examinations. The interview should ascertain the patient's history of enuresis, urinary infection, urinary calculi, surgery, medications, bowel dysfunction, and dyspareunia. The patient's current urological symptoms should be elicited in detail.

The physical examination of the patient with neuropathic bladder should include analysis of the sacral reflexes and sensations subserved by the sacral segments. The bulbocavernosus reflex is usually tested in the female by digitally palpating a contraction of the anal sphincter. The reflex may be elicited through the vesical mucosa by tugging on an indwelling catheter (trigonal reflex). Likewise, this reflex pathway may be tested by cutaneous stimulation of the perianal skin, which will produce external anal sphincter contraction (anal wink). The spinal cord segments involved in these reflexes are primarily S2 to S4, but higher segments in the lumbar cord may be involved.

Sensory loss in the perineum or perianal area is associated with S2 to S4 dermatomes. Involvement of higher dermatomes such as S1 and S2 produces sensory loss in the lateral border of the foot, where-

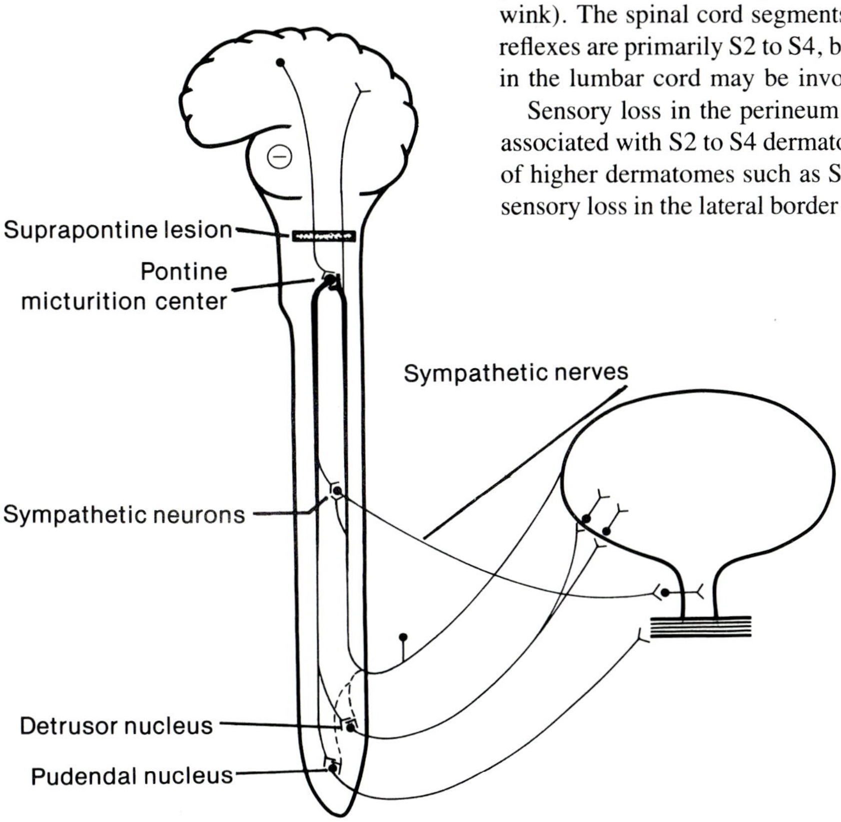

Figure 18.3 Schematic representation of suprapontine lesion, which will result in decreased inhibition from higher centers on pontine micturition center and therefore detrusor hyperreflexia. However, detrusor hyperreflexia will be accompanied by preservation of coordinated sphincteric activity. (From Krane, R.J., and Siroky, M.B., editors. 1979. Clinical neuro-urology, Boston. Little, Brown & Co.)

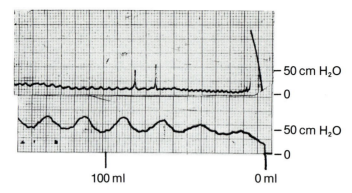

Figure 18.4 Bethanecol supersensitivity test (BST). Upper cystometrogram illustrates detrusor areflexia. At volume of 100 ml, intravesical pressure is 10 cm H_2O. Lower tracing was recorded approximately 15 minutes after 5 mg of bethanecol hydrochloride was injected subcutaneously. At 100 ml volume, intravesical pressure has risen to about 50 cm H_2O. This represents positive BST.

as L4 and L5 lesions produce a loss of sensation in the lateral aspect of the lower leg.

Finally, the examiner should evaluate deep tendon reflexes in the lower extremities, clonus, and plantar responses.

Cystometry. Urodynamic examination in neuropathic bladder rests heavily on combined cystometrography–sphincter electromyography. The cystometrogram consists of continuous monitoring of intravesical pressure during filling and contraction. The relative merits of various methods used in performing cystometry are beyond the scope of this discussion. However, assessment of denervation supersensitivity of the bladder has obvious importance in neuropathic disorders and deserves further comment.

When filling of the bladder fails to elicit a detrusor contraction, the possibility of neuropathic detrusor areflexia may be assessed by bethanecol chloride supersensitivity testing (BST)(Figure 18.4). This test is based on Cannon's law, which states that a denervated muscle develops supersensitivity to its natural neurotransmitter (Lapides et al., 1962). Thus, when significant bladder neuropathy exists, a supersensitive response to bethanecol would be confirmatory, but lack of such a response is not particularly meaningful.

In our laboratory, the test is performed by measuring intervesical pressure at a volume of 100 ml. Bethanecol chloride (5 mg for most patients; 2.5 mg for those with body weight below 40 kg) is injected subcutaneously. This drug must not be injected intradermally or intramuscularly. When the patient reports a flushed feeling and increased salivation, cystometry is repeated and intravesical pressure at a volume of 100 ml again measured. An increase of 15 cm H_2O pressure was suggested by Lapides et al., but we prefer 20 cm H_2O as the minimum pressure rise indicative of supersensitivity. Since it is impossible to predict absorption from the injection site, the test must be performed at the time of autonomic effect, which varies from as little as 7 minutes to as much as 25 minutes. Atropine should be available to reverse untoward effects such as bradycardia, bronchospasm, and gastrointestinal spasm. Such reactions are extremely rare.

In our experience, bethanecol supersensitivity was observed in 98% of 63 patients with neuropathic detrusor areflexia caused by cauda equina or peripheral neuropathy but in none of 15 control patients (Pavlakis, Siroky, and Krane, 1982). Based on these findings, diagnosis of bladder neuropathy should not be attempted without a positive bethanecol test as corroboration in most instances.

Electromyography. Assessment of perineal floor innervation and control is performed by electromyography. Depolarization of muscle membranes by neural activity results in characteristic electrical potentials that may be picked up by an appropriately placed surface or needle electrode in the pelvic floor. Needle electrodes produce the highest-quality electromyographic recordings because they are placed at the site of depolarization, that is, the muscle itself.

Two types of information are provided by electromyography. Characteristic changes in the number and type of potentials occur in neuropathies of diverse cause such as alcoholism, diabetes mellitus, and trauma (Blaivas et al., 1977; Dibenedetto and Yalla, 1979). The diagnosis of neuropathy requires the use of needle electrodes. Second, co-ordination between the detrusor and pelvic striated muscles during filling as well as during voiding can be assessed. A gross determination of whether the striated muscles contract during voiding can be done with surface electrodes. Perineal electromyography can only assess the activity of the particular muscle closest to the electrode. If the anal sphincter is being used, activity of the external urethral sphincter is assessed by inference. Perineal electromyography cannot determine smooth muscle sphincter activity.

CLASSIFICATION AND NOMENCLATURE

With newer modalities of urodynamic examination, classification schemes have changed to incorporate abnormalities of both the bladder and the sphincter. With few exceptions, previous classification schemes were based on detrusor dysfunction alone or the anatomical location of neurological lesions. Current classification schemes concern themselves with abnormal bladder states and concomitant sphincteric dysfunction.

With the use of cystometry two abnormal bladder states can be diagnosed. Vesical or detrusor hyperreflexia is characterized by involuntary detrusor contractions in excess of 15 cm H_2O that occur during bladder filling and cannot consciously be suppressed by the patient. The inability to inhibit is characterized by a short latency period between the urge to void and detrusor contraction. In many cases, the patient reports an urge to void only after the detrusor contraction is well under way. The sine qua non of detrusor hyperreflexia is that the patient cannot prevent the detrusor contraction, regardless of the volume at which it occurs, although it usually occurs at less than 200 ml. Detrusor areflexia is defined as the inability to elicit a detrusor reflex during cystometry despite the presence of sensory urge or discomfort. However, lack of detrusor contraction need not imply the presence of a neurological lesion, since a large number of normal individuals will have bladder areflexia during testing as a result of psychological inhibition. In addition, detrusor areflexia may be caused by chronic infravesical obstruction.

The status of the smooth and striated sphincters may be assessed by intraurethral pressure measurements, perineal electromyography, or combined techniques. Two abnormal sphincter states are recognized currently using sphincter electro-

myography: sphincter hyperactivity and sphincter neuropathy. Normally during bladder filling there is a gradual increase in the perineal muscle activity until the time of voiding (guarding reflex) (Figure 18.5). Before the bladder contraction, the electrical activity of the perineal floor decreases, producing what is called electrical silence (Figure 18.6). Normally the proximal smooth muscle of the urethra relaxes and funnels before a detrusor contraction. With sphincter hyperactivity there may be no decrease or an increase in electrical activity during voiding contractions. When this is associated with detrusor hyperreflexia, it is called *vesicosphincter dyssynergia* (Figure 18.7). When associated with vesical areflexia, vesicosphincter dyssynergia is more accurately called *nonrelaxing external sphincter* (Figure 18.8).

In contrast, sphincter neuropathy is characterized by abnormal potentials during sphincter electromyography that are indicative of partial or complete denervation. The characteristic changes evident with electromyography include fibrillation potentials, positive sharp waves, decreased interference pattern, and increased polyphasic potentials (Figure 18.9). These findings on sphincter electromyography almost always indicate a neurological lesion of the sacral cord, cauda equina, or peripheral nerves. Rarely there appears to be isolated nonrelaxation of the smooth muscle sphincter, which may be sufficient to cause outflow obstruction.

Thus a classification may be developed in which the vesical abnormalities are combined with the various possible sphincter abnormalities:

I. Detrusor hyperreflexia
   A. Sphincter coordination
   B. Vesicosphincter dyssynergia
   C. Smooth muscle sphincter dyssynergia
II. Detrusor areflexia
   A. Striated muscle sphincter
     1. Denervated
     2. Nonrelaxing
   B. Smooth muscle sphincter
     1. Nonrelaxing
   C. Coordinated sphincters

Each of the various categories will be described in terms of its clinical and urodynamic characteristics and appropriate treatment.

Detrusor hyperreflexia

Patients with detrusor hyperreflexia are troubled by frequency, urgency, and urgency incontinence.

Normal external sphincter EMG

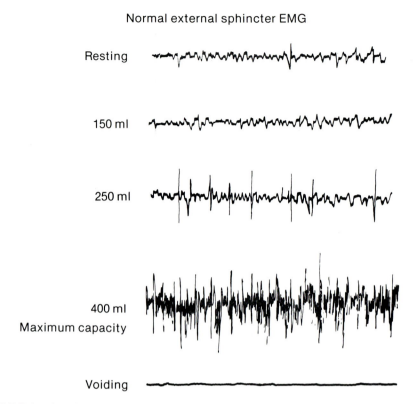

Resting

150 ml

250 ml

400 ml
Maximum capacity

Voiding

Figure 18.5 Striated sphincter electromyogram as seen on oscilloscope. With increasing intravesical volume there is increasing sphincteric electrical activity (guarding reflex). During voiding electrical silence occurs.

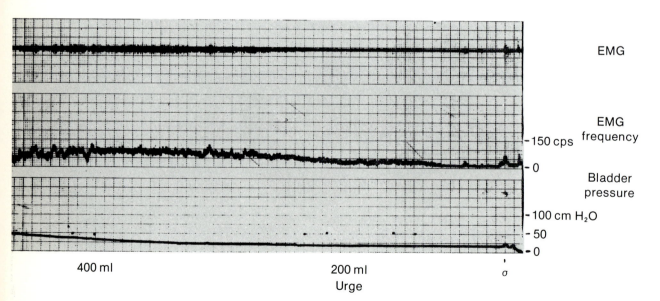

EMG

EMG frequency

-150 cps

-0

Bladder pressure

-100 cm H_2O

-50

-0

400 ml   200 ml   σ
                Urge

Figure 18.6 Combined cystometry and pelvic floor electromyography showing normal interaction between bladder and external sphincter. Immediately before voiding contraction, relaxation begins to occur in striated pelvic floor.

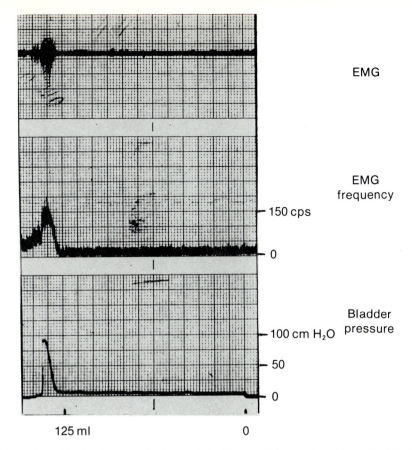

EMG

EMG
frequency

— 150 cps

— 0

Bladder
— 100 cm H₂O pressure

— 50

— 0

125 ml   0

Figure 18.7 Vesicosphincter dyssynergia demonstrated by combined cystometric and pelvic floor electro-myographic study. During uninhibited bladder contraction, which occurs at approximately 130 ml of intravesical volume, there is inappropriate firing of striated sphincter. Guarding, which is usually characteristic of patients with sphincter dyssynergia and complete spinal cord injury, is absent.

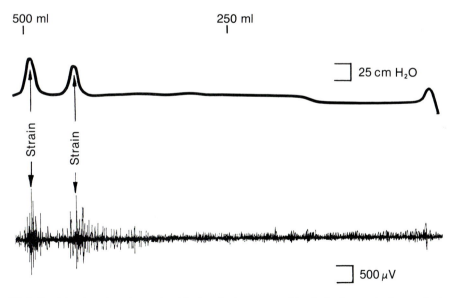

500 ml   250 ml

25 cm H₂O

Strain   Strain

500 µV

Figure 18.8 Combined cystometry and sphincter electromyographic study demonstrating vesical areflexia with nonrelaxation of external striated sphincter. These urodynamic findings may be seen with neurological disease as well as with functional problems.

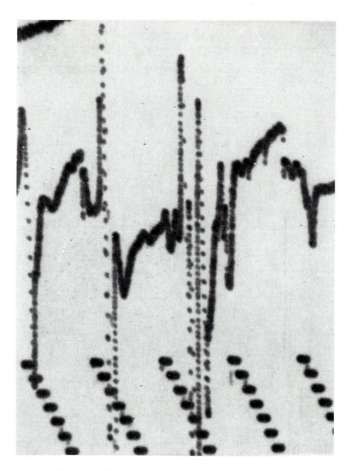

Figure 18.9 Electromyographic recording of polyphasic potentials associated with neuropathy. Potentials were recorded from pelvic striated muscles in patient with cauda equina syndrome. (Polyphasic potentials can be seen only on oscilloscopic recording.)

Obstructive symptoms such as hesitancy, weak stream, incomplete emptying, and straining to void may occur depending on the status of the outflow tract and sphincters. These symptoms may also be present in the absence of obstruction, simply because of constant urgency despite an empty bladder.

The differential diagnosis of detrusor hyperreflexia includes psychogenic frequency, cystitis of any origin, outflow obstruction (rare in females), and carcinoma in situ. Thus the diagnosis of neuropathic detrusor hyperreflexia requires evidence of an appropriate neurological lesion as well as exclusion of other possible causes. Detrusor hyperreflexia typically occurs in cerebrovascular disease, parkinsonism, and incomplete spinal cord transection. The status of the sphincters may be one of complete coordination, striated sphincter obstruction (vesicosphincter dyssynergia), or smooth muscle sphincter obstruction.

Sphincter coordination. A hyperreflexic detrusor with coordinated sphincters (Figure 18.10) occurs when the pontine micturition center is no longer under the control of higher centers. It may also occur when the pontine center is partially separated from the lower spinal cord by incomplete spinal transection. Neurological conditions most commonly associated with this finding are dementia, cerebrovascular disease, brain tumors, parkinsonism, multiple sclerosis, cervical myelopathy resulting from herniated intervertebral disk, and spondylosis.

Because of normal sphincter coordination, residual urine is minimum to absent. Endoscopy may show significant trabeculation. Radiological examination reveals normal upper tracts in most cases.

Vesicosphincter dyssynergia. Striated sphincter obstruction, or vesicosphincter dyssynergia, typically occurs in patients with complete supra-

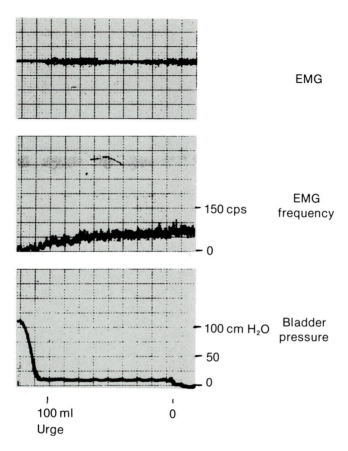

EMG

EMG frequency

— 150 cps

— 0

— 100 cm H₂O

Bladder pressure

— 50

— 0

100 ml   0

Urge

Figure 18.10 Combined cystometry and electromyographic study demonstrating detrusor hyperreflexia with appropriate relaxation of striated sphincter. As stated in text, this pattern of interaction is seen in patients with suprapontine lesions and incomplete suprasacral cord lesions.

sacral spinal cord transection. This pattern may result from traumatic injury, advanced multiple sclerosis, transverse myelitis, or vascular compromise of the spinal cord. Immediately after suprasacral spinal transection, during the period of *spinal shock,* reflexes below the level of injury are lost. Urodynamic findings are vesical areflexia and absence of bladder sensation. If untreated, these will produce overflow incontinence.

Over a period of 2 to 3 months (occasionally as long as 6 months) the deep tendon reflexes mediated by the isolated cord gradually return. During this recovery period, cystometry will likewise show the return of the detrusor reflex. In a small proportion (about 5%) of patients with suprasacral spinal transections, detrusor areflexia persists after recovery from spinal shock for reasons that are unclear.

The urodynamic findings of vesicosphincter dyssynergia are involuntary detrusor contractions ac-

companied by bursts of electrical activity in the external urethral sphincter (Figure 18.7). Clinically, patients with vesicosphincter dyssynergia have evidence of outflow obstruction including high residual ("paradoxical residual") urine volumes and occasionally bilateral hydronephrosis. Although sphincteric dyssynergia is a true obstructive phenomenon, these patients also suffer from detrusor contractions that are short-lived, uncoordinated, and therefore ineffective despite the generation of high intravesical pressures. This additional factor tends to tip the balance in favor of outflow obstruction. Over time, there is a relatively high incidence of upper urinary tract deterioration as a result of this combination of abnormalities including ureterovesical obstruction, vesicoureteral reflux, and stone formation.

Patients with combined vesical hyperreflexia and sphincter dyssynergia are particularly prone to *autonomic dysreflexia*. This syndrome occurs primarily in spinal lesions above T6 and is characterized by hypertension, flushing, headache, and reflex bradycardia as a result of bladder or bowel distension. In severe cases, cerebral hemorrhage may occur.

Smooth muscle sphincter dyssynergia. In a small percentage of spinal cord–injured patients, detrusor hyperreflexia may be associated with proximal sphincter obstruction. Most often this is associated with or may be a constituent of the syndrome of autonomic dysreflexia.

Treatment. Treatment in cases of detrusor hyperreflexia with coordinated sphincters is primarily medical. The objective of pharmacological therapy is to decrease hypercontractility of the detrusor muscle. Drugs that are useful in this regard may be divided into three categories: (1) pure anticholinergic agents such as propantheline, (2) anticholinergic and direct smooth muscle relaxants such as oxybutynin or dicyclomine, and (3) direct smooth muscle relaxants, such as flavoxate. Despite the large number of therapeutic agents, propantheline remains the preferred drug for several reasons: it has both muscarinic and nicotinic blocking activity and a wide range of dosage schedules. The proper dosage of propantheline must be individualized. Our practice is to begin at 60 mg divided into four doses a day and gradually increase the dose until the appropriate effect is achieved (that is, suppression of incontinence of patient reports of maximum side effects). The earliest side effect is dryness of the mouth, which is followed by constipation and finally visual changes. Occasionally a useful adjunct to propantheline is imipramine, which itself has anticholinergic activity and acts synergistically with propantheline to produce a more complete blockage of the bladder. The usual dosage of imipramine is 25 mg four times a day. This drug should be used with caution in patients with hypertension and cardiac arrhythmias because it may cause tachycardia.

Oxybutynin is a newer drug that has the theoretical advantage of combining anticholinergic activity and direct smooth muscle relaxation. It is unclear, however, whether it has a clinical advantage over propantheline at present. Intramuscular injection of propantheline in conjunction with cystometry can predict the effectiveness of the oral medication in the treatment of detrusor hyperreflexia. Flavoxate is the archetypal drug for direct smooth muscle inhibition and has been found to be useful in the treatment of detrusor hyperreflexia.

When medical therapy fails to abolish detrusor contractions and incontinence or irritative symptoms persist, treatment options include chronic catheterization (which is often limited by the persistence of leakage around the catheter), bladder denervation procedures such as sacral rhizotomy or phenol blocks of the sacral roots, and bladder augmentation procedures such as ileocystoplasty or cecocystoplasty. Further details of such treatments may be obtained by referring to textbooks of anesthesiology or neurosurgery. When no vesicoureteral reflux is present, a bladder augmentation procedure can be accomplished simply by augmenting bladder capacity with a piece of ileum (ileocystoplasty). In situations involving vesicoureteral reflux, bladder augmentation should proceed along the lines of an ileocecocystoplasty with an antireflex reimplantation technique.

The S3 nerve root is mainly concerned with bladder contractions; blocking this root may be an effective treatment for vesical hyperreflexia (Torrens, 1975; Rockswold and Bradley, 1977). Our practice is to selectively block the sacral nerve roots at the sacral foramina with a short-acting anesthetic such as xylocaine in conjunction with cystometric analysis before and after injection. When the nerve root or roots required to control hyperreflexia are ascertained by this means, a more permanent block with phenol or alcohol or surgical division of the root may be accomplished. Sacral rhizotomy should be considered particularly in spinal cord–injured patients with detrusor hyperreflexia that is not amenable to treatment by other means. In one series a complete bilateral resection of the anterior and posterior roots of S2 to S4 in 28 patients resulted in areflexia of the bladder in 25 with adequate capacity, and 23 were able to empty their bladders without use of a catheter (Misak et al., 1962).

Detrusor hyperreflexia may also be suppressed by electrical stimulation of the perineal skeletal muscles. In this method the sacral reflex arc is apparently activated by intrarectal or intravaginal electrical stimulation. This results in contraction of the external urinary sphincter mediated by the pudendal nerve and also suppression of bladder contractions by a possible reflex mechanism (Godec, Cass, and Ayala, 1975; Teague and Merrill, 1977).

The treatment of choice for vesicosphincter dyssynergia in the female patient, when possible, is conversion of the hyperreflexic bladder into an areflexic bladder by pharmacological or neurosurgical means with self-intermittent catheterization or Credé's maneuver. In this situation the dyssynergic external sphincter may be used as a continence mechanism, allowing for the success of intermittent self-catheterization. This option is not realistic in the quadriplegic patient. If this treatment is unsuccessful, few options remain aside from chronic indwelling catheters or supravesical diversion. This is in great contrast to the situation in male patients, in whom treatment of the external sphincter obstruction by sphincterotomy is usually successful and condom catheter drainage can be instituted.

In cases of less complete spinal cord transection in which some control of the bladder remains, treatment of the obstructing external sphincter component by medical means may be successful. Available pharmacological agents include dantrolene sodium, baclofen, and diazepam. Dantrolene acts at a level of the skeletal muscle itself (sarcoplasmic reticulum) to inhibit the release of calcium. The mechanism of action of baclofen is unknown, although it was originally thought to decrease γ-efferent activity in the spastic spinal cord. Diazepam is thought to relieve spasticity by preferentially blocking polysynaptic pathways in the spinal cord. In our experience, pharmacological therapy with any of these agents is relatively unsuccessful. In cases of smooth muscle sphincter obstruction and detrusor hyperreflexia, the preferred treatment is a combination of anticholinergic and α-adrenergic blocking agents (phenoxybenzamine).

Detrusor areflexia

Detrusor areflexia is lack of detrusor contraction resulting from a neurological lesion, usually one of the conus medullaris, cauda equina, or peripheral nerves. However, neurological lesions higher in the central nervous system, for example, those which result in bladder paralysis during spinal shock, may be causative. The patient more often has overflow incontinence than obstruction symptoms, since the urge to void is lost. The stream is weak, and the patient voids by suprapubic pressure or abdominal straining.

In the differential diagnosis, neuropathic detrusor areflexia must be distinguished from nonneuropathic causes, primarily functional urinary retention, as well as anatomical causes such as urethral prolapse, a ureterocele prolapsing through the urethra, and urethral carcinoma. Among neurological causes, early multiple sclerosis and herpes genitalis are especially significant, since they occur in the younger female and may easily be mistaken for hysterical urinary retention.

Examination will reveal absent or decreased cu-taneous sensation in the perineum and/or lower extremities and diminished bulbocavernosus reflex, anal sphincter tone, and deep tendon reflexes. Radiography may show a vertebral fracture, spina bifida, or congenital absence of the sacrum (best seen on lateral view). Sacral agenesis is associated with lower limb malformations in almost 50% of cases (Koff and Deridder, 1977).

Striated muscle sphincter. Evidence of affected innervation of the striated sphincter may be obtained by sphincter electromyography. In a recent study of 63 patients with cauda equina or peripheral neuropathy and neuropathic detrusor areflexia (Pavlakis, Siroky, and Krane, 1982), about 67% of patients exhibited neuropathic changes on perineal electromyography. However, such changes do not necessarily imply that the external sphincter becomes incapable of contraction, since the neuropathy may be minor in degree.

In fact, the most common situation is one in which the external sphincter remains active during attempts at voiding by Credé's maneuver of abdominal straining and constitute an obstructive factor. This situation occasionally has been misnamed vesicosphincter dyssynergia. We prefer the term *nonrelaxation of the striated sphincter.*

Smooth muscle sphincter obstruction. Although a rare occurrence, detrusor areflexia may be associated with isolated proximal sphincteric obstruction (Abel et al., 1974). This phenomenon is assumed to be caused by overactivity (possibly supersensitivity) of the α-adrenergic receptors in the proximal smooth muscle sphincter (Krane and Olsson, 1073). Unfortunately it is difficult to obtain direct evidence of such neuropathic dysfunction, although the use of phentolamine has been described for this purpose (Olsson, Siroky, and Krane, 1977).

Treatment. In cases of incomplete lesions, pharmacological therapy may be able to improve bladder emptying. The rationale of drug therapy is the mimicking, modification, or blockage of naturally occurring neuroactive substances such as acetylcholine, norepinephrine (noradrenaline), histamine, and prostaglandins. In the restoration of the detrusor reflex, the mechanism and even the efficacy of many commonly used agents is still in doubt.

Our knowledge of autonomic neuroreceptor distribution has increased greatly in recent years. Muscarinic cholinergic receptors predominate in the bladder body and base; they are far less numerous in the proximal urethra. When activated, these receptors cause smooth muscle contraction. Adrenergic receptors in the lower urinary tract are of two types: α-receptors, which are stimulatory, and β-receptors, which are inhibitory. The former type predominate in the bladder base, bladder neck, and proximal urethra. The latter type are primarily found in the bladder body with a far less dense distribution in bladder neck and proximal urethra.

Thus increased urethral pressure will result from either α-adrenergic stimulation (phenylephrine) or β-adrenergic blockage (propranolol). Conversely, decreased urethral pressure follows administration of α-adrenergic blocking agents (phenoxybenzamine) or β-adrenergic stimulation (isoproterenol). Since there are β-adrenergic receptors in the bladder body, isoproterenol also causes impaired bladder emptying. Cholinergic agents (bethanecol) cause detrusor contraction, whereas cholinergic blockage (propantheline) impairs contractions.

In the treatment of detrusor areflexia, bethanecol chloride is the most frequently used agent. The effect is the same as that of acetylcholine, except that it is relatively resistant to acetylcholinesterase. Bethanecol has a predominately muscarinic effect

with little nicotinic effect. Thus there is little effect on heart rate or blood pressure with therapeutic doses of 40 to 200 mg daily. Higher doses can cause bradycardia.

There are surprisingly few controlled studies of the efficacy of bethanecol administered orally. Certainly one must doubt any therapeutic effect attributed to oral doses of less than 100 mg daily, since this has been shown to have no effect on the cystometrogram of the normal male (Wein et al., 1978). Even the injection of 5 mg bethanecol subcutaneously, which increases intravesical pressure, has no effect on clinical voiding parameters such as flow rate and residual urine (Wein et al., 1980).

It has been suggested that therapeutic results with bethanecol are poor because of nicotinic effects on the urethral smooth muscle, which are mediated by norepinephrine (Khanna, 1976) (Figure 18.11). This has led to the use of phenoxybenzamine in doses of 10 to 40 mg daily in combination with bethanecol. Khanna (1979) has reported significant improvement in 26 of 31 patients treated in this way.

Nonrelaxing external sphincter. As mentioned,

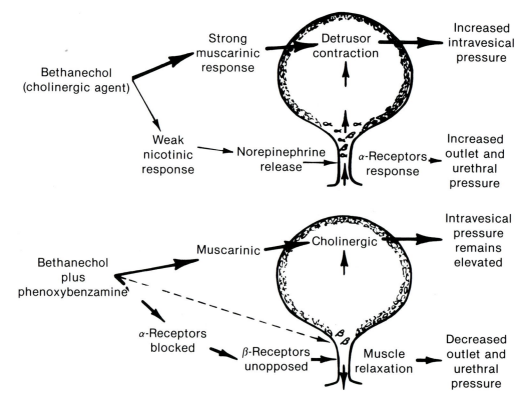

Figure 18.11 *Top,* Effects of bethanecol on bladder and urethra. *Bottom,* Effect of bethanecol plus phenoxybenzamine. (From Khanna, O.P. 1976. Urology **8:**316-338.)

some cases demonstrate external sphincter activity during abdominal straining or Credé's maneuver, which may further compromise emptying. Drug therapy aimed at reducing external sphincter spasm includes agents such as dantrolene, baclofen, and diazepam. In general, these agents fail to achieve urological efficacy except at high doses with significant toxicity. In addition, the long-term safety of some agents (for example, dantrolene) has not been established. In cases in which perineal anesthesia can be accepted, bilateral pudendal nerve block or neurectomy may be a valuable technique.

External stimulation. Many attempts have been made to develop an implantable bladder stimulator for the treatment of neuropathic detrusor areflexia. Halverstadt and Parry (1975) have pointed out several problems with such a device, including the following: (1) stimulation tends to be painful with incomplete lesions, (2) current spread may cause spasm of distant muscles, (3) electrodes may migrate from the original site of implantation, and (4) infection may supervene, necessitating removal. Implantation of electrodes directly into the conus medullaris (Grimes, Nashold, and Anderson, 1975) or the sacral roots is currently being investigated as an alternative to the bladder pacemaker.

Self-intermittent catheterization. The renaissance of this method of emptying the bladder (first mentioned by Stromeyer in 1844) has vastly increased the number of therapeutic options. Aseptic intermittent catheterization was popularized by Guttman for patients with spinal cord injuries. The results reported by Guttman and Frankel (1966) demonstrated unequivocally the value of this technique in achieving a sterile, catheter-free state in more than half of their patients. The relative adequacy of clean (as opposed to sterile) intermittent catheterization was established by Lapides et al. (1971, 1973).

There is no doubt that self-intermittent catheterization is preferable to indwelling catheter drainage. Sterile urine is maintained in from 45% to 90% of cases with the aseptic technique and in from 39% to 65% of cases by the clean method. Better results are obtained when suppressive antimicrobial agents are used. The teaching of self-intermittent catheterization in the female without manual or visual impairment takes about half an hour. Even blind persons have little difficulty in properly performing the procedure. Disposable, inexpensive catheters are readily available commercially.*

Our practice is to instruct the patient in the clean self-catheterization technique. More important than the technique, however, is the attitude toward the treatment displayed by every member of the health care team, particularly the physician. The patient must be constantly encouraged to learn and accept the treatment program. Sources of patient anxiety should be addressed directly and factually: pain should not occur, infection will be treated promptly if it occurs, no harm is done to the urethra, and so on. The advantages inherent in self-intermittent catheterization —for example, avoidance of surgery, no requirement for an external appliance, and preservation of renal function— should be stressed.

Surgical therapy to promote emptying of the neuropathic bladder has lost its former preeminence, especially with the advent of self-intermittent catheterization. Transurethral resection of the bladder neck has been reported to be successful in approximately 90% of patients with detrusor areflexia (Bunts, 1970). Bladder neck contracture may occur as a complication. In the female, the risk of total incontinence is always present, especially with external sphincter neuropathy. This unfortunate occurrence would convert a situation manageable by self-intermittent catheterization to one that may require supravesical diversion. In our practice, this procedure no longer fills a useful purpose in the female patient with detrusor areflexia.

The use of a prosthetic urinary sphincter to achieve continence offers possibilities in patients with detrusor areflexia (Furlow, 1976). Patients with detrusor hyperreflexia that cannot be controlled by some means are not candidates for an artificial sphincter. If residual urine is present, outflow resistance must be eliminated before reimplantation. The best location for placement of the artificial sphincter is at the vesical neck. The rate of complications including component failure and urethral erosion has been high.

COMPLICATIONS

Urethral complications. Complications involving the urethra almost always result from an indwelling Foley catheter and include urethrovaginal fistula, periurethral abscess, and urethral divertic-

---

*Mentor Corporation, 1499 West River Road North, Minneapolis, Minn. 55411.

ulum (occasionally containing one or several stones). Management of these complications should center on removal of the cause, that is, the indwelling catheter. For example, self-intermittent catheterization should be instituted as soon as possible after treatment of the acute urethral problem.

Bladder complications. Infection is by far the most common complication of neuropathic bladder. It must be treated in the context of a program intended to reduce residual urine and remove foreign bodies (that is, catheters and stones). Asymptomatic bacteriuria in the absence of vesicoureteral reflux is generally of no clinical importance and may be treated orally with urinary antimicrobial agents (nitrofurantroin) or by periodic bladder irrigation during self-catheterization. *Candida albicans* may be found in significant numbers in some patients who have received multiple broad-spectrum antibiotics. This infection may be treated by alkalinizing the urine or local bladder irrigation with nystatin solution. Septic episodes associated with bacteriuria require investigation as to the organism's source of access to the bloodstream (usually renal), as well as specific intravenous antimicrobial therapy.

Bladder calculi occur for the same reasons that tend to cause infection (for example, residual urine and foreign bodies) but can also be caused by hypercalciuria as a result of skeletal demineralization. Infection by urea-splitting organisms (*Proteus* species) causes an alkaline urine in which calcium ions are much less soluble. For small stones, transurethral cystolitholapaxy will usually be successful. Large struvite stones, which predominate among spinal cord–injured patients, may be broken by electrohydraulic lithotripsy, and the fragments irrigated from the bladder (Raney, 1976). Thus the need for suprapubic cystolithotomy is rare.

Finally, one should bear in mind the increased incidence of squamous cell carcinoma of the bladder in patients with indwelling catheters and recurrent infection.

Vesicoureteral reflux. The incidence of vesicoureteral reflux in spinal cord–injured patients gradually rises to about 15% after 20 years (Donnelly, Hackler, and Bunts, 1972). The presence of reflux, especially if bilateral and associated with detrusor hyperreflexia, is highly deleterious to renal function and is probably the most common cause of renal failure and death (Marchetti and Gonick, 1970). Bilateral ureteral reimplantation is successful in about 50% of patients with adequate bladder capacity (at least 200 ml) and upper tracts that have not yet deteriorated. If these criteria cannot be met, serious consideration should be given to supravesical diversion in an attempt to preserve renal function.

Hydronephrosis. Even in the absence of reflux, significant hydronephrosis may result from obstruction of the ureter by the greatly thickened detrusor muscle. This complication is less frequent with current management of the neuropathic bladder, occurring in about 5% of spinal cord–injured patients. When all conservative measures aimed at relieving the hydronephrosis have failed, supravesical diversion should be attempted in this group of patients (Koziol and Hackler, 1975).

Renal calculi. The presence of infection, hydronephrosis, reflux, and hypercalciuria all contribute to the noticeable propensity of patients with neuropathic bladders to form renal calculi. The treatment of renal calculosis in the presence of neuropathic bladder does not differ significantly from the usual medical and surgical management of this condition.

SUMMARY

The neuropathic bladder may affect the patient in a wide variety of ways, ranging from inconvenience (frequent urination) and embarrassment (incontinence) to death (renal failure, squamous cell carcinoma). Modern treatment has greatly decreased the morbidity and mortality of this condition. Such treatment, in turn, rests on accurate identification of the micturition abnormality by appropriate urodynamic techniques.

REFERENCES

Abel, B.J., et al. 1974. The neuropathic urethra. Lancet **4:**1229-1230.

Barrington, F.J.F. 1914. The nervous mechanism of micturition. Q. J. Exp. Physiol. **8:**33-71.

Blaivas, J.G., et al. 1977. A new approach to electromyography of the external urethral sphincter. J. Urol. **117:**773-777.

Bunts, R.C. 1970. Surgery of urinary tract dysfunction due to disease or injury of the nervous system, In Dodson, A.I., Jr., editor. Urological surgery. ed. 4. St. Louis. The C.V. Mosby Co.

DeGroat, W.C. 1975. Nervous control of the urinary bladder of the cat. Brain Res. **87:**201-211.

Dibenedetto, M., and Yalla, S.V. 1979. Electrodiagnosis of striated urethral sphincter dysfunction. J. Urol. **122:**361-365.

Donnelly, J., Hackler, R.H., and Bunts, R.C. 1972. Present urologic status of the World War II paraplegic: 25-year follow-up comparison with status of the 20-year Korean war paraplegic and 5-year Vietnam paraplegic. J. Urol. **108:**558-562.

Ek, A., et al. 1977. Adrenergic and cholinergic nerves of the human urethra and urinary bladder: a histochemical study. Acta Physiol. Scand. **99:**345-352.

Furlow, W.L. 1976. The implantable artificial genitourinary sphincter in the management of total urinary incontinence. Mayo Clin. Proc. **51**:341-345.

Godec, C., Cass, A.S., and Ayala, G.F. 1975. Bladder inhibition with functional electrical stimulation. Urology **6**:663-666.

Goldstein, I., et al. 1982. Neurologic abnormalities in multiple sclerosis. J. Urol. **128**:541-545.

Gosling, J.A., Dixon, J.S., and Lendon, R.G. 1977. The autonomic innervation of the human male and female bladder neck and proximal urethra. J. Urol. **118**:302-305.

Grimes, J.H., Nashold, B.S., and Anderson, E.E. 1975. Clinical application of electronic bladder stimulation in paraplegics. J. Urol. **113**:338-340.

Guttmann, L., and Frankel, A. 1966. The value of intermittent catheterization in the early management of traumatic paraplegia and tetraplegia. Paraplegia **4**:63-84.

Halverstadt, D.B., and Parry, W.L. 1975. Electronic stimulation of the human bladder: 9 years later. J. Urol. **113**:341-344.

Iggo, A. 1955. Tension receptors in the stomach and urinary bladder. J. Physiol. **128**:593-607.

Khanna, O.P. 1976. Disorders of micturition: neuropharmacologic basis and results of drug therapy. Urology **8**:316-338.

Khanna, O.P. 1979. Non-surgical therapeutic modalities. In Krane, R.J., and Siroky, M.B., editors. Clinical neurourology. Boston. Little, Brown & Co.

Koff, S.A., and DeRidder, P.A. 1977. Patterns of neurogenic bladder dysfunction in sacral agenesis. J. Urol. **118**:87-89.

Koziol, I., and Hackler, R.H. 1975. Cutaneous ureteroileostomy in the spinal cord injured patient: a 15-year experience. J. Urol. **114**:709-711.

Lapides, J., et al. 1962. Denervation supersensitivity as a test for neurogenic bladder. Surg. Gynecol. Obstet. **114**:241-244.

Lapides, J., et al. 1971. Clean, intermittent self-catheterization in the treatment of urinary tract disease. Trans. Am. Assoc. Genitourin. Surg. **63**:92-96.

Lapides, J., et al. 1973. Follow-up on unsterile, intermittent self-catheterization. Trans. Am. Assoc. Genitourin. Surg. **65**:44-50.

Marchetti, L.F., and Gonick, P. 1970. A comparison of renal function in spinal cord injury patients with and without reflux. J. Urol. **104**:365-367.

Misak, S.J., et al. 1962. Nerve interruption procedures in the urologic management of paraplegic patients. J. Urol. **88**:392-401.

Olsson, C.A., and Krane, R.J.1973. Phenoxybenzamine in neurogenic bladder dysfunction. II. Clinical considerations. J. Urol. **110**:653-666.

Olsson, C.A., Siroky, M.B., and Krane, R.J. 1977. The phentolamine test in neurogenic bladder dysfunction. J. Urol. **111**:481-485.

Pavlakis, A., Siroky, M.B., and Krane, R.J. 1982. Neurogenic detrusor areflexia: correlation of bethanecol supersensitivity and perineal electromyography. J. Urol. (In Press.)

Raezer, D.M., et al. 1973. Autonomic innervation of canine urinary bladder: cholinergic and adrenergic contributions and interaction of sympathetic and parasympathetic systems in bladder function. Urology **2**:211-221.

Raney, A.M. 1976. Electrohydraulic cystolithotripsy. Urology **8**:379-381.

Rockswold, G.L., and Bradley, W.E. 1977. The use of sacral nerve blocks in the evaluation and treatment of neurologic bladder disease. J. Urol. **118**:415-417.

Siroky, M.B., and Krane, R.J. 1981. Neurologic aspects of detrusor-sphincter dyssynergia with special reference to the guarding reflex. J. Urol. **127**:953-957.

Tanagho, E.A. 1981. Neuropathic bladder disorders. In Smith, D.R., editor. General urology. Los Altos, Calif. Lange Medical Publishers.

Teague, C.T., and Merrill, D.C. 1977. Electric pelvic floor stimulation: mechanism of action. Invest. Urol. **15**:65-69.

Torrens, M.J. 1975. Urodynamic analysis of differential sacral nerve blocks and sacral neurectomy. Urol. Int. **30**:85-91.

Wein, A.J., et al. 1978. The effect of oral bethanecol chloride on the cystometrogram of the normal male adult. J. Urol. **120**:330-331.

Wein, A.J., et al. 1980. The effects of bethanecol chloride on urodynamic parameters in normal women and in women with significant residual urine volumes. J. Urol. **124**:397-399.

chapter 19

Bladder after radical pelvic surgery

ECKHARD PETRI

In 1898 Wertheim first reported the extensive dissection of both ureters and the bladder during abdominal hysterectomy for cervical carcinoma to facilitate the wide removal of paracervical and parametrial tissue. Radiation therapy was applied to the treatment of cervical carcinoma in the early years of this century. Rapid improvement in the radiographic equipment, the clinical use of radium, and the uniformity of dosimetry far outstripped advances in surgery, so that by the late 1920s radiation therapy had replaced surgery in many countries. American, Japanese, and European surgeons progressed and made their operative techniques more radical. Surgery is now performed for earlier stages of cervical carcinoma, generally limited to patients with stage Ib and IIa lesions.

Radical hysterectomy requires mobilization of the bladder to allow removal of the upper vagina to ensure an adequate margin of resection. Radical hysterectomy therefore places the bladder at considerable risk. While intraoperative injury to the urinary tract is rare, urinary problems continue to be the most significant complications following radical hysterectomy. These postoperative complications include vesicovaginal fistulae (see Chapter 18) and bladder dysfunction. The incidence of bladder disturbances following radical hysterectomy ranges from 16% to 80% (Bors and Comarr, 1971).

With more extensive surgery within the small pelvis, such as abdominoperineal resection or posterior exenteration in selected cases of carcinoma of the cervix, vagina, or vulva, a higher incidence of voiding disorders has to be expected.

The literature on urological problems after radical pelvic surgery is numerous. Different indications, different surgical techniques (abdominal route with extensive lymphadenectomy and large resection of the vagina: limited procedures, for example, TeLinde; vaginal procedures, for example, Schauta), different forms of radiation therapy (preoperative, postoperative, radium, cesium, telecobalt, betatron), and different types of postoperative management of bladder drainage make a comparison of published data almost impossible. Because of changes in surgical technique and postoperative regimes, comparison of long-term results is difficult.

PATHOPHYSIOLOGY

The causes of disorders of the lower urinary tract after radical pelvic surgery range from calculated

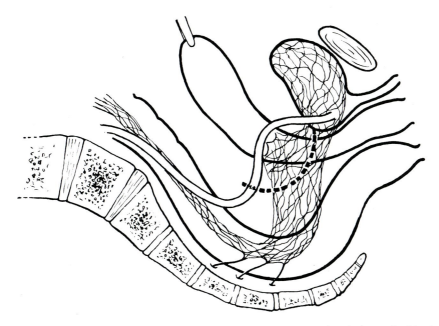

Figure 19.1 Distortion of relationships of ureter and pelvic plexus by traction during radical hysterectomy. Interrupted line indicates portion of plexus usually excised.

injuries to the pelvic nerves and postural changes of the bladder in an empty pelvic cavity to accidental lesions caused by inadequate postoperative bladder drainage and urinary tract infection.

The majority of the nerves from the pelvic plexus supplying the bladder pass over and around the vagina. It is therefore apparent that any operation that involves excision of the paracervical and paravaginal web of retroperitoneal tissue will interrupt some portion of the bladder innervation (Figure 19.1). Some of the fibers pass around the lateral aspect of the vagina; however, it is evident that unless the dissection is carried fairly deep, that is, to include a major segment of the paravaginal portion of the web, complete interruption of the innervation is unlikely. It is also evident that in the operation as usually performed, this is the only site at which the parasympathetic nerves to the bladder enter the field of dissection (Twombly and Landers, 1956). Complete interruption of the parasympathetic innervation can take place during abdominoperineal resection of the rectum and in posterior exenteration. In these cases an additional lesion of the somatic pudendal nerve may occur. We can classify three types of surgical lesions of the lower urinary tract that lead to different disorders in filling and voiding phases (Figures 19.2 to 19.5):

Type I—Isolated lesion of the parasympathetic nerve (pelvic nerve) innervating the detrusor. Bladder sensation (hypogastric nerve) and pudendal nerves are unharmed. There is no spontaneous micturition, because the detrusor is acontractile.

Type II—Partial lesion of the pelvic ganglia with the pudendal nerve unharmed. The bladder is hypertonic with low compliance and contains residual urine because of a functional bladder outlet obstruction.

Type III—Complete destruction of the pelvic ganglia. The bladder is acontractile with sensory loss and additional sphincter incompetence because of an atonic urethra.

All three types of postoperative sequences can be seen after radical hysterectomy. Besides these, direct nerve lesions, changes in blood supply, and lymphatic drainage play decisive roles in bladder dysfunction. During the extended Wertheim-Meigs procedure, several branches of the hypogastric artery are ligated and dissected, including the uterine artery at its origin, the inferior vesical artery, the vaginal artery, the medial hemorrhoidal artery, and sometimes even the whole hypogastric artery. Removing all structures of connective tissue and vessels of the pelvis together with the lymph nodes leads to an interruption of lymphatic drainage. The

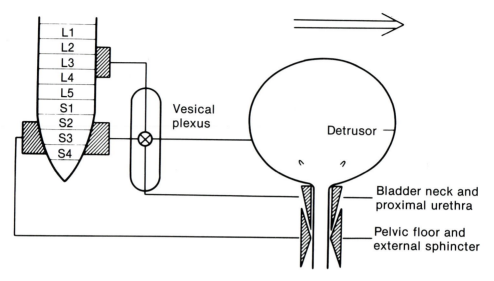

Figure 19.2 Functional segments of reservoir and voiding function and their nervous control.

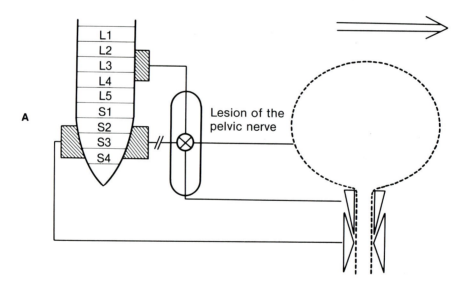

Figure 19.3 A, Surgical lesion type I: isolated lesion of parasympathetic pelvic nerve supplying detrusor. Hypogastric nerve (sensation) and pudendal nerve (motor somatic) are unharmed.

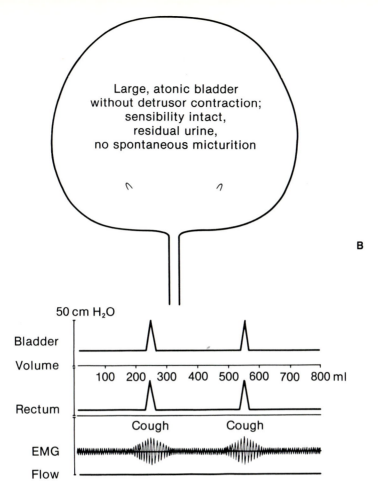

Large, atonic bladder
without detrusor contraction;
sensibility intact,
residual urine,
no spontaneous micturition

50 cm H$_2$O

Bladder

Volume

100 200 300 400 500 600 700 800 ml

Rectum

Cough   Cough

EMG

Flow

B

Figure 19.3, cont'd. B, Cystometry. There is large atonic bladder with residual urine and no detrusor contraction. Sensation is intact. There is no spontaneous micturition.

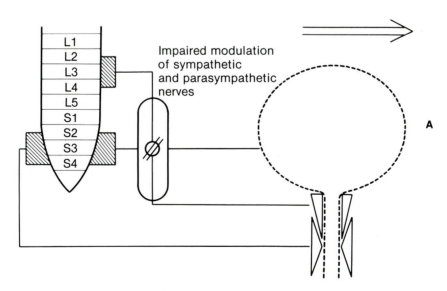

L1
L2
L3
L4
L5
S1
S2
S3
S4

Impaired modulation
of sympathetic
and parasympathetic
nerves

A

Figure 19.4 A, Surgical lesion type II: partial lesion of pelvic ganglion. Pudendal nerve is unharmed; pelvic floor electromyogram is undisturbed.

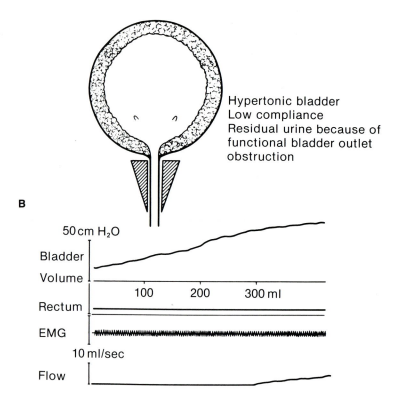

Hypertonic bladder
Low compliance
Residual urine because of
functional bladder outlet
obstruction

Figure 19.4, cont'd. B, Hypertonic low compliance bladder with residual urine because of functional bladder outlet obstruction.

interruption of lymphatic and blood circulation of the bladder is inevitable. Although collateral vessels are good, there is a phase of adaptation leading to transitory local ischemia and lymphostasis and followed by damage to the tissue and functional disorders.

Bilateral oopherectomy in premenopausal women induces typical changes in the mucosa of the bladder, urethra, and vagina. An estrogen deficit results, which is known to induce reduction of urethral closure pressure, pressure transmission to the urethra, and alterations in sensibility and contractility of the bladder.

Voiding disorders because of functional outlet obstruction have usually been treated by transurethral catheterization, which is a known cause of urethritis and ascending infection occurring within 2 to 3 days. After a variable period of time (6 to 50 days), depending in the surgeons's preference and when micturition can resume, the catheter is removed. Voiding problems may result from overdistension as a result of persistent residual urine (without a desire to void because of the sensory loss) or from repeated catheterization to detect re-

sidual urine. Thus the causes of micturition disorders after radical pelvic surgery are multifactorial and comprise surgical lesions to nerve, vascular, and lymphatic supply; dislocation of the bladder into the wound cavity; and iatrogenic lesions caused by repeated catheterization during the postoperative course.

INCIDENCE

The great number of surgical modifications, new discussions on lesser or greater radical surgery (Ober, 1978; Burghardt, 1981), radical vaginal techniques still in use (Barclay and Roman-Lopez, 1975; Fischer, Selig, and Lamm, 1978; Pflüger et al., 1980), different forms of preoperative or postoperative radiation therapy, and different types of intraoperative management together with small numbers of patients make objective comparison of the literature difficult.

Differentiation between postoperative data and long-term results is necessary. There are only a few prospective studies (Seski and Diokno, 1977; Christ and Gunselmann, 1980) or control series. Only preoperative assessment of subjective mic-

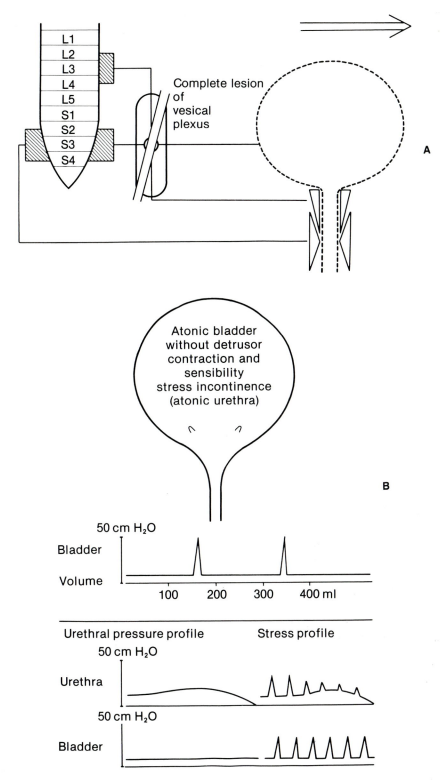

Figure 19.5 A, Surgical lesion type III: complete lesion of pelvic ganglion. Bladder is atonic; there is sensory denervation and possible sphincter incompetence. **B,** Cystometry and urethral pressure profile. Cystometry shows atonic bladder without detrusor contraction and loss of sensation. Resting urethral pressure profile is reduced.

TABLE 19.1   Urinary tract symptoms after radical pelvic surgery (literature)

	Vesical dysfunction	Incontinence	Diminished sensation
Lewington (1956)	43%	28%	34%
Busse and Muth (1957)	—	—	36% postoperative 13% 1 yr postoperative
Green et al. (1962)	16%	10%	—
Fraser (1966)	59%	24%	22%
Schmid and Baumann (1967)	70% postoperative 38% 2 yr postoperative	41%	15% postoperative 5% 1 yr postoperative
Gaudenz (1977)	52%	52%	
Buchsbaum (1983)	21%	—	—
Christ and Gunselmann (1980)	71%	—	—
Pflüger et al. (1980)	87%		13%
Articus, Staufer, and Lochmüller (1980)	52%	21%	5%
Manzl et al. (1981)	—	Wertheim: 10% postoperative 3.7% 1 yr postoperative	27.3% postoperative 18% 1 yr postoperative
		Latzko: 21% postoperative 27% 1 yr postoperative	90% postoperative 45% 1 yr postoperative

turition problems and urodynamic data would be able to bring postoperative problems into correct perspective. Christ and Gunselmann (1980) performed a controlled prospective study with preoperative urodynamic assessment that indicated preexisting bladder dysfunction in 10 of 35 patients. Most published data deal with subjective complaints and would need exact confirmation (Table 19.1).

Additional radiotherapy does not apparently influence bladder symptoms; there is evidence that the shorter the vaginal remnant, the greater the chance of the patient having urinary symptoms. Lewington (1956) demonstrated that 69% of patients with a vaginal length shorter than 4 cm had symptoms in comparison with 21% of patients with a vagina longer than 4 cm. Fraser (1966) found that 73% of patients with a shorter vaginal length compared with 52% with a longer length were symptomatic, whereas Christ and Gunselmann (1980) did not find a significant difference.

Urinary incontinence is the most frequent symptom, demonstrated in 96% of patients with bladder symptoms in our own material (that of my colleagues and myself). Introduction of modern urodynamic investigations allows a further differentiation of the basic disorders. Functional infravesical obstruction is of clinical importance as possible sequelae to all three types of surgical lesions. It was described by Fraser (1966) in 22% of patients, by Pflüger et al. (1980) in 45% of patients, and by Articus, Staufer, and Lochmüller (1980) in 25% of patients and could be demonstrated in 32% of our patients by urodynamic-radiological investigation, being located mainly in the bladder neck region.

PREVENTION

To reduce the frequency of bladder dysfunction after radical pelvic surgery, detailed preoperative examination of the urinary tract is necessary. While intravenous urography and urethrocystoscopy are sine qua non, other preoperative urodynamic investigations have to be performed if the findings of these procedures are abnormal or when there are subjective complaints, for example, incontinence, urgency, dysuria, or infravesical obstruction that could be corrected during surgery. Christ and Gunselmann (1980) showed a high percentage of pre-operative voiding difficulties that were only slightly increased by the surgical procedure.

Accurate dissection is a matter of course. To minimize the symptoms resulting from nerve damage to the bladder, the following dissection during removal of pelvic lymph nodes and radical hysterectomy by Asmussen may be used. The amount of success will depend on the extent to which lymph nodes are involved and their ease of removal. The standard lateral procedure was described by Asmussen in 1981. After ligation of the round ligaments and the infundibulopelvic ligaments, the perivesical and perirectal spaces are opened by blunt dissection down to the pelvic floor (Figure 19.6). The structure running from the pelvic floor into the uterus and vagina, separating these two spaces, is the lateral retinaculum (the cardinal ligament, the web, Mackenrodt's ligament, and the parametrium). When the common iliac, internal iliac, obturator, and external iliac lymph nodes have been removed, the uterine artery and obliterated umbilical arteries are identified where they originate from the internal iliac (hypogastric) artery. As much fat as possible is removed, exposing normally three to four veins running from the pelvic wall to the vagina and bladder (Figure 19.7). These veins are ligated individually as laterally as possible. Hereafter the part of the hypogastric plexus that supplies the lower urinary tract with sensory and motor fibers is exposed (Figure 19.8). The surgical procedure is then continued by tunneling and free dissection of the ureters (Figure 19.9). Finally the specimen is removed with as good a margin as possible. The technique outlined here spares a major part of the hypogastric nerve plexus without interfering with the radical nature of the surgical procedure. A suprapubic catheter is left for 1 week after the operation, and bilateral extraperitoneal drainage is used for 5 to 10 days.

Efficient drainage of wound cavities (to remove blood and lymph and prevent adhesions and infection) and of the bladder plays a decisive role. Bladder drainage is best accomplished with a suprapubic catheter because of:

Good patient tolerance

Reduction of incidence of urinary infection

Early return to spontaneous micturition

Possible control of residual urine without further catheterization

Avoidance of urethral trauma and discomfort

In addition, reduction of the incidence of fistula formation seems possible by effective suprapubic drainage (Van Nagell, Penny, and Roddick, 1972; Petri and Jonas, 1980).

Whether less radical surgery as proposed by some clinicians (Ober, 1978) may reduce the incidence of bladder dysfunction is open to question. During the postoperative period, prophylaxis against urinary tract infection, early bladder activity (using the suprapubic catheter), and adjuvant pharmacotherapy will accelerate bladder rehabilitation. Estimation of residual urine should be carried out by ultrasound to avoid continuous urethral trauma. Should severe voiding disorders persist in spite of this regime, early urodynamic investigation will enable specific therapy to be adopted.

TREATMENT
Routine

It is necessary, in treating postoperative bladder dysfunction, to differentiate between routine postoperative measures and specific treatment. Since the report of Green et al. (1962), prolonged postoperative bladder drainage is in use in most departments dealing with radical pelvic surgery. My colleagues and I use a suprapubic catheter placed in the bladder at the completion of the operation (Figures 19.10 and 19.11) and agree with van Nagell, Penny, and Roddick (1972), who reported satisfactory results with this technique. Since 1977 we have performed more than 150 radical pelvic operations without a vesicovaginal fistula and were able to discharge all patients without a catheter (residual urine below 100 ml) between day 8 and day 14. We allow continuous drainage for 5 days, then clamp the catheter and ask the patient to void every 3 to 4 hours, whether or not there is any desire to void. Being aware of the high percentage of functional infravesical obstruction (32% in our patient material), we give phenoxybenzamine, starting at 10 mg in the evening for several days. Should micturition be insufficient with residual urine being over 100 ml, we increase the phenoxybenzamine to 5 mg in the morning, 5 mg in the afternoon, and 10 mg in the evening. With this management our patients who have undergone the Wertheim-Meigs operation have avoided difficulty in micturition.

Specific

Indications for the use of physical, medical, or surgical action is not determined by the classification of the neurological or structural lesion but by subjective complaints and urodynamic findings.

Text continued on p. 233.

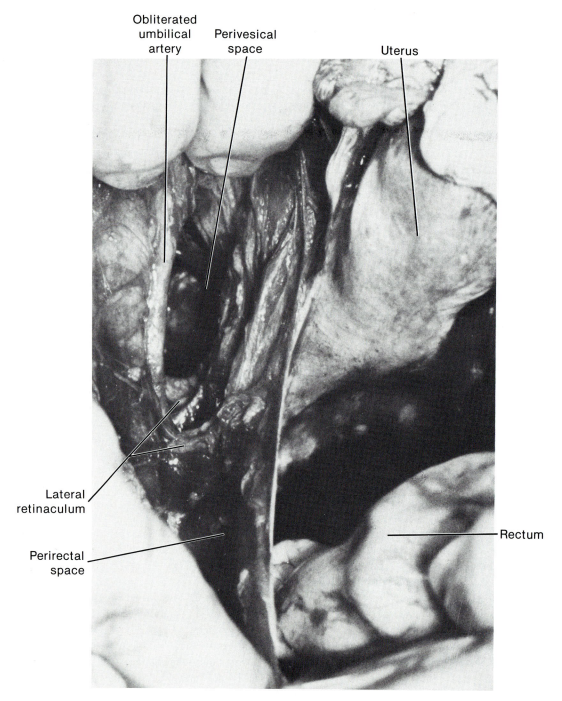

Figure 19.6 Standardized lateral procedure dissection: lateral retinaculum and perivesical and perirectal spaces are displayed. (From Asmussen, M. 1981. Radical hysterectomy with lymph node dissection without denervating the lower urinary tract. Proceedings from the fifth annual International Urologists and Gynecologists Association meeting. Stockholm.)

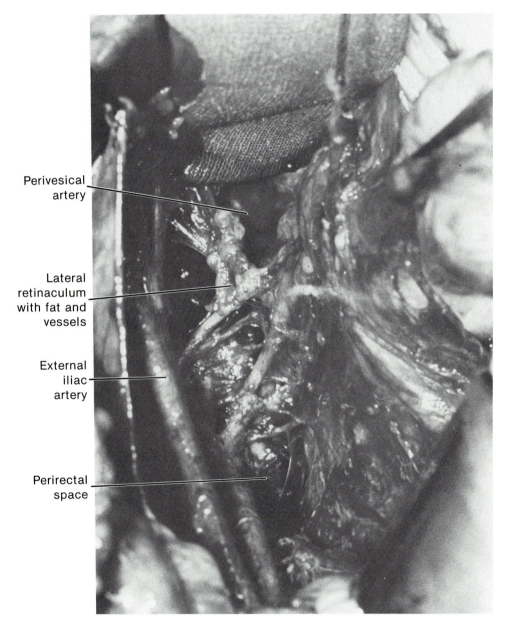

Perivesical
artery

Lateral
retinaculum
with fat and
vessels

External
iliac
artery

Perirectal
space

Figure 19.7 Vessels in lateral retinaculum. (From Asmussen, M. 1981. Radical hysterectomy with lymph node dissection without denervating the lower urinary tract. Proceedings from the fifth annual International Urologists and Gynecologists Association meeting. Stockholm.)

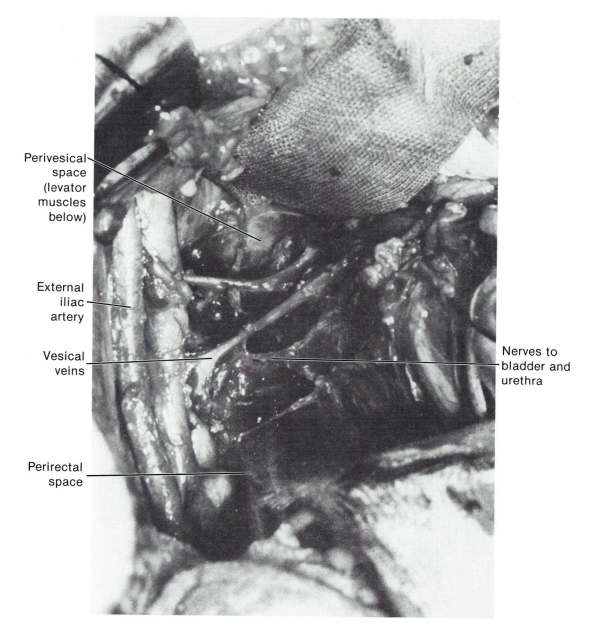

Perivesical space (levator muscles below)

External iliac artery

Vesical veins

Perirectal space

Nerves to bladder and urethra

Figure 19.8 Hypogastric plexus with nerves to bladder and urethra are displayed. (From Asmussen, M. 1981. Radical hysterectomy with lymph node dissection without denervating the lower urinary tract. Proceedings from the fifth annual International Urologists and Gynecologists Association meeting. Stockholm.)

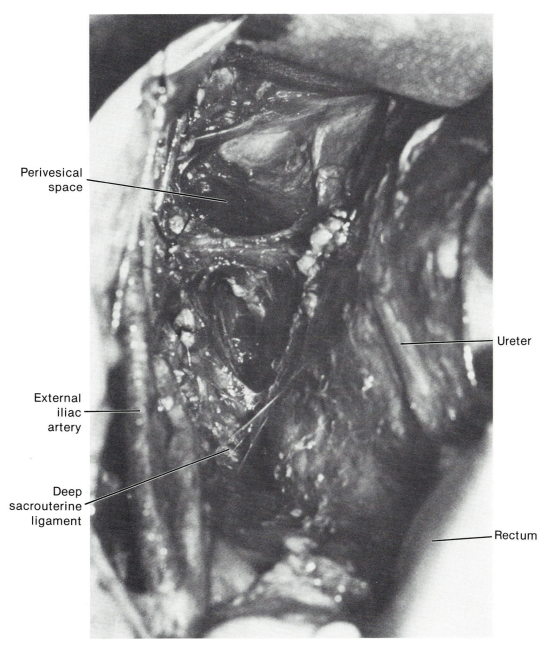

Perivesical space

Ureter

External iliac artery

Deep sacrouterine ligament

Rectum

Figure 19.9 Continuation of dissection with display of ureter. (From Asmussen, M. 1981. Radical hysterectomy with lymph node dissection without denervating the lower urinary tract. Proceedings from the fifth annual International Urologists and Gynecologists Association meeting. Stockholm.)

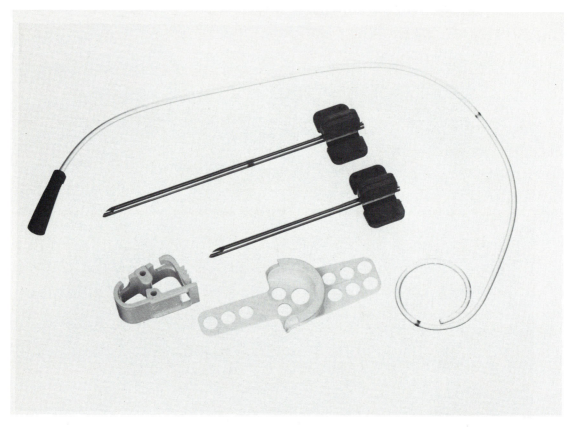

Figure 19.10 Suprapubic catheter (Cystofix) with bisected trochar, Silastic catheter (No. 7 Fr) with memory curve and multiple perforations at tip, plate for fixation, and clamp. (Courtesy of B. Braun Co., Melsungen, West Germany.)

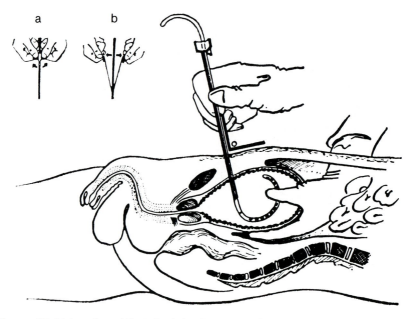

Figure 19.11 Insertion of Cystofix during laparotomy for suprapubic bladder drainage.

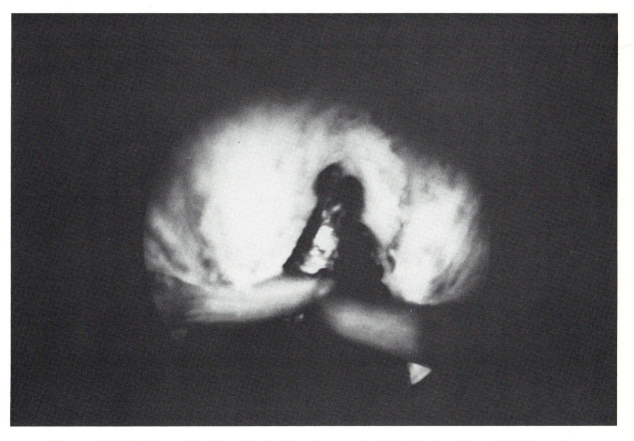

Figure 19.12 Bladder neck incision with electric cautery needle at 12 o'clock position until bladder neck opens and funnels.

As explained in the section on pathophysiology, functional or morphological infravesical obstruction is a common complication of radical pelvic surgery. As well as using phenoxybenzamine to decrease urethral pressure, a cholinergic agent to increase the bladder tone (see Chapter 39) is also used. If suprapubic drainage is not available, clean intermittent catheterization is performed to control the residual urine. If effective voiding is not achieved within 7 to 10 days, a urodynamic evaluation will give objective data, for example, flow rate, micturition pressure, provocation of detrusor contractions, and morphological appearance of the lower urinary tract during voiding, such as funneling of the bladder neck and ballooning of the proximal urethra.

Bladder neck incision using the technique of Turner-Warwick et al. (1973) has been the method fo choice in our department in the event that pharmacological therapy is unsuccessful (Petri, Walz, and Jonas, 1978; Jonas, Petri, and Hohenfellner,

TABLE 19.2 Results following bladder neck incision (maximum flow of urine)

	Preoperative	Postoperative
Mean	8.2 ml/sec	21.5 ml/sec
Range	5-15 ml/sec	15-40 ml/sec

1979). The bladder neck incision is performed with an electric cautery needle (Figure 19.12) at the 5, 7, and 12 o'clock positions until the bladder neck opens widely and funnels sufficiently. An indwelling urethral catheter is left in place for 1 postoperative day. Of 30 women with postoperative voiding problems, 28 were cured or improved with this procedure (Table 19.2). Postoperative urodynamic investigation including cinéradiography showed good funneling of the bladder neck and reduction of urethral closure pressure (Figures 19.13 and 19.14).

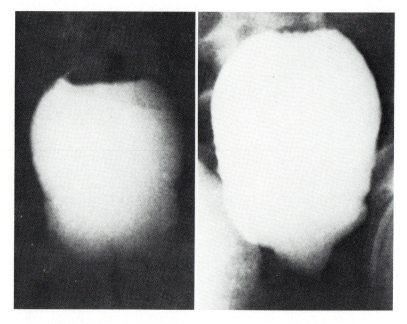

Figure 19.13 Micturition cystogram: before incision *(left)* bladder neck remains closed, impeding good voiding stream; following incision *(right)* good funneling is visible, guaranteeing normal flow.

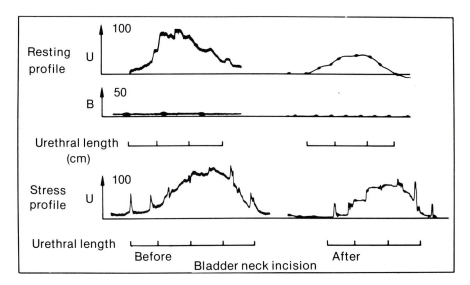

Figure 19.14 Recording of urethral profile (resting and stress profile) before and after bladder neck incision. Note shortening of functional length and lowering of amplitude following incision.

With attention to the effective emptying of the bladder and additional pharmacotherapy, most patients will establish satisfactory voiding within 3 months without urinary tract infection. Extreme surgical procedures for treatment of voiding disorders remain for selected patients only. These include bladder stimulation by means of a pacemaker, which has several disadvantages:

Device failure

Migration of the electrodes, leading to reduced effectiveness

Infection, necessitating removal of the device

Inadvertent stimulation of adjacent nerves, producing spasms of the legs, abdominal musculature, and pelvic floor muscles

Pain associated wtih bladder stimulation in the case of an incomplete lesion, such as occurs after radical pelvic surgery (Hackler, 1979)

Our own experience with this procedure is limited, since we have implanted only two pacemakers after pelvic surgery, leading to adequate voiding by stimulation in one patient and reflex voiding in the other (Jonas and Hohenfellner, 1978).

Some patients with incontinence as a result of neuropathic dysfunction after radical pelvic surgery may benefit from an artificial urinary sphincter (Figure 16.18). This device, employing an inflatable cuff, has been beneficial in properly selected cases. The complication rate has been significant owing to the amount of foreign material involved and the complexities of the system (see Chapter 16).

POSTERIOR EXENTERATION

In selected cases of squamous cell carcinoma of the cervix, vagina, or vulva, posterior exenteration is performed to perserve the bladder and to restrict the psychosocial trauma to a bearable state. In ad-

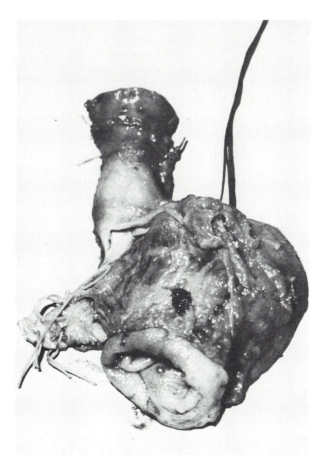

Figure 19.15 Surgical specimen from posterior exenteration for treatment of squamous cell carcinoma of posterior vaginal wall.

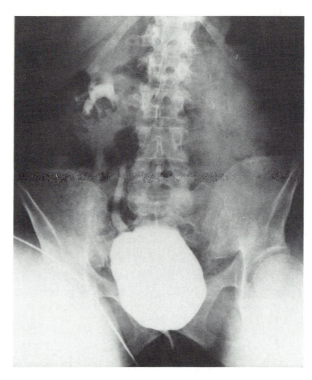

Figure 19.16 Same patient as in Figure 19.15 1 year postoperatively: voiding cystourethrogram demonstrates residual urine, vesicoureteric reflux, and deviation of bladder neck because of extensive scarring. Clinically this patient had persistent urinary tract infection together with stress incontinence.

dition, reduction of the extent of surgery should lower morbidity and mortality. Reviewing our 2-year survival rate, this seems to be true (70% in comparison with 55% of patients with anterior or total exenteration), but because of intense denervation (type III) and tilting of the bladder into the empty sacral wound cavity (as in abdominoperineal resection), severe micturition disorders result. Lesions of the pelvic and hypogastric plexuses lead to an atonic bladder with residual urine and loss of sensation with additional sphincter incompetence caused by a hypotonic urethra. Despite some incontinence, emptying of the bladder is insufficient and intermittent catheterization or suprapubic drainage is necessary. In our patients, all forms of bladder training, pharmacotherapy, and urethral surgery were insufficient. In younger patients with a good prognosis for the primary disease, we now recommend total exenteration; we think managing a wet stoma is easier to learn and bear than permanent incontinence, catheterization, and urinary tract infection (Figures 19.15 and 19.16).

SUMMARY

Radical pelvic surgery results in various bladder disturbances because of damage to pelvic nerves,

interruption of blood supply, and lymphatic drainage. Dislocation of the bladder into the wound cavity and iatrogenic lesions of the urethra during the postoperative period augment these disorders. The therapeutic regime cannot be decided schematically but is influenced by clinical findings and urodynamic data. If, in spite of suprapubic drainage and adjuvant pharmacotherapy, adequate voiding cannot be established, specific drugs (see Chapter 39), bladder retraining (see Chapter 35), bladder neck incision, or, in selected cases, implantation of an artificial sphincter or a bladder stimulator may be helpful.

REFERENCES

Articus, M., Staufer, F., and Lochmüller, H. 1980. Ergebnisse urodynamischer Untersuchungen nach abdominaler operativer Beseitigung des Zervixkarzinoms. Gebursthilfe Frauenheilkd. **40:**237-241.

Asmussen, M. 1981. Radical hysterectomy with lymph node dissection without denervating the lower urinary tract. Proceedings from the fifth annual International Urologists and Gynecologists Association meeting. Stockholm.

Barclay, D.I., and Roman-Lopez, J.J. 1975. Bladder dysfunction after Schauta hysterectomy. Am. J. Obstet. Gynecol. **123:**519-526.

Bors, E., and Comarr, A.E. 1971. Neurological urology. Basel. S. Karger.

Buchsbaum, H.J. 1983. The urinary tract and radical hysterectomy. In Buchsbaum, H.J., and Schmidt, J.D., editors. Gynecologic and obstetric urology. Ed. 2. Philadelphia. W.B. Saunders Co.

Burghardt, E. 1981. Zur Frage der sogenannten konservativen Behandlung des atypischen Zervixepithels. Geburtshilfe Frauenheilkd. **41:**330-334.

Busse, O., and Muth, H. 1957. Über Funktionsstörungen von Ureter und Blase nach der Wertheimschen Operation. Zentralbl. Gynaekol. **79:**114-127.

Christ, F., and Gunselmann, W. 1980. Untersuchungen zur Urodynamik von Harnblase und Harnröhre nach Zervixkrebsoperationen. Gubertshilfe Frauenheilkd. **40:**610-618.

Fischer, W., Selig, V., and Lamm, D. 1978. Fortschritte bei der Verhütung und Bekämpfung urologischer Komplikationen des Zervixkarzinoms. Zentralbl. Gynaekol. **100:**1320-1331.

Fraser, A.C. 1966. The late effects of Wertheim's hysterectomy on the urinary tract. Br. J. Obstet. Gynaecol. **73:**1002-1007.

Gaudenz, R. 1977. Spätstörungen der Blasenfunktion nach erweiterter Hysterektomie, ohne Nachbestrahlung, wegen eines Kollumkarzinoms. Eine urodynamische Nachuntersuchung. Geburtschilfe Frauenheilkd. **37:**19-26.

Green, T.H., et al. 1962. Urologic complications of radical Wertheim hysterectomy: incidence, etiology, management, and prevention. Obstet. Gynecol. **20:**293-312.

Hackler, R. 1979. Surgical treatment of the adult neurogenic bladder dysfunction. In Krane, R.J., and Siroky, M.B., editors. Clinical neuro-urology. Boston. Little, Brown & Co.

Jonas, U., and Heidler, H. 1979. Ursachen und Therapie postoperativer Harnverhaltungen. Gynaekol. Rundsch. **19**(suppl. 1):97-106.

Jonas, U., and Hohenfellner, R. 1978. Late results of bladder stimulation in 11 patients: followup to 4 years. J. Urol. **120:**565-568.

Jonas, U., Petri, E., and Hohenfellner, R. 1979. Indication and value of bladder neck incision. Urol. Int. **34:**260-265.

Lewington, W. 1956. Disturbances of micturition following Wertheim hysterectomy. J. Obstet. Gynaecol. Br. Emp. **63:**861-864.

Manzl, J., et al. 1981. Funtionelle Störungen des unteren Harntraktes nach Radikaloperation des Kollumkarzinoms. Geburtshilfe Frauenheilkd. **41:**145-150.

Ober, K.G. 1978. Die abgestufte Therapie des Zervixkarzinoms. Geburtshilfe Frauenheilkd. **38:**671-684.

Petri, E., and Jonas, U. 1980. Indikationen der transurethralen und suprapubischen Harnableitung. Urologe (B) **20:**164-165.

Petri, E., Walz, P.H., and Jonas, U. 1978. Transurethral bladder neck operation in neurogenic bladder, Eur. Urol. **4:**189-191.

Pflüger, H., et al. 1980. Diagnostik und Therapie postoperativer Blasenentleerungsstörungen nach gynäkologischer Radikaloperation. Gynaekol. Rundsch. **20**(suppl. 2):191-194.

Schmid, I., and Baumann, U. 1967. Blasenkomplikationen nach abdominaler erweiterter Hysterektomie mit Lymphonodektomie und Nachbestrahlung. Geburtshilfe Frauenheilkd. **24:**954-969.

Seski, J.C., and Diokno, A.C. 1977. Bladder dysfunction after radical abdominal hysterectomy. Am. J. Obstet. Gynecol. **128:**643-651.

Turner-Warwick, R., et al. 1973. A urodynamic view of the clinical problems associated with bladder neck dysfunction and its treatment by endoscopic incision. Br. J. Urol. **45:**44-59.

Twombly, G.H., and Landers, D. 1956. The innervation of the bladder with reference to radical hysterectomy. Am. J. Obstet. Gynecol. **71:**1291-1300.

Van Nagell, J.R., Penny, R.M., and Roddick, J.W. 1972. Suprapubic bladder drainage following radical hysterectomy. Am. J. Obstet. Gynecol. **113:**849-850.

chapter 20

Genitourinary fistulae

UDO JONAS and ECKHARD PETRI

Since the first successful closures of vesicovaginal fistulae in 1845 by Sims and the first description of vesicouterine-vaginal fistulae by Jobert de Lamballe in 1852, many vaginal and abdominal approaches have been described to solve a serious problem of which Sims himself wrote in June 1849, "I realise that at least my efforts were blessed by success and that I had made perhaps one of the most important discoveries of the age for the relief of suffering humanity."

Sim's fundamental directives that finally led to a successful closure were:

1. Allowance of sufficient time for spontaneous healing and maturation of the fistula
2. Union of broad raw surfaces without tension
3. Use of fine suture material
4. Maintenance of free postoperative urinary drainage

Goodwin and Scardino (1980) found that "one of the few remaining pleasant romances between urological and gynaecological surgery relate to fistulae between the urinary tract and the vagina" and stated that until today we had little to suggest that we could improve on Sims' basic technique in the treatment of vesicovaginal and ureterovaginal fistulae.

Fallon and Culp (1983) found that the formation of urinary fistulae was one of the dreaded complications of gynecological surgery for benign and malignant conditions. They further stated that the more frequent the surgery, the more likely it was that fistulae would occur.

CLASSIFICATION

Gynecological-urinary fistulae are classified according to the organs between which the fistulae are established and are divided into simple and mixed forms (see list below). This classification will be used further in discussing causes, diagnosis, treatment, and results (Figure 20.1).

Genitourinary fistulae

I. Simple fistulae
  A. Urethrovaginal
  B. Vesicovaginal
  C. Ureterovaginal
  D. Vesicouterine
  E. Ureterouterine
II. Mixed fistulae
  A. Vesicoureterovaginal
  B. Vesicoureterouterine
  C. Vesicovaginorectal

SIMPLE FISTULAE
Urethrovaginal fistulae

Urethrovaginal fistulae occur following surgical repair (for example, cystocele or urethral diverticulum) or obstetrical trauma. In addition, they can occur after irradiation for neoplasia of the cervix, uterus, and vagina.

Vesicovaginal fistulae

Vesicovaginal fistulae are generally located in the posterior bladder wall or in the trigone. They very often occur after complicated childbirth or following pelvic surgery, especially abdominal hysterectomy. Extensive plevic trauma and irradiation are additional etiological factors. Apart from gynecological surgery, urological surgery, particularly ureteroneocystostomy, may be causative.

Ureterovaginal fistulae

In 1967 Higgins stated, ''The venial sin is injury to the ureter but the mortal sin is failure of recognition.'' Ureterovaginal fistulae may occur following radical hysterectomy, transvaginal ureterolithotomy, pelvic surgery, or pelvic irradiation. Gynecological surgery is responsible for the majority of these lesions. Urological surgery, including operations for calculi, partial cystectomy, and partial nephrectomy with ureterectomy in a duplicated system, are also etiological factors (Goodwin and Scardino, 1980). Obstetrical trauma is of lesser importance here.

Vesicouterine fistulae

Because of improved obstetrical practice, the incidence of vesicouterine fistulae has decreased. Therefore prolonged labor, difficult forceps delivery, and breech presentations are less important etiological factors in the causation of vesicouterine fistulae. However, a full bladder at the time of labor may predispose the patient to fistula formation. In recent years uterine procedures for therapeutic abortions have become a significant etiological factor.

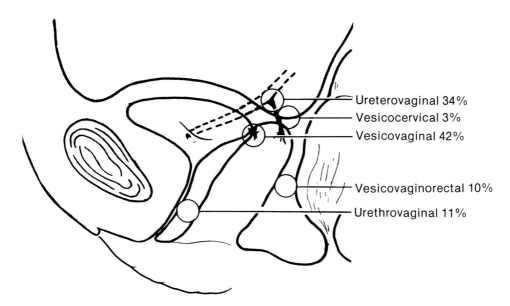

Ureterovaginal 34%
Vesicocervical 3%
Vesicovaginal 42%
Vesicovaginorectal 10%
Urethrovaginal 11%

Figure 20.1 Incidence and site of genitourinary fistulae.

Vesicouterine fistulae are rare but are occasionally seen as a complication following cesarean section through a transverse incision into the lower segment (Henriksen, 1981). These fistulae have an incidence of less than 4% (Petri, 1981) and are therefore of minor importance.

Ureterouterine fistulae

Ureterouterine fistulae may occur following those operations that are also responsible for vesicouterine fistulae. The risk of a ureteric lesion leading to a ureterouterine fistula increases in repeat operations where the ureter is too close to the uterine incision, for example, repeat cesarean sections. Fisher and Lamm (1972) observed 2 ureterocervical fistulae in 570 urogenital fistulae.

MIXED FISTULAE

Mixed fistulae are classified according to the organs that become connected via the fistulae. Three different types are known:

1. Vesicoureterovaginal fistulae
2. Vesicoureterouterine fistulae
3. Vesicovaginorectal fistulae

The causes of these more complicated fistulae are similar to those named previously.

CAUSES

The main causes of fistulae are extensive and repeated surgery, obstetrical trauma, and irradiation. Other recognized predisposing causes include arteriosclerosis, hypertension, diabetes mellitus, obesity, and pelvic inflammatory disease (Van Nagell, Donaldson, and Wood, 1983). Vesicovaginal fistulae are the most common, and the majority are caused by gynecological surgery (Landes, 1979; Goodwin and Scardino, 1980; Patil, Waterhouse, and Laungani, 1980; Tancer, 1980) followed by obstetrical trauma, urological operations, and irradiation.

PREVENTION

In most cases fistulae are not recognized during surgery, especially with recurrent operations. Failure of closure is then a common cause for the fistula. Hutch and Noll (1970) suggest the following guide for prevention of fistulae:

1. Immediate detection of any vesical injury
2. Watertight closure of the defect in the vesical wall
3. Proper drainage
4. An alternative plan (to avoid opening the vagina)

5. Prolonged postoperative vesical training

To facilitate detection of a fistula, staining of the urine with indigo carmine or methylene blue will make an accidental opening of the bladder immediately evident. Besides the recognition of direct extravasation, even accidental dissection of the vesical musculature can be easily seen by the bluish color of the mucosa.

The best way to prevent urterovaginal fistulae is to avoid using blind ligation, especially that involving large portions of unidentified tissue. Therefore identification of the distal ureter is mandatory.

Another cause of fistula development is the accidental lateral uterine tear with bleeding of the uterine vessels during cesarean section. The ureter is frequently harmed by those ligatures required to control the bleeding.

To prevent fistula formation, careful closure of the bladder in two inverted layers together with long-term drainage of the paravesical space and 3 weeks of bladder drainage are recommended.

SYMPTOMS AND SIGNS

The classical symptom of vesicovaginal and ureterovaginal fistulae is continuous incontinence, which has to be distinguished from stress and urge incontinence as well as from incontinence caused by an ectopic ureter. The typical sign is a constant urinary loss day and night, without any symptoms of urge or bladder instability.

The typical sign of a vesicouterine or a ureterouterine fistula is cyclic hematuria and secondary vaginal amenorrhea, to be distinguished from bladder endometriosis (Petri, 1981), with or without incontinence. Iatrogenic ureterovaginal fistulae mainly start with prolonged wound drainage postoperatively, obstruction of the upper urinary tract (with symptoms of obstruction), and secondary wound healing and incontinence.

Urethrovaginal fistulae distal to the sphincteric mechanism may lead to urethral obstruction and inflammation and are often difficult to identify. The most likely symptom of a proximal urethrovaginal fistula is stress incontinence, whereas a fistula in the distal two thirds of the urethra is manifested mainly by postmicturition dribbling.

INVESTIGATION AND DIAGNOSIS

In all cases where a genitourinary fistula is suspect, an intravenous urogram with delayed films in the supine (and also in the oblique or lateral) position is mandatory (see list on opposite page).

Diagnostic aids for vesicourinary fistulae

1. Intravenous urogram + delayed films (+ lateral and oblique positions)
2. Urethrocystoscopy
   Vaginoscopy
3. Retrograde urethrogram
   Retrograde ureterogram
4. Hysterosalpingography ⎫
   Hysteroscopy   ⎬ In vesicouterine and
                        ⎭ ureterouterine fistu-
                          lae
5. Dye test: methylene ⎫
   blue or indigo carmine
   Double-dye test: in-
   travesical carmine ⎬ With sterile swabs in
   solution and intrave- ⎰ vagina
   nous indigo carmine
   (*Cave*: vesicoureteric
   reflux)   ⎭

Urethrocystoscopy and vaginoscopy are both basic diagnostic procedures. Care has to be taken to identify double or combined fistulae, for example, vesicoureterovaginal fistulae. Therefore it is important to use a combination of intravenous urogram and retrograde studies as well as different dye tests (O'Conor, 1980; Petri, 1981; Petri and Hohenfellner, 1981). Our own experiences using the dye test or the double-dye test have been identical to those described by Raghavaiah (1974) and generally have led to the correct diagnosis. Urethrocystoscolporectography (Kümper, Richer, and Koch, 1976) does not seem to be necessary in the diagnosis of genitourinary fistulae. To diagnose uterine fistulae, a hysterosalpingogram and, in exceptional cases, hysteroscopy may be necessary.

In the case of a urethrovaginal fistula, vaginal examination, urethroscopy, and vaginoscopy are helpful. A catheter may be passed through the fistula to aid visualization.

In the case of a vesicovaginal fistula, besides the swab test, cystoscopy and vaginoscopy, especially in the knee-chest position, may be helpful. O'Conor (1975) described the air bubbles that may be seen escaping from the fistulous canal. To facilitate vaginoscopy, Diaz-Ball and Moore (1969) used a balloon catheter to occlude the vaginal introitus for improved filling of the vagina and therefore better visualization of the fistula. A cystoscope was inserted through the side hole of the catheter, and when the catheter balloon was inflated, water distended the vagina, allowing improved visualization. To diagnose ureterovaginal fistulae in cases of mixed fistulae, the double-dye test is of value.

Especially with these types of fistulae, the intravenous urogram with documentation of obstruction or extravasation is very helpful.

PREOPERATIVE MANAGEMENT

The most important factor in preoperative management of genitourinary fistulae is to wait before having the patient undergo surgical repair. This time varies in the literature from 6 weeks to 1½ years (Gonzalez and Fraley, 1976; Landes 1979; O'Conor, 1980; Patil, Waterhouse, and Laungani, 1980; Petri and Hohenfellner, 1981). The conclusion from these suggestions is that a waiting period of 2 to 3 months for surgical lesions and 6 to 12 months for postirradiation fistulae should be observed. The use of local estrogen cream to improve tissue quality and the use of cortisone therapy are controversial. Collins et al. (1967) believed that edema and fibrosis diminished faster with the use of cortisone. Symmonds (1980), however, refutes this therapy because it inhibits wound healing. In general, it may be stated that the exact date of fistula closure depends on the cause, site, and size of the fistula and especially on the quality of the surrounding tissue.

In this waiting phase before surgery, spontaneous fistula closure may happen with catheter drainage or following cystoscopic coagulation of the fistula tract, a technique first described in 1938 (O'Conor, 1980).

Only after inspection of the fistula shows that edema and inflammation have disappeared and that there is good vascularization and good epithelialization of the fistula canal should closure of the fistula be attempted. The most important treatment in this waiting period is kind and sympathetic support for the patient, along with assurance that an optimum time for closure will enhance the eventual success rate. To make this period easier for the patient and socially more acceptable, Landes (1979) suggests using the Wolff-Gilliland vaginal diaphragm catheter, which consists of gluing a Pezzer catheter to a fitted contraceptive diaphragm using rubber cement. This procedure keeps the patient fairly dry and does not interfere with healing of the fistula. Furthermore, it allows the patient freedom of movement.

Another possibility for easing the preoperative waiting period is the use of linking vesical catheters (Magee, 1979). This consists of a self-retaining balloon catheter, inserted via the urethra, linked to a similar catheter inserted via the fistula (Figure 20.2).

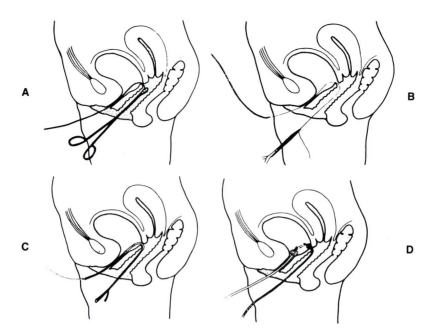

Figure 20.2 Use of linked catheters to obtain continence before fistula repair. **A,** Bougie is introduced via urethra into bladder and exits via fistula. **B,** Fistula catheter is attached to bougie and drawn into fistula. **C,** Fistula catheter is in place. **D,** Urethral and fistula catheters are linked and in place. (From Magee, M. The changing social implications of vesicovaginal fistulas: linking vesical catheters—a useful adjunct. J. Urol. **122**(2):260-262. Copyright 1979, The Williams & Wilkins Co. Reproduced by permission.)

The social situation in this period is best described by Sims, who wrote, "The size of the fistula makes no difference. . . . urine will escape as readily and as rapidly from an opening the size of a goose quill as it will when the whole base of the bladder is destroyed."

O'Conor (1980) wrote, "The exact time for repair depends to a great extent on how the tissues feel and appear when examined cystoscopically and vaginally." During this period he kept the patient free of a catheter and prepared the vagina for operation with an estrogen cream.

TECHNIQUES OF CLOSURE

The controversy over the best route for a fistula operation, such as transvaginal, transvesical, transperitoneal, or combined, depends on the individual situation. Marshall's statement (1979), "Try the best operation the first time" should be remembered. It seems that the vaginal approach is easier to perform with less risk, and from the point of view of morbidity, it is superior to the other approaches. However, the frequent disadvantage of the vaginal approach is loss of functional length of the vagina and possible stress incontinence caused by a decrease in the important mobility of the lower

urinary tract as a result of scar tissue formation. Stress incontinence is encountered postoperatively in 7% to 25% of patients.

Fundamental indications for the use of the abdominal approach are:

1. Fistulae with a diameter greater than 2 cm
2. Fistulae affecting the ureteric orifices
3. Multiple fistulae
4. Vesicocervical fistulae
5. Recurrence of a fistula
6. Poor quality of local tissues (for example, following irradiation, chronic infection, or in diabetes mellitus)

Transvaginal approach

The vaginal approach has advantages in cases of small anteriorly located vesicovaginal fistulae (Eisen et al., 1974). It is a minor procedure that is well tolerated and results in an uneventful recovery. Ueda et al. (1978) suggest the use of a vaginal flap in closure of a vesicovaginal fistula. A Foley catheter is inserted into the bladder via the fistula and pulled to expose the area to be denuded (Figure 20.3, *A*). After denudation, a flap of vaginal mucosa is used to cover the fistula opening, and the remaining surrounding vaginal mucosa is

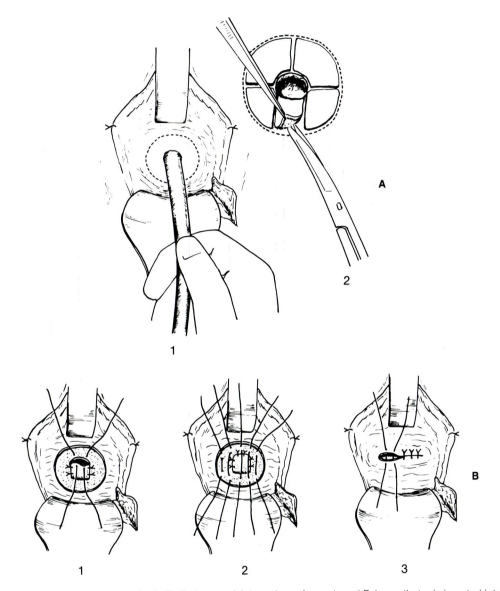

Figure 20.3 Transvaginal repair. **A,** Preliminary episiotomy is performed, and Foley catheter is inserted into fistula, *1.* Vaginal mucosa is removed, *2.* **B,** Vaginal flap is prepared and used to cover fistula, *1.* Submucosa is approximated, *2.* Vaginal mucosa is closed, *3.* (**A** and **B** from Ueda, E., et al. Closure of a vesicovaginal fistula using a vaginal flap. J. Urol. **119**(6):742-743. Copyright 1978, The Williams & Wilkins Co. Reproduced by permission.)   *Continued.*

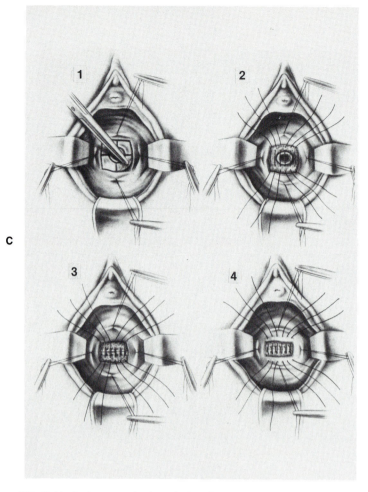

Figure 20.3, cont'd. C, Vaginal mucosa is denuded, *1.* Sutures are inserted into bladder wall, and fistula is closed, *2.* Submucosa sutures are inserted and tied, *3.* Vaginal mucosa sutures are inserted before closure of vaginal defect, *4.* (**C** from Marshall, V.F. Vesicovaginal fistulas on one urological service. J. Urol. **121**(1):25-29. Copyright 1979, The Williams & Wilkins Co. Reproduced by permission.)

removed. After closure of the fistula by the mucosal flap, the submucosal tissue is approximated, followed by closure of the vagina (Figure 20.3, *B*). Rader (1975) suggests closure of vesicovaginal fistulae by partial colpocleisis. He believes that the Latzko partial colpocleisis is easy, fast, and less traumatic, attended by a success rate of 100%. All fistulae are closed with a single operation.

The same technique has been used by Trotnow (1977), who suggests this technique as the method of choice for treatment of posthysterectomy fistula. The interposition of viable gracilis muscle or labial fatty tissue in the management of difficult vesicovaginal and urethrovaginal fistulae is suggested by Patil, Waterhouse, and Laungani (1980). Six of

nine of their patients underwent this repair with a good result.

An interesting modification of the Latzko operation was published by Hribar (1977), who treated a postirradiation fistula with a fascia lata patch and Histoacryl in combination with the Latzko operation. Another vaginal operative technique described by Sims (1852) and by Simon (1854) is excision of the fistula followed by a double-layer closure. This is similar to the technique described by Füth (1918). An important step during this operation is the wide denudation of vaginal mucosa so that the bladder is sufficiently mobilized to permit a multilayer closure of the bladder defect.

Another modification of the vaginal fistula clo-

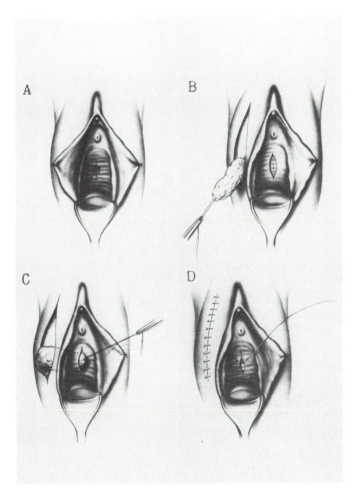

Figure 20.4 Use of labial fat graft. **A,** Fistula is exposed. **B,** Right labial fat graft is prepared. **C,** Graft is slid subcutaneously to site of fistula. **D,** Labial wound and fistula are closed. (From Brikhoff, J.D., et al. Urinary fistulas: vaginal repair using a labial fat pad. J. Urol. **117**(5):595-597. Copyright 1977, The Williams & Wilkins Co. Reproduced by permission.)

sure is interposition of a myocutaneous flap or labial fat pad (Figure 20.4), which is seen as a good alternative to the pedicled omental flap or the pedicled myocutaneous gracilis muscle flap, both of which require a synchronous transabdominal operation (Tölle et al., 1981).

It may be concluded that the indication for vaginal repair of vesicovaginal and ureterovaginal fistulae still depends on the size of the fistula at the first operation. Larger fistulae close to the ureteric orifices, and recurrent fistulae should be closed by a combined or transvesical approach. No attempt should be made, however, to close a postirradiation fistula by the vaginal approach (Trotnow, 1977).

Abdominal closure approach

Indications for the abdominal closure approach have already been outlined (p. 242). There are three different modifications of the transabdominal approach:

1. Simple closure (Figure 20.5)
2. Peritoneal flap interposition (Figure 20.6)
3. Omentum interposition (Figure 20.7)

Besides these three modifications, a combined vaginal-abdominal closure can be used. The patient is placed in the supine position on the operating table with her legs apart, and the vagina is packed tightly with gauze (Gonzalez and Fraley, 1976). The abdominal cavity is opened through a midline

Text continued on p. 250.

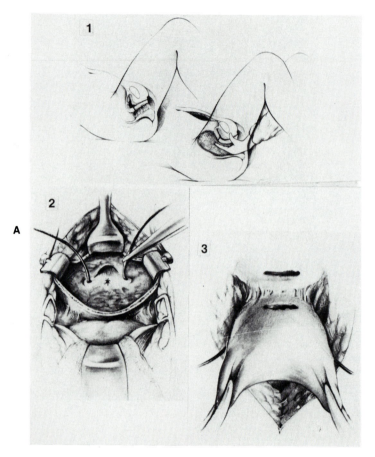

Figure 20.5 Transabdominal repair. **A,** Vagina is packed, *1.* Ureteric catheters are inserted, *2.* Bladder is dissected off vagina to expose fistulous track, *3.* (From Gonzalez, R., and Fraley, E. Surgical repair of post-hysterectomy vesicovaginal fistulas. J. Urol. **115**(6):660-663. Copyright 1976, The Williams & Wilkins Co. Reproduced by permission.)

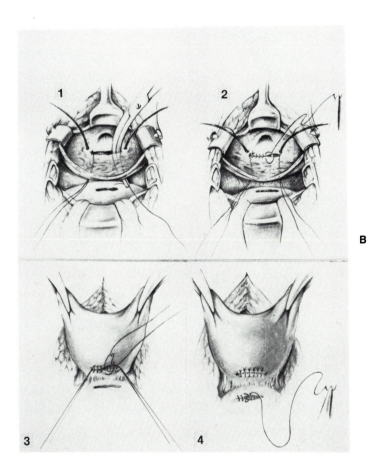

Figure 20.5, cont'd. B, Bladder defect is closed, *1* and *2*. Vaginal defect is closed, *3*. Further layer of bladder sutures is inserted, *4*.

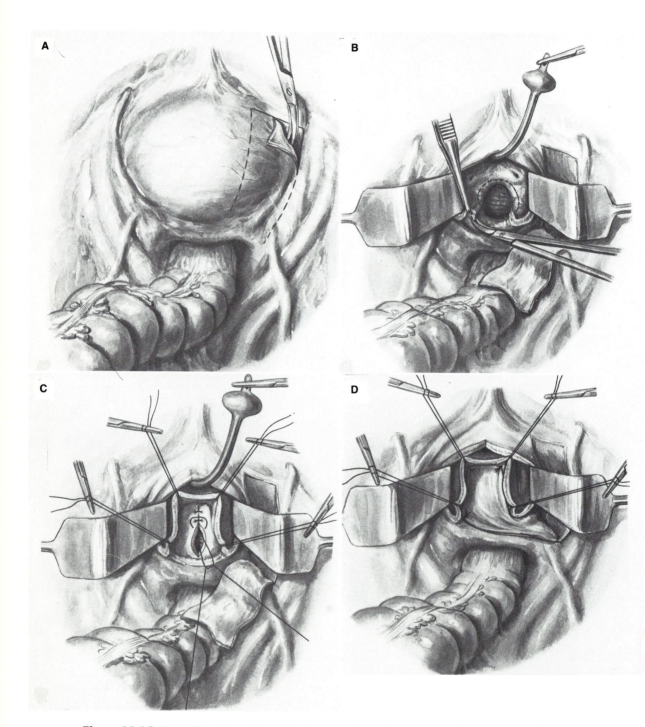

Figure 20.6 Peritoneal flap interposition. **A,** Pedicled peritoneal flap is prepared from paravesical peritoneum. **B,** Scar tissue is removed from around fistula. **C,** Vaginal defect is closed. **D,** Peritoneal flap is placed over vaginal suture line. **E,** Bladder is closed.

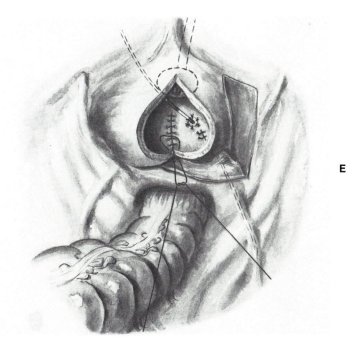

E

Figure 20.6, cont'd. For legend see opposite page.

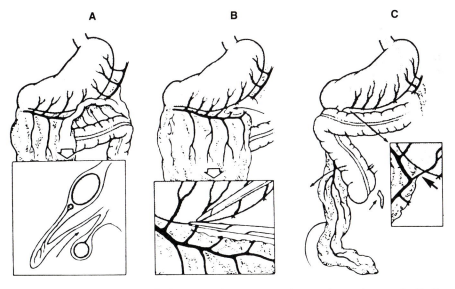

A   B   C

Figure 20.7 Omentum interposition. **A,** Anatomy of greater omentum and vascular supply. **B,** Omentum is dissected, and each short gastric vessel is ligated. **C,** Omentum is rotated on right gastroepiploic artery. *Inset,* Complete mobilization of gastroepiploic arch to its origin from gastroduodenal pedicle avoids traction on last undivided gastric branch. Omental pedicle is positioned behind ascending colon. Prophylactic appendectomy is optional. (From Petri, E., and Hohenfellner. 1981. Der Gynaekologe Heidelberg. Springer-Verlag.)   *Continued.*

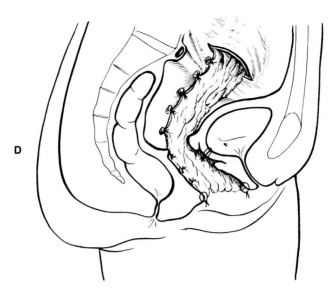

Figure 20.7, cont'd. D, Omentum is in position behind repaired vesical fistula.

or Pfannenstiel's incision. The peritoneum is opened, the bladder carefully identified, and its posterior wall dissected caudally until the fistula track is entered. All authors strongly recommend the careful identification of the bladder, wide mobilization of the bladder and vagina (O'Conor, 1980), and adequate dissection as far as possible to free the posterior wall of the bladder. The fistula track is excised with the help of instruments such as a Young prostatic retractor and two half metal balls (Mobilio and Cosciani Cunico, 1977) (Figure 20.8) or a sponge rubber ball (Landes, 1979) to pull the vagina into the operative field, allowing a more complete excision of the fibrous and necrotic tissue. After generous excision of the fistula track, vaginal closure is perfomed using fresh viable tissue in two layers, followed by a double-layered closure of the bladder. Adequate drainage of the bladder by a suprapubic cystostomy and/or an indwelling urethral catheter for at least 10 days and good wound drainage are mandatory. With recurrent fistulae, however, and in the case of postirradiation fistulae, interposition of a peritoneal flap or omentum is recommended.

Peritoneal flap interposition (Figure 20.6). Peritoneal flap interposition is seen as a method of choice and consists of preparation of a 4 × 6 cm pedicled peritoneal flap from the paravesical peritoneum (Petri and Hohenfellner, 1981). The bladder is widely exposed in the midline down to the fistula track, and as much scarred and necrotic tissue as possible is excised. The vaginal wall is closed as

mentioned previously, and the peritoneal flap is rotated to cover the vaginal suture line. It is of no importance if the serosa is turned to face the vagina or the bladder. Bladder closure follows as described previously.

Omental patch graft reconstruction (Figure 20.7). Omental patch graft reconstruction is especially advocated by Turner-Warwick (1976), who describes omentum as "the only body tissue specifically developed for the resolution of infected processes." The greater omentum is mobilized on the right gastroepiploic artery and rotated down to use as an additional layer between the bladder and the vagina. Since the preparation of the omentum requires extensive dissection with some morbidity (for example, ileus), this technique should be used more specifically for the closure of larger defects, in cases of poor-quality tissue (for example, following irradiation or in cases of chronic infection, necrosis, or diabetes), and in cases where it is difficult to obtain an adequate dissection of the bladder and vagina. This type of operation seems to be the method of choice in the case of extended vesicovaginorectal fistulae (Petri and Hohenfellner, 1981). Omentum and surrounding tissue heal satisfactorily, leading to good occlusion between the vagina and the bladder.

Combined closure approach

Marshall (1979) favors the combined technique in large fistulae, especially those caused by irradiation. A liberal excision of the vaginal mucosa

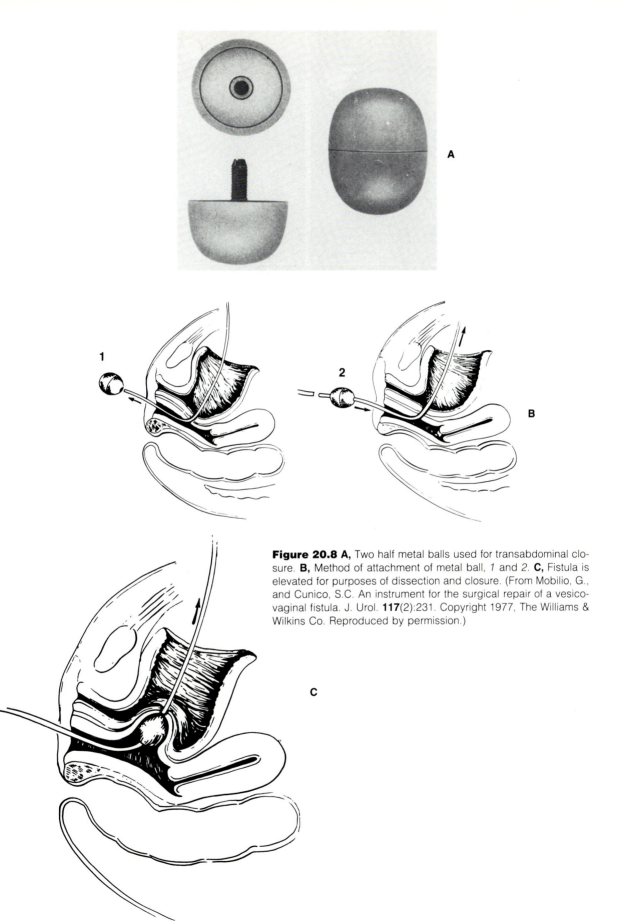

Figure 20.8 A, Two half metal balls used for transabdominal closure. **B,** Method of attachment of metal ball, *1* and *2.* **C,** Fistula is elevated for purposes of dissection and closure. (From Mobilio, G., and Cunico, S.C. An instrument for the surgical repair of a vesico-vaginal fistula. J. Urol. **117**(2):231. Copyright 1977, The Williams & Wilkins Co. Reproduced by permission.)

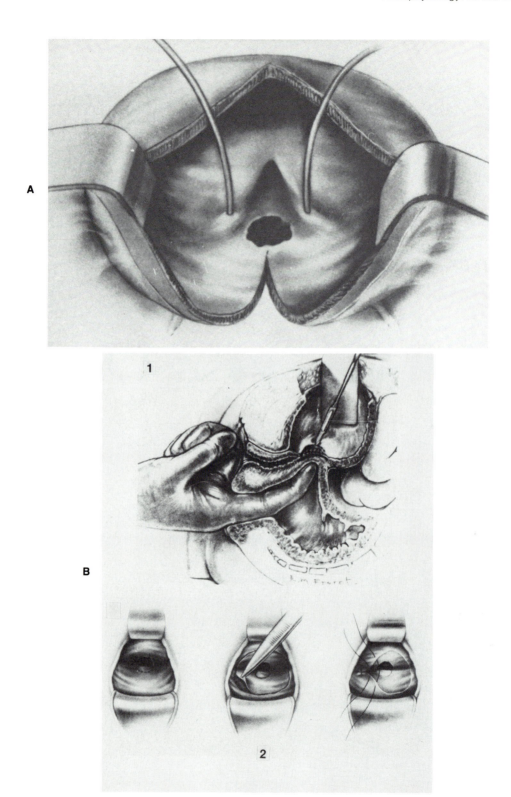

Figure 20.9 Combined closure. **A,** Midline section of posterior bladder wall is performed to expose fistula. **B,** Fistula is dissected from bladder aspect, *1*. Fistula is dissected and closed from vaginal aspect, *2*. (From Marshall, V.F. Vesicovaginal fistulas on one urological service. J. Urol. **121**(1):25-29. Copyright 1979, The Williams & Wilkins Co. Reproduced by permission.)

with colpocleisis is performed via the vagina in combination with a transvesical closure of the vesical defect (Figure 20.9).

In the case of fistulae that are very close to the ureteric orifices, ureteric reimplantation may become necessary during closure. The technique reported by Politano and Leadbetter (1958) seems to be the method of choice.

With ureterovaginal fistulae, a Boari flap plasty (1894) or a psoas hitch procedure may be necessary. Furthermore, in the case of a combined vesicoureterovaginal fistula or vesicoureteric reflux, closure of the defect in the urinary bladder or the distal ureteric stump becomes necessary.

Closure of vesicoureterouterine fistula. The technique described by Jobert de Lamballe in 1852 wherein the cervical canal is covered with part of the portio vaginalis, leading to diversion of menstrual blood via the bladder, was the first attempt at treating vesicouterine fistulae. Single cases of conservative treatment have been reported in which hormonally induced amenorrhea led to spontaneous closure. Other spontaneous closures have been observed following transurethral or transrenal urinary drainage.

Low vesicocervical fistulae can be treated vaginally via colpotomy. The bladder and cervix are separated and closed in two layers. However, for better identification, a transperitoneal transvesical approach seems to be in favor. Hysterectomy is not mandatory, but it can be performed. Again, peritoneal flap interposition and omental flap interposition are methods of choice.

POSTOPERATIVE CARE

The most important feature of the postoperative management is the maintenance of good urinary drainage by means of an indwelling urethral catheter and/or a suprapubic catheter. Suggestions on the duration of catheter drainage vary from 2 to 14 days (Rader, 1975; Tancer, 1980). The technique recommended is to leave an indwelling urethral catheter for a few days and maintain good urinary drainage via the suprapubic cystostomy for 2 weeks. This combined suprapubic and transurethral urinary drainage avoids postoperative retention caused by blood clot.

Low-pressure suction as suggested by Marshall (1979), which is automatically interrupted (bubble suction), may also be used.

Suprapubic drainage allows early removal of the transurethral catheter with less danger of ascending infection and without urethral irritation.

Ureteric catheters are used only when ureteric reimplantation becomes necessary because of extended fistulae or ureterovaginal fistulae.

Wound drainage from the retroperitoneal space is necessary. Penrose or suction drains are favored. The duration is generally 3 to 4 days, depending on the volume that is drained.

The use of broad-spectrum antibiotics is recommended. The vaginal pack is left for no longer than 3 days. The patient is mobilized after 1 week, and stool softeners may be given. Sexual activity should be prohibited for at least 3 to 4 months following surgery (Patil, Waterhouse, and Laungani, 1980).

TABLE 20.1 First-attempt closure of vesicovaginal fistulae according to technique

Route	Technique	Closure (%)	No.	Author
Vaginal	Füth-Mayo	76	34	Lange and Hardt, 1977
	Sims	94	157	Keettel et al., 1978
	Döderlein	96	29	Massoudnia, 1974
	Latzko	92	38	Käser, 1977
	Moir	70	40	Steg, Vialatte, and Olier, 1977
Abdominal	Bladder rotation flap	87	56	Carl and Praetorius, 1974
	Omental pedicle graft	100	27	Kiricuta and Goldstein, 1971
	O'Conor	75	20	O'Conor et al., 1973
	Peritoneal flap	90	54	Petri and Hohenfellner, 1981

From Petri, E., and Hohenfellner, R. 1981. Gynakologe **14**:177-182.

COMPLICATIONS

Fistula recurrence is the most important complication. With the Latzko procedure, reduction of the functional vaginal length may occur. Scar tissue formation following closure may lead to stress incontinence in 7% to 25% of patients. Reoperation should be performed using the abdominal route. This approach is mandatory when the ureters are affected. Only in the case of recurrent failure is urinary diversion using an ileal conduit, colon conduit, or ureterosigmoidostomy indicated (Goodwin and Scardino, 1980).

RESULTS

The percentage of success using the vaginal route varies from 70% to 94% (Table 20.1) (Petri and Hohenfellner, 1981). Similar results are to be expected using the abdominal approach; Petri and Hohenfellner (1981) found the percentage of success to be from 75% to 100%. O'Conor (1980) described a spontaneous fistula closure in 6 of 42 patients following catheter drainage. Spontaneous fistula closure in a vesicouterine fistula by producing hormonally induced amenorrhea was described by Rubino (1981).

REFERENCES

Boari, A., 1894. Contributo sperimentale alla plastica dell' uretere. Atti Accad. Sci. Med. Nat. Ferrara. **68**:149-154.

Carl, P., and Praetorius, M. 1974. Der transvesikale Verschluss von Blasenscheidenfisteln. Geburtshilfe Frauenheilkd **34**:699-705.

Collins, C.G., et al.: 1971. Early repair of vesicovaginal fistula. Am. J. Obstet Gynecol. **111**:524-528.

Diaz-Ball, F.L., and Moore, C.A. 1969. A diagnostic aid for vesicovaginal fistula. J. Urol. **102**:424-426.

Eisen, M., et al. 1974. Management of vesico-vaginal fistulas with peritoneal flap interposition. J. Urol. **112**:195-198.

Fallon, B., and Culp, D. 1983. The urologic examination. In Buchsbaum, H.J., and Schmidt, J.D., editors. Gynaecologic and obstetric urology. Ed. 2. Philadelphia. W.B. Saunders Co.

Fisher, W., and Lamm, D. 1972. 30 Jahre Urogenitalfisteln an der Berliner Universitats-Frauenklinik (1941 bis 1970). Zentralbl. Gynaekol. **94**:1603-1622.

Füth, H. 1918. Zur Operation der Blasenscheidenfisteln. Arch. Gynaekol. **109**:489-497.

Gonzalez, R., and Fraley, E.E., 1976. Surgical repair of posthysterectomy vesicovaginal fistulas. J. Urol. **115**:660-663.

Goodwin, W.E., and Scardino, P.T. 1980. Vesico-vaginal and uretervaginal fistulas: a summary of 25 years of experience. J. Urol **123**:370-374.

Henriksen, H.M. 1981. Vesico-uterine fistula following caesarean section. J. Urol. **125**:884.

Higgins, C.C. 1967. Ureteral injuries during surgery: a review of 87 cases. JAMA **199**:82-88.

Hribar, I. 1977. Der interessante Fall: Verschluss einer Vesicovaginalfistel mit Hilfe eines aufgeklebten Patches. Altern Urologie **8**:221-223.

Hutch, J.A., and Noll, L.E., 1970. Prevention of vesico-vaginal fistulas. Obstet. Gynecol. **35**:924-927.

Käser, O. 1977. The Latzko operation for vesico-vaginal fistulae. Acta Obstet. Gynecol. Scand. **56**:427-431.

de Lamballe, J. 1852. Traité des fistules vésico-utérines, vésicoutéro-vaginales, etc. Paris. Cited in Bardescu, N. 1900. Ein neues vefahren für die Operation der tiefen Blasen-Uterus-Scheidenfisteln. Zentralbl. Gynaekol. **6**:170-182.

Keettel, W.C., et al. 1978. Surgical management of urethrovaginal and vesicovaginal fistulas. Am. J. Obstet. Gynecol. **131**:425-431.

Kiricuta, I., and Goldstein, A.M.B. 1972. The repair of extensive vesicovaginal fistulas with pedicles omentum: a review of 27 cases. J. Urol. **108**:724-727.

Kümper, H.J., Richer, K., and Koch, J. 1976. Darstellung gynäkologischer Fisteln im Docht-Urethrozystokolporektogramm. Urol. Int. **31**:401-409.

Landes, R.R. 1979. Simple transvesical repair of vesico-vaginal fistula. J. Urol. **122**:604-606.

Lange, J., and Hardt, W. 1977. Ergebnisse bei der Behandlung von Fisteln und Stenosen der unteren Harnwege in Gynäkologie und Geburtshilfe. Geburtshilfe Frauenheilkd **37**: 322-326.

Magee, M.C. 1979. The changing social implications of vesicovaginal fistulas: linking vesical catheters—a useful adjunct. J. Urol. **122**:260-262.

Marshall, V.F. 1979. Veisco-vaginal fistulas on the urological service. J. Urol. **121**:25-29.

Massoudnia, N. 1974. Ein Beitrag zur "Einrollplastik" nach G. D'auoderlein zur operativen Behandlung grober Blasen—und Harnröhrenscheidenfisteln. Zentralbl. Gynaekol. **96**:624-629.

Mobilio, G., and Cosciani-Cunico, S. 1977. An instrument for the surgical repair of a vesico-vaginal fistula. J. Urol. **117**:231.

O'Conor, V.J., Jr. 1975. Female urinary incontinence and vesico-vaginal fistula. In Glenn, J.F., editor. Urologic surgery. New York. Harper & Row, Publishers, Inc.

O'Conor, V.J., Jr. 1980. Review of experience with vesicovaginal fistula repair. J. Urol. **123**:367-369.

O'Conor, V.J., Jr., et al. 1973. Suprapubic closure of vesicovaginal fistulas. J. Urol. **109**:51-54.

Patil, U., Waterhouse, K., and Laungani, G. 1980. Management of 18 difficult vesico-vaginal and urethro-vaginal fistulas wtih modified Infelman-Sundberg and Martius operations. J. Urol. **123**:653-656.

Petri, E., 1981. Vesiko und uretero-uterine Fisteln (editorial). Aktuel. Urol. **12**:265-266.

Petri, E., and Hohenfellner, R. 1981. Zur Therapie komplizierter Blasenscheidenfisteln. Gynakologe **14**:177-182.

Politano, V.A., and Leadbetter, W.F. 1958. An operative technique for the correction of vesico-urethral reflux. J. Urol. **79**:932-941.

Rader, E.S. 1975. Post-hysterectomy vesicovaginal fistula: treatment by partial colpocleisis. J. Urol. **114**:389-390.

Raghavaiah, N.V., 1974. Double-dye test to diagnose various types of vaginal fistulas. J. Urol. **112**:811-812.

Rubino, S.M. 1980. Vesico-uterine fistula treated by amenorrhea induced with contraceptive steroids. Br. J. Obstet. Gynaecol. **87:**343-344.

Simon, G. 1854. Ueber die Heilung der Blasenscheidenfisteln. Giessen.

Sims, J.M. 1852. The treatment of vesicovaginal fistula. Am. J. Med. Sci. **23:**59-83.

Steg, A., Vialatte, P., and Olier, C. 1977. Le traitement des fistules vésico-vaginales par la technique Chassar-Moir. Ann. Urol. **11:**103-107.

Symmonds, R.E., 1980. Verhutung und Behandlung von Urogenital-fisteln. Extracta Gyneacol. **4:**103-116.

Tancer, M.L. 1980. The post-total hysterectomy (vault) vesicovaginal fistula. J. Urol. **123:**839-840.

Tölle, E., et al.: 1981. Verschluss eines grossen Blasen-Harnröhren-Scheidenwanddefektes durch gestielten myokutanen Musculus-gracilis-Lappen. Urologe (1) 274-277.

Trotnow, S. 1977. Fruh und Spatergebnisse bei der Behandlung von Blases-Scheiden-Fisteln durch vaginale Operationsverfahren. Urologe (A) **16:**267-271.

Turner-Warwick, R. 1976. The use of the omentum pedicle graft in urinary tract reconstruction. J. Urol. **116:**341-347.

Ueda, T., et al. 1978. Closure of a vesico-vaginal fistula using a vaginal flap. J. Urol. **119:**742-743.

Van Nagell, J.R., Jr., Donaldson, E.S., and Wood, E.G. 1983. Urinary tract involvement by invasive cervical cancer. In Buchsbaum, H.J., and Schmidt, J.O., editors. Gynaecologic and obstetric urology. Ed. 2. Philadelphia. W.B. Saunders Co.

chapter 21

Voiding difficulties and retention

STUART L. STANTON

Voiding difficulties and retention represent a gradation of failure of bladder emptying. In the woman, it is a poorly documented condition mainly because it is frequently misdiagnosed. Since it rarely progresses to upper tract dilatation and renal failure, it is not associated with mortality, but its morbidity is significant. The disorders are a spectrum, ranging from an asymptomatic condition diagnosed on the basis of urodynamic studies to an acute condition with chronic retention, which is recurrent with a familiar but sometimes confusing clinical presentation.

Most gynecological and urological textbooks fail to mention voiding difficulties and retention as separate entities. Any reference made is usually to the treatment of retention, with scant attention paid to cause or investigation.

The absence of clear definitions presents a further difficulty in attempting to classify and clarify these disorders. Fox, Jarvis, and Henry (1976) and

Farrar and Turner-Warwick (1979), when discussing chronic retention and outflow obstruction, fail to define the conditions at all. Doran and Roberts (1976) define acute retention in women as "a painful and acute onset with less than 1 litre of urine obtained on catheterisation." In men, Abrams, Dunn, and George (1978) define chronic retention as "a residual urine over 300 ml, the minimum volume at which the bladder becomes palpable suprapubically." Neither of these definitions are wholly satisfactory. Concerning acute retention, the onset may be painless, for example, following an epidural anesthetic or in spinal shock, and in such circumstances the amount of urine may be much larger than 1 L. It is reasonable that the need for catheterization be introduced into the definition to enable the history of voiding difficulty to be interpreted correctly, to allow for objective measurement of the amount of urine withdrawn, and to distinguish this condition from chronic retention. The amount of urine that needs to be present to qualify for "acute" or "chronic" retention is controversial and should be a mimimum rather than a maximum amount. The reason for imposing a lower limit is to avoid including patients who claim to have retention, yet on catheterization have small amounts removed, well below the maximum cystometric capacity (International Continence Society definition). It is unrealistic to propose a volume without referring to the maximum cystometric capacity.

DEFINITIONS AND CLASSIFICATION
(Table 21.1)

The most common terms are acute retention and chronic retention. I would define these as follows:

Acute retention—A sudden painful or painless inability to void over a 24-hour period, requiring catheterization, which yields at least 50% of the maximum cystometric capacity.

Chronic retention—An insidious failure of bladder emptying that results in at least 50% of the maximum cystometric capacity being retained. There are two phases: in the earlier phase the patient is able to control voiding although it is impaired; there may be straining, a poor stream, and frequency. In the later stage voiding is uncontrolled, and overflow incontinence occurs.

TABLE 21.1   Classification of voiding difficulty

Condition	Symptom	Sign	Urodynamic data
Asymptomatic voiding difficulty	Urgency and frequency caused by urinary tract infection	± Palpable bladder	Peak flow rate < 15 cm H_2O Maximum voiding pressure may be elevated ± Residual urine
Symptomatic voiding difficulty	Poor stream Incomplete emptying Straining to void ± Symptoms of urinary tract infection	± Palpable bladder	Peak flow rate < 15 cm H_2O Maximum voiding pressure may be elevated ± Residual urine
Chronic retention ± overflow	Poor stream Incomplete emptying Straining to void Frequency ± Incontinence ± Symptoms of urinary tract infection	Palpable bladder	Peak flow rate may be reduced Residual urine ± Upper tract dilatation ± Acontractile
Acute retention	Painful or painless symptoms of primary cause	Palpable bladder	Residual urine
Acute with chronic retention	Painful or painless symptoms of primary cause Past history of chronic retention ± Incontinence ± Frequency	Palpable bladder	Residual urine ± Upper tract dilatation ± Acontractile

There are two phases through which patients may pass before encountering either acute or chronic retention: asymptomatic voiding difficulty and symptomatic voiding difficulty.

Asymptomatic voiding difficulty is a situation wherein the patient is unaware of impaired bladder emptying. The urinary stream is reduced, and the peak flow rate is below 15 ml/sec. The maximum voiding pressure is usually normal, and there may not be any residual urine. Urinary tract infection may be present.

The next stage in bladder decompensation is when symptoms of voiding difficulty appear, for example, a poor stream, straining to void, and incomplete emptying. The urinary flow rate is reduced to below 15 ml/sec, and the maximum voiding pressure may be elevated. There may be residual urine, as well as associated urinary tract infection. Of 600 women attending a urodynamic clinic with lower urinary tract symptoms of bladder dysfunction, 12 patients (2%) had proved to be asymptomatic and 87 patients (14%) had proved to have symptomatic voiding difficulties. In the asymptomatic group the patients were older and had a higher incidence of pelvic surgery and psychiatric illness. The residual urine volume was appreciably greater in the symptomatic group. When these patients with voiding difficulties were analyzed, the ones who complained directly of a voiding difficulty had a greater residual urine volume than those patients in whom symptoms of voiding difficulty were not as distressing, as for instance, symptoms of stress incontinence, urgency, or frequency (Stanton, Ozsoy, and Hilton, 1983).

ETIOLOGY AND PATHOPHYSIOLOGY

Voiding occurs in the woman when the intravesical pressure exceeds the intraurethral pressure. This is accomplished by relaxation of the urethral sphincter mechanism and pelvic floor, with or without detrusor contraction or with the help of abdominal straining.

The causes of voiding difficulties are varied, as indicated below.

Causes of voiding difficulties and retention

I. Neurological
   A. Upper motor neuron lesion
   B. Lower motor neuron lesion
   C. Autonomic lesion
   D. Local pain reflex
II. Pharmacological
   A. Tricyclic antidepressants
   B. Anticholinergic agents
   C. α-Adrenertic stimulating agents
   D. Ganglionic blocking agents
   E. Epidural anesthesia
III. Acute inflammation
   A. Acute urethritis
   B. Acute vulvovaginitis
   C. Acute anogenital infection
IV. Obstruction
   A. Distal urethral stenosis
   B. Acute urethral edema of surgery
   C. Chronic urethral fibrosis
   D. Foreign body, calculus
   E. Impacted pelvic mass
      1. Retroverted gravid uterus
      2. Hematocolpos
      3. Uterine fibroid
      4. Ovarian cyst
   F. Urethral distortion with cystocele
   G. Ectopic ureterocele
V. Endocrine
   A. Hypothyroidism
   B. Diabetic neuropathy
VI. Overdistention: acontractile or hypotonic detrusor
VII. Psychogenic

Neurological lesions

Neurological lesions either cause failure of detrusor contraction or failure of the urethral spincter mechanism and pelvic floor to relax, or they may result in an incoordinate action between the detrusor and the sphincter, called detrusor sphincter dyssynergia. These conditions occur when there is a lesion or interruption in the coordinating center for micturition, in the brainstem, or in the afferent and efferent pathways between the brainstem, sacral spinal cord, or parasympathetic and sympathetic systems supplying the bladder and urethra.

Lesions of discrete areas of the brain (frontal lobes, internal capsule, reticular formation of the pons, and cerebellum) can produce voiding difficulty and urinary retention as well as other disorders of micturition. Lesions lower down the micturition pathway, for example, in the cord or affecting autonomic innervation, are more likely to lead to voiding difficulties and retention. If hypertonic or hyperreflexic activity occurs, continence or retention will depend on whether the tone in the urethral sphincter mechanism and outlet resistance is greater than or less than the pressure developed within the bladder.

Pharmacological causes

Drugs that interfere with the release and action of acetylcholine at cholinergic synapses or neuromuscular junctions, such as tricyclic antidepressants, anticholinergic agents (for example, atropine or propantheline bromide), and ganglionic blocking agents may produce voiding difficulties, usually when voiding is already impaired. The α-stimulating drugs can produce voiding difficulties by increasing bladder outflow resistance. Epidural anesthesia, by preventing transmission of nerve impulses in the afferent and efferent supply to the bladder, leads to temporary retention.

Acute inflammation

Voiding difficulties can result from painful stimuli produced by urine coming into contact with inflamed mucosa of either the urethra or vagina. This may be aggravated by local edema of urethral mucosa. Urethritis, vulvovaginitis, and anogenital herpetic infection may all produce retention. It has been suggested that genital herpes is associated with sacral meningomyelitis and radiculitis and that this is the cause for retention (Oates and Greenhouse, 1978).

Obstruction

There are a variety of conditions that will cause outflow obstruction. Distal urethral stenosis, usually a menopausal condition, is detected on attempting endoscopy or passing a catheter for cystometry or videocystourethrography. Acute urethral edema may be a result of bladder neck surgery, such as anterior colporrhaphy, and will resolve within 2 to 3 days: it is difficult to evaluate the role of pain following surgery in the genesis of retention. Urethral edema secondary to premenstrual fluid retention, resulting in acute urinary retention proceding each period, has occurred in one patient whom I have seen.

Chronic urethral fibrosis, probably complicated by urethritis, is a long-term effect of bladder neck and urethral surgery. The urethra becomes converted into a narrow and almost rigid tube. Foreign bodies and calculi are rare causes of urethral obstruction in women.

Extrinsic causes of obstruction include impaction of a retroverted gravid uterus at about 14 weeks' gestation, as well as impaction of uterine fibroids and ovarian cysts. Hematocolpos is a rare condition that can cause retention if it becomes impacted in the pelvis; it usually is manifested by primary amenorrhea, monthly low abdominal pain, and pelvic swelling that may be palpable abdominally.

Urethral distortion associated with a cystocele is an uncommon cause of voiding difficulty (Figure 21.1).

Finally, an ectopic ureterocele is a cause of lower

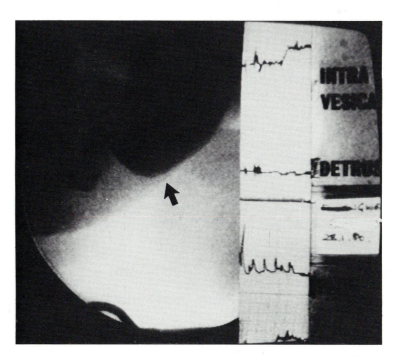

Figure 21.1 Videocystourethrogram image showing large cystocele.

urinary tract obstruction in children and will cause urinary retention if it prolapses through the bladder neck.

Endocrine causes

Both hypothyroidism and diabetes mellitus can cause peripheral neuropathy and in turn urinary retention as a result of detrusor atony or acontractility.

Overdistention

Bladder overdistension as a result of mismanagement of acute or chronic retention or of idiopathic origin will compound any preexistent voiding difficulty; often voiding disorders in the elderly woman are a result of an acontractile or hypotonic bladder of large capacity and unknown cause. This does not imply that all large bladders are functionally abnormal. Weir and Jacques (1974) noted that in a series of 52 women with a bladder capacity greater than 800 ml, 33% were normal on urodynamic testing and only 13% had an atonic or acontractile detrusor.

Psychogenic causes

Psychogenic causes of urinary retention are well recognized (Barrett, 1978; Krane and Siroky, 1979). Criteria for this diagnosis are an absence of neurological and other significant organic disease, correlation of psychological disturbance with the onset of symptoms, and a significant response to psychotherapy and psychopharmacological treatment. Because the diagnosis of psychiatric illness may be misapplied to any subsequent symptom or condition and because this diagnosis still carries a social stigma, it should be made only after careful evaluation of the case and exclusion of all other diagnoses. Psychiatric diagnosis includes hysteria, depression, and schizophrenia, the majority of patients being neurotic rather than psychotic.

The consequences of failure of bladder emptying are overflow incontinence, recurrent urinary tract infection, and sometimes upper tract dilatation. The latter occurs partly as a result of a high pressure system developing within the obstructed bladder and partly as a result of passive vesicoureteric reflux. It is less common in women than in men.

PRESENTATION
Symptoms

In a few patients impaired voiding may be asymptomatic, but in the majority it is associated with a variety of lower urinary tract symptoms. The most reliable symptom is the complaint of a poor stream, then incomplete emptying, and straining to void (Stanton, Ozsoy, and Hilton, 1983). Where there is residual urine (more than 50% of the maximum cystometric capacity), there may be a complaint of frequency. Overflow incontinence may occur with chronic retention, and if the residual urine becomes infected, the symptoms of urinary tract infection will be present.

In addition, there may be symptoms referable to the primary cause of the voiding difficulty; therefore the history should be directed to detecting this. A drug history should always be taken and note made of any recent genital or urinary tract infection. Recent past pelvic surgery, particularly around the bladder neck, should be enquired about; there is good objective evidence that anterior colporrhaphy does not cause voiding difficulty (Stanton et al., 1982; Walter et al., 1982), but the colposuspension (Stanton and Cardozo, 1979) and sling procedures (Beck, 1978) are known to produce them.

Signs

The patient should be examined for signs of the primary cause of impaired voiding, according to the outline on p. 258. A neurological examination should be performed and the back examined for stigmata of an underlying spinal cord disorder. After the patient voids, a pelvic examination is carried out to exclude residual urine. Bimanual palpation will detect a residual volume of 200 ml or more, and simple suprapubic palpation will detect a bladder with 300 ml or more. It is also important to exclude other pelvic masses, such as uterine fibroids, early pregnancy, and an ovarian cyst. The latter is sometimes mistaken for a full bladder and vice versa. Not infrequently, a patient may be taken to the operating room for removal of an "ovarian cyst" that disappears on catheterization.

Any urethral or vulvovaginal inflammation is noted. The urethra is palpated for tenderness, and scarring and prolapse should be demonstrated.

Finally, the patient's demeanor should be carefully noted to detect any sign of abnormal psychiatric behavior.

INVESTIGATIONS

The two fundamental investigations are uroflowmetry and cystometry, both of which define the condition and quantify it. The remaining investigations will identify the cause and help quantify the voiding difficulty.

Urinary diary

It is necessary to have a record of urinary output when a patient with frequency and incomplete emptying is being managed and certainly when catheterization has been performed. It is vital to note the amount removed from the bladder at the initial catheterization. The diary or fluid balance chart can be maintained by the patient herself when not in hospital; otherwise, this is an important function of the nursing staff. During the recovery phase following treatment of a voiding difficulty, the urinary diary is a useful method of assessing progress.

Uroflowmetry

Uroflowmetry (see Chapter 11) is the most important initial screening procedure and is simple and noninvasive. The measurement should be made in privacy, and the patient should have a comfortably full bladder. A lower limit of 15 ml/sec, for a voided volume of at least 150 ml, is accepted as normal in women. Values below this require further measurement to exclude artifacts. The flow rate depends on several factors, including the volume voided, the state of the detrusor, and outflow resistance. The effect of the volume voided is shown in Figure 21.2. Urine flow rates for volumes below 150 ml are unreliable. Many patients will record volumes below their peak flow rate when voiding

at maximum bladder capacity, so the patient should be encouraged to attend with a comfortably full bladder.

A normal flow pattern is shown in Figure 21.3, in comparison with reduced flow rates associated with unsustained detrusor contractions and abdominal straining, as illustrated in Figure 21.4. Other than these two examples, it is not possible to distinguish among further causes of reduced flow rate by using uroflowmetry alone.

Some patients with outflow obstruction may void in excess of 15 ml/sec, and this is accomplished by a higher than normal maximum voiding pressure; to detect this, it is necessary to simultaneously measure the maximum voiding pressure and urine flow rate during cystometry (Figure 21.5). When these values are represented graphically, a more complete view of micturition is obtained (Figure 21.6).

Cystometry

The filling phase of cystometry may indicate a lower or upper motor neuron lesion. The voiding phase of cystometry will confirm any disorder of bladder emptying.

The following cystometric changes may be found in cases of voiding difficulty and retention:

Residual urine—Increased above 50 ml

First sensation—Earlier if upper motor neuron lesion, otherwise (including lower motor neuron lesion) may be greatly delayed (500 to 600 ml)

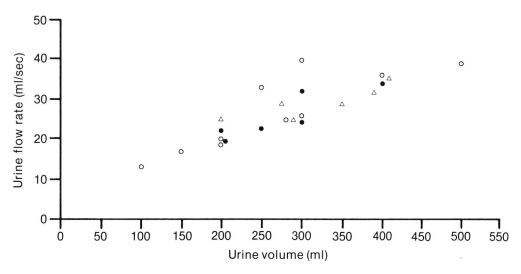

Figure 21.2 Effect of increasing bladder volume on peak flow rate in three asymptomatic and urodynamically normal young nulliparas.

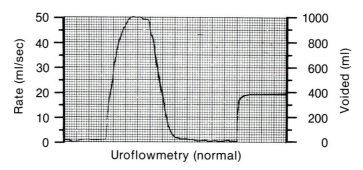

Figure 21.3 Normal peak urine flow rate, showing "bell-shaped" curve rising to maximum flow rate of 50 ml/sec for volume voided of 400 ml in 14 seconds.

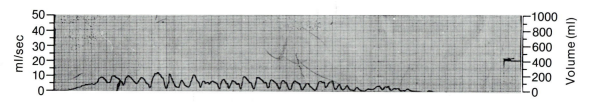

Figure 21.4 Reduced peak urine flow rate with straining.

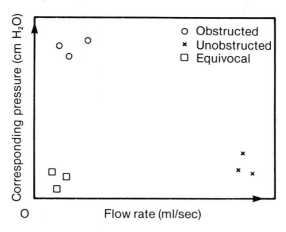

Figure 21.5 Relationship between maximum voiding pressure and flow rate.

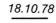

18.10.78

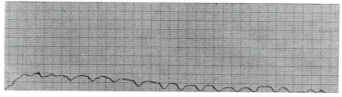

10/440 (90 sec)

Urethrotomy 5.12.78

4.1.79

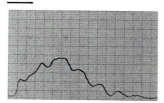

23/310 (40 sec)

9.8.79

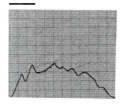

20/340 (30 sec)

3.1.80

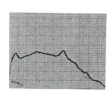

22/300 (27 sec)

Figure 21.6 Several uroflow recordings showing progress after initial low uroflow *(top)* and subsequently following urethrotomy.

Capacity—Smaller with upper motor neuron lesion, otherwise (including lower motor neuron lesion) may be greatly extended

Pressure rise on filling and on standing—Elevated with an upper motor neuron lesion, otherwise may be normal

Isometric pressure—May be decreased (below 15 cm H_2O)

Maximum voiding pressure—May be raised if the bladder is not decompensated; if the bladder is decompensated, it may be within the normal range.

The residual urine volume is a good indicator of bladder efficiency, provided the patient has voided normally and in privacy beforehand. While absence of residual urine does not exclude a voiding disorder or outflow obstruction (Farrar and Turner-Warwick, 1979), the presence of a residual urine volume of more than 50 ml is not normal, and interpretation and management will depend on the clinical situation and remainder of the urodynamic data. An isolated instance of residual urine is usually not of significance.

Measurement of the isometric contraction pressure (P_{iso}) may give some indication of the reserve potential of the detrusor. To calculate this pressure, the patient is asked to stop micturition during the voiding phase. If the urethral sphincter mechanism can close and arrest the urinary stream while the detrusor contraction is present, the detrusor pressure rises. A pressure above 15 cm H_2O is believed to be evidence of the normal potential of detrusor function, but there is much need for further scientific evidence concerning this. Values below 15 cm H_2O may indicate early detrusor failure.

The presence of a lower motor neuron lesion may be detected by use of the bethanechol supersensitivity denervation test. This is based on Cannon's law, that denervated smooth muscle is supersensitive to its natural transmitter. Cystometry is performed, and the bladder pressure is noted at 100 ml bladder volume. A subcutaneous injection of 2.5 mg of bethanechol is given and cystometry repeated after 30 minutes. An increase in detrusor pressure to greater than 15 cm H_2O is indicative of denervation. The test is, however, not entirely reliable, and caution and clinical judgment are needed in its interpretation.

Radiology

Plain abdominal radiograph. A plain abdominal radiograph will disclose a full bladder (see Figure 16.6). Occasional evidence of past indiscretions, such as injections of heavy metal to cure tabes dorsalis, which will cause loss of bladder sensation and contractility of the detrusor, may be found (see Figure 9.2).

Lumbosacral spine radiograph. A lumbosacral spine radiograph will disclose anatomical lesions of the spinal column, such as the congenital lesion of spina bifida occulta with diastomatomyelia and tethering of the filum terminale (see Figure 9.6), sacral agenesis (see Figure 9.5), disk space narrowing and prolapse of the intervertebral disk (see Figiure 9.10), and spondylolisthesis (see Figure 9.11).

Videocystourethrography. The combination of radiological screening of the bladder and cystometry usually involves the patient's voiding in the sitting or standing position; both require micturition in as much privacy as possible. If the patient cannot void erect during screening, there should be easy access to a private room where voiding can occur over a flowmeter, with pressure lines in situ.

The main value of radiological screening is to show whether outflow obstruction is at the bladder neck (which is rare in women) or in the distal urethra—distal urethral stenosis (see Figure 9.34). Detrusor activity will be indicated by detrusor pressure measurements, which allow a distinction to be made between an acontractile detrusor and an unsustained voiding contraction. The presence of vesicoureteric reflux may be demonstrated.

Intravenous urogram. Upper tract dilatation (hydronephrosis and hydroureter) can occur with outflow obstruction and may be relatively asymptomatic. Fortunately, these conditions are rare in women. The rare condition of an ectopic ureterocele, bilateral in 10% of patients, may show a filling defect in the bladder and dysplasia of the associated renal unit.

Endoscopy

Initial difficulty in passing an endoscope may indicate distal urethral stenosis.

It is not possible to confirm or refute bladder neck obstruction in women on the basis of endoscopy alone (Farrar and Turner-Warwick, 1979). Videocystourethrography is needed for this.

Trabeculation, a frequent finding in women, may occur in cases of outlet obstruction and detrusor instability and is not necessarily a diagnostic feature of either. The value of endoscopy lies in the elucidation of such symptoms as accompany voiding difficulty, such as frequency and urgency, which result from bladder calculi, foreign bodies (intentionally or otherwise introduced), or mucosal lesions such as papillomata. Occasionally a rare condition such as ectopic ureterocele may be found.

Electromyography

Detection of spasticity or increased tone in the urethral sphincter mechanism is desirable but difficult to achieve in practice. Use of external anal sphincter electromyographic activity is commonplace (Blaivas and Labib, 1977); the innervation is similar to that of the periurethral striated component of the urethral sphincter mechanism, and since most women can pass water and not wind simultaneously, the technique lacks accuracy.

The urethral sphincter is composed of differing smooth and striated muscles, and the practical difficulties of being able to accurately sample any one of these components are great. The periurethral striated muscle is the easiest to record. Single-fiber electromyography using an oscilloscope to accurately locate the needle in the muscle group is the most likely method of achieving success, but the fundamental difficulty of knowing exactly in which muscle the needle is placed still remains.

TREATMENT
Prophylactic measures

It is known that difficulty in resuming spontaneous voiding occurs in over 45% of patients after radical pelvic surgery for gynecological malignancy (Fraser, 1966; Smith et al., 1969) in over 60% of patients undergoing vaginal surgery for incontinence and cystocele (Cameron, 1966), in patients undergoing sling operations (Beck, 1978), in elderly patients undergoing incontinence operations (Stanton and Cardozo, 1980), and, finally, following the use of epidural anesthesia for gynecological or obstetrical procedures. This indicates a preemptive need to drain the bladder after all these maneuvers. Whether a urethral or suprapubic catheter should be used is discussed elsewhere (see Chapter 37). Obtaining a preoperative flow rate to detect asymptomatic voiding difficulties is important before embarking on any of these operations. If found, the likelihood of postoperative delayed voiding should be explained to all patients. The indications for some nonmalignant operations may require revision if a significant voiding difficulty is detected, since undoubtedly some procedures (for example, sling operations) will certainly aggravate

the condition and lead to retention. Concerning epidural anesthesia, either the patient is catheterized at the time of the epidural anesthesia and the catheter is then removed 24 hours later, or, if voiding has not occurred 6 hours following epidural anesthesia, the patient is then catheterized. Either way, the medical and nursing staff should be responsible for ensuring that normal micturition is resumed.

Definitive treatment

The cause and effect should be treated simultaneously. When acute retention is present, there is clearly some urgency to institute bladder drainage promptly. The following modes of treatment may be used.

Drug therapy. Detrusor-stimulating drugs include acetylcholine-like preparations, for example, bethanechol (Myotonine) given 5 to 10 mg subcutaneously or 25 mg q.d.s. orally, increasing by 25 mg q.d.s. until side effects (gastrointestinal colic) or voiding occurs, prostaglandin E_2 (Bultitude, Hills, and Shuttleworth, 1976; Stanton, Cardozo, and Kerr-Wilson, 1979), and prostaglandin $F_{2\alpha}$ (Vaidyanathan et al., 1981). Anticholinesterase compounds, such as distigmine bromide (Ubretid), which act as parasympathomimetic agents, stimulate the detrusor to contract by inactivating cholinesterase, which destroys the endogenous acetylcholine. The dosage is 0.5 mg intramuscularly daily or a 5 mg tablet daily.

To diminish urethral resistance, an α-adrenergic blocking agent such as phenoxybenzamine (Dibenzyline) is given 10 mg orally initially, increasing by 10 mg q.d.s. until side effects (faintness or hypotension) or voiding occurs. (Before these drugs are given, lying and standing blood pressures and an electrocardiogram should be taken).

Diazepam (Valium), which is a muscle relaxant and an anxiolytic, can be given as night sedation (in a dose of 10 to 20 mg) for patients undergoing surgery, and this has been found to be effective in initiating voiding postoperatively (Stanton, Cardozo, and Kerr-Wilson, 1979).

Urethral dilatation. Urethral dilatation is a time-honored method of increasing the urethral caliber and facilitating voiding. It seems to lack precision and consistency because of the variations in the types and sizes of dilators that are available. However, some clinicians believe that there is less fibrosis formed after dilatation than after urethrotomy.

Internal Otis urethrotomy. Urethrotomy is car-

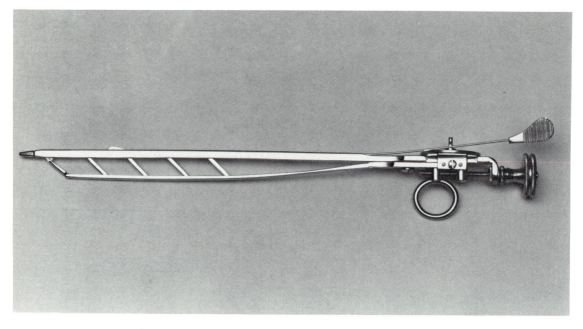

Figure 21.7 Otis urethrotome partially open with blade in place.

ried out using an Otis urethrotome (Figure 21.7). This produces longitudinal cuts that are 2 mm deep. Three of these are made at the 4, 8, and 12 o'clock positions while the patient is anesthetized, starting with the calibration, for example, at 38 and increasing to 40 or 42 with each successive cut. An indwelling Foley catheter of 26 to 28 gauge is left in place for 2 to 5 days of continuous drainage (Worth, 1980). Urethrotomy performed in the presence of uninhibited detrusor contractions or a high detrusor pressure may result in incontinence. Postoperative progress can be assessed by means of a urinary diary (which will indicate increased voiding volumes) and uroflowmetry.

Intermittent self-catheterization. Intermittent self-catheterization was first described by Lapides et al. (1972), principally for neurogenic bladder disorders, but it is now used for chronic retention, including that caused by psychogenic factors. The patient has to be reasonably dexterous and is taught by the nursing staff using a clean technique and a mirror: the patient lies down initially, and when she becomes proficient using a mirror, she is taught to catheterize the external urethral meatus by feel without using a mirror, when sitting or standing over a toilet. For those patients preferring visual aids, a metal catheter with an attached mirror has been devised. As well as catheterization, the patient is encouraged to reflexively empty the bladder and use straining and Credé's maneuver. The daily frequency of catheterization will vary; the aim is to avoid incontinence and keep the bladder empty.

Specific conditions

Asymptomatic voiding difficulty. There is no active treatment for asymptomatic voiding difficulty unless these is a urinary tract infection associated with a residual urine volume. The treatment is then use of an appropriate antibiotic combined with drug therapy and urethrotomy to try to diminish the residual urine. Uninfected residual urine, in the absence of upper tract dilatation, does not normally require treatment.

Symptomatic voiding difficulty. For treatment of symptomatic voiding difficulty, the same principles apply as stated previously except that symptoms indicate a deterioration in bladder function; therefore drug therapy or urethrotomy is needed to facilitate emptying and relieve the symptoms.

Chronic retention with overflow. Treatment of chronic retention with overflow is required on the principle that the symptoms and the presence of recurrent urinary tract infection and deterioration in the upper urinary tract are of concern. Appropriate antibiotic therapy according to culture and sensitivity should be used. Drug therapy to decrease urethral resistance or increase detrusor contractility may be helpful and should be tried. Intermittent self-catheterization probably has most to offer here and should be used. If that fails, internal urethrotomy or urethral dilatation is indicated.

Acute retention. In the treatment of acute retention, it is particularly important that both the cause of retention is searched for (see outline below) and the bladder is drained. Concerning the cause, neurological conditions will require consultation with a neurologist or neurosurgeon and may require prolonged care. Retention caused by drug therapy may be reversed if the dosage of the particular drug can be reduced or curtailed. Inflammatory causes should respond to appropriate antibiotic therapy and will require catheter drainage during the acute inflammatory phase. Obstructive causes are treated by the appropriate surgical procedure. An impacted retroverted gravid uterus can be gently anteverted with the patient under light general anesthesia with little risk of miscarriage or of continued retention. Recovery from the peripheral neuropathy of hypothyroidism or diabetes may take many weeks, but usually it is eventually reversible. Thyroid replacement will be needed for hypothyroidism.

Neurological disorders causing voiding difficulty and retention

I. Lesions of the brain
   A. Cerebrovascular disease
   B. Parkinsonism
   C. Multiple sclerosis
II. Lesions of the spinal cord
   A. Spinovascular disease
   B. Conus medullaris or cauda equina tumors
   C. Prolapsed intervertebral disk
   D. Spinal stenosis
   E. Spinal arachnoiditis
   F. Tabes dorsalis
   G. Multiple sclerosis
   H. Spinal cord injury
   I. Dysraphic lesions
III. Lesions of autonomic innervation
   A. Autonomic neuropathy
   B. Sacral agenesis
   C. Corda equina tumors
   D. Spinal cord injury

The chances of recovery in a thin-walled hypotonic overdistended bladder are slight. The female bladder responds poorly to obstruction, and overdistension occurs readily. Operations to reduce the capacity of the bladder are theoretically dubious and in practice rarely work. Finally, acute retention from psychogenic causes will require psychiatric help.

The controversy of suprapubic versus urethral catheter drainage is referred to in Chapter 37. If it is thought that a single catheterization will relieve retention, a No. 12 or 14 French urethral catheter should be inserted, the bladder drained and the amount noted, and the catheter withdrawn. An accurate fluid balance chart must be maintained over the next 24 hours to confirm normal voiding. If single catheterization is not thought to be likely to succeed or has been tried already, a self-retaining urethral Foley catheter of the same gauge may be left in place for 48 hours and then removed.

Catheterization for longer than 48 hours is best managed with a suprapubic catheter such as a Bonnano, which permits voiding via the urethra and avoids recourse to repeated urethral catheterization if the patient is unable to void spontaneously. Regular catheter specimens of urine for culture and sensitivity should be sent, and antibiotic treatment is necessary only if bacteriuria is associated with evidence of tissue invasion, that is, fever or suprapubic or loin pain (see Chapter 26).

Acute on chronic retention. The main difference between acute retention and the foregoing condition is its chronicity and likelihood of recurrence. Therefore simple indwelling catheterization is unlikely to be successful, and suprapubic catheterization combined with drug therapy should be tried. Once voiding resumes, the treatment of chronic retention should then be adopted.

CONCLUSION

Voiding difficulties in women are still poorly understood. Prompt treatment of acute retention and the need to detect early impairment of bladder function before certain types of surgery must be emphasized.

REFERENCES

Abram, P.H., Dunn, M., and George, N. 1978. Urodynamic findings in chronic retention of urine and their relevance to results of surgery. Br. Med. J. **2:**1258-1260.

Barrett, D. 1978. Evaluation of psychogenic urinary retention. J. Urol. **120:**191-192.

Beck, R.P. 1978. The sling operation. In Buchsbaum, H.J., and Schmidt, J.D., editors. Gynecologic and obstetric urology. Philadelphia. W.B. Saunders Co.

Blaivas, J.G., and Labib, K. 1977. Acute urinary retention. Urology **10:**383-389.

Bultitude, M., Hills, N., and Shuttleworth, K. 1976. Clinical and experimental studies on the action of prostaglandin and the synthesis inhibitors on detrusor muscle in vitro and in vivo. Br. J. Urol. **48:**631-637.

Cameron, M.D. 1966. Distigmine bromide (Ubretid) in the prevention of post-operative retention of urine. Br. J. Obstet. Gynaecol. **73:**847-848.

Farrar, D., and Turner-Warwick, R. 1979. Outflow obstruction in the female. In Turner-Warwick, R., and Whiteside, C.G. Clinical urodynamics. Urol. Clin. North Am. **6:**217-225.

Fox, M.J., Jarvis, G., and Henry, L. 1976. Idiopathic chronic urinary retention in the female. Br. J. Urol. **47:**797-813.

Fraser, A.C. 1966. The late effects of Wertheim's hysterectomy on the urinary tract. Br. J. Obstet. Gynaecol. **73:**1002-1007.

Krane, R., and Siroky, M. 1979. Psychogenic voiding dysfunction. In Krane, R., and Siroky, M., editors. Clinical Neuro-urology. Boston. Little, Brown & Co.

Lapides, J., et al. 1972. Clean intermittent self-catheterization in the treatment of urinary tract disease. J. Urol. **107:**458-461.

Oates, J., and Greenhouse, P.R. 1978. Retention of urine in ano-genital herpetic infection. Lancet **1:**691-692.

Smith, P.H., et al. 1969. The urological complications of Wertheim's hysterectomy. Br. J. Urol. **41:**685-688.

Stanton, S.L., and Cardozo, L. 1979. A comparison of vaginal and suprapubic surgery in the correction of incontinence due to urethral sphincter incontinence. Br. J. Urol. **51:**497-499.

Stanton, S.L., and Cardozo, L. 1980. Surgical treatment of incontinence in elderly women. Surg. Gynecol. Obstet. **150:**555-557.

Stanton, S.L., Cardozo, L., and Kerr-Wilson, R. 1979. Treatment of delayed onset of spontaneous voiding after surgery for incontinence. Urology **13:**494-496.

Stanton, S.L., Ozsoy, C., and Hilton, P. 1983. Voiding difficulties in the female: prevalence, clinical and urodynamic review. Obstet. Gynecol. **61:**144-147.

Stanton, S.L., et al. 1982. Clinical and urodynamic effects of the anterior colporrhaphy and vaginal hysterectomy for prolapse with and without incontinence. Br. J. Obstet. Gynaecol. **89:**459-463.

Vaidyanathan, S., et al. 1981. Study of intravesical instillation of 15(S)–15 methyl prostaglandin $F_{2\alpha}$ in patients with neurogenic bladder dysfunction. J. Urol. **126:**81-85.

Walter, S., et al. 1982. Urodynamic evaluation after vaginal repair and colposuspension. Br. J. Urol. **54:**377-380.

Weir, J., and Jacques, P. 1974. Large capacity bladder, Urology **4:**544-548.

Worth, P. 1980. Urethrotomy. In Stanton, S., and Tanagho, E., editors. Surgery of female incontinence. Heidelberg. Springer-Verlag.

chapter 22

Congenital anomalies

PETER H.L. WORTH and SIR JOHN DEWHURST

part one UROLOGICAL ASPECTS

part two GYNECOLOGICAL ASPECTS

part one
UROLOGICAL ASPECTS

Peter H.L. Worth

The development of the kidney and ureter is a complex matter, and it is not surprising that there are many congenital anomalies. It is always difficult to be certain of the true incidence of congenital anomalies of the urinary tract, because they tend to be associated with a high incidence of disease, making the clinical incidence higher than the postmortem incidence. It is fair to say that finding a congenital abnormality does not necessarily mean that it is the cause of a particular symptom, and not infrequently one finds a duplicated system on the contralateral side to a patient's pain. Since ab-

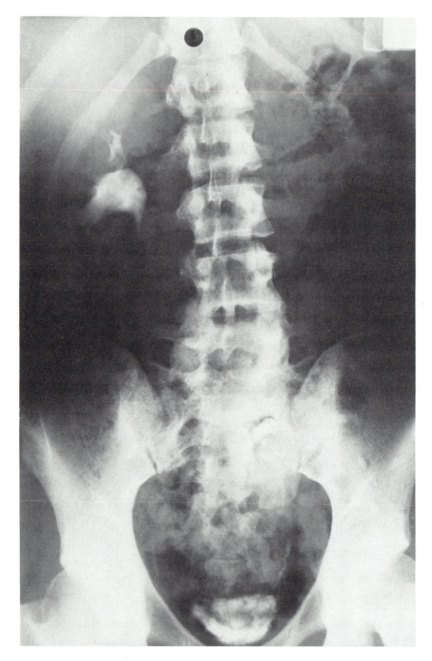

Figure 22.1 Intravenous urogram showing left pelvic kidney. Note absence of left kidney from its normal anatomical site. Lower left ureter can be seen, and there is contrast in calyx overlying sacrum.

normal genitalia are said to be associated with upper tract anomalies in a third of cases, it would be wise to do an intravenous urogram in such a situation.

CONDITIONS ASSOCIATED WITH ABNORMAL KIDNEY POSITION OR WITH FUSION
Pelvic kidney

The incidence of a pelvic kidney (Figure 22.1) is about 1 in 800, and 1 in 2000 if there is only one kidney. It may present as a pelvic mass on vaginal examination and is a rare cause of obstruction in labor. A solitary pelvic kidney often has multiple blood vessels and may cause hypertension. A pelvic kidney may be missed on a routine intravenous urogram, because the calyces overlie the sacrum and the contrast may merge imperceptibly with the bone. If the diagnosis of a pelvic kidney is not entertained, serious problems can be encountered if a laparotomy is undertaken. No attempt should ever be made to remove a pelvic kidney without having full information about the contralateral kidney.

Crossed ectopia

Crossed ectopia has an incidence of about 1 in 2000. The kidney may be in close proximity or fused with the opposite kidney (Figure 22.2). The ureter usually opens in the normal position. This kidney, as with other forms of ectopia, may be more easily palpable, therefore the investigation of any abdominal mass should include an intravenous urogram before laparotomy or laparoscopy is undertaken. No specific treatment is indicated unless some disease is present.

Horseshoe kidney

The incidence of a horseshoe kidney is approximately 1 in 6000. These kidneys are usually fused across their lower elements and may therefore be easily palpable. They are often associated with other congenital abnormalities, especially cardiac problems. They also have a high incidence or urological problems, for instance, pelviureteric junction obstruction, which may be accompanied by pain and urinary infection. The intravenous urogram is characteristic, with malrotation of both kidneys, and the lower calyx usually lies medial to the ureter (Figure 22.3). When surgery is required, there is nothing to be gained by dividing the bridge, because these kidneys often have multiple blood

vessels and the kidneys will not fall back into their normal position if the bridge is divided.

RENAL MASS

Although there are many causes of renal enlargement, there are two that should be discussed.

Hydronephrosis

Hydronephrosis is secondary to pelviureteric junction obstruction and is caused by an abnormality at the pelviureteric junction that fails to allow propulsion of urine down the ureter. As a result, the pelvis and calyces enlarge and in some cases may contain more than a liter of urine. In 10% of cases the condition is bilateral. The severity of the obstruction will dictate at what age the individual becomes symptomatic. Symptoms may be vague loin pain, intermittent in nature and often worse at night. The pain may be precipitated by a large fluid load. If infection develops in the presence of this obstruction, the patient may be quite ill, with a high fever associated with abdominal pain and vomiting, and it is certainly a condition to be considered in a pregnant patient with severe loin pain.

The intravenous urogram may be very abnormal (Figure 22.4), but if it is performed on a patient in a dehydrated state, the kidney may occasionally appear normal. Where there is a strong suspicion that the diagnosis has been missed on standard radiology, the intravenous urogram should be repeated, with the patient hydrated following the injection of contrast medium and given a diuretic. This may then cause the pelvis to distend. A diuretic renogram will also show whether the isotope leaves the kidney or is held up.

Treatment is by some form of pyeloplasty, which either removes the obstruction, such as the Anderson-Hynes procedure, or opens it out, such as the Culp procedure. Nephrectomy is rarely necessary, but, if carried out, close follow-up of the remaining kidney is necessary because a subclinical obstruction at the pelviureteric junction may become real, since the remaining kidney has to cope with an increased urine output. An obstructed kidney loses its concentrating ability; therefore its removal may more than double the urine output of the remaining kidney.

Polycystic disease

Polycystic disease (Figure 22.5) is an important condition in women because there are two types.

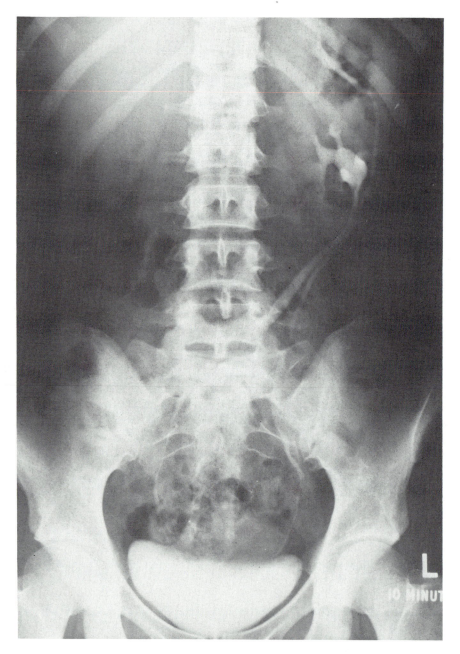

Figure 22.2 Intravenous urogram showing crossed ectopia. Both kidneys can be seen on left side, but one ureter crosses over to right side.

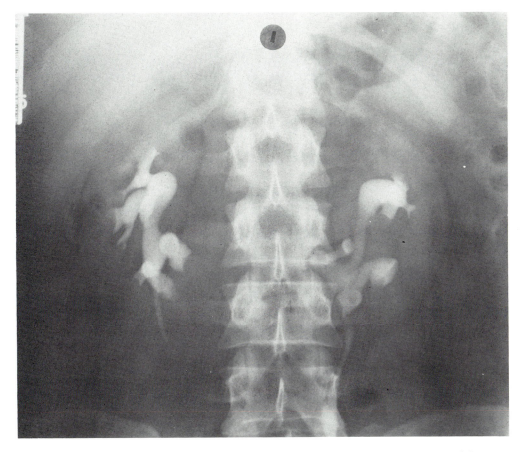

Figure 22.3 Intravenous urogram showing horseshoe kidney. Note that lower calyces lie medial to ureters and that lower border of kidney can be traced across vertebrae.

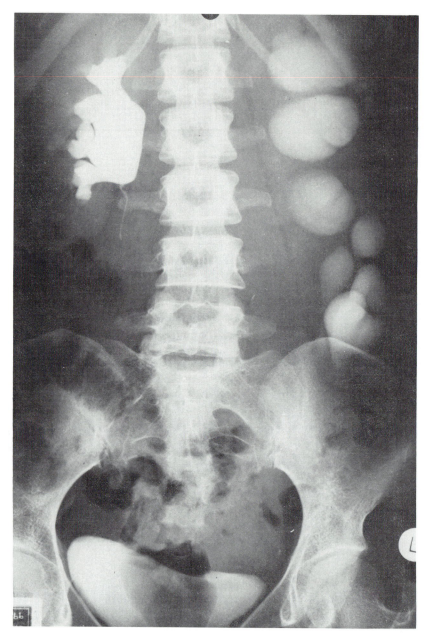

Figure 22.4 Intravenous urogram showing pelviureteric junction obstruction. Note gross hydronephrosis on left side. There is also distended pelvis on right side with narrow upper ureter.

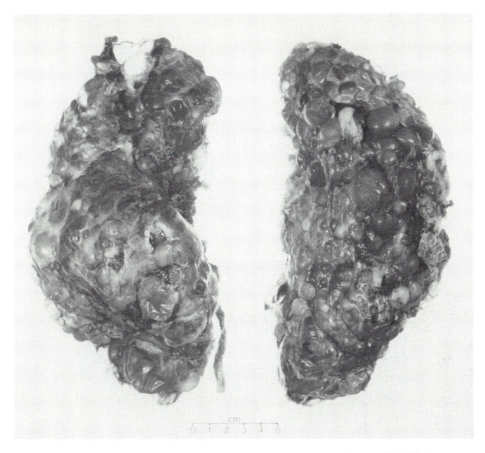

Figure 22.5 Typical polycystic kidney with gross deformity of substance showing fluid-filled cysts, some of which contain blood.

First, there is the congenital variety, which may interfere with labor and cause problems not only to the fetus but also to the mother, and second, there is the adult form of the disease, which is inherited. This type may not appear until middle age, which is usually after childbearing, and one cannot give a guarantee to an individual even in the presence of a normal intravenous urogram that she will not manifest the condition. More severe forms manifest themselves earlier, and pregnancy may be contraindicated because of renal failure. Associated hepatic and pancreatic cystic disease may also be present. The congenital variety is autosomal recessive, and the adult form is autosomal dominant. There is an abnormality of the development of the collecting ducts and tubules, which also fail to fuse. In adults, 95% are bilateral; therefore the finding of bilateral renal swelling should suggest the diagnosis. Patients often have bouts of pain, infection, and hematuria and may have hypertension.

The disease is readily diagnosed on the basis of intravenous urogram but must be distinguished from other forms of cystic disease that in fact are often unilateral. Until the patient is symptomatic or uremic, no specific treatment is necessary. Life expectancy is usually 5 to 10 years after the diagnosis has been made, but these patients are considered for transplantation. Unlike other patients with renal failure, they are not usually anemic; therefore at least one kidney should be preserved until the time of transplantation.

EXSTROPHY

Bladder exstrophy and its variants are easily recognized. However, female epispadias is difficult to identify, and occasionally the only problem is an incompetent bladder neck. This may be recognized on an intravenous urogram with a slightly wide symphysis and contrast in the proximal urethra (Figure 22.6).

Exstrophy is obvious, and the diagnosis is easy

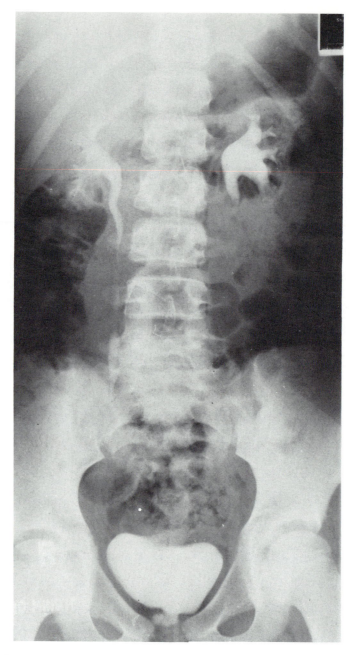

Figure 22.6 Female epispadias, with contrast in proximal urethra and widening of symphysis pubis.

(Figure 22.7). Treatment will depend on the potential bladder capacity. If it appears adequate (this is assessed by pressing in the defect with the patient under anesthesia), it can be closed in a complex way. The bladder neck and the urethra will need to be reconstructed using a Young-Dees procedure. Muscle closure is obtained by Z-plasties, and skin closure is achieved by rotation flaps. Whether os-

teotomies of the sacroiliac joints are necessary is very debatable, but some authors favor it, especially in the younger child. Ureteric reflux often occurs later, and subsequent reimplantation may be indicated.

If the bladder capacity is thought to be too small, diversion is necessary. This should not be done until about the age of 3, when the potential function

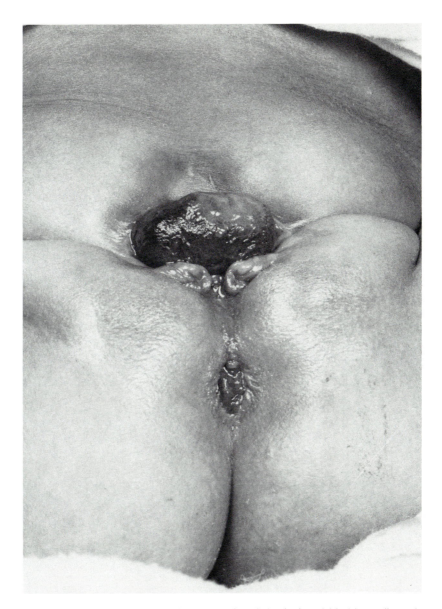

Figure 22.7 Bladder exstrophy showing absent anterior abdominal and bladder walls and exposure of posterior bladder wall. Clitoris is separated and anus is anteriorly placed.

of the anal sphincter can be assessed. Ureterosigmoidostomy has been popular in this condition and has resulted in good sphincter control. There are problems with this diversion, but if it works well, it is very satisfactory. Hyperchloremic acidosis can be controlled with sodium bicarbonate supplements but often results in poor growth. Pyelonephritis can be controlled with antibiotics. Hypokalemia, which results from diarrhea and tubular damage, is corrected with potassium supplements. What has emerged over the years is that there is a real chance of carcinoma of the colon developing at the site of the ureteric anastomoses. If the intravenous urogram shows an obstructed upper tract when previously it had been all right, or if rectal bleeding occurs, colonoscopy should be done. The latent interval for a tumor to develop is on the order of 20 to 30 years, so that if diversion was done at the age of 3 years, there is a real risk of cancer occurring in the young patient. Surgical excision of the tumor is necessary with conversion to an ileal conduit.

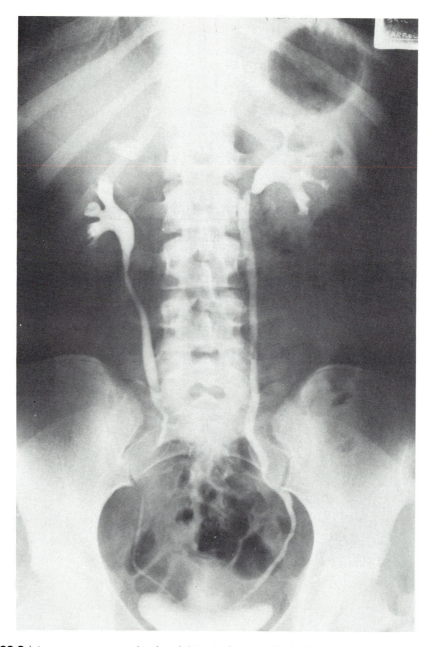

Figure 22.8 Intravenous urogram showing right ectopic ureter in duplex system. Note contrast in upper calyx and displacement of lower calyces.

An alternative initial diversion could be a colonic or ileal conduit. There is a real risk of decreasing renal function over the years with intestinal conduits, and there is no real evidence to suggest that colonic conduits, with their potentially lower pressure, have a better prognosis than ileal conduits. It is important to have a reflux preventing ureteric anastomosis and a free draining conduit without stomal stenosis.

URETERIC DUPLICATION

Degrees of duplication vary from a bifid pelvis to a completely double ureter opening separately into the bladder. Duplication occurs as a result of premature division of the metanephric bud and is relatively common. It may be asymptomatic, and certainly it should not be assumed that it is responsible for symptoms just because it is found. Incomplete duplication may cause pyelonephritis

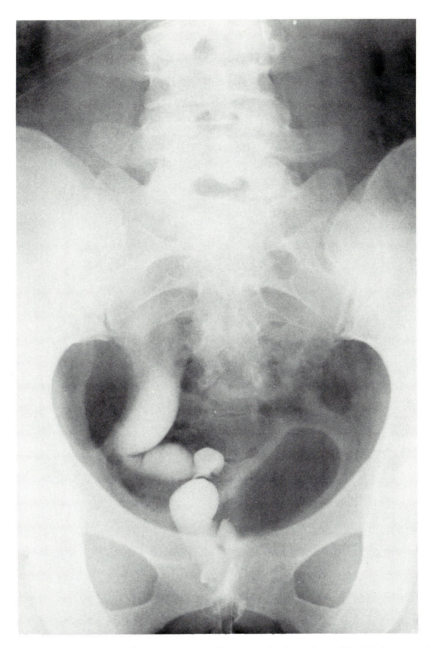

Figure 22.9 Right ascending ureterogram showing ectopic ureter outlined in lower part.

by means of the so-called yo-yo phenomenon, wherein reflux occurs from one to the other because of a slightly abnormal segment just below where they join. In complete duplication, it is usually the lower pole ureter with the higher insertion that is likely to reflux, because it has a shorter course through the bladder wall; therefore it is the lower pole that may be scarred.

An ectopic ureter may be single or part of a

duplex system (Figure 22.8). The single ectopic ureter will result in incontinence because the bladder neck and trigone are usually deficient. This can usually be seen on an intravenous urogram with low insertions of the ureter and a wide-open bladder neck. Treatment is difficult, because not only will bladder neck reconstruction be necessary, but both ureters will need to be reimplanted.

An ectopic ureter that is part of a duplex system

usually is manifested by dribbling incontinence, that is, the patient passes urine quite normally but is always a little damp in between times. Patients do not always admit to this symptom, and the diagnosis may then be difficult. One woman I saw only admitted to the symptom after her daughter had been cured of her incontinence by removal of an ectopic ureter. Some patients are not affected by dribbling incontinence until they are in their late teens, and sometimes their initial symptom is a kidney infection with the onset of sexual intercourse. This late appearance of symptoms may be a result of the fact that the terminal part of the ureter is intimately related to the bladder neck muscle, and if the ureter opens into the urethra, the distal mechanism may have sufficient strength to control the leakage. These ureters may open anywhere from the bladder neck down to the urethra or in the perineal skin or in the vagina, and the opening may be very difficult to identify (Figure 22.9). It is not essential to find the opening, but it is helpful to do so. The intravenous urogram has a classical appearance, with the lower part of the kidney lying laterally, with the pelvis flattened and the ureter displaced laterally (Figure 22.8). It may be possible to see the outline of the kidney, and the giveaway (if the upper pole calyx is not visualized) is the long distance from the edge of the uppermost calyx to the renal border. With high-dose tomography some excretion may be seen. Occasionally the intravenous urogram may look normal. If a duplex system is obvious or suspected on one side, the other kidney should be carefully inspected in case there is a similar problem that is not so obvious.

As already mentioned, it may be difficult to identify the ectopic ureter, even if the urine is stained with Pyridium or methylene blue. A catheter can be inserted into the ectopic ureter under direct vision and into the other ureter through a cystoscope. Contrast is then injected through both catheters so that a rewarding radiograph can be obtained. Occasionally the opening may be quite big, and an ectopic ureter has been catheterized by a urethral catheter in the course of a micturating cystogram.

Treatment involves removing that part of the kidney draining into the ectopic ureter (Figure 22.10). The kidney usually has more than one artery and vein; therefore the abnormal ureter should be carefully freed from the lower pole ureter. The branch of the renal artery going to the apex of the kidney should be isolated and tied and an upper pole partial

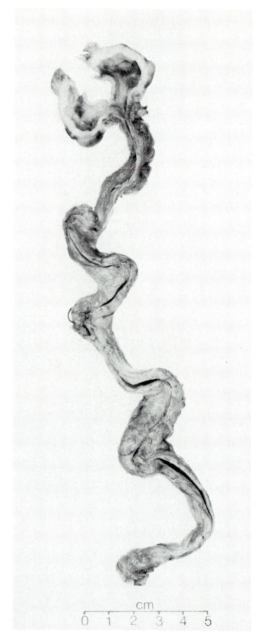

Figure 22.10 Heminephroureterectomy specimen showing typical dilated and tortuous ureter with small part of kidney attached.

nephrectomy performed. Usually the portion of kidney that has to be removed is quite small and often dysplastic. A separate incision must be made to explore the lower end. As the ureters get near the bladder, they run in the same sheath, so that the normal ureter can be easily damaged. The ectopic ureter is intimately connected to the muscle at the base of the bladder and bladder neck, and it

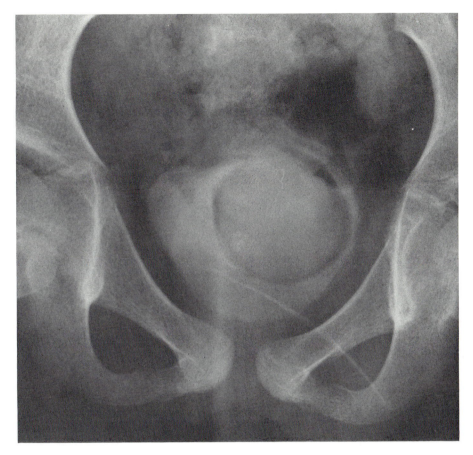

Figure 22.11 Appearance on intravenous urogram of left-sided ureterocele. (From Kasby, C.B., and Parsons, K.E. 1980, Br. J. Obstet. Gynaecol. **87:**1178-1180.)

should be divided as low as possible. The stump needs to be removed at a later date only if the patient develops problems from it. If it is connected to the urethra, reflux may occur into it and the patient may get recurrent infections, or still have some incontinence. Removal of this lower segment may be quite difficult.

URETEROCELE

A ureterocele is an outpouching of the distal ureter into the bladder, causing an obstruction. It may be single and orthotopic, but in 75% of cases it is associated with a duplication. The complex ones will usually be symptomatic in young children, but occasionally they may not be detected until the late teens.

A ureterocele may cause a variety of symptoms. If large, it may cause incomplete bladder emptying, and in young girls it has even presented as a lesion at the external urethral orifice (see Part Two of this

chapter). The ureterocele may obstruct its own ureter (it is the upper part of the kidney that is obstructed), but in addition, because of dilatation, the ipsilateral ureter may either be obstructed or develop reflux. The contralateral ureter may also be obstructed.

The diagnosis of a ureterocele is made by means of an intravenous urogram and micturating cystography (Figure 22.11). If the function in the affected portion is very poor, details may be seen on the intravenous urogram only after the use of large doses of contrast and delayed film. The position of the remaining calyces of the middle and lower parts are characteristically displaced, as in an ectopic ureter. As mentioned in the preceding clinical presentation, there may be changes in the contralateral kidney as well. The ureterocele may be seen as a negative shadow in the bladder. If the ureterocele is compressible or has ruptured, the cystogram will show reflux.

The treatment depends on a number of factors: if there is very poor function in the upper pole of the kidney, it is usually necessary to consider a heminephroureterectomy. If the ureterocele is complex, it will usually be necessary to consider reimplantation of the remaining ipsilateral ureter, and there may be a lot of reconstruction to do to the bladder wall where the ureterocele lay. If the ureterocele extends below the bladder neck, it may be a formidable undertaking. In a young child in a very toxic state, it may be possible to drain the obstructed ureter only until the general condition improves; definitive surgery is undertaken later. Single orthotopic ureteroceles should be treated only if there is obstruction with or without infection. Simple endoscopic uncapping is likely to lead to reflux, so that primary reimplantation is probably indicated.

part two
GYNECOLOGICAL ASPECTS
Sir John Dewhurst

Many congenital abnormalities of the genital tract exist alongside other malformations of the urinary tract or have important urinary tract associations. Sometimes the urological aspects are the more important, and sometimes the gynecological ones are. Both aspects are discussed in this part of the chapter, the major gynecological lesions are considered first, followed by the gynecological aspects of the major urological lesions.

HYDROCOLPOS

Hydrocolpos and hematocolpos, which will be considered later, usually arise as a result of the lower vagina being obstructed by an imperforate membrane. This membrane is commonly referred to as an imperforate hymen, but careful inspection usually reveals the hymen to be a separate structure closely applied to the superficial aspect of the imperforate membrane. Rarely, the obstruction is not membranous but consists of a length of uncanalized vagina.

Hydrocolpos is apparent clinically in only a minority of newborn children; most cases go unrecognized until puberty, when the addition of menstrual blood to the fluid that has already accumulated causes symptoms and physical signs. Whether or not hydrocolpos does become evident during the

neonatal period probably depends on the amount of fluid that has collected. The fluid is evidently produced as a result of passive hormone stimulation, to which the fetus in utero in late pregnancy is always subjected. If the quantity of fluid is small, as it generally is, the condition may well escape detection; if much more fluid is present, clinical features become evident.

When hydrocolpos is seen as a clinical phenomenon, it is usually seen in a newborn child of a day or so of age. The child may then be found to have a cystic lower abdominal mass. The infant may also be fretful and perhaps sometimes pyrexial. Initially, there is retention of urine, but since overflow incontinence develops rapidly, this feature goes unrecognized.

Examination reveals a cystic mass that is usually confined to the lower abdomen but may be so large as to almost fill it. The mass is the grossly overdistended bladder perched on top of a vagina full of blood. If the vulva is inspected—and this important step is sometimes omitted—the tense, bulging membrane should be easily visible (Figure 22-12). A rectal examination performed with a little finger will disclose a tense, cystic swelling in front of the examining finger.

Despite the fact that these physical signs are clear-cut and easy to detect, mistakes in diagnosis are not uncommon. These arise for several reasons: the condition of hydrocolpos may not be known to the physician, since it is uncommon; the vulva may not be inspected; or the size of the abdominal swelling may lead the medical attendant to the diagnosis of an ovarian tumor. If the latter diagnosis is made, the abdomen may be opened and an unnecessary hysterectomy performed, perhaps with fatal results (Joseph, Nayar, and Kannankutty, 1966).

In reality, treatment is extremely easy. All that is required is that the membrane be incised and the retained fluid released. The redundant portions of the membrane may then be snipped away with scissors, and nothing else need or should be done. The character of the retained fluid is illustrated in Figure 22.13.

Later an intravenous urogram should be performed, since there may be associated abnormalities of the urinary tract. I have encountered a double renal element on one or both sides several times, and on one occasion the two ureters opened into the posterior urethra instead of the bladder. During the obstructive phase of the disorder, it is likely that in addition to the enormous distension of the

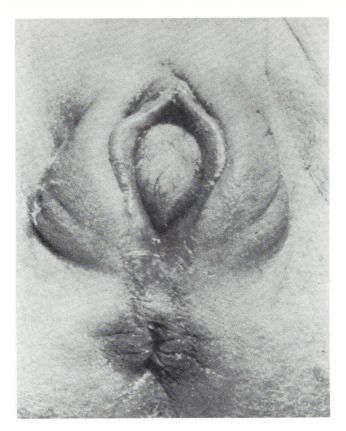

Figure 22.12 Bulging, imperforate membrane at vulva of newborn child with hydrocolpos. (From Dewhurst, J. 1968. Br. J. Obstet. Gynaecol. **75:**388.)

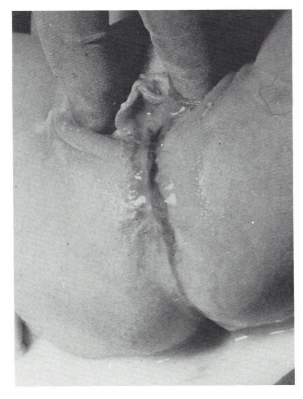

Figure 22.13 Imperforate membrane seen in Figure 22.12 has been incised and quantity of milky fluid, seen in lower part of picture, released. (Reprinted from Dewhurst, J. 1980. Practical pediatric and adolescent gynecology, New York. By courtesy of Marcel Dekker, Inc.)

bladder there will be reflux present. Investigation of the immediate urological situation is not necessary, however, since the diagnosis can readily be made clinically; treatment at once is required.

HEMATOCOLPOS
Uncomplicated forms

Hematocolpos is the counterpart of hydrocolpos and occurs about the time of puberty. Since the outflow of the menstrual blood is obstructed, this collects within the vagina (hematocolpos). The vagina is capable of considerable distension, but if no treatment is carried out, sooner or later some blood begins to collect in the uterus (hematometra) or even in the fallopian tubes (hematosalpinx).

The gradual collection of blood in the blocked vagina is associated with pain each time there is internal menstruation. Although it is frequently stated that these pains occur at monthly intervals, they usually do not. Early menstrual cycles are seldom regular; therefore the pain is similarly irregular. Sooner or later, sufficient blood collects to obstruct the bladder neck and there is acute retention of urine.

The patient seen with these features is usually a 13-, 14-, or 15-year-old girl with good secondary sexual development who has never menstruated. Examination will reveal features similar in all respects to those described for hydrocolpos—a lower abdominal cystic swelling (Figure 22.14), a bulging membrane at the introitus (Fig. 22.15), and a cystic mass palpable on rectal examination. This diagnosis could scarcely be more straightforward. Treatment is equally easy, since the membrane merely requires incision (Fig. 22.16) with removal of the redundant portions as already described.

It should be emphasized that douching, or examination or instrumentation within the vagina, is neither necessary nor advisable, since these procedures can achieve nothing and may introduce infection.

The urological aspects of hematocolpos are usually minor during the more acute phase of the disorder, but as with hydrocolpos, malformations of the urinary tract frequently coexist, and appropriate investigation to confirm or refute them should be undertaken later.

Complicated forms

Straightforward though the clinical features and the management of hematocolpos are in the majority of instances, much more complex forms do exist, in which case the diagnosis and treatment are a great deal more difficult.

If the obstruction is an uncanalized length of vagina instead of an imperforate membrane, there

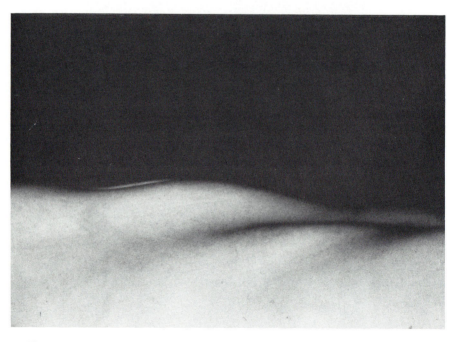

Figure 22.14 Lower abdominal cystic swelling in pubertal child with hematocolpos.

will be differences in the clinical presentation and in the physical signs. The intermittent abdominal pain is present, but urinary obstruction is usually absent, since the majority of the blood collects above the bladder neck level. There will be no lower abdominal swelling until a later stage in the disease, when perhaps there is significant hematometra or hematosalpinx present. On rectal examination the retained blood will be evident at a higher level (Figure 22.17). Moreover, if most of the vagina is absent, it may be difficult to be certain of the presence of a pelvic mass or to know in which organ the blood is collecting.

These cases seldom present symptoms so acutely as do straightforward forms of hematocolpos, so that investigation to detect the presence and nature of the obstruction can be undertaken. It is extremely important, if at all possible, to be precise about how much of the vagina is absent, where the blood is retained, and whether the uterus is single or double so that treatment can be correctly undertaken.

Apart from careful clinical examination, an ultrasound scan of the pelvis is likely to be helpful. If this is undertaken with a full bladder, the blood retained in the upper vagina and uterus can usually be detected (Figure 22.18), and with care an impression may be gained of the portion of the vagina likely to be uncanalized. An intravenous urogram should be undertaken to avoid surgical injury to, perhaps, a single pelvic kidney, which is a distinct risk if laparoscopy is undertaken. Laparoscopy is of limited value and is distinctly dangerous in complex forms of hematocolpos; it should seldom be performed (p. 297).

The aim of treatment is to let out the retained blood and then maintain drainage—the latter being more difficult than the former.

During the dissection to release the blood, injury to the bowel or bladder or both is a distinct risk, and care must be exercised. If it is thought that there is only a small portion of the vagina absent, for example, 2 to 3 cm, a careful dissection may be undertaken from below. If the collection of

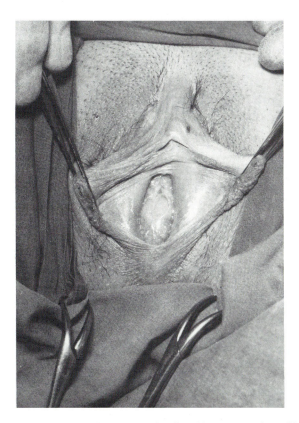

Figure 22.15 Intact membrane at vulva in a pubertal child with hematocolpos. Note that hymen can be clearly distinguished from imperforate membrane.

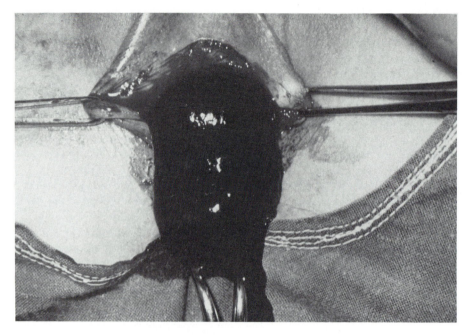

Figure 22.16 Release of retained blood following simple incision of imperforate membrane in patient with hematocolpos.

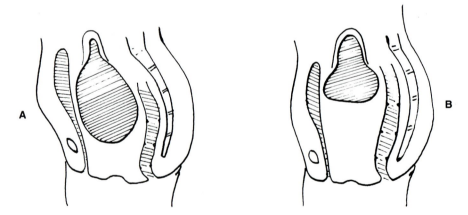

Figure 22.17 Diagrammatic representation of hematocolpos associated with absence of, **A,** smaller or, **B,** larger part of vagina. (From Dewhurst, J. 1972. Br. J. Obstet. Gynaecol. **16**:39.)

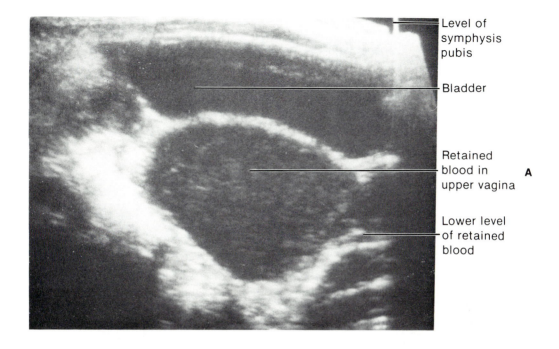

- Level of symphysis pubis
- Bladder
- Retained blood in upper vagina
- Lower level of retained blood

A

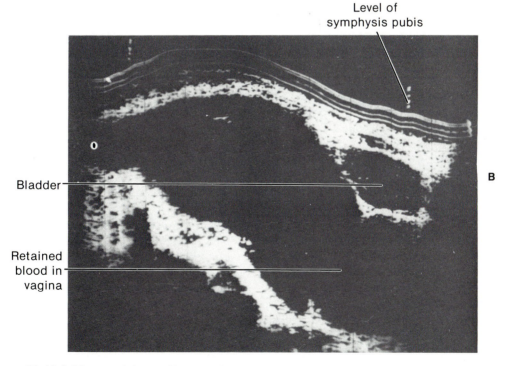

- Level of symphysis pubis
- Bladder
- Retained blood in vagina

B

Figure 22.18 A, Ultrasound picture of hematocolpos in which approximately lower half of vagina was absent. Collection of retained blood extends downwards to approximate level of symphysis pubis, below which is undilated vagina. **B,** Ultrasound picture of hematocolpos associated with imperforate membrane at vulva. Note that retained blood extends much lower than in **A.**

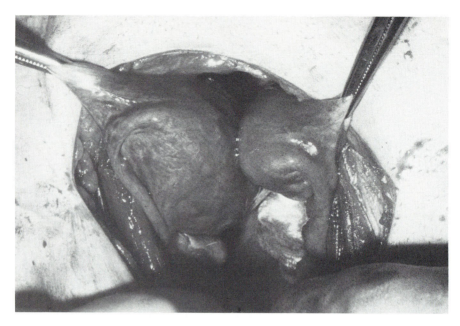

Figure 22.19 Abdominal appearance in patient with double genital tract, left part of which is obstructed. Note that left uterine horn is larger than right one because of quantity of blood within it (hematometra).

blood is entered soon, well and good; if it is not, and dissection is required higher and higher up the blind vagina, the abdomen should be opened so that palpation from above and below can identify the precise situation of the blood and permit it to be drained without injury to nearby structures. Release of blood retained high in the vagina is very difficult, partly because the irritation of the blood poured out at each period causes considerable fibrosis in the nearby tissues, so that the lower border of the hematocolpos will be thick and fibrous and difficult to penetrate with safety.

Unfortunately, letting out the blood is only part of the treatment. If nothing else is done, the vagina is certain to contract, perhaps to an extent sufficient to cause menstrual blood to be retained again. To avoid this, it is recommended that 1 week or so after the initial drainage the patient be examined again under anesthesia, the track of the new "vagina" dilated to a sufficient size, and a firm hollow mold inserted and sewn into place. This allows the new tract of the dissection to epithelialize from above and below, which will take a varying amount of time, depending on the extent of the vagina absent; the mold may need to be worn for 2 to 3 months. During this time it is advisable to have the patient take continuously a combined oral contraceptive to prevent further breakdown of endometrium. When the mold is finally removed and

epithelialization has occurred, the patient must wear the mold as often as possible and must get used to removing it, cleansing it, and replacing it. Once intercourse is undertaken, no further risk of contraction exists.

A further form of complicated hematocolpos that can also cause real difficulties is when half of the double genital tract is imperforate (Figures 22.19 and 22.20). Again, the clinical features are different from straightforward forms of the condition. There is no amenorrhea, since the patient menstruated from the patent vagina. There is intermittent pelvic pain, but probably no urinary obstruction. A pelvic swelling may not be detectable on abdominal examination or may be detectable only with difficulty, but vaginal examination will show the presence of a cystic swelling bulging into the patent vagina and perhaps reaching a low level. In these difficult cases an ultrasonic scan may help to clarify the picture. An intravenous urogram should also be performed.

Treatment consists of incising the retained collection of blood so that the blind vagina drains into the patent one. However, unless much of the septum between the two vaginas is excised, there may be difficulty later; if treatment is limited to a simple incision, this is liable to close again with recurrence of symptoms; thus once the blood has drained away, as much of the septum between the vaginas

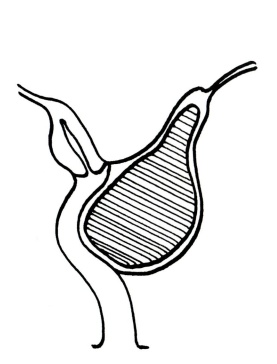

Figure 22.20 Diagrammatic representation of findings illustrated in Figure 22.19. (From Dewhurst, J. 1972. Br. J. Obstet. Gynaecol. **16**:39.)

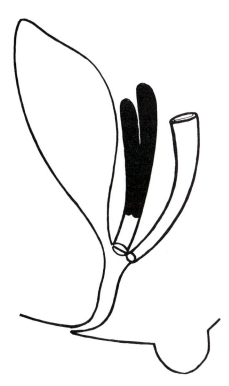

Figure 22.21 Diagrammatic appearance of patient with persistent cloaca. Note double genital tract, which is a common associated finding in such cases, and very narrow external opening of cloaca.

as possible should be removed. Usually this cannot be done at the time of the incision, since the upper vagina is filled with so much old blood, which takes some time to drain away, that the field is completely obscured. It is advisable to undertake it a week or so later.

For further consideration of these difficult cases, Dewhurst (1976, 1980) should be consulted.

PERSISTENT CLOACA

Persistence of the cloaca is a very serious fault that gives rise to incontinence of urine and feces (Figure 22.21). Other malformations may be found elsewhere in the body, and some of these may be so serious as to demand treatment first (Klugo, Fisher, and Retik, 1974). Other local pelvic abnormalities that may accompany persistence of the cloaca include sacral agenesis with lack of neurological control of pelvic floor muscles, hydrocolpos, vesicoureteric reflux, and hydronephrosis; sometimes the external opening of the cloaca is much reduced in size by excessive fusion of the genital folds (Gough, 1959; Dewhurst, 1972, 1978).

The initial management of this abnormality is unlikely to involve the gynecologist unless there is associated hydrocolpos. Provided there is a possibility that good spincter control might ultimately be established, a perineal pull-through procedure may be undertaken once the bowel has been separated from the other elements of the cloaca; to allow this to be done satisfactorily, a temporary colostomy may be required. The likelihood of the patient acquiring satisfactory urinary control will also influence the choice of management of the vesicouterine part of the cloaca. Should good urinary control seem possible, the patient may be treated in the manner referred to below, when persistence of the urogenital sinus is considered. If a hydrocolpos is present, this should be drained, since the longer there is retained fluid, the more likely it is that vesicoureteric reflux will occur.

These are rare and serious cases and, perhaps not surprisingly, different views have been expressed on the priorities in management. Snyder (1966), Stephens and Smith (1971), and Bill (1972) prefer a colostomy initially, after which the case may be thoroughly assessed and the most appropriate surgical approach decided. Raffensperger and Ramenofsky (1973), however, favor early separation of the three systems—urinary, genital, and gastrointestinal—during the neonatal period. They believe that temporizing procedures such as a colostomy predispose the patient to urinary tract sepsis and that satisfactory separation of all three tracts is possible at a very early stage. These authors also point out that although in some cases the outlook is poor, more favorable results may be achieved than seem likely at first sight.

PERSISTENT UROGENITAL SINUS
Normal sexuality

Persistence of the urogenital sinus (Figure 22.22) is not so serious an abnormality as persistence of the cloaca and, unless hydrocolpos is a complicating feature, seldom demands early intervention. In most patients, even those in whom the vagina enters the urogenital sinus at a very high level (close to the bladder base), urinary control may be achieved.

The problem in these patients is therefore seldom immediate, but the ultimate problem, which is likely to present the gynecologist with real difficulty, is to make it possible for the patient to live a normal sexual life and to be fertile. The ultimate aim would be to separate the vagina from the sinus and to construct an artificial vagina between the bowel and the bladder to meet the upper vaginal fragment at some point. Such a procedure is far from easy, and there may be damage to nearby structures unless great care is exercised. As always, one problem presented by such cases is not so much constructing the track of the artificial vagina, but keeping it open. For this reason, since cooperation of the patient would be required to keep the vagina open, the procedure should not be undertaken during childhood. Menstruation is likely to continue satisfactorily for a time into the upper urethra, so that there is no need for early gynecological surgery. Once the patient is postpuberal and her tissues

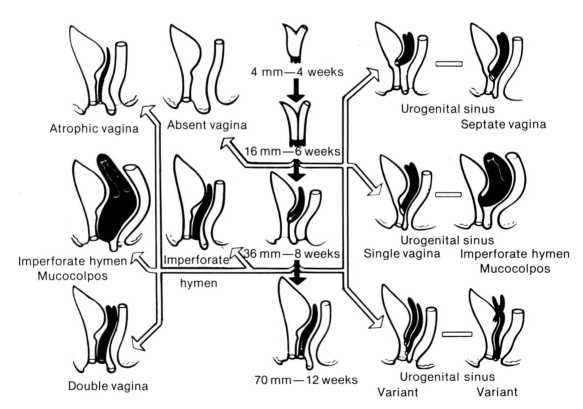

Figure 22.22 Diagrammatic representation of normal and abnormal development of genital tract. Normal development is indicated by black arrows in center of picture and abnormal development by white arrows. On right side, various forms of malformation associated with persistent urogenital sinus are illustrated. (From Dewhurst, J. 1968. Br. J. Obstet. Gynaecol. **75**:378. After Stephens 1966.)

well estrogenized, surgery, although still far from simple, is less difficult. An approach using a hollow mold similar to that already described for treatment of complicated hematocolpos is likely to be the most satisfactory form of treatment.

If good urinary control cannot be established, perhaps because of a marked degree of sacral agenesis, the formation of an ileal loop into which ureters are implanted will almost certainly need to be undertaken. This has one advantage in that the urogenital sinus is left behind and can be made to function as a vagina after being enlarged in later life. Since the urethra is capable of considerable distension, it is possible that in such a case dilatation may be all that is required.

Intersexuality

One form of persistent urogenital sinus that is amenable in most instances to much simpler treatment is that seen in female patients with congenital adrenal hyperplasia. These cases normally are symptomatic at birth, with the sex of the child in doubt. Appropriate and urgent investigation will usually disclose without difficulty that the child is genetically female and that the masculinization of the external genitalia (Figure 22.23) has arisen as a result of the excessive production of androgens during early intrauterine life by the adrenal gland; these androgens cause enlargement of the clitoris and excessive fusion of the genital folds that come together in front of the urethra and vagina. The abnormality is illustrated in diagrammatic form in Figure 22.24.

Female patients with congenital adrenal hyperplasia, provided they are recognized early in life, should always be brought up in the female role, since surgical correction of the external genital abnormality can be successfully undertaken. Once the diagnosis has been made and treatment with cortisol or one of its synthetic analogs instituted (Dewhurst, 1980, 1981), attention may be paid to this surgical correction. Reduction in the size of the phallus should be undertaken early in life, even during the neonatal period. The clitoris may simply be amputated at a deep level, so as not to leave too much erectile tissue, and its base clamped and ligated. It is doubtful that there are serious difficulties associated with this simple procedure, although it sometimes causes parental concern that in later life enjoyment of sexual intercourse may be curtailed. It seems probable that this does not happen in the majority of cases, but is has led to

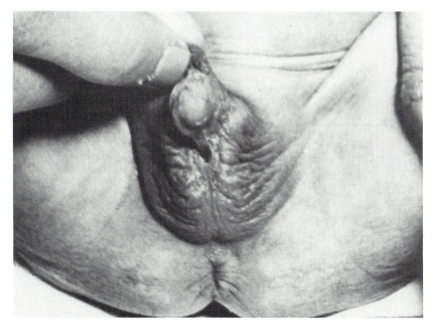

Figure 22.23 Marked masculinization of external genitalia of female child with congenital adrenal hyperplasia. Note enlarged clitoris and markedly rugose genital folds that resemble scrotum and that have fused in midline. Single opening evident at base of phallus is that of urogenital sinus. (From Dewhurst, J. 1968. Br. J. Obstet. Gynaecol. **75**:385.)

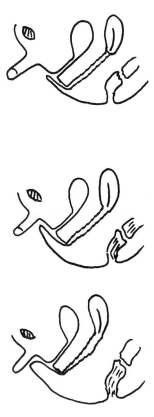

Figure 22.24 Diagrammatic representation of abnormality found in congenital adrenal hyperplasia. Note that in each drawing urethral and vaginal orifices are obscured by fused genital folds that create urogenital sinus with single external opening. Extent of fusion and thickness of genital folds increase from above downward. (From Dewhurst, J. 1978. In Stanton, S.L., editor. Clin. Obstet. Gynaecol. **5:**51-65.)

a variety of procedures being devised in an attempt to preserve the function of the glans. The most satisfactory procedure for this is probably that devised by Allen (1979). Allen points out that the nerve supply to the glans, which clearly must be preserved if the organ is to retain its erotic function, runs in the sheath of the corpora cavernosa. He recommends a vertical incision on the dorsum of the clitoris that is carried through the sheath, the right and left portions of which are then retracted laterally with the nerves intact. The erectile tissue of the corpora cavernosa is then excised and the glans stitched back in place (Dewhurst, 1980). This procedure gives a good cosmetic result, since the loose clitoral skin can be formed into the appearance of labia minora.

Although the neonatal period is an ideal time for

this procedure to be carried out, it is not an ideal time for surgery to be directed at the urogenital sinus. Unless the fused genital folds are very thin, surgery on the young child may be very difficult, scar tissue may result, and a further and more difficult procedure may need to be carried out later in life. I am strongly in favor of leaving the surgical treatment of the fused genital folds until after puberty, when the patient is fully grown and the tissues estrogenized. At that time the fused folds may be divided and, provided they are thin, the vaginal epithelium can be brought down to the perineal skin and a normal introitus formed (Figure 22.25). If the fused genital folds are very thick, however, it may be necessary to bring extra skin flaps into the lower vagina so that intercourse will be satisfactory later. These surgical procedures are considered in more detail by Federman (1968), Jones and Scott (1971), and Dewhurst (1980).

BLADDER EXSTROPHY

Bladder exstrophy is another serious condition that, although having gynecological associations, is initially a problem—often a formidable one—for the pediatric surgeon or urologist (see Part One of this chapter). Recent advances in treatment, however, have made it more likely that an individual so afflicted may be able to live an almost normal existence and may be fertile.

The gynecological associations of the various forms of bladder exstrophy include stricture of the vaginal introitus, genital prolapse, perhaps at a very early age, and occasionally concern about the ugly defect that the bifid clitoris can give rise to. These abnormalities have been reviewed by Jones (1973), Stanton (1974), Dewhurst (1978, 1980), and Blakeley and Mills (1981).

Treatment of these cases is the concern of the pediatric surgeon or urologist during the early stages of the disorder. It is sometimes possible to reconstruct the bladder and anterior abdominal wall, particularly in cases of minor degrees of the abnormality; even though the anterior defect in the bladder may be successfully repaired, urinary control may remain imperfect. The gynecologist may have an involvement in the treatment of those patients with minor degrees of abnormality in whom there is imperfect urinary control. Some kind of plastic urethral repair procedure may be undertaken, but in view of the large defect to the anterior part of the pelvis (Figure 22.26), which is asso-

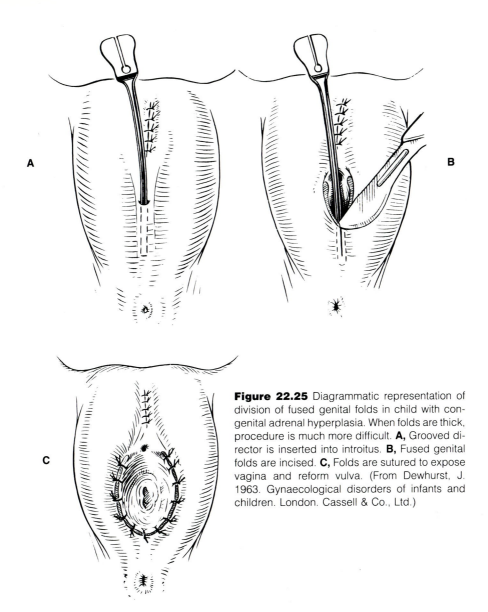

Figure 22.25 Diagrammatic representation of division of fused genital folds in child with congenital adrenal hyperplasia. When folds are thick, procedure is much more difficult. **A,** Grooved director is inserted into introitus. **B,** Fused genital folds are incised. **C,** Folds are sutured to expose vagina and reform vulva. (From Dewhurst, J. 1963. Gynaecological disorders of infants and children. London. Cassell & Co., Ltd.)

ciated with a similar defect in the pubocervical fascia and the levator ani muscles, less may be achieved by the ordinary suburethral repair procedure than usual. If sufficient tissue cannot be found in the periurethral area, it will be necessary to find tissue elsewhere and bring it into the area; the gracilis muscle may be used as a means of support or a sling procedure undertaken. The likelihood of success of these operations is probably small, and eventually a decision may be required as to whether or not urinary diversion should be performed.

If the problem of incontinence is eventually solved, the services of the gynecologist may be required in later life for one of the gynecological conditions already mentioned that are associated with such cases.

Treatment of a constricted vaginal introitus (Figure 22.27) is very simple. All that is required is that an incision be made posteriorly from the contracted orifice, and the vagina will be found to be normal underneath. It must be emphasized, however, that if too large an incision is made (Figure 22.28), the tendency that already exists for a prolapse to occur may be aggravated. This can be seen in Figure 22.28, in which a considerable bulge of the lower part of the anterior vaginal wall is already evident, a bulge that has previously been contained

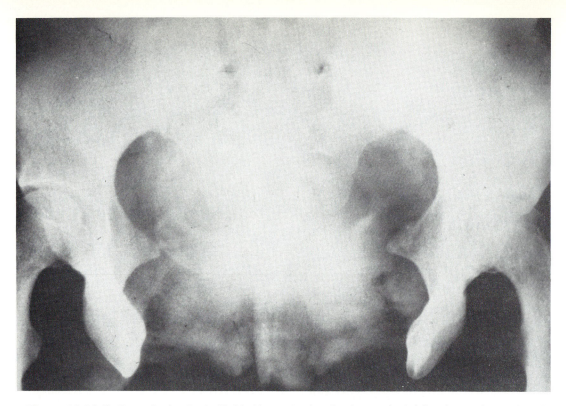

Figure 22.26 Radiograph of patient with bladder exstrophy showing marked defect in anterior portion of pelvis.

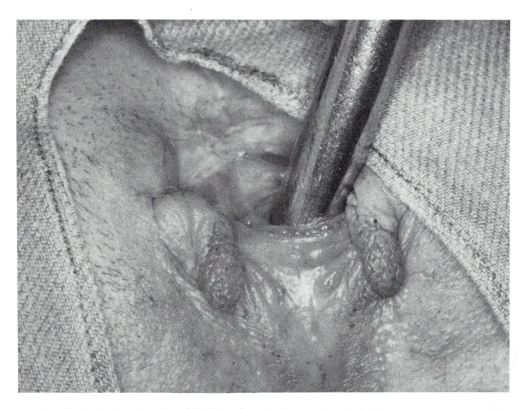

Figure 22.27 Marked contraction of introitus of vagina in patient with bladder exstrophy that was treated by excision during early childhood. Note bifid nature of clitoris and fact that introitus admits only comparatively fine probe. (From Dewhurst, J. 1968. Br. J. Obstet. Gynaecol. **75**:382.)

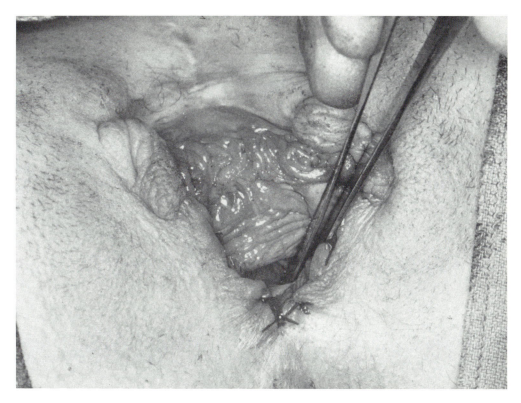

Figure 22.28 Same patient as in Figure 22.27 following posterior division of fused genital folds that have narrowed the introitus of vagina. Note that already a distinct cystocele seems to be forming. (From Dewhurst, J. 1968. Br. J. Obstet. Gynaecol. **75**:382.)

by the fused genital folds. This tendency to prolapse should be borne in mind when a posterior incision is being made, and the incision should be restricted to only what is essential to permit intercourse to occur.

The management of prolapse associated with bladder exstrophy presents a difficult problem, since the normal structures that are used to support a vault of the vagina and the bladder are absent or grossly deficient. For this reason it is unlikely that a standard form of pelvic floor repair will succeed, since the operator will be attempting to support the prolapse with inadequate tissues. An alternative approach to the problem is to attempt to fix the uterus posteriorly to the periosteum on the anterior surface of the sacrum. Provided there is sufficient mobility and the uterus can be brought into direct proximity with the sacrum, this will not present a difficult surgical problem. However, it may be possible in most cases to bring the uterus so far backward, and I have attempted to solve this problem by using an Ivalon sponge to bridge the gap between the posterior surface of the upper part of the cervix and the anterior portion of the sacrum (Dew-

hurst, 1980). This sponge is rapidly infiltrated with fibroblasts and may be able to form a sufficiently strong fibrous band to retain the uterus in position.

Should the deformity of the lower anterior abdominal wall and the anterior part of the vagina remain a problem, either physical or psychological, in relation to the patient's ultimate enjoyment of sexual activity, a plastic repair procedure to correct the ugly deformity may be indicated. These repairs are discussed more fully in Erich (1959), Dewhurst (1972), and Weed and McKee (1974).

HYPOSPADIAS

Hypospadias is not so common a condition in women as it is in men. It is manifested by imperfect urinary control. There is a defect that involves the lower part of the posterior urethral wall (Figure 22.29), and there is likely to be some interference with micturition, such as stress incontinence or even almost complete incontinence in more severe cases. Rarely, very minor degrees of the abnormality may leave the patient with effective control of micturition. There is no associated defect in the pubic bones or levator ani muscles, as there may

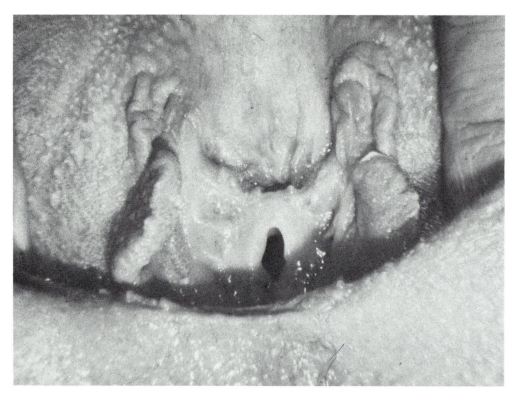

Figure 22.29 Hypospadias in 17-year-old girl. Bifid clitoris is clearly evident, and grooved roof of urethra can be seen. Urethral floor is deficient for most of its length. (From Dewhurst, J. 1978. In Stanton, S.L., editor. Clin. Obstet. Gynaecol. **5:**51-65.)

be in epispadias and bladder exstrophy, and the condition is rather more amenable to successful surgical treatment. The technique of repair, as described by Moir (1961) and Russell (1962), for refashioning the urethra damaged at childbirth may also be used for patients with hypospadias. In this technique a U-shaped incision is made to encircle the margins of the urethral defect. Undercutting the edges is then carried out with care taken that neither the urethral nor the skin margin is devitalized by dissecting flaps that are too thin and that the blood supply is not damaged. The urethral incisions are then brought together, thus folding up the urethra as a tube once more. Once this has been done, further suburethral dissection may be carried out and the supporting stitches inserted as in the standard urethroplasty. Finally, the vaginal skin is closed to complete the procedure.

EPISPADIAS

Rarely, the gynecologist may be consulted about the most minor form of bladder exstrophy—epispadias. Here the roof of the urethra may be absent (Figure 22.30) throughout its whole length or in part. If a sufficient portion of the proximal urethra is left intact, incontinence may be minimal or absent; if the proximal urethra is affected, however, serious incontinence is likely. This problem is usually dealt with by the pediatric surgeon, but if the gynecologist in a particular center is considered to be the most important person to undertake treatment, an approach similar to that described previously for hypospadias may successfully reconstitute the urethral tube. Even if this is successfully accomplished, however, incontinence may remain as a result of inadequacy of sphincter control; if this is so, suburethral repair at a later time may be effective in reestablishing continence.

ASSOCIATED URINARY TRACT ANOMALIES

We have already seen that malformations of the genital tract and those of the urinary tract frequently coexist. While treatment of urinary tract lesions comes within the jurisdiction of the urologist or pediatric surgeon and is considered in Part One of

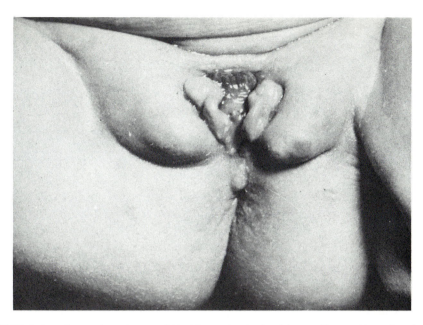

Figure 22.30 Epispadias—minor degree of bladder exstrophy involving urethra and lowest part of bladder. (From Dewhurst, J. 1963. Gynaecological disorders of infants and children. London. Cassell & Co., Ltd.)

this chapter, it is important for the gynecologist to be aware of their presence, since they may influence treatment of the genital tract abnormality. Recognition of such lesions as congenital absence of the vagina, partial or complete hydrocolpos, or hematocolpos should indicate an intravenous urogram to confirm or refute the presence of a urinary tract lesion.

Pelvic kidney

Various urinary tract malformations such as a single kidney, a duplex kidney, a horseshoe kidney, or a pelvic kidney may be discovered. Treatment may be required, although usually not until the gynecological lesion has been dealt with. One abnormality of particular importance to the gynecologist is the pelvic kidney. The kidney in this position or its ureter, which will almost certainly pursue an abnormal course, is at risk during gynecological surgery. The kidney itself is most in danger during laparoscopy, which is a method of investigation not infrequently employed by the gynecologist who encounters one or another of the malformations discussed earlier. It is debatable, however, to what extent laparoscopy is of value in such cases. Congenital absence of the vagina, for example, is, in the majority of instances, associated with congenital absence of the uterus, so that if there are no clinical features pointing to blood col-

lecting in the pelvis in a postpuberal patient, the absence of the uterus may be assumed with confidence and laparoscopy omitted. Furthermore, if the uterus is present and functioning, as in the complicated forms of hematocolpos already discussed, laparoscopy becomes a more dangerous procedure that is unlikely to give really helpful information. Such complicated forms of hematocolpos are often associated with sizable lower abdominal (as distinct from pelvic) masses, which are vulnerable to injury during insertion of the trochar; adhesions resulting from the irritation of the collections of blood are also common, so that the view through a laparoscope may be obscured by them or by bleeding caused by injury to blood vessels. All in all, laparoscopy is seldom indicated in such cases and should never be undertaken without a preliminary intravenous urogram to exclude a pelvic kidney and careful examination to exclude the presence of an abdominal mass liable to injury.

Certain urinary tract anomalies are liable to be seen as apparent gynecological faults, and much gynecological investigation is sometimes undertaken before the true nature of the condition is determined.

Ectopic ureter

The ectopic ureter may open into some part of the lower genital tract, and the patient may be trou-

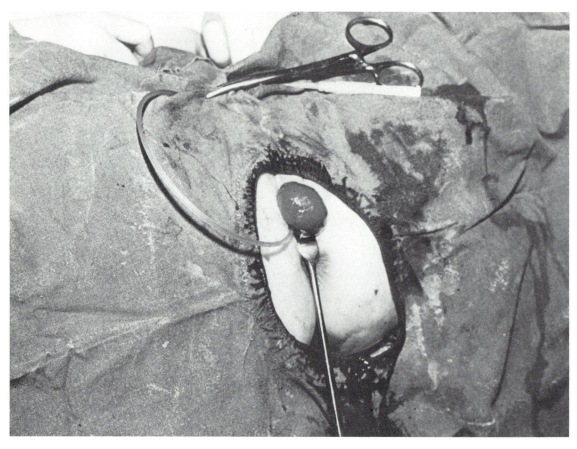

Figure 22.31 A, Prolapsed ureterocele at vaginal introitus. (From Kasby, C.B., and Parsons, K.F., 1980. Br. J. Obstet. Gynaecol. **87:**1178-1180.)

bled by constant or intermittent wetness, the cause of which may not be obvious. Sometimes diagnosis may not be made until after puberty, when the presence of a fluid vaginal discharge may be considered to have a gynecological explanation; repeated swabs may be taken for bacteriological study and numerous treatments prescribed without improvement. In cases of vaginal discharge and vulval soreness that are resistant to treatment, especially if these are encountered in childhood, the possibility of an ectopic ureter dribbling urine should be borne in mind. The investigation and management of such cases is described in Part One of this chapter.

Ectopic ureterocele

The ectopic ureter may also be the cause of a most unusual type of abnormality that can be seen in highly mysterious circumstances as a possible gynecological fault. The patient, often a child, is brought in for advice because of the sudden appearance of vulval swelling. By the time the patient and her parent reach the physician's office, however, there is nothing to be seen, so they are thought to be making an unnecessary fuss and are sent home. The abnormality may recur again and again before the swelling is actually seen or its explanation suspected even in its absence.

The cause of such a disappearing vulval tumor is likely to be a prolapsing ectopic ureterocele (Kasby and Parsons, 1980) (Figure 22.31). The ureterocele (discussed in more detail in Part One of this Chapter), which exists at the lower end of the ectopic ureter at the point where it enters the bladder or urethra, prolapses through the urethra to be clearly visible externally until it retracts and there is no fault to be seen. This history should always lead to further urological examination, and since such cases are difficult to recognize and to treat, the help of a urologist should always be requested.

REFERENCES

Allen, H. 1979. Personal communication.

Bill, A.H. 1972. Clinical aspects of female patients with high anorectal agenesis. Surg. Gynecol. Obstet. **135:**411-416.

Blakeley, C.R., and Mills, W.G. 1981. The obstetric and gynaecological complications of bladder exstrophy and epispadias. Br. J. Obstet. Gyneacol. **88:**167-173.

Dewhurst, C.J. 1963. Gynaecological disorders of infants and children. London. Ballière Tindall.

Dewhurst, C.J. 1972. The surgical treatment of genital tract malformations (Margaret Orford Memorial Lecture for 1972). Trans. Coll Med. S. Afr. **16:**39-53.

Dewhurst, C.J. 1978. Congenital malformations of the lower urinary tract. In Stanton, S.L., editor. Clin. Obstet. Gynaecol. **5:**51-65.

Dewhurst, J. 1980. Practical pediatric and adolescent gynecology. New York. Marcel Dekker, Inc.

Dewhurst, J. 1981. Genetic and congenital sexual disorders. In Hawkins, D.F., editor. Gynaecological therapeutics. London. Ballière Tindall.

Erich, J.B. 1959. Plastic repair of the female perineum in a case of exstrophy of the bladder. Proc. Staff Mtgs. Mayo Clin. **34:**235-246.

Federman, D.D., 1968. Abnormal sexual development: a genetic and endocrine approach to differential diagnosis. Philadelphia. W.B. Saunders Co.

Gough, M.H. 1959. Anorectal agenesis with persistence of cloaca. Proc. R. Soc. Med. **52:**886-889.

Jones, H.W. 1973. An anomaly of the external genitalia in female patients with exstrophy of the bladder. Am. J. Obstet. Gynecol. **117:**748-765.

Jones, H.W., and Scott, W.W., editors. 1971. Hermaphroditism, genital anomalies and related endocrine disorders. Baltimore, The Williams and Wilkins Co.

Joseph, M.K., Nayar, B.J., and Kannankutty, M. 1966. Hydrohaematocolpos. Br. Med. J. **1:**89-90.

Kasby, C.B., and Parsons, K.F. 1980. Prolapsed ureterocele presenting as a vulvular mass in a child. Br. J. Obstet. Gynaecol. **87:**1178-1180.

Klugo, R.C., Fisher, J.H., and Retik, A.B. 1974. Management of urogenital anomalies in cloacal dysgenesis. J. Urol. **112:**832-835.

Moir, J.C. 1961. The vesico-vaginal fistula. London. Ballière Tindall.

Raffensperger, J.G., and Ramenofsky, M.L. 1973. The management of a cloaca. J. Pediatr. Surg. **8:**647-657.

Russell, C.S. 1962. Vesico-vaginal fistulas and related matters. Springfield, Ill. Charles C Thomas, Publisher.

Synder, W.H. 1966. Some unusual forms of imperforate anus in female infants. Am. J. Surg. **111:**319-325.

Stanton, S.L. 1974. Gynecologic complications of epispadias and bladder exstrophy. Am. J. Obstet. Gynecol. **119:**749-754.

Stephens, F.S., and Smith, E.D. 1971. Ano-rectal malformations in children. Chicago. Year Book Medical Publishers, Inc.

Weed, J.C., and McKee, D.M. 1974. Vulvoplasty in cases of exstrophy of the bladder. Obstet. Gynecol. **43:**512-516.

SUGGESTED READING

Harrison, J.H., et al. 1979. Campbell's urology. ed 4., vol. 2. Philadelphia. W.B. Saunders Co.

chapter 23

Urinary urgency and frequency

LINDA CARDOZO

DEFINITION AND PREVALENCE

Frequency and urgency of micturition are common symptoms that may occur together or independently and may be associated with other urinary symptoms. Diurnal frequency is the passage of urine every 2 hours or more than seven times during the day; nocturnal frequency, or nocturia, is the interruption of sleep more than once each night for micturition. Some people void several times during the night because they suffer from insomnia or broken sleep for other reasons, but this behavior does not constitute nocturia. Urinary urgency is a strong and sudden desire to void, which, if not relieved immediately, may lead to urge incontinence.

In an epidemiological study, Bungay, Vessey, and McPherson (1980) assessed the prevalence of various symptoms in 1120 women and 510 men between 30 and 65 years of age. They found that approximately 20% of women admitted to frequency and that this did not alter significantly with age. However, less than 10% of men below age 50 complained of frequency, but above that age there was a marked increase in the incidence of urinary frequency. Urgency showed a similar pattern: about 15% of women reported this symptom irrespective of age, whereas very few men under 50 years old had urgency, but nearly 30% of men complained of urgency by the age of 65.

Common causes of urgency and frequency	
Urinary tract infection	Small-capacity bladder
Urethral syndrome	Pelvic mass
Detrusor instability	Previous pelvic
Upper motor neuron	surgery
lesion	Radiation cystitis or
Habit	fibrosis
Large fluid intake	Chronic residual or
Diuretic therapy	retained urine
Pregnancy	Urethritis
Bladder mucosal lesion	Genital warts
(for example,	Impaired renal function
papilloma)	Diabetes mellitus
Bladder calculus	Diabetes insipidus
Urethral diverticulum	Hypothyroidism
Urethral caruncle	

ETIOLOGY

Frequency and urgency are only symptoms for which there are many causes. The more common causes are shown in the box above.

PRESENTATION
History

A thorough history would exclude many of the more common disorders and should include the patient's specific complaint and any additional urological symptoms, especially stress incontinence, dysuria, or voiding difficulties such as straining to void, poor stream, or incomplete bladder emptying. A past history of recurrent urinary tract infections, childhood enuresis, or episodes of urine retention may be relevant.

The gynecological history should include symptoms of prolapse, abnormal vaginal discharge, and details of the menstrual cycle or menopause if they are related to the urological symptoms. Previous trauma, pelvic surgery, and pelvic irradiation involving the bladder neck are important factors.

Neurological symptoms, including leg weakness, paresthesias, rectal soiling, or backache, may indicate a neuropathy, which could also be responsible for the symptoms of frequency and urgency.

Details of the patient's drinking habits should be recorded, and she should be questioned about diabetes, past renal disease, and psychiatric disorders. A drug history is important because diuretics will cause frequency of micturition. The time of drug administration should be noted.

Examination

A simple neurological examination is performed to detect nystagmus, change in balance, and lower limb reflexes, power, and sensation. Particular reference is made to the second, third, and fourth sacral nerves. If a neuropathy is suspected, the patient should be referred to a neurologist.

A gynecological examination will exclude pregnancy, pelvis mass, or a chronic large residual urine volume as a cause of the symptoms. A urethral caruncle or genital warts will be obvious on examination of the vulva.

INVESTIGATION
Initial procedures

Before extensive time-consuming investigations are undertaken, certain simple causes can be excluded. Urine should be tested for sugar and a midstream specimen sent for culture and sensitivity in all cases of frequency or urgency to detect and enable treatment of any infection. This is important because a urinary tract infection may be the sole cause of these symptoms. Three early morning urine specimens should be sent for acid-fast bacilli culture. If an abnormal vaginal discharge is present, high vaginal, urethral, and cervical swabs should be sent for culture organisms, including *Chlamydia* organisms.

Urinary diary

All patients complaining of frequency and urgency should be given a urinary diary or frequency/volume chart to complete for a week. This will provide information about the patient's drinking habits and the volumes voided and differentiate between true frequency of micturition and polyuria. A urinary diary will also reveal certain bad habits such as regular voiding two or three times before going out, which the patient may feel is necessary to avoid embarrassing incontinence.

Urethrocystoscopy

Endoscopy, with the patient under local or general anesthesia, should be performed on all patients in whom there is no obvious cause for frequency of micturition. The residual volume should be noted (normally less than 50 ml) and bladder capacity (normally 400 to 800 ml) recorded. True small-capacity bladders are rare, but they may be caused by interstitial cystitis, which is diagnosed by the appearance of small hemorrhagic patches appearing on filling, followed by the development of shallow, irregular, linear ulcers in the vault of the bladder. The bladder should be inspected for trabeculation, sacculation, diverticuli, mucosal injection, papillomata, neoplasms, or calculi. Urethroscopy will exclude urethritis or a urethral diverticulum.

Cystometry and videocystourethrography

Subtracted cystometry will detect detrusor instability, which is a major cause of urgency and frequency. First sensation and bladder capacity should be noted. Videocystourethrography with pressure and flow studies is necessary only when incontinence is also a symptom. It will demonstrate ureteric reflux, trabeculation or sacculation of the bladder, and a urethral diverticulum.

Miscellaneous procedures

Any patient with hematuria, loin or groin pain, a large residual urine volume, or suspected impairment of renal function should have a plain radiograph of the abdomen and lumbosacral spine, an intravenous urogram, and estimation of serum urea, electrolytes, creatinine clearance, and urine osmolality.

NEGATIVE FINDINGS

In a large proportion of cases, no obvious cause will be found for the symptoms of frequency and urgency. Some patients with negative findings void frequently through habit which usually develops following an acute urinary tract infection or an episode of incontinence. Alternatively, the bad habit may have been present since childhood, especially if one parent voided frequently; it is interesting that often several family members suffer from similar urinary complaints.

Another common cause of frequency in women with negative findings is the urethral syndrome, which is defined as recurrent episodes of frequent, painful micturition not associated with any abnormality of the lower female genital tract. This is a broad definition that may include urinary infection and urethral hypersensitivity (Powell et al., 1981), a condition that has only recently been elucidated. The urethral syndrome may occur at any age, and it is important that an organic cause be excluded before the diagnosis is made.

TREATMENT
General therapy

Any underlying causes should be treated. Difficult cases are those where there is no obvious organic disease. All patients with frequency should be advised to limit their fluid intake to less than 2 L a day and to avoid drinking at times when they feel the problem is worse. Certain drinks such as coffee or tea may precipitate nocturia and should be avoided in the evening. Some patients are helped by a urinary diary alone. Once it has been pointed out to a patient that the volume voided early in the morning is far greater than the volume at any other time of the day and therefore that bladder sensation is unreliable, he or she may be able to increase the time between voidings without any other specific treatment.

Drug therapy

When no cause can be found for frequency of micturition, drugs are not particularly helpful, but propantheline, 15 mg t.d.s., will be effective in some cases. Imipramine, 50 mg b.d., is sometimes helpful, especially if nocturia is a problem. Hilton and Stanton (1980) have shown that Desmopressin (a synthetic analog of vasopressin) produces a significant reduction in nocturia, which can be a problem, especially in elderly patients. It is administered in a measured intranasal dose given before the patient retires for the night. Hypertension and ischemic heart disease should be excluded before Desmopressin is prescribed. This drug cannot simultaneously be used to alleviate diurnal frequency.

Bladder drill

A group of patients exist who have urgency and frequency of micturition, with or without incontinence, but have stable bladders and sterile urine. This condition has been described as sensory urgency and is particularly refractory to treatment. Jarvis (1981) has described the use of inpatient bladder drill for such patients. The results of treatment were not as good as for patients with detrusor instability. In a study of 33 patients, 54% were symptom free after 6 months, and there was significant urodynamic improvement in first sensation and cystometric capacity.

Cystodistension

Various methods of treatment have been employed for frequency caused by interstitial cystitis. These include bladder instillation with silver nitrate, local injection with heparin and saline, and numerous drugs. Turner-Warwick and Ashken (1967) have recommended cystocystoplasty or cecocystoplasty, and Worth and Turner-Warwick

(1973) have assessed cystolysis: all were found satisfactory for pain relief. Dunn et al. (1977) used one or more prolonged hydrostatic bladder distensions to treat 25 patients with interstitial cystitis. Sixteen were initially symptomatically cured, and there was a significant improvement in cystometric capacity. However, relapses are known to occur with this treatment, and there is a significant risk of bladder rupture.

Therapy for urethral syndrome

There are believed to be two basic causative factors in the urethral syndrome, a bacterial and a urethral element. The bacterial element has always been thought to be caused by migration of *Escherichia coli* across the urethra, for which Smith (1981) has recommended perineal hygiene, especially after sexual intercourse. In the case of an acute attack, he suggests high fluid intake combined with bicarbonate to alter the pH of the urine and short courses of antibiotics such as co-trimoxazole (Septrin) or nitrofurantoin (Furadantin). Prolonged low-dose chemotherapy is sometimes necessary for relapsing or chronic cases.

In a recent study Stamm et al. (1981) found that 71% of young women with the urethral syndrome had abnormal pyuria (defined as eight or more leukocytes per cubic millimeter of midstream urine), and 88% of these had a lower urinary infection with less than 10^5 coliforms, staphylococci, or *C. trachomatis*. In a randomized double-blind trial of doxycycline and placebo, they found that doxycycline was significantly more effective than placebo in eradicating urinary symptoms, pyuria, and the infecting microorganisms. They did not recommend antibiotic therapy for women with the acute urethral syndrome without pyuria. These results stress the need for repeated culture and sensitivity of clean specimens of urine. If there is any doubt regarding contamination, suprapubic aspiration of urine should be employed. Although it is still not always possible to culture chlamydia, it should be borne in mind as a causative organism when antibiotics are prescribed.

Various surgical methods of treatment have been tried for resistant cases of the urethral syndrome. Urethral dilatation is often employed, but there is no rationale behind its use, since it is rare to find outflow obstruction in these women. Similarly, urethrotomy is sometimes employed; however, it is not indicated, and it may cause incontinence. Rees et al. (1975) have found that less than 8% of 156 women with the urethral syndrome had outflow obstruction and that the results of urethral dilatation or internal urethrotomy were no better than medication alone.

In some women, attacks of the urethral syndrome are closely associated with sexual intercourse, and on examination the urethral meatus is sometimes seen to open far back along the anterior vaginal wall, where it is vulnerable to trauma during intercourse. Symptoms in such women may be relieved by a urethrovaginoplasty with freeing and advancement of the urethra or urethrolysis (Smith et al., 1981).

Smith (1977) has defined another group of women who experience the urethral syndrome for the first time after menopause. He blames atrophic changes on the distal urethra, which is sensitive to estrogens and responds in the same way as the vagina to estrogen deficiency. He recommends treatment with oral estrogens together with a progestogen to prevent endometrial hyperplasia.

CONCLUSION

In assessing frequency and urgency of micturition, one must be aware that they are only symptoms that may be caused by many different diseases. After organic disease is excluded, there remains a group of patients whose symptoms are psychosomatic and who will benefit from psychiatric referral. For the rest, treatment must unfortunately be empirical, and there will undoubtedly be a proportion of sufferers resistant to all currently available therapy.

REFERENCES

Bungay, G., Vessey, M.P., and McPherson, C.K. 1980. Study of symptoms in middle life with special reference to the menopause. Br. Med. J. **281**:181-183.

Dunn, M., et al. 1977. Interstitial cystitis, treated by prolonged bladder distension. Br. J. Urol. **49**:641-645.

Hilton, P., and Stanton, S.L., 1982. Use of Desmopressin for nocturia in the female. Br. J. Urol. **54**:252-255.

Jarvis, G. 1981. The management of urinary incontinence due to vesical sensory urgency by bladder drill. Proceedings of the eleventh annual meeting of the International Continence Society. Lund. 123-124.

Powell, P.H., et al. 1981. The hypersensitive female urethra—a cause of recurrent frequency and dysuria. Proceedings of the eleventh annual meeting of the International Continence Society. Lund. 81-82.

Rees, D.L., et al. 1975. Urodynamic findings in the adult female with frequency and dysuria. Br. J. Urol. **47**:853-860.

Smith, P.J., 1977. The menopause and the lower urinary tract—another case for hormonal replacement therapy. Practitioner **218**:97-99.

Smith, P.J., 1981. The urethral syndrome. In Fisher, A.M., and Gordon, H., editors. Gynaecological enigmata. Clin. Obstet. Gynaecol. **8**(1):161-172.

Smith, P.J., et al. 1981. Urethrolysis in the management of females with recurrent frequency and dysuria. Br. J. Urol. **53:**634-636.

Stamm, W.E., et al. 1981. Treatment of the acute urethral syndrome. N. Engl. J. Med. **304**(16):956-958.

Turner-Warwick, R.T., and Ashken, M.H., 1967. The functional results of partial, sub-total and total cystoplasty with special reference to ureterocystoplasty, selective sphincterotomy and cystocystoplasty. Br. J. Urol. **39:**3-12.

Worth, P.H., and Turner-Warwick, R.T., 1973. The treatment of interstitial cystitis by cystolysis with observations on cystoplasty. Br. J. Urol. **45:**65-71.

chapter 24

Urinary tract infection

WILLIAM ROSS CATTELL

The past quarter of a century has seen major advances in knowledge of the criteria for diagnosis, the significance, and the treatment of urinary tract infection such that effective treatment of single or recurrent infection is now possible in most patients. Unfortunately, the management of such patients in general remains unsatisfactory, and very many suffer quite unnecessary misery.

Although the treatment of urinary tract infection is now possible, there is no room for complacency. Prevention of infection in the first place remains poorly defined. In addition, effective treatment of infection has revealed a population of patients with symptoms commonly attributed to infection in whom this cannot be demonstrated by conventional methods: patients with the so-called urethral syndrome. The treatment of these latter individuals remains singularly unsatisfactory.

DIAGNOSIS

If we accept the definition of urinary tract infection as the "establishment and multiplication of microorganisms within the urinary tract," it follows that the diagnosis must be based on bacteriological assessment. Urinary tract infections cannot be positively diagnosed on the basis of symptoms. Patients with urinary tract infections may have typical symptoms (Figure 24.1), atypical symptoms, or no symptoms. Conversely, patients with symptoms suggestive of urinary tract infections, for example, frequency and/or dysuria, may have no evidence of infection.

Pyuria

The time-honored use of an excess of pus cells in the urine as a criterion for the diagnosis of urinary tract infection is unsatisfactory. Pyuria reflects inflammation within the urinary tract that may or may not be caused by infection. Thus pyuria in the absence of bacteriuria is a common finding in patients with stones or papillary necrosis and must always stimulate the search for tuberculous infection. Many patients with bacteriologically proven infection do not have pyuria. Its presence or absence is thus no criterion for the diagnosis of urinary tract infection. In patients with previously proven bacteriuria, it is valuable as evidence of continuing inflammation and should stimulate the search for atypical infecting organisms.

Bacteriuria

The diagnosis of urinary tract infection is now firmly based on the demonstration of bladder bacteriuria by bacteriological methods (Sussman and Asscher, 1979). Such is the potential for urine to sustain bacterial multiplication that bladder urine is rarely if ever sterile when there are bacteria present within the kidney or urinary tract. The few exceptions include cortical—usually staphylococcal—abscess of the kidney and, rarely, the presence of a totally obstructed upper tract. In patients with relapsing infection, bladder urine may be temporarily sterile following antibacterial treatment, but bacteriuria will always recur within 7 to 14 days. Contrary to former opinion, foci of infection do not persist in the kidney in the continuing absence of bacteriuria. Conversely, persistently sterile bladder urine excludes the diagnosis of urinary tract infection. The diagnosis of bladder bacteriuria is most commonly based on the demonstration of significant bacteriuria on quantitative bacteriological culture of a clean-catch midstream sample of urine. By "significant" is meant the presence of more than 100,000 (10^5) of the same organism per mil-

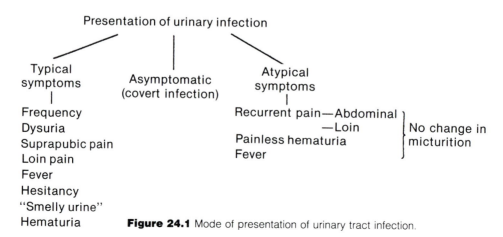

Figure 24.1 Mode of presentation of urinary tract infection.

liliter of freshly plated urine. Counts below 10,000 (10^4), especially those made up of mixed organisms, generally indicate contamination of the urine sample during collection. Counts in the range of 10^4 to 10^5 are equivocal and require repetition.

In the interpretation of bacterial counts, however, it is essential that there not be too rigid adherence to absolute values: bladder bacteriuria may be present with bacterial counts of less than 10^5 of the same organism. Thus in women with normal urinary tracts, a high fluid intake with frequent voiding can result in a dramatic reduction in bacterial counts (Cattell et al., 1970). Failure to recognize this can result in failure to identify and treat genuine infection. A safeguard is to obtain urine samples for culture from the first voiding in the morning, since a low urine flow at night with infrequent bladder voiding allows multiplication of bacteria within the bladder. False-negative urine cultures may be obtained if the patient has already started antibiotic therapy or if disinfectant has been used during the collection of midstream urine and has contaminated the collecting vessel.

Suprapubic aspiration of urine

When there is doubt regarding the significance of low bacterial counts, bladder urine must be obtained by suprapubic aspiration (Kunin, 1979). Bladder urine is normally sterile. The isolation of bacteria in suprapubic aspiration samples is thus always significant whatever the count. In symptomatic patients with low bacterial counts in clean-catch midstream urine samples, bladder bacteriuria can never be confidently excluded without the culture of urine obtained by suprapubic aspiration. Some clinics, including antenatal clinics, make routine use of suprapubic aspiration in all patients. In my experience this is not necessary if nursing staff members are familiar with the correct practices for obtaining clean-catch midstream urine samples.

Bladder catheterization with the sole object of obtaining a urine sample for bacteriological examination is rarely justified. Not only can catheterization itself introduce bacteria into the bladder and make interpretation of urine culture difficult, but even with the greatest care, it may lead to urinary tract infection.

Bacteriological methods

Space precludes any detailed review of laboratory methods. Excellent reviews of these have ap-

peared in the recent literature (Sussman and Asscher, 1979; PHLS, 1978). It must be emphasized, however, that no laboratory can be expected to produce meaningful reports if urine samples are badly collected and neither refrigerated nor sent to the laboratory immediately.

Dip inoculation

Special mention must be made of techniques such as the Dipspoon or Dipslide kits for obtaining midstream urine samples (Mackey and Sandys, 1966; Guttmann and Naylor, 1967) (Figure 24.2). Various modifications of these techniques are immensely valuable in the diagnosis of urinary infection and especially recurrent urinary infection. Their availability allows both family physician and patient to obtain urine for culture at any time.

Chemical methods

Several chemical methods have been introduced for the diagnosis of bacteriuria (Kunin, 1979). While possibly of some value in very large screening programs, none have proved satisfactory for routine clinical use. The principal objection is that they yield an unacceptable level of false-negative results.

CAUSATIVE ORGANISMS

The most common bacterial species isolated from patients with symptomatic or asymptomatic bacteriuria is *Escherichia coli*. This is followed in frequency by *Proteus mirabilis* and other coliform organisms that are not *E. coli*. In recent years it has also been recognized that certain coagulase-negative staphylococci are an important cause of urinary tract infections especially in young women.

Less common pathogens include *Klebsiella aerogenes*, *Pseudomonas* organisms, and *Streptococcus faecalis*. Primary, domiciliary infection with these organisms is unusual. They are most often encountered in hospital practice, especially where there has been instrumentation or catheterization of the bladder and where there is some anatomical abnormality such as stones or a neuropathic bladder. Isolation of such organisms demands careful review of the anatomical situation within the urinary tract.

Anaerobic and fastidious organisms

The isolation of pathogenic bacteria does, of course, require the use of appropriate culture tech-

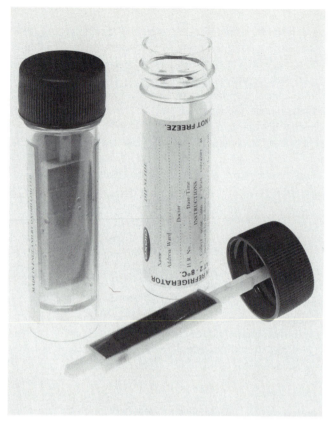

Figure 24.2 Dip inoculation slide used for urine culture in domiciliary practice. "Slide" is coated with culture medium, inoculated by dipping into urine, and sent to laboratory in empty container.

niques. It has been argued that symptomatic "abacteriuric" patients may be infected with organisms requiring special cultural conditions. Thus Maskell, Pead, and Allen (1979) have recently reported the isolation of fastidious organisms requiring prolonged incubation in 7% carbon dioxide—lactobacilli, corynebacteria, and *Streptococcus milleri*—from symptomatic patients who were cured by appropriate antibacterial therapy. More recently, Stamm et al. (1980, 1981) have reported similar findings in regard to *Chlamydia trachomatis*. These observations remain to be confirmed. At present, it is suggested that such organisms be sought in abacteriuric symptomatic patients, especially if they are pyuric. Urine must be obtained by suprapubic aspiration.

CLINICAL SIGNIFICANCE

Urinary tract infection is primarily a condition that affects women. Thus, apart from the first few weeks of life and in later life with the development of prostatism, urinary tract infections are always more common in women than in men (Kunin, 1979). Many population surveys indicate that the prevalence of bacteriuria in women increases with age from 1% to 2% in schoolgirls to 5% in women, becoming even more common with advancing years and parity. It has been calculated that approximately 50% of all women will at some time in their lives develop bacteriuria. Not all will have symptoms, and many will lose their bacteriuria spontaneously.

Clinical concern relates to the potential for urinary tract infection to lead to distressing symptoms on the one hand and to damage to the urinary tract, especially the kidney, on the other. Twenty years ago it was generally believed that recurrent or persistent infection of the urinary tract led to progressive kidney damage and the development of chronic pyelonephritis. This is now known to be false. Chronic or atrophic pyelonephritis (sometimes called reflux nephropathy) is now known to result from vesicoureteric reflux plus infection in the first few years of life or even in utero. Conversely, it

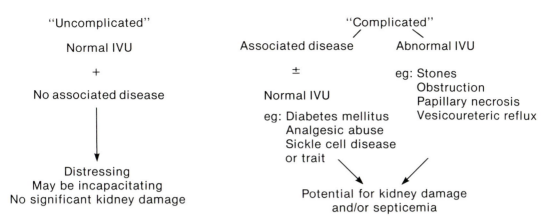

Figure 24.3 Significance of persistent or recurrent urinary tract infection.

is accepted that recurrent or persistent bacteriuria in women with normal urinary tracts and no associated disease seldom if ever results in significant kidney damage. In such women infection may be a cause of great morbidity, but it is not life threatening. The same is not true in cases where there is an abnormality of the urinary tract, such as stones, obstruction, or vesicoureteric reflux. Mixed infected stones may result from infection, an inflammatory proteinaceous matrix providing the nidus for stone formation. The problem is compounded by infection with *P. mirabilis,* where the urea-splitting capability of the organism leads to alkalinization of the urine and facilitates the deposition of triple phosphates. Such stones may damage the kidney by their size but more often by causing urinary tract obstruction. The combination of infection and obstruction, whether caused by stones, pelviureteric junction stenosis, ureteric stenosis, or even bladder outflow obstruction, is especially damaging to the kidney. Few conditions cause renal destruction more rapidly than an obstructed pyonephrosis. This is also one of the most common causes of life-threatening gram-negative septicemia in hospital practice. Vesicoureteric reflux plus infection is most commonly found in children, reflux usually ceasing spontaneously around the age of puberty with growth of the bladder base and a more oblique entry of the ureters into the bladder, leading to competence of the valve mechanism. Reflux may, however, persist into adult life and indeed may develop in adult life if there is damage (surgical or as a consequence of radiotherapy) to the vesicoureteric junction. Uncontrolled infection in the presence of high-pressure reflux is undoubtedly damaging to the kidney.

Other "nonsurgical" conditions may determine the potential for renal damage as a result of infection. Thus diabetes mellitus, analgesic abuse, and sickle cell disease or trait may, of themselves, be associated with renal damage. There is good evidence that in such patients infection aggravates the potential for kidney damage.

It is now conventional and convenient to classify urinary tract infections in adults as complicated or uncomplicated (Figure 24.3).

SIGNIFICANCE OF SYMPTOMS

The continuing confusion in the management of urinary tract infections largely revolves around the interpretation of symptoms, especially frequency and/or dysuria, and loin pain.

Single, isolated episodes of frequency and/or dysuria in nonpregnant women, whether or not they are caused by urinary tract infection, are of small importance provided that the patient is subsequently shown to be abacteriuric and have no clinical symptoms or signs of renal tract disease—no proteinuria and normal urine microscopy. Problems arise with women who have recurrent or persistent symptoms. Most often, the symptoms are frequency and/or dysuria, but they also include intermittent loin pain and intermittent hematuria. Failure to employ a simple but systematic approach to unraveling this problem invariably leads to confusion and poor treatment.

A careful long-term study of several thousand women with symptoms suggestive of urinary tract infection has shown that they fall into three main groups (Figure 24.4) (O'Grady et al., 1972). There are those who, when they have symptoms, are always bacteriuric (group A); those who despite re-

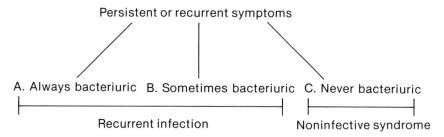

Figure 24.4 Symptomatic groups in patients with or without bacteriuria.

peated urine culture (including urine obtained by suprapubic aspiration while symptomatic and examination for fastidious organisms) are never bacteriuric (group C); and those who, when symptomatic, are sometimes bacteriuric but at other times are not (group B). Groups A and B belong to a population of women who undoubtedly develop recurrent urinary tract infections and should be treated as such. Women in group B do not have urinary tract infections as the cause of their symptoms. The unfortunate term *urethral syndrome* has been introduced to describe this last group of patients: those with recurrent loin pain or hematuria who, on repeated examination, do not have bacteriuria and thus do not have infection as the cause of their symptoms.

To effect this distinction between patients who have bacteriuria and those who do not, it is essential to follow certain basic rules. Thus in patients with intermittent symptoms, urine cultures must be done as soon after the onset of symptoms as possible. Thus bacteriuria may be transient, whereas symptoms—as a result of the secondary inflammation—are more persistent (Cattell et al., 1975). This is especially true in young women who embark on a high-fluid intake at the onset of symptoms. In patients with recurrent symptoms, antibacterial therapy should not be begun until two urine samples have been sent for culture, one preferably obtained on the first voiding in the morning. This can now readily be done by providing such patients with Dipslides to keep at home in the refrigerator. Pending antibacterial therapy, symptoms can be assuaged by symptomatic treatment. In patients with recurrent or persistent symptoms in whom conventional bacteriological examination of midstream urine samples yields negative or equivocal results, urine samples must be obtained by suprapubic aspiration and subjected to more sophisticated bacteriological examination to exclude the presence of organisms with special growth re-

quirements (p. 308). This is especially important in patients with pyuria, in whom urine should also be cultures for *Mycobacterium tuberculosis*.

Strict adherence to these ground rules should allow clear-cut distinction between patients with recurrent infection and those without. By definition, urinary tract infection cannot be diagnosed in the continuing absence of bacteriuria. Symptomatic patients who never have bacteriuria have some other cause for their symptoms, which must be sought.

NATURAL HISTORY

The natural history of bacteriuria (Figure 24.5), whether symptomatic or asymptomatic, follows four main patterns.

Isolated episode

The isolated episode of a urinary tract infection is the most common occurrence and clears spontaneously or readily responds to treatment. There is no recurrence. A considerable proportion of women will experience such an episode at some time in their life. Apart from the distress at the time of the episode, however, this is not a significant problem.

Recurrent infection

Much more important in terms of morbidity are those patients who have recurrent symptomatic infection. Recurrent infection can be classified into two subdivisions: relapse and reinfection.

Relapse. Some patients who develop bacteriuria become abacteriuric when treated with an appropriate antibiotic. However, bacteriuria with the same organism recurs within 7 to 14 days of completion of treatment. This situation is called relapse or persistence of infection. Antibacterial treatment has "sterilized" the urine but has failed to eradicate the infecting organism from the urinary tract. This most often occurs in patients with stones; in those

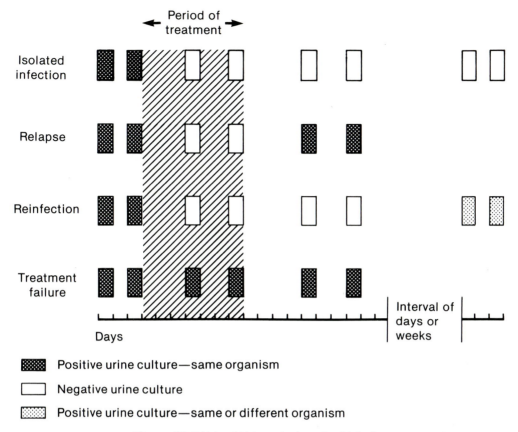

Figure 24.5 Natural history of urinary tract infection.

with scarred, damaged, or cystic kidneys; and occasionally in those with diverticuli or ureteric stumps. There is difficulty in achieving effective levels of antibiotic in the stones or scarred tissue, so that while the urine is "sterilized" during treatment, bacteria persist to reemerge and establish themselves within the urine when it no longer contains antibiotics. While often difficult to treat, this situation is not a common cause of recurrent bacteriuria.

Reinfection. Reinfection is much the more common type of recurrent infection (more than 80% of cases). Bacteriuria is eradicated by appropriate treatment, and the patient remains abacteriuric for weeks or months. She then has a new episode of infection with the same or a different organism. This is not a failure to eradicate the infection but repeated reinfection of a susceptible urinary tract.

Treatment failure

In the case of treatment failure, the bacteriuric patient is given an appropriate antibiotic but during treatment the urine remains infected with the same organism. The causes of this are limited. Rarely, there is laboratory error in defining antibacterial sensitivities and an inappropriate antibacterial agent has been used. Occasionally there is patient noncompliance in taking the drug or persistent vomiting—as, for example, with nitrofurantoin—resulting in limited absorption of drug from the gut. Most often it is caused by severe impairment of renal function such that effective antibacterial concentrations cannot be achieved in the urine.

CYSTITIS, PYELITIS, AND PYELONEPHRITIS

In the past, the terms *cystitis, pyelitis,* and *pyelonephritis* have been used to describe clinical syndromes believed to reflect infection confined to the bladder (cystitis) or ascending to the upper tract (pyelitis) and finally to the kidney (pyelonephritis). There has also been the implication of an ascending order of severity of illness and potential for renal damage. While in general a severe illness with fever, loin pain, and systemic illness does indicate extension of the infection to the upper tract, it is clear that the level of infection cannot be accurately diagnosed on the basis of symptoms. Further, in uncomplicated urinary tract infection the prognosis and management are much the same.

SIGNIFICANCE OF URINARY TRACT INFECTION IN PREGNANCY

The prevalence of asymptomatic bacteriuria is very similar in pregnant and nonpregnant women. In both, prevalence increases with age and parity and may also be increased in socioeconomically deprived groups (Kunin, 1979). These factors are themselves interdependent, and no special weight should be given to one. These observations imply that pregnancy per se does not predispose women to the acquisition of urinary tract infection. By contrast, there is now an abundance of evidence that women with asymptomatic bacteriuria in early pregnancy have a low spontaneous clearance rate and a very high incidence of acute, symptomatic urinary tract infection later in their pregnancy. Thus the pregnant state, while not predisposing women to the acquisition of infection, does predispose them to acute infection (usually upper tract) should bladder bacteriuria be present or develop. This fact alone demands careful attention to and treatment of pregnant women with asymptomatic bacteriuria and women known to have had a history of bacteriuria before pregnancy.

Much more controversial is the effect of urinary tract infection on the course of the pregnancy and on the development of the fetus (Asscher, 1980). Many investigators have claimed that the presence of asymptomatic bacteriuria during pregnancy predisposes women to develop anemia, preeclamptic toxemia, and premature labor, and to give birth to small infants. An equal number of reports deny these associations. The situation is confused by the failure of many studies to distinguish between bacteriuria in women with normal urinary tracts and bacteriuria in women with preexisting renal damage. This distinction is important, since preexisting renal damage can certainly predispose women to develop hypertension and anemia during pregnancy and lead to the birth of small infants. This is a consequence of the established renal disease and is not attributable to infection during pregnancy.

The argument surrounding these points is somewhat academic, since bacteriuria in pregnancy should always, when possible, be treated and be shown to remain eradicated because of its potential for producing acute pyelonephritis. In terms of

practical management, all pregnant women should have urine cultures performed at the first visit to identify those with asymptomatic bacteriuria, and all women with a history of recurrent symptomatic bacteriuria must be considered at high risk for acquiring bacteriuria during pregnancy.

Finally, there is the question of whether urinary tract infection in pregnancy affects the life expectancy of the mother and whether it is hazardous for patients with recurrent urinary tract infections to become pregnant. There is no evidence that uncomplicated urinary tract infections in pregnancy causes permanent kidney damage or alters the life expectancy of the patient. In women with a previous history of recurrent infection, the risk of acute pyelonephritis in pregnancy should be explained to the patient, and if she is prepared to have regular supervision and treatment, pregnancy need not be forbidden.

PATHOGENESIS

The successful management of patients with recurrent urinary tract infections demands a clear understanding of present knowledge of the pathogenesis of urinary tract infection.

Source of infection

There is now general agreement that the organisms causing urinary tract infection in domiciliary practice come from the patient's own fecal flora. There is also general agreement that the frequency with which *E. coli* is recovered from the urinary tract reflects the frequency with which these organisms are present in the feces—implying no particular uropathogenicity (Grüneberg, Leigh, and Brumfitt, 1968). Recently, however, there has been increasing evidence that a high proportion of these organisms isolated from women and children with urinary tract infections have a special faculty for adhering to uroepithelial surfaces (Svanborg-Edén, Lidin-Janson, and Lindberg, 1979). This appears to depend on surface pili on the organism attaching to receptor sites on the epithelial cells. It may thus be that one factor determining an organism's ability to invade the urinary tract is its degree of pilation and thus adhesiveness. Many other biological characteristics of *E. coli* have been studied, including O and K antigenicity, hemolytic capacity, and resistance to the bactericidal effect of normal serum. Some association with infection can be shown, but overall it is unimpressive (Brooks et al., 1980). In practical terms, all women carry bacteria in their fecal flora that are capable of causing urinary tract infection, and to date no method is available for altering this reservoir of potential infection.

The source of infection and the nature of the organisms in hospitalized patients is different. In this situation organisms are commonly introduced into the bladder by instrumentation or catheterization and may come from the local environment rather than the patient's gut. Cross-infection or drug treatment may also alter the patient's gut flora to yield a higher proportion of potentially invasive organisms.

Route of infection

Bacteria may gain access to the urinary tract by four potential routes: direct extension from the gut, lymphatic spread, via the bloodstream, or by the ascending transurethral route from the perineum. Direct extension does occasionally occur and is almost always associated with vesicocolic or (more rarely) vesicovaginal fistulae. This can usually be diagnosed on the basis of pneumaturia, evidence of gross contamination on microscopy of the urine, or culture of mixed organisms, including anaerobic bacteria. Lymphatic spread of infection is speculative and highly unlikely. Blood-borne infection is the route of infection for renal carbuncles and tuberculosis of the kidney, conditions not dealt with in this chapter. It is difficult to establish how often blood-borne infection occurs in more conventional cases of enterobacterial urinary tract infection, but it is probably uncommon and most likely to occur when there is established renal disease, such as obstruction of renal cysts. There is now a great deal of evidence that urinary tract infection most often results from ascending infection of the bladder via the urethra (Table 24.1). A series of steps are involved.

Periurethral colonization. The first requirement is colonization of the perineum and periurethral area with pathogenic organisms from the gut. There is some controversy regarding this. Stamey (1972) has claimed that in normal women there is no significant carriage of bacteria on the perineum. Preceding an episode of infection there is a period of heavy colonization that he attributes to some biological characteristic of the perineal surface allowing colonization to occur. My colleagues and I (Cattell et al., 1974) and others have failed to show any significant difference in periurethral carriage of *E. coli* between normal and recurrently infected women when the latter are studied between episodes of infection; in other words, pathogenic bacteria can regularly be recovered from all women. We would agree with Stamey, however, that there is a buildup in colonization preceding infection. We suggest that this is more likely to be caused by biological characteristics of the bacteria, for ex-

---

TABLE 24.1 Ascending bladder infection

Sequential steps	Conditioning factors	Prophylactic measures
Fecal reservoir of organisms	No special uropathogenicity *but* (?) piliated forms	Cannot modify
↓		
Perineal or periurethral colonization	Organism always present Buildup preceding infection (?) Bacterial adhesion (pili)	No effective local treatment Avoid bubble baths
↓		

Transurethral passage to bladder	Facilitated by
	  Catheterization
	  Instrumentation
	  Vaginal massage
	  Coitus
		Vaginal lubricants
		Postcoital voiding
		Avoid bubble baths

↓		

Establishment in bladder	Facilitated by
	  Infrequent and impaired bladder emptying
	  Low urine flow rate
	  Impaired bladder wall defenses
	  (?) Previous inflammation
		Ensure high fluid intake
		Regular voiding
		Double micturition
		Surgery to improve emptying

ample, adhesiveness, than by the periurethral surface. To date there is no effective method of altering periurethral carriage other than oral prophylactic antibacterial therapy.

Urethral passage. The second step toward infection is the transfer of bacteria along the urethra and into the bladder. The distance to traverse in the short female urethra is small, and it is not difficult to understand how what are often motile organisms can reach the bladder. The passage of bacteria is facilitated by catheterization and instrumentation and has been shown to follow vaginal massage. It is probably facilitated by coitus—an important factor in the development of postcoital infection (Kunin, 1978). The position of the external urethral orifice in relation to the opening of the vagina has been considered a possible factor in the pathogenesis of postcoital bacteriuria. In some women the external urethral orifice is on the anterior lip of the vagina. During intercourse, with ascent of the vault, the orifice may become an "intravaginal" opening. It has been suggested that this may facilitate the entry of organisms during coitus and their transfer to the bladder. While of interest, there is no good evidence that this is true and, more importantly, no evidence that surgery to this area to separate the external urethral orifice and the vagina is of any value. Concerning the role of coitus, it does seem that in individual patients symptoms do appear to be more common with one form of contraception than with another. There is, however, little evidence that, in general, one form of contraception is more likely to predispose women to urinary tract infection than another with the possible exception of methods associated with drying up of vaginal secretion, as is sometimes experienced by women taking oral contraceptives. Lack of vaginal secretion does appear to encourage bladder bacteriuria.

In men, prostatic secretions contain antibacterial material, and this may well be an important factor in preventing ascending urethral infection. Whether similar secretions are present in women is unknown, although many authorities believe that women possess paraurethral glands, which are the equivalent of the prostate.

Establishment of bladder bacteriuria

The entry of bacteria into bladder urine is not synonymous with the development of infection. For this to occur, the bacteria must multiply and become established. It seems entirely probable that organisms frequently enter the female bladder but do not become established; that is, there is spontaneous elimination. Spontaneous clearance has been demonstrated by Cox and Hinman (1961), who deliberately infected the bladders of healthy young female subjects and showed bacterial clearance within 48 hours. What are the factors that determine bladder bacteriuria?

Urine as a culture medium

Lacking both humoral and cellular defense mechanisms, human urine is an excellent medium for bacterial growth. While at the physiological extremes of pH (less than 5.5 and more than 7.5) there is inhibition of the growth of *E. coli*, as there is at the extremes of urine osmolality (less than 300 and more than 1200 mosm/kg), urine in general supports vigorous bacterial growth. There is statistical evidence that female urine, especially pregnant female urine, supports bacterial growth more readily than does male urine. While of interest, it is doubtful whether this has any important relevance to the pathogenicity and prophylaxis of urinary tract infection. Despite these observations, in most women the bladder is sterile.

Bladder defense mechanisms

Given the ready availability of pathogenic bacteria, the short female urethra, and the excellence of urine as a culture medium, it seems inescapable that the major factor preventing bladder infection must be intrinsic defense mechanisms within the bladder. Some of these are understood and some are not.

Hydrokinetic bacterial clearance. The importance of urine flow rate, frequency and completeness of voiding, and dilatation of the urinary tract has been extensively studied in vivo and in vitro (O'Grady and Cattell, 1966a; 1966b; O'Grady, 1976) and is of immense relevance to an understanding of both the pathogenesis and the management of urinary tract infection. In summary, it is now well established that high rates of urine flow along with frequent and complete voiding result in "bacterial washout," causing the population of bacteria to diminish dramatically. Conversely, low rates of urine flow along with infrequent and incomplete voiding predispose the bladder to bacterial multiplication and establishment. The same applies to dilated and distended urinary systems wherein the volume of the space is large in relation to urine flow. Underperfused diverticuli are excellent sites for bacterial multiplication, as are large, poorly emptying systems, such as neuropathic bladders or ileal conduits (Figure 24.6). Impaired bladder emptying is especially important. Recurrent infection in patients with vesicoureteric reflux is in part conditioned by the postvoiding residual urine that had refluxed at the time of voiding.

Bladder wall defense mechanisms. In addition to hydrokinetic clearance, there is good evidence for a further mucosal defense system. The nature of this is unknown, although speculation has

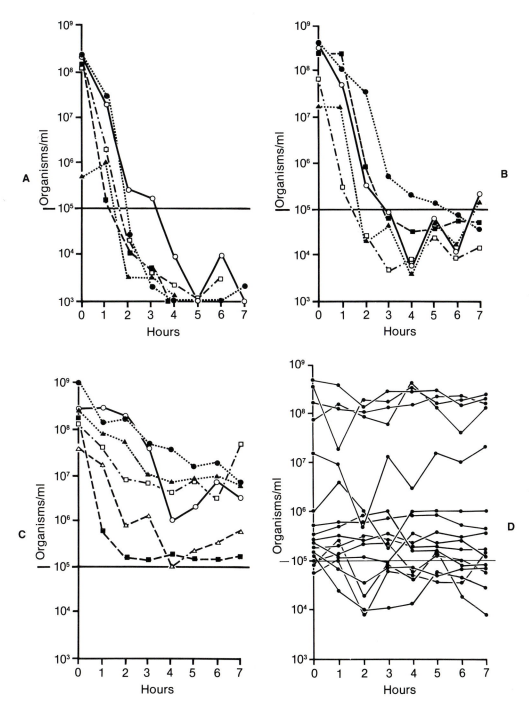

Figure 24.6 A, Effect of high (300 ml/hr) fluid intake and hourly voiding on bacterial content of urine in patients with normal urinary tracts. **B,** to **D,** Effect of increasing dilatation of system and/or impaired bladder emptying. (From Cattell, W.R., et al. 1970. Br. Med. J. **1:**377-379.)

centered on some phagocytic or bactericidal property of the lining cells. The urine from patients
with urinary tract infection contains IgG, IgM, and
IgA immunoglobulins. Urine, however, lacks the
components of complement and is itself anticom-
plementary. It seems that only bladder-produced
secretory IgA may be of importance. It is still unclear as to how it works, but it may block adherence
of bacteria to epithelial cells, that is, it is part of
the mucosal defense system.

Upper tract infection

Fundamental to an understanding of the management of urinary tract infection is the realization
that establishment of bacteria within the bladder is
the first critical step in the development of urinary
tract infection. If established, infection may be
confined to the bladder or extend upward into the
ureters and thus to the kidney. Several factors determine this. Most important is vesicoureteric reflux, which if severe can lead to intrarenal reflux.
Characteristics of the bacteria themselves, such as
motility and K antigen, play a part (Brooks et al.,
1980). Impaired ureteric motility with dilated systems such as occurs in pregnancy facilitates ascending infection. This probably accounts for the
high incidence of acute pyelonephritis in pregnant
women. Bacterial endotoxin itself can also reduce
ureteric motility. Just as impaired bladder emptying
predisposes women to bladder bacteriuria, so too
do dilated upper tracts predispose them to ascending infection.

INVESTIGATION

The diagnosis of urinary tract infection must be
based on urine culture, and the most important
investigation for successful management is careful
sequential urine culture. Only by doing this can
the natural history of the situation be defined and
the need for further investigation and treatment assessed. In general, special investigations are of value only in predicting the significance of recurrent
infection or in defining potentially correctable anatomical or functional abnormalities of the urinary
tract. There is no place for special investigations
in the woman who has had an isolated episode of
urinary tract infection provided urine cultures taken
after treatment are negative and she has no symptoms or clinical signs of urinary tract disease.
Women with two or more illnesses thought to be
caused by infection must be investigated in detail.
The first critical step is to establish whether or not
such illnesses are associated with bacteriuria and,

if so, whether the infection is relapsing or recurrent. In all instances an intravenous urogram will
be necessary.

Asymptomatic infection in pregnant women demands treatment and careful sequential urine culture. Further investigation during pregnancy is
rarely necessary except in patients with relapsing
bacteriuria, in which case a plain radiograph may
be required to define the presence or absence of
stones. In asymptomatic nonpregnant women with
persisting or recurrent bacteriuria, it is my practice
to carry out an intravenous urogram primarily to
establish whether the urinary tract infection is complicated or uncomplicated. If it is uncomplicated,
there is no indication for further investigation.

Intravenous urography

Excretion urography is always associated with
some discomfort for the patient and some risk of
untoward reactions. It should never be carried out
casually. When requested, the purpose of and justification for the intravenous urogram must be considered. The purpose of the intravenous urogram
in patients with recurrent urinary tract infection is
to define predisposing anatomical or functional abnormalities that may be correctable. Second, it will
identify patients in whom there are complicated
factors (p. 306) that affect the natural history and
significance of recurrent infection. Finally, the intravenous urogram has a role in the management
of patients with symptoms suggestive of urinary
tract infection but in whom bacteriuria cannot be
demonstrated, for example, recurrent loin pain and
fever.

It follows from this that there is no justification
for an intravenous urogram in women with a single,
isolated, and uncomplicated episode of proven or
suspected urinary tract infection. It is required in
all women with recurrent infection, principally to
define bladder emptying but equally important, to
allow reassurance of the patient that her upper urinary tract is normal and that there is minimum
likelihood of renal damage in the future. It should
not be repeated in patients already shown to have
a normal intravenous urogram unless some new
situation is anticipated, for example, the development of low-density renal stones. In patients with
relapsing bacteriuria, the intravenous urogram is
undertaken to define the presence or absence of
such problems as stones, renal scarring, or cystic
disease, with predisposition to difficulty in eradicating infection. Initial plain tomograms of the renal areas will help exclude low-density stones.

If these rules are followed, there will be a dramatic reduction in the number of unnecessary intravenous urograms carried out.

Cystoscopy

Few investigations are so badly abused as cystoscopy in patients with frequency and/or dysuria. There is virtually no place for cystoscopy in women with recurrent documented bacteriuria who have a normal intravenous urogram without a significant postmicturition bladder residual. In these circumstances it contributes nothing to the management. The indications for cystoscopy are impaired bladder emptying on intravenous urogram in patients shown to have bladder outflow obstruction by urodynamic studies; unexplained overt hematuria in abacteriuric patients or in patients between 30 and 40 years of age whether they are bacteriuric or not; and recurrent frequency and/or dysuria in abacteriuric patients. Cystoscopy should be avoided if at all possible while patients are bacteriuric.

Micturating cystourethrography and urodynamic studies

There is a limited role for micturating cystourethrography and urodynamic studies in women shown to be bacteriuric. They are required primarily to evaluate impaired bladder emptying whether it is caused by outflow obstruction or by detrusor failure of vesicoureteric reflux. In the latter instance bladder urine refluxed during voiding returns to the bladder at the end of micturition, and its volume may constitute a considerable and significant postmicturition residual. In most instances this can be eliminated by training in double or triple micturition. Ureteric reimplantation to control reflux is rarely required in adults except when there is difficulty in controlling recurrent infection, when there is gross reflux with evidence of upper tract damage, or when there is ipsilateral loin pain during micturition. In the absence of these, undertaking a micturating cystourethrography to establish whether or not minor reflux occurs makes no contribution to management.

Localization studies

Clinical criteria are in general a poor guide to the localization of infection within the urinary tract. Thus patients with purely bladder symptoms may be shown to have bacteriuria in the upper urinary tract, and in patients with loin pain symptoms may be confined to the bladder. Since it was at one time considered essential to define the localization of infection to permit correct treatment, localization studies enjoyed a brief vogue. The methods most commonly used were both direct and indirect. Of the direct tests, the most accurate is that of ureteric catheterization and collection of separate bladder and ureteric urine samples (Stamey, Govan, and Palmer, 1965). It is, however, invasive and time consuming. A direct technique of bladder washout without ureteric catheterization devised by Fairley et al. (1967) is much simpler but fails to lateralize reinfection. The most popular of the indirect tests has been measurement of the humoral immune response to infection, including antibodies to O antigens of gram-negative bacteria (Percival, Brumfitt, and de Louvois, 1964) and local production of antibody in the urinary tract as evidenced by coating of bacteria by antibody (Thomas, Shelokov, and Forland, 1954). Such indirect tests have given conflicting results in different hands, and all tests give false-positive and false-negative results.

While localization studies have contributed greatly to our understanding of the natural history of urinary tract infection, it is now clear that they have little place in the management of infection (Turck, 1978). It may be argued they are of help in defining the source of relapsing bacteriuria, but the necessary management information can usually be obtained by intravenous urogram (Cattell et al., 1972). Rarely, ureteric catheterization may be desired before nephrectomy is done when all other treatment has failed.

Bladder residue

Measurement of the postvoiding bladder urine residue by isotopic techniques has also proved useful in the evolution of management policies. It is, however, rarely required in practice, since as much information as is necessary can be obtained from a carefully conducted intravenous urogram with satisfactory postmicturition bladder radiographs. Recently, ultrasonography has been used to measure postmicturition bladder residuals, but in my experience it has not been very satisfactory.

TREATMENT

For management, patients should be classified as being symptomatic or asymptomatic (Figure 24.7). Symptomatic infections must then be subclassified as a single, isolated episode or recurrent. The latter is further classified as relapsing or reinfecting. Asymptomatic or "covert" bacteriuria must be subclassified as occurring in pregnant or in nonpregnant women.

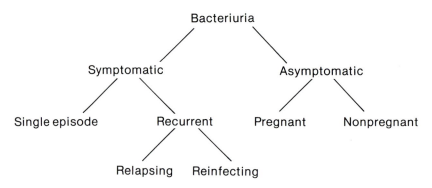

Figure 24.7 Classification of patients with urinary tract infection for management purposes.

Symptomatic infections

Single attack. Acute symptoms suggestive of urinary tract infection should be treated with a high fluid intake (2 L or 4 pints a day) and a "best bet" antibacterial drug, such as cotrimoxazole tablets, 2 b.d.; ampicillin, 500 mg t.d.s.; or nitrofuratoin, 100 mg t.d.s. A pretreatment midstream urine sample should be obtained, but antibiotic treatment should not be delayed if symptoms are disabling. Time-honored symptomatic treatment such as potassium citrate or flavoxate hydrochloride (Urispas) can be of value. The duration of treatment is subject to debate. There is little advantage in having the patient take drugs for more than 5 to 7 days. Several studies have shown excellent results in young women given only 3 days of treatment (Charlton et al., 1976), and even a single 3 g dose of amoxicillin gives a high cure rate in uncomplicated cases (Bailey and Abbott, 1977). At present, a reasonable median is 5 days of treatment. Symptoms usually improve within 48 hours, and if not, the result of the pretreatment urine culture, including sensitivity testing, should be available. Both the diagnosis and choice of drug should be reviewed. A midstream urine sample should be obtained 7 days after treatment and the patient advised to maintain a liberal fluid intake for some weeks.

Relapsing infection. Patients who have recurrence of bacteriuria with the same organism and/or symptoms within 7 to 10 days of completing treatment have, by definition, relapsed. In terms of practicality, it is worth giving a more prolonged course (10 to 14 days) of an appropriate oral antibiotic, obtaining midstream urine samples during treatment to ensure compliance and sterilization of the urine. If further relapse occurs, the patient must have an intravenous urogram to identify the cause. If stones are present, surgical removal should be considered. If there is no surgically treatable le-

sion, a 5- to 7-day course of high-dose treatment with drugs such as one of the aminoglycosides (gentamicin, tobramycin, or kanamycin) or carbenicillin should be given. The intention is to achieve high blood levels and hopefully deliver sufficient antibiotic to the persisting nidus of infection to eradicate the organisms. If this fails, consideration should be given to long-term, low-dose suppressive therapy to control symptoms and reduce the potential for stone formation or acute pyelonephritis. The treatment schedule is as for prophylactic treatment. Rarely, where infection is confined to one kidney that makes no significant contribution to total renal function, nephrectomy may be considered. In some cases further treatment to eradicate infection is not indicated.

Reinfection. Reinfection is the most common cause of recurrent infection in women and young girls. The problem is not one of eradicating infection but of preventing reestablishment of bacteriuria. The first step is to explain to the patient the nature of the problem and recruit her active participation in preventing infection. Without positive, informed self-help, treatment is difficult. It must also be explained that active prophylactic measures must be maintained for at least 12 months after the last episode of infection.

Prophylaxis should first be attempted without drugs. Thus after, if necessary, a short course of antibiotics to eradicate any current infection, patients must adhere strictly to the following regime:

1. They must have a high fluid intake (at least 4 pints of liquid daily) to achieve a high rate of urine flow.
2. They must void every 2 to 3 hours during the day and always before going to bed.
3. They should be taught and should practice double or triple micturition. This is especially important in patients with reflux. Patients

with a neuropathic bladder should be taught to manually assist voiding by pressing downward and backward over the suprapubic area during voiding.

4. They must be taught to void following intercourse. Some women may find the use of a vaginal lubricant such as KY jelly helpful.

The value of other measures is to a considerable extent anecdotal. Obsessional perineal toilet is not necessary, and it may be harmful. The use of bubble baths or disinfectants in bathwater should be discouraged. Constipation should be avoided, since a full rectum can impair bladder emptying. Coexisting vaginitis should be treated if possible.

On this regime a considerable proportion of patients have no or very rare recurrence. If, despite this regime, patients develop reinfection twice or more within 6 months, they should be given longterm, low-dose antibacterial prophylaxis.

Low-dose prophylaxis. Following a short course of treatment the patient continues to take one dose of an antibacterial drug immediately before retiring. The drugs of choice are nitrofurantoin, 50 to 100 mg; cotrimoxazole, 1 tablet; or trimethoprim, 100 mg. Treatment should be continued for at least 12 months after the last infection. The dosage may be reduced to alternate nights after 3 months but can only rarely be reduced further (Cattell et al., 1971). In the very few patients in whom there is a clear-cut relationship between coitus and infection, one dose of antibacterial drug after intercourse may suffice, and this may allow a significant reduction in dosage. Should superinfection occur with a different (and resistant) organism, a short course of an appropriate alternative antibiotic should be given and the patient then returned to low-dose treatment for a further 12 months. At the end of 12 months patients should be encouraged to maintain their high fluid intake. Most will have no further trouble. Some will have recurrence of problems and must return to lowdose treatment for a period of 2 years, again stopping to see if they are cured. Some may require lifelong prophylaxis.

Role of surgery in recurrent reinfection. Tempting as it may be, there is a very limited role for surgery in these patients, and it relates primarily to measures to improve bladder emptying. There is no good evidence that urethral dilatation is of any value except as a means of giving temporary symptomatic relief. Bladder outflow obstruction can be dealt with. Reconstructive operations to improve bladder emptying are dealt with elsewhere

in this book but all too often do not achieve their objective. Surgery to the upper urinary tract, except where there is free reflux and an uncontrollable postmicturition bladder residue, plays no part in preventing the acquisition of bladder bacteriuria.

Low-dose suppressive treatment. The same regime is used as for prophylaxis, but it is unusual to reduce the dosage to less than once nightly.

Asymptomatic patients

The management of women found to be bacteriuric on routine urine culture varies depending on whether or not they are pregnant and also on whether or not they have a previous history of infection, renal disease, or hypertension. It also depends on whether or not they are truly symptom free. Thus many women with covert infection may not seek medical advice yet have symptoms attributable to the infection. These include nocturia, urgency incontinence, vague backache, and general malaise or tiredness.

Nonpregnant women. It is my practice in the first instance to treat covert infection is the same manner as for symptomatic infection. If there is recurrent asymptomatic bacteriuria, such patients are investigated by intravenous urogram primarily to exclude some potentially harmful urinary tract disease and to allow advice to be given to the patient. If no significant abnormality is found, further covert infection is not treated. We do, however, pay special attention to patients with *Proteus* bacteriuria because of the special potential for stone formation. If bacteriuria is persistent, such patients should have a plain radiograph of the abdomen taken at 2-year intervals to exclude stone formation.

Pregnant women. Pregnant women must be treated and followed with serial urine cultures throughout the pregnancy. Patients with recurrent bacteriuria (if frequent) should be treated with lowdose therapy and require full investigation after the pregnancy. In patients with relapsing recurrence, a single plain abdominal radiograph is indicated to exclude stones. High-dose treatment is rarely necessary during pregnancy.

Certain antibacterial drugs should be avoided in pregnancy. Thus tetracycline is best avoided because of pigmentation of the teeth of the child. Intravenous tetracycline can cause fatal liver necrosis. Sulfonamides (including cotrimoxazole) should be avoided in the third trimester, since they may precipitate or exacerbate kernicterus. Nalidixic acid should be avoided in late pregnancy, since it may produce hydrocephalus. The evidence of harm to the fetus from other drugs is scanty, but in general all drugs should be avoided unless clearly indicated. Nitrofurantoin is probably the safest of all antibacterials to use during pregnancy.

When not to treat. Treatment is not indicated in asymptomatic patients when it is likely to be ineffective or even harmful. This applies particularly to patients with dilated and poor emptying systems, for example, ileal conduit and neurogenic bladder, and to patients with multiple calculi that cannot be removed. The potential for eradicating infection and maintaining the system sterile is often small. Conversely, the use of multiple antibacterial agents increases the potential for the emergence of polyresistant strains. In general, if there is a low pressure within the urinary tract, the potential for serious kidney damage is small. In these patients it is my practice not to continue attempts at treatment if there is rapid recurrence of infection or infection with drug-resistant organisms. Rather, I warn them to report immediately should they develop symptoms, especially those of loin pain or fever. Patients are then treated for this symptomatic attack.

BLADDER CATHETERIZATION

The only certain way to avoid catheter-induced urinary tract infection is to avoid catheterization. Even with meticulous techniques there is always the potential for the establishment of bacteriuria. This risk increases with indwelling catheters. Thus every catheterization must be justified and the hazards recognized. The principal indication for isolated catheterization is to relieve a temporary obstruction or inability to void. Rarely, it is required to obtain a urine sample for culture in the elderly or infirm. It is, of course, required for micturating cystourography and urodynamic studies, and these investigations must be clearly justified. A strict aseptic technique must be employed, and catheters must be passed gently. There is little evidence that lubricants containing antibacterial agents are of much value. In high-risk patients, for example, those suspected of having acute oliguric renal failure, diagnostic bladder catheterization should include the instillation of 30 ml of a 1% to 2% solution of noxythiolin before removal of the catheter.

Intermittent catheterization

Intermittent catheterization in the spinal cord–injured patient and in patients with neuropathic bladders from other causes has been shown to be safe and effective by dedicated teams, both in the United Kingdom and in the United States (Guttman and Frankel, 1966; Lapides, Diokno, and Gould, 1975). It does, however, demand close attention to detail and should not be practiced casually.

Self-catheterization

Self-catheterization has also revolutionized the care of patients with neuropathic bladders (Lapides, Diokno, and Gould, 1975) but again requires training and supervision by a dedicated team (see Chapter 37).

Suprapubic drainage

Suprapubic drainage is gaining in popularity. Although not widely practiced in the United Kingdom, it is likely to become more widespread with the development of new and better catheters.

Indwelling urethral catheter

Use of the indwelling catheter remains the safest technique for patients who cannot void, are grossly incontinent, or require continuous drainage for surgical reasons. It must be used conservatively and be practiced carefully. A closed catheter drainage system is mandatory. The perineum must be washed twice daily and kept dry. There is little evidence that prophylactic intermittent or continuous irrigation with antibacterial agents has any significant advantage. Similarly, the application of antibacterials to the perineum has no proven advantage except possibly in the use of a plastic sponge that is placed around the catheter and that abuts against the external urethral orifice; such a sponge is kept impregnated with antiseptic solution (Gillespie, Lennon, and Linton, 1964).

Prophylactic oral antibiotics should not be given to patients on a regime of continuous drainage. Should bacteriuria develop, provided there is free drainage, this need not be treated unless there is clinical evidence of tissue invasion: fever, suprapubic pain, or loin pain. The need for the catheter should be reviewed and treatment given after it is removed. A detailed review of catheter care has been done superbly and at length by Kunin (1979).

ABACTERIURIC FREQUENCY AND/OR DYSURIA

The major clinical problem in women with symptoms referable to the urinary tract is recurrent or persistent frequency and/or dysuria despite persistently negative urine cultures. In these patients it is essential to obtain midstream urine samples at the outset of symptoms and subject the urine to sophisticated bacteriological examination if they are not to be wrongly designated as abacteriuric. They cannot be given this designation without being studied over some period of time. The term *urethral syndrome* is not helpful, since there is no evidence of infection or inflammation of the urethral lumen. It is my experience and that of others (Stamm et al., 1980) that the majority of patients referred with a diagnosis of urethral syndrome can subsequently be shown to be intermittently bacteriuric.

Elucidation of the nature of the problem in the truly abacteriuric patient demands careful history taking and examination. In many of these patients the dominant problem is frequency, often only during the day. If the problem is dysuria, close questioning should be done to try to establish whether urethral or vulval pain is involved, since the latter is often referred to as dysuria. If symptoms are intermittent, some pattern should be sought in relation to menstruation, intercourse, or wearing tight clothes. Patients must be asked about the use of bubble baths and the addition of chemicals such as Dettol or Sudol to bathwater, all of which may be associated with dysuria. Examination must include careful examination of the vulva and vagina to exclude vulvovaginitis or genital herpes. In older women evidence of hormone-deficient vaginitis should be sought. All patients require detailed examination of the bladder by cystoscopy to exclude interstitial cystitis and urodynamic studies, including radiographic visualization, to exclude neuropathic bladder and bladder outflow obstruction.

When investigated in this way, patients fall into various groups. A small number have obvious vulvovaginitis and respond to treatment for this. In some patients the problem relates to the use of bubble baths, and so on. A number of elderly women with atrophic vaginitis respond to treatment with local or, preferably, systemic hormone replacement. A very small number of patients have interstitial cystitis and respond to bladder dilatation with or without the use of steroids or azathioprine. A considerable number have frequency during the day as their main problem, whereas the remainder have frequency and dysuria without obvious cause. Despite a plethora of urodynamic studies and an increasing complexity of labels such as "irritable bladder," "unstable bladder," and "detrusor instability," there is little clear understanding as to why some patients develop frequency during the day and others both frequency and discomfort during voiding. A pragmatic approach for those with frequency is to arrange with the patient to measure and record the time of all fluid intake throughout each day for several days and to do the same thing with urine output. Commonly it will be found that patients are capable of voiding 300 to 400 ml of urine on waking but by day pass volumes of 50 to 75 ml. Patently these patients have a bladder capable of containing normal volumes, and voiding during the day is "inappropriate." When this is demonstrated to the patient, her help must be recruited in "retraining" her bladder by trying to defer voiding as long as possible. Such patients may be helped with the use of drugs such as emepronium bromide (Cetiprin) or diazepam (Valium). Documentation may, of course, demonstrate that the frequency relates to polydipsia and consequent polyuria. A restriction of fluid intake can then often resolve the problem.

Patients with frequency and dysuria are the most difficult to manage. In many there may be psychological or psychosexual factors. Treatment is unsatisfactory and demands a great deal of careful and sympathetic history taking plus the judicious use of drugs such as diazepam or flavoxate hydrochloride. At present there is no simple solution.

REFERENCES

Asscher, A.W. 1980. The challenge of urinary tract infections. London, Academic Press, Inc., Ltd.

Bailey, R.R., and Abbott, G.D. 1977. Treatment of urinary tract infection with a single dose of amoxycillin. Nephron **18**:316-318.

Brooks, H.J.L., et al. 1980. Uropathogenic properties of *Escherichia coli* in recurrent urinary tract infection. J. Med. Microbiol. **13**:57-68.

Cattell, W.R., et al. 1970. Effect of diuresis and frequent micturition on the bacterial content of infected urine. Br. J. Urol. **42**:290-295.

Cattell, W.R., et al. 1971. Long-term control of bacteriuria with trimethoprim-sulphonamide. Br. Med. J. **1**:377-379.

Cattell, W.R., et al. 1972. The localisation of urinary tract infection and its relationship to relapse, reinfection and treatment. In Brumfitt, W., and Asscher, A.W., editors. Urinary tract infection. London. Oxford University Press.

Cattell, W.R., et al. 1974. Periurethral enterobacterial carriage in pathogenesis of recurrent urinary infection. Br. Med. J. **4**:136-139.

Cattell, W.R., et al. 1975. Approach to the frequency and dysuria syndrome. Kidney Int. **8**:S138-143.

Charlton, C.A.C., et al. 1976. Three day and ten day chemotherapy for urinary tract infection in general practice. Br. Med. J. **1**:124-126.

Cox, C.E., and Hinman, F., Jr. 1961. Experiments with induced bacteriuria, vesical emptying and bacterial growth on the mechanism of bladder defence to infection. J. Urol. **86**:739-748.

Fairley, K.F., et al. 1967. Simple test to determine the site of urinary tract infection. Lancet **2:**427-428.

Gillespie, W.A., Lennon, G.G., and Linton, K.B. 1964. Prevention of urinary infection in gynaecology. Br. Med. J. **2:**423-425.

Grüneberg, R.N., Leigh, D.A., and Brumfitt, W. 1968. *Escherichia coli* serotypes in urinary tract infection: studies in domiciliary, antenatal and hospital practice. In O'Grady, F., and Brumfitt, W., editors. Urinary tract infection. London, Oxford University Press.

Guttman, L., and Frankel, H. 1966. The value of intermittent catheterisation in the early management of traumatic paraplegia and tetraplegia. Paraplegia **4:**63-84.

Guttmann, D.E., and Naylor, G.R.E. 1967. Dip-slide: an aid to quantitative urine culture in general practice. Br. Med. J. **3:**343-345.

Kunin, C.M. 1978. Sexual intercourse and urinary infection. N. Engl. J. Med. **278:**336-338.

Kunin, C.M. 1979. Detection, prevention and management of urinary tract infection. ed. 3. Philadelphia. Lea & Febiger.

Lapides, J., Diokno, A.C., and Gould, F.R. 1975. Further observation on self-catheterisation. Am. Assoc. Genito-Urinary Surgeons **67:**15-17.

Mackey, J.P., and Sandys, G.H. 1966. Diagnosis of urinary infection. Br. Med. J. **1:**1173.

Maskell, R., Pead, L., and Allen, J. 1979. The puzzle of "urethral syndrome"; a possible answer? Lancet **1:**1058-1059.

O'Grady, F. 1976. Initiation and ascent of urinary tract infection. In Williams, D.I., and Chisholm, G.D., editors. Scientific foundations of urology. vol. 1. London. Heinemann Medical Books, Ltd.

O'Grady, F., and Cattell, W.R. 1966a. Kinetics of urinary tract infection. I. Upper urinary tract. Br. J. Urol. **38:**149-155.

O'Grady, F., and Cattell, W.R. 1966b. Kinetics of urinary tract infection. II. The bladder. Br. J. Urol. **38:**156-162.

O'Grady, F.W., et al. 1972. Natural history of intractable 'cystitis' in women referred to a special clinic. In Brumfitt, W., and Asscher, A.W., editors. Urinary tract infection. London. Oxford University Press.

Percival, A., Brumfitt, W., and de Louvois, J. 1964. Serum antibody levels as an indication of clinically inapparent pyelonephritis. Lancet **2:**1027-1033.

PHLS Monograph Series No. 10. 1978. In Meers, P.D., editor. The bacteriological examination of urine. London. Her Majesty's Stationery Office.

Stamey, T.A., 1972. Urinary infections. Baltimore. The Williams & Wilkins Co.

Stamey, T.A., Govan, D.E., and Palmer, J.M. 1965. The localisation and treatment of urinary tract infection. Medicine **44:**1-36.

Stamm, W.E., et al. 1980. Cause of the acute urethral syndrome in women. N. Engl. J. Med. **303:**409-415.

Stamm, W.E., et al. 1981. Treatment of the acute urethral syndrome. N. Engl. J. Med. **304:**956-958.

Sussman, M., and Asscher, A.W. 1979. Urinary tract infection. In Black, D., and Jones, N.F., editors. Renal disease. ed. 4. Oxford. Blackwell Scientific Publications, Ltd.

Svanborg-Edén, C., Lidin-Janson, G., and Lindberg, U. 1979. Adhesiveness to urinary tract epithelial cells of fecal and urinary *Escherichia coli* isolates from patients with symptomatic urinary tract infection. J. Urol. **122:**185-188.

Thomas, V., Shelokov, A., and Forland, M. 1974. Antibody coated bacteria in urine and the sight of urinary tract infection. N. Engl. J. Med. **29:**588-590.

Turck, M. 1978. Importance of localization of urinary tract infection in women. In Kass, E.H., and Brumfitt, W., editors. Infections of the urinary tract. Chicago. University of Chicago Press.

chapter 25

Urethral lesions

JACK R. ROBERTSON

The female urethra is said to be short on anatomy but long on function. It is a short, complex extension from the bladder that functions as a biological valve. The proximal urethra is a mesodermal structure lined by transitional epithelium. The terminal urethra is an ectodermal structure lined by squamous epithelium.

The urethra is subject to trauma, anomalies, pathologic conditions, and the influence of hormones. It is surrounded by a plexus of interanastomotic ducts and glands. Skene's glands are usually located at the 5 and 7 o'clock positions, just inside the external meatus.

The urethra and bladder function as a unit. Malfunction of the urethra interferes with the storing or voiding phase of the lower urinary tract.

TRAUMA

Urethral trauma is uncommon since the urethra is partly protected by the symphysis pubis and is not as firmly anchored as the male urethra. Obstetrical trauma has almost disappeared as a result of the increased use of cesarean section. Automobile injuries resulting in pelvic fractures may cause laceration or transection of the urethra. Straddle injuries and the insertion of foreign bodies are more common in children. Separation or diastasis of the symphysis pubis (see Figure 16.3) following pelvic fracture leads to rupture of the posterior pubourethral ligament with loss of support for the bladder neck. These patients may complain of incontinence when mobilization begins during recovery from their injury.

Iatrogenic injury to the urethra is not uncommon. It is often a result of surgical enucleation of a diverticulum and may lead to almost total incontinence.

Urethral injury usually is seen as sudden incontinence or difficulty in voiding and may be accompanied by hematuria, dysuria, and pain. The diagnosis is established by radiographs or urethroscopy. The latter is easy to perform and localizes the lesion.

Most urethral lacerations require suturing. A fistula will require specialized surgery (Chapter 20) and may need a Martius fat-pad graft from a labium majus to give the increased blood supply for healing. If the urethra is destroyed, a new urethra can be formed from an anterior bladder flap. If continence is not obtained, an artificial urinary sphincter may be needed in addition (Furlow, 1980).

Urethral coitus is associated with ignorance of local anatomy or presence of vaginal agenesis. Continence of urine may be adversely affected; the patient usually complains of incontinence just after intercourse. She may be continent at other times. The urethra, although admitting two to three fingers, usually retains its contractility.

CARUNCLE

A caruncle is a common lesion. It is a small red growth characteristically seen at the 6 o'clock position on the external meatus, often as a result of estrogen deficiency found during menopause. It is a benign growth covered by transitional epithelium. It is usually asymptomatic, but symptoms may consist of pain, bleeding, and dysuria. Treatment is estrogen vaginal cream. The response is good, but the caruncle may recur. If bleeding or pain occurs, the caruncle should be removed by excision biopsy, since it can be confused with carcinoma. The biopsy can be complicated by the formation of a tender neuroma (Figure 25.1).

DIVERTICULUM

A urethral diverticulum may be congenital or acquired (Glassman, Weinerth, and Glenn, 1975). Infection, with subsequent obstruction of urethral glands, results in cyst formation. The cyst may rupture into the urethral lumen causing formation of a diverticulum.

Diverticuli vary in size from a few millimeters to as large as 8 cm. Ostia vary in size from 1 mm to more than 1 cm. The majority of ostia are located in the middle third of the urethra lying on the posterior wall between the 5 and 7 o'clock positions. Occasionally calculi or carcinoma occurs in a diverticulum, but the latter is rare (Allen and Nelson, 1978).

The typical patient is between 30 and 60 years of age and has a long history of recurrent urinary complaints. She commonly has had a chronic urinary tract infection. She may have difficulty in initiating voiding after intercourse. Massaging the urethra occasionally produces pus or a spurt of urine. I have seen patients with as many as three diverticuli who had no signs of a diverticulum during massaging the urethra.

The diagnosis is made by voiding cystogram (Figure 25.2), urethrography (using a Davis-Te-Linde or Tratner catheter), ultrasound, or urethroscopy (Robertson, 1978; Pliskow and Silver, 1980). During urethroscopy the vesical neck is compressed against the symphysis pubis by a finger in the vagina. This distends the diverticular sac. The urethra is massaged and the examiner looks for urine or pus escaping from the ostium.

The conventional surgical treatment of a urethral diverticulum has a high complication rate (Figure 25.3). When the fragile infected sac is partially removed, it may be difficult to adequately close the urethra.

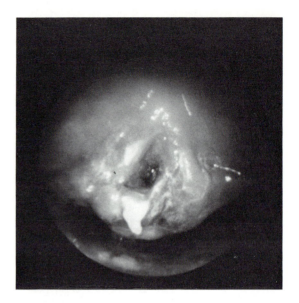

Figure 25.1 Urethral caruncle. Subsequent biopsy led to exquisite tenderness and apareunia for 2 years.

In 1970 Spence and Duckett reported a simplified technique. A deliberate incision is made through the floor of the urethra, extending from the external meatus into the mouth of the diverticulum. This saucerizes the diverticular sac. A running locking stitch of 3.0 polyglycolic acid suture takes in the margins of the urethral mucosa, the sac, and the vaginal mucosa. The complication rate is low compared with the conventional surgical treatment (Lichtman and Robertson, 1976). A urethral pressure profile may help in determining the location of the orifice in relationship to the continence zone ; Robertson, 1980).

In my opinion, the Spence procedure is the best operation when the diverticular opening is distal to the continence zone, that is, in the distal urethra. If more proximal, conventional surgical enucleation is carried out.

The complication rate with conventional surgery is nearly 20%. I have performed over 100 Spence procedures with a complication rate of 4%. Following this procedure, the patients neither complain of dysparenunia nor of recurrent urinary tract infection and void without spraying.

CARCINOMA

Primary carcinoma of the female urethra is rare. In 1952 McCrea collected 546 cases of primary carcinoma of the urethra. By 1970 Ziegerman and Gordon had collected 768 primary malignant tumors of the urethra in female patients. The total reported cases number about 1000.

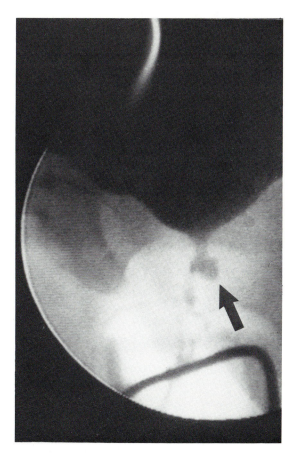

Figure 25.2 Anteroposterior radiograph taken during videocystourethrography showing urethral diverticulum.

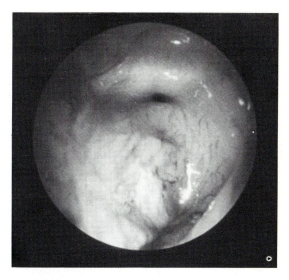

Figure 25.3 Urethral fistula. Patient had persistent vaginitis and recurrent urinary tract infection for 8 years. She had had two operations for urethral diverticula and had been assured that she did not have a fistula.

Neoplasms of the urethra may be benign or malignant. The former are uncommon and are usually papillomas (Figure 25.4). Malignant lesions may be primary or secondary, the latter arising from adenocarcinoma of the endometrium, transitional cell carcinoma of the bladder, and squamous cell carcinoma of the vulva and vagina. Primary carcinomas are commonly epidermoid; transitional cell carcinoma is the most common in the proximal urethra. Approximately 12% to 20% are adenocarcnoma. Staging of the disease is based on the classification of Chau and Green (1965):

Stage I
Disease limited to the distal half of the urethra
Stage II
Disease involving the entire urethra with periurethral extension but *not* involving the vulva or bladder neck.
Stage III
A. Disease involving the urethra and vulva.
B. Disease invading the vaginal mucosa.
C. Disease involving the urethra and bladder neck.

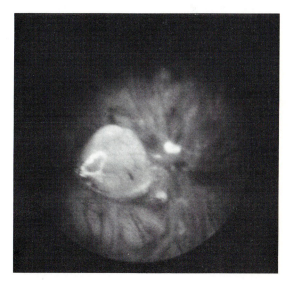

Figure 25.4 Benign tumor of urethral mucosa.

Stage IV
A. Disease involving the parametrium and/or the paracolpium.
B. Metastasis
   1. Inguinal lymph nodes.
   2. Pelvic nodes.
   3. Paraaortic nodes.
   4. Distant.

The symptoms are nonspecifc. Vaginal bleeding including hematuria is the most common initial symptom seen (Grabstald et al., 1966). Hematuria may not be an early symptom. Frequency, burning

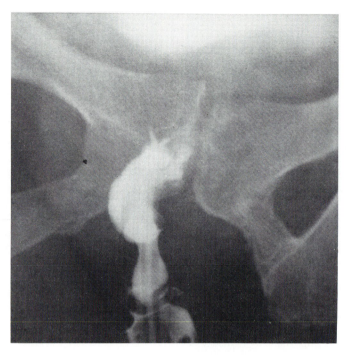

Figure 25.5 Davis double-balloon urethrogram showing carcinoma in urethral diverticulum. Patient had already been treated with external beam and interstitial irradiation. (Courtesy of Dr. W. James.)

on urination, incontinence, tenesmus, and recurrent urinary tract infections may occur. Necrosis tends to produce foul vaginal discharge. Urinary retention may be the first symptom seen (Staubitz et al., 1955). It may be seen in association with a diverticulum, and therefore symptoms caused by a diverticulum should always be investigated (Figure 25.5). An advanced tumor may be present as a palpable or visible mass.

Lesions at the meatus are readily inspected, palpated, and biopsis simple, making diagnosis easy. Urethroscopy is the easiest and most reliable method of diagnosis. A biopsy must be taken of any suspicious lesion.

As with other malignant tumors, early diagnosis is essential for cure. For this reason the prognosis for lesions of the distal third of the urethra is better than a 50% 5-year survival. When the tumor involves the entire urethra, treatment, whether by radical excision, irradiation, or exenteration, has a poor prognosis. Because of small numbers, the optimum method and results of treating carcinoma of the female urethra are unclear. Treatment is related to the size and extent of the lesion and is usually a combination of surgery and radiotherapy. Surgery consists of urethrectomy, cystourethrectomy with

lymph node dissection, radical vulvectomy, and anterior exenteration, depending on the location and extent of the disease.

Irradiation is indicated in small lesions located in the anterior urethra. Irradiation gives poor results in posterior urethral tumors and also with large tumors that extend into periurethral tissues, the bladder, or vulva (Taggart, Castro, and Rutledge, 1972). Observation that cancer of the urethra is usually a regional disease, coupled with the high incidence of local recurrence and the poor prospect of survival in patients with recurrence or tumors of the entire urethra, has led to an aggressive surgical approach, including exenteration (Peterson et al., 1973).

Bracken et al, (1976) report survival rates for tumors of all sites to be 45% for stage I, 41% for stage II, 26% for stage III, and 18% for stage IV lesions.

URETHRAL STENOSIS

Urethral stenosis may occur anywhere from the vesical neck to the external meatus. Obstruction of the vesical neck is rare. Most stenosis leading to obstruction is located at midurethra or at the external meatus. Symptoms of urethral obstruction are similar to those in patients who are not obstructed. A poor urinary flow may or may not be related to urethral obstruction. A history of recurrent urinary tract infections is common. The striated voluntary sphincter becomes spastic, and a cycle of infection and spasm is begun.

The following investigations may be used in the diagnosis of this condition. Uroflowmetry is a helpful noninvasive procedure but may not be diagnostic. Synchronous videocystourethrography is diagnostic but may not differentiate between mechanical and functional stenosis (detrusor sphincter dyssynergia) unless electromyography is used as well. The "stop-test" is helpful in evaluating those patients whose voiding is largely accompanied by straining (Moolgaoker et al., 1972). These patients have difficulty in initiating voiding. They void with a poor stream and are able to inhibit voiding instantly. Most patients have significant residual urine. Urethroscopy is essential in differentiating between mechanical and functional stenosis (Figure 25.6). Bougies-à-boules are designed for urethral dilatation and calibration. This is a static procedure to evaluate a dynamic phenomenon (Gleason, Bottaccini, and Lattimer, 1969).

Treatment may include the following: Urethral dilatation is a controversial empirical procedure commonly practiced (Stamey, 1979). I dilate the urethra with a female endoscope that has a No. 24 Fr sheath. Two fingers are placed in the vagina to elevate the vesical neck against the symphysis pubis. In this manner gas or fluid is trapped in the urethra while the examiner massages the anterior vaginal wall as the endoscope is withdrawn through the urethra.

The Otis urethrotome was developed as an improvement to urethral dilatation (see Figure 21.7). I have seen several incontinent patients following vigorous urethrotomy. Tanagho and Lyon (1971) showed that internal urethrotomy always results in scarring and dense fibrosis.

Bladder neck incision under direct vision for bladder neck dysfunction is carried out by some clinicians (Turner-Warwick, Whiteside, and Worth, 1973).

Estrogen cream applied to the vulva and vagina is beneficial in those patients at or past the menopause, provided no contraindications exist. The estrogen is well absorbed systemically and should be used daily for 3 out of 4 weeks for at least 3 months before the full effects are realized. If the uterus has not been removed, cyclical progestogens should be

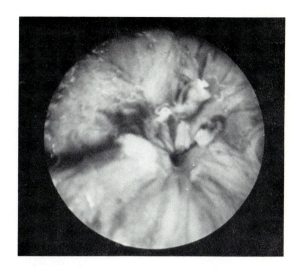

Figure 25.6 Urethral stenosis. Patient had received innumerable antibiotics for recurrent urinary tract infection. Following urethral dilatations and 6 months of antibiotic therapy, she was symptom free.

administered to avoid the development of cystic and adenomatous endometrial hyperplasia.

Finally, it should be noted that vesical prolapse may cause functional obstruction of the bladder neck. This is corrected by surgery to cure the cystocele.

ENDOMETRIOSIS

Endometriosis is a condition in which endometrial tissue is found outside the endometrium. That endometriosis occurs in the urinary tract demonstrates the close relationship of the genital and urinary tracts in women. The incidence of cesarean section has now markedly increased, which raises the risk of bladder injuries and the potential for development of endometriosis of the urinary tract.

The symptoms of endometriosis in the urethra are not well established, since only one case has been published (Palagiri, 1978). The patient had severe dyspareunia and burning with urination 2 weeks before seeking medical attention. She had postmicturition dribbling but no history of hematuria. Examination revealed a bulging mass in the anterior vaginal wall. A diverticulum was diagnosed by a urethrogram. Vaginal resection of the diverticulum was accomplished, and endometrial stroma and glands were found in the wall of the diverticulum.

I have seen three patients with urethral endometriosis. I am familiar with one other patient with urethral endometriosis (White, 1981). All these pa-

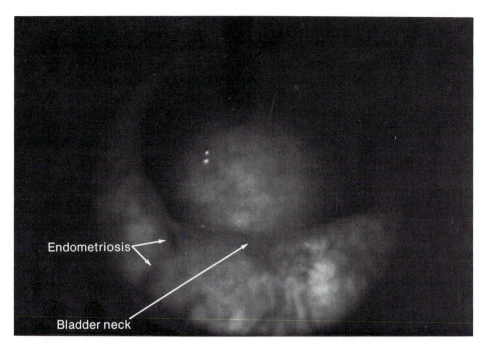

Figure 25.7 Urethral endometriosis: Urethroscopy shows two deposits at bladder neck

tients had microscopic hematuria, urgency, and dysuria just before and during menses. One patient was lost to follow-up; two patients had total abdominal hysterectomies and bilateral salpingo-oophrectomies, and both are asymptomatic. The fourth patient refused surgery and was treated with a routine of oral contraceptives for 6 months. After return of menses, she no longer had dyspareunia, urgency, or dysuria. Four months after discontinuing all medication, she was asymptomatic.

The diagnosis of this condition is by urethroscopy (Figure 25.7). This is enhanced if the patient is examined during her menses as is true with pelvic endometriosis. Ultimate diagnosis is by biopsy.

MUCOSAL PROLAPSE

Urethral mucosal prolapse is congenital or results from aging or atrophy. It occurs at the extremes of life, childhood and old age. It is an eversion of the entire circumference of the urethral mucosa.

Because of venous congestion the mucosa appears dusky. If thrombosis occurs, it appears blue and may even become gangrenous. Childhood urethral prolapse occurs primarily in black children (Esposito, 1968). It is seen more commonly in older patients. It is not painful, and symptoms include bleeding, dysuria, and serous discharge. The

onset may be insidious, but commonly the onset is sudden.

The diagnosis is established by inserting a catheter or sound through the center of what looks like a tumor mass. The treatment may take any of the following forms:

1. Incision: retraction of the urethral mucosa during excision may be avoided by placing fixation sutures and trimming in quadrants until all the prolapsed tissue is removed.
2. Linear cautery may be accomplished by hot cautery or cryosurgery (Livermore, 1921).
3. A Foley catheter may be inserted through the prolapse and the tissue teased down the urethra (Peters, 1962). The suture is placed around the base of the prolapse and tied. This causes amputation of the prolapsed mucosa, and the catheter is removed in 3 to 4 days.

REFERENCES

Allen, R., and Nelson, R.P. 1978. Primary urethral malignancy: review of 22 cases. South Med. J. **71:**547-550.

Bracken, R.B., Johnson, D.E., Miller, L.S., Ayala, A.G., Gomez, J.J., and Rutledge, F. 1976. Primary carcinoma of the female urethra. J. Urol. **116:**188-192.

Chau, P.M., and Green, A.E. 1965. Radiotherapeutic management of malignant tumors of the vagina. Prog. Clin. Cancer, 1:728-750.

Esposito, J.M. 1968. Circular prolapse of the urethra in children: a cause of vaginal bleeding. Obstet. Gynecol. **31:**363-367.

Furlow, W.L. 1980. Artificial sphincter. In Stanton, S.L., and Tanagho, E.A., editors. Surgery of female incontinence. Berlin. Springer-Verlag.

Glassman, T.A., Weinerth, J.L., and Glenn, J.F. 1975. Neonatal female urethral diverticulum. Urology **5:**249-251.

Gleason, D.M., Bottacini, M.R., and Lattimer, J.K. 1969. What does the bougie-à-boule calibrate? J. Urol. **101:**114-116.

Grabstald, H., Hilaris, B., Henschke, U., and Whitmore, W.F., Jr. 1966. Cancer of the female urethra. J.A.M.A. **197:**835-842.

Lichtman, A.S., and Robertson, J.R. 1976. Suburethral diverticula treated by marsupialization. Obstet. Gynecol. **47:**203-206.

Livermore, G.R. 1921. The treatment of prolapse of the urethra: with report of a case. Surg. Gynecol. Obstet. **32:**557-559.

McCrea, L.E. 1952. Carcinoma of the female urethra. Urol. Survey **2:**85-149.

Moolgaoker, A.S., Ardran, G.M., Smith, J.C., and Stallworthy, J.A. 1972. The diagnosis and management of urinary incontinence in the female. Br. J. Obstet. Gynaecol. **79:**481-497.

Palagiri, A. 1978. Urethral diverticulum with endometriosis. Urology **11:**271-272.

Peters, W.A., Jr. 1962. Prolapse of the urethral mucosa. Am. J. Obstet. Gynecol. **84:**862-866.

Peterson, D.T., Dockerty, M.B., Utz, D.C., and Symmonds, R.E. 1973. The peril of primary carcinoma of the urethra in women. J. Urol. **110:**72-75.

Pliskow, N., and Silver, T.M. 1980. Ultrasonic diagnosis of urethral diverticulum. Urology **15:**625-626.

Robertson, J.R. 1978. Carbon dioxide urethroscopy in gynecologic urologic problems. Clin. Obstet. Gynecol. **21:**737-758.

Robertson, J.R. 1980. Urethral diverticula. In Ostergard, D.R., Gynecological urology and urodynamics: theory and practice. Baltimore. The Williams & Wilkins Co.

Spence, H.M., and Duckett, J.W., Jr. 1970. Diverticulum of the female urethra: clinical aspects and presentation of a simple operative technique for cure. J. Urol. **104:**432-437.

Stamey, T.A. 1979. Urinary incontinence in the female. In Harrison, J.H., and Campbell, M.F., editors. Urology. Vol 3. Philadelphia. W.B. Saunders. Co.

Staubitz, W.J., Carden, L.M., Oberkircher, O.J., Lent, M.H., and Murphy, W.T. 1955. Management of urethral carcinoma in the female. J. Urol. **73:**1045-1053.

Taggart, C.G., Castro, J.R., and Rutledge, F.N. 1972. Carcinoma of the female urethra. Am. J. Roentgenol. Radium Ther. Nucl. Med. **114:**145-151.

Tanagho, E.A., and Lyon, R.P. 1971. Urethral dilatation versus internal urethrotomy. J. Urol. **105:**242-244.

Turner-Warwick, R.T., Whiteside, C.G., and Worth, P.H.L. 1973. A urodynamic view of the clinical problems associated with bladder neck dysfunction and its treatment by endoscopic incision. Br. J. Urol. **45:**44-59.

White, R. 1981. Personal communication.

Zeigerman, J.H., and Gordon, S.F. 1970. Cancer of the female urethra: a curable disease. Obstet. Gynecol. **36:**785-789.

chapter 26

Vaginal prolapse

STUART L. STANTON

CLASSIFICATION

Vaginal prolapse may be defined as descent of urethra (urethrocele); bladder (cystocele); uterus, cervix, and small bowel (enterocele); and rectum (rectocele) into the vagina and sometimes beyond. Sometimes an enterocele may contain omentum as well. Some amount of vaginal wall laxity is normal so that rather than being absolute, prolapse is a matter of degree.

Prolapse can be classified according to its anatomical location, and it is convenient to start from the anterior and move to the posterior vaginal wall. It may be graded according to whether it is slight, where there is some movement on coughing, or marked, where the prolapse appears at or beyond the introitus. Uterine descent is graded differently in that first degree refers to some descent within the vagina, second degree indicates that the cervix appears at the introitus, and third degree, or procidentia, indicates that the uterus is entirely outside

the introitus. When a hysterectomy has been performed and there is descent of the vaginal vault, this may be called vault prolapse.

The condition of prolapse is common and may be associated with urinary symptoms. It is usually benign, but third-degree uterine prolapse with a cystocele can cause ureteric obstruction and therefore is potentially fatal. The ureters are also at risk of being traumatized during vaginal hysterectomy and anterior colporrhaphy.

INCIDENCE

Cystourethrocele is the most common prolapse, followed by uterine descent and rectocele. A urethrocele occurring on its own is rare. Enteroceles are more common following abdominal or vaginal hysterectomy or colposuspension.

Approximately 20% of patients waiting for gynecological surgery are due to have repair of prolapse (Stallworthy, 1971). The incidence rises in the elderly, constituting 59% in one series of patients who underwent major gynecological surgery (Lewis, 1968). With improved general health, better care in labor (particularly shorter duration of the first and second stages), and a tendency toward smaller families, it is likely that prolapse may become less common.

PELVIC ANATOMY

The pelvic viscera are supported by the pelvic floor, which is composed of muscle, fasciae, and ligamentous supports.

Pelvic floor

The pelvic floor includes the levator ani, coccygeal, internal obturator, and piriform muscles and superficial and deep perineal muscles (Figure 26.1). The levator ani (which is in two parts—pubococcygeal and iliococcygeal) is covered by pelvic fascia and arises from the pelvic surface of the pubic bone (lateral to the symphysis pubis) and posteriorly from the ischial spine. In between, it

takes origin from the internal obturator fascia (tendinous arch). The pubococcygeal muscle fans out and forms two parts, which are inserted differently. The anterior fibers decussate around the vagina and pass to the perineal body and anal canal. Although anteriorly the fibers of the pubococcygeal muscle are in close relation to the urethra, they are not structurally attached to it (Gosling, 1981). Posterior fibers join the raphe formed by the iliococcygeal muscle. The deeper fibers of each side unite behind the anorectal junction to form the puborectal muscle, which slings the anorectal junction from the pubic bone. The fibers of the iliococcygeal muscle proceed downward medially and backward to be inserted into the last two pieces of the coccyx and into a median fibrous raphe that extends from the tip of the coccyx to the anus. The muscle is supplied by the anterior primary rami of S3 and S4.

The coccygeal muscle is a flat, triangular muscle arising from the ischial spine and in the same plane as the iliococcygeal muscle. It is inserted into the lateral margin of the lower two pieces of the sacrum

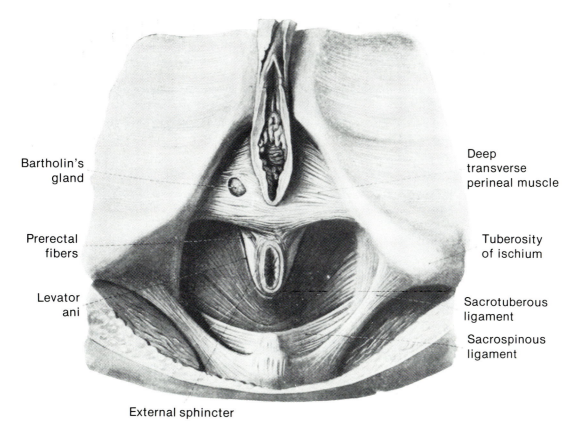

Bartholin's gland

Prerectal fibers

Levator ani

External sphincter

Deep transverse perineal muscle

Tuberosity of ischium

Sacrotuberous ligament

Sacrospinous ligament

Figure 26.1 Perineal surface of pelvic floor structures. (From Howkins, J. 1971. Shaw's textbook of gynaecology. ed. 9. Edinburgh. Churchill-Livingstone.)

and upper two pieces of the coccyx. Its nerve supply is the anterior primary rami of S3 and S4.

Both of these muscles act as supports for the pelvic viscera and as sphincters for the rectum and vagina. Contraction of the pubococcygeal muscle will also arrest the urinary stream.

These muscles are aided by the muscles of the urogenital diaphragm—the superficial and deep perineal muscles that originate from the ischial ramus and are inserted into the perineal body. They are supplied by the perineal branch of the pudendal nerve (S2 to S4) and brace the perineum against the downward pressure from the pelvic floor. The muscles are covered superiorly by fascia continuous with that over the levator ani and internal obturator muscles and inferiorly by fascia called the perineal membrane.

Pelvic ligaments

The pelvic ligaments are condensations of pelvic fascia that sling the cervix, uterus, and upper part of the vagina from the walls of the pelvis. They include the following:

1. The pubocervical ligament (pubocervical fascia) extends from the anterior aspect of the cervix to the back of the body of the pubis.
2. The lateral cervical ligament (transverse cervical, Mackenrodt, or cardinal ligaments) extends from the lateral aspect of the cervix and upper vagina to the pelvic side walls. It is the lower part of the broad ligament, and

nerves and vessels pass through from the pelvic side walls to the uterus. The ureter passes underneath it to the ureterovesical junction. The upper edge of the broad ligament contains the ovarian vessels.
3. The uterosacral ligaments extend from the back of the uterus to the front of the sacrum, keeping the uterus anteverted.
4. The posterior pubourethral ligaments extend from the posteroinferior aspect of the symphysis to the anterior aspect of the middle third of the urethra and onto the bladder. They maintain elevation of the bladder neck and prevent excess posterior displacement of the urethra (Gosling, 1981). They may facilitate micturition and are important in the maintenance of continence.
5. The round ligament, which is not ligamentous but is formed of smooth muscle, passes from the uterine cornu through the inguinal canal to the labium majus. It is believed to keep the uterus anteflexed but probably plays little part in actually supporting the uterus.

Structures involved in prolapse

A cystocele represents descent of the bladder through the pubocervical fascia with attenuation of the overlying vaginal skin (Figure 26.2). A large cystocele will carry both the uterovesical junctions and the lower end of the ureters with it, so that these protrude outside the vagina. This can result

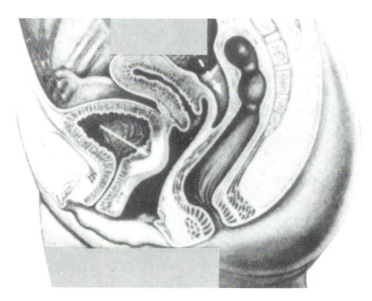

Figure 26.2 Sagittal section of pelvis indicating site of cystocele. (From Howkins, J. 1971. Shaw's textbook of gynaecology. ed. 9. Edinburgh. Churchill-Livingstone.)

in ureteric obstruction, and ureteric damage can occur when these structures are not recognized (Figure 26.3).

The urethrocele represents loss of support by the pubocervical fascia and posterior pubourethral ligaments (Figure 26.4). Indeed, the latter are prob-

ably the single most important structures supporting the urethrovesical junction and helping maintain continence.

Descent of the uterus and cervix occurs when the lateral cervical ligaments become weakened (Figure 26.5). Sometimes, particularly in prolapse

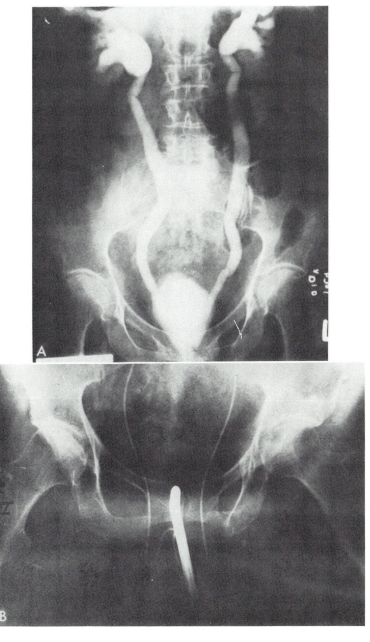

Figure 26.3 A, Preoperative intravenous urogram in patient with uterine prolapse showing bilateral hydronephrosis. **B,** Ureteric catheters demonstrating caudal displacement of ureterovesical junctions. (From Buchsbaum, H.J., and Schmidt, J.D. 1982. Gynecologic and obstetric urology. Philadelphia. W.B. Saunders Co.)

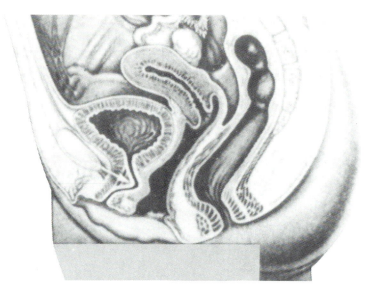

Figure 26.4 Sagittal section of pelvis. Arrow indicates site of urethrocele. (From Howkins, J. 1971. Shaw's textbook of gynaecology. ed. 9. Edinburgh. Churchill-Livingstone.)

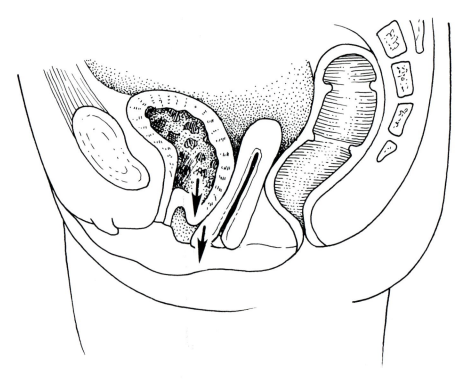

Figure 26.5 Sagittal section of pelvis. Arrows indicate second-degree uterine descent and cystocele. (From Howkins, J. 1971. Shaw's textbook of gynaecology. ed. 9. Edinburgh. Churchill-Livingstone.)

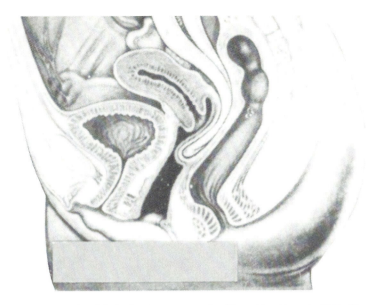

Figure 26.6 Sagittal section of pelvis indicating enterocele. (From Howkins, J. 1971. Shaw's textbook of gynaecology. ed. 9. Edinburgh. Churchill-Livingstone.)

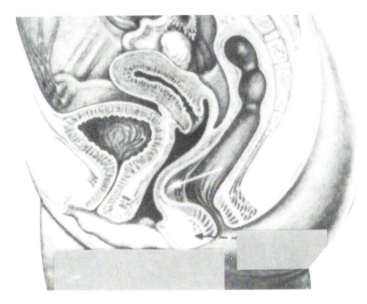

Figure 26.7 Sagittal section of pelvis. Arrows indicate rectocele. (From Howkins, J. 1971. Shaw's textbook of gynaecology. ed. 9. Edinburgh. Churchill-Livingstone.)

associated with nulliparity, the cervix elongates and the uterus descends without any cystocele but with an enterocele. The pelvic fascia condensations are inadequately developed and lack their normal resilience. Following vaginal or abdominal hysterectomy, descent of the vaginal vault can occur because of inadequacy of its remaining supports.

An enterocele usually contains small bowel or omentum and may accompany uterine descent or follow abdominal or vaginal hysterectomy or colposuspension (Figure 26.6). It used to be a common sequel to vaginal hysterectomy until its prevalence was noted and a prophylactic high fascial repair performed (Hawskworth and Roux, 1958). Failure despite this may be caused by the presence of deep uterovesical and uterorectal peritoneal pouches.

Finally, a rectocele represents weakness in the posterior vaginal wall allowing protrusion of the rectum into the vaginal canal (Figure 26.7). The rectum descends through the rectovaginal septum and carries attenuated vaginal wall in front of it. There is separation of the posterior fibers of the pubococcygeal muscle.

ETIOLOGY

Congenital weakness of pelvic fascia and ligaments can account for a small percentage of prolapse, especially when spina bifida or bladder exstrophy is present. Congenital shortness of the vagina or deep uterovesical or uterorectal peritoneal pouches are also responsible (Jeffcoate, 1967). However, the most common factors are antecedent childbirth and the menopause. Prolapse can occur during pregnancy. Keettel (1941) has reported an incidence of between 1 in 10,000 and 1 in 15,000 pregnancies. Factors include prolonged and difficult labor, bearing down before full dilatation, multiparity, laceration of the lower genital tract in the second stage, forceful delivery of the placenta during the third stage, and inadequate repair of pelvic floor injuries.

After childbirth, menopause (with estrogen deficiency) is probably the most significant factor. Lacking estrogen, the tissues of the female genital tract become atrophic and weakened. This condition may be aggravated by anything that raises the intraabdominal pressure, for example, chronic cough, constipation, or heavy lifting.

PRESENTATION
Symptoms

Symptoms of prolapse will depend not necessarily on the size but on the site and type of prolapse. Discomfort experienced with prolapse is usually caused by abnormal tension on nerves in the tissues that are being stretched.

Cystocele and cystourethrocele. Prolapse of the bladder and urethra may lead to dragging discomfort, sensation of a lump experienced in the vagina, and urinary symptoms, the most common of which is stress incontinence, which will be present if there is undue mobility and descent of the urethrovesical junction or if repeated operations have produced scarring around the urethra and bladder neck, resulting in inadequate urethral closure. About 50% of patients with urethral sphincter incompetence and stress incontinence have a cystourethrocele; therefore a prolapse is not the sole

cause of this condition. Retention of urine can occur if a large cystocele is present and the bladder neck is anchored normally. This leads to overflow incontinence and misdiagnosis of retention. It can be corrected temporarily by manually replacing the prolapse. If sufficient urine is being voided but there remains a chronic residual volume, the patient may complain of frequency and inadequate emptying, and urinary tract infection may supervene.

Urgency and frequency are found in association with cystocele, and its correction may relieve these symptoms but not invariably. It is therefore unwise to perform a repair operation just for these symptoms, especially without the exclusion of other causes of urgency and frequency (for example, instability of the detrusor) beforehand. It is important to realize that a patient with incontinence may develop frequency and urgency as "a self-induced habit" to keep the bladder empty. The patient voids at frequent intervals, believing that incontinence will be better controlled if the bladder is kept as empty as possible. From time to time, while endeavoring unsuccessfully to find a toilet, she may experience urgency. If this pattern is repeated, urgency becomes an established symptom. Certainly these symptoms are often linked, and cure of one may lead to cure of both (Stanton, Williams, and Ritchie, 1976).

Uterine descent. First- and second-degree uterine descent may cause low backache, which is relieved by lying flat or by temporarily using a ring pessary, which will support the prolapse. A patient with procidentia may complain of protrusion of the cervix and a blood-stained, sometimes purulent, vaginal discharge.

Enterocele. An enterocele may produce only vague symptoms of vaginal discomfort. Since an enterocele is often associated with other prolapse, it can be difficult to ascribe separate symptoms to it. Rarely, dehiscence of an enterocele may occur; the patient complains of acute pain, and small bowel may be seen at the vulva.

Rectocele. A rectocele gives rise to symptoms of backache, a lump in the vagina, and incomplete bowel emptying: the patient may have discovered that digital reduction of her rectocele allows completion of bowel action.

Signs

Certain predisposing conditions to prolapse such as chronic cough and constipation may be noted. The patient complaining of prolapse should be ex-

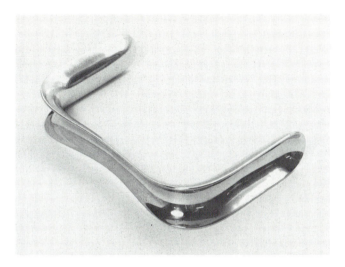

Figure 26.8 Sims' vaginal speculum.

amined in the dorsal position and also in the left lateral position by using a Sims' speculum (Figure 26.8). Stress incontinence is most likely to be demonstrated if the bladder is full. The patient is asked to cough or bear down, and any anterior vaginal wall prolapse or uterine descent will be demonstrated by retracting the posterior vaginal wall. An estimate of the extent of prolapse should be made. Sometimes the patient may have to stand up to show prolapse descent. Enterocele and rectocele can be demonstrated by using the speculum to retract the anterior vaginal wall. If the rectocele protrudes and obscures an enterocele, it can be reduced by the examining finger, and an enterocele will either be seen at the tip of the examining finger or felt as an impulse on coughing. Further differentiation can be made by asking the patient to cough and simultaneously examining the rectum and vagina. If the cervix protrudes outside the vagina, it may be ulcerated and hypertrophied, with thickening of the epithelium and keratinization. Carcinoma of the cervix is not a sequel to long-standing procidentia but may be a coincidental finding. A full pelvic examination should always be performed to exclude a pelvic mass that might cause prolapse.

Differential diagnosis

A variety of conditions can occur and mimic prolapse of the anterior vaginal wall, such as a congenital anterior vaginal wall cyst (remnant of the mesonephric duct system, for example, Gartner's duct), a urethral diverticulum, metastasis from a uterine tumor (for example, choriocarci-

noma or adenocarcinoma), and an inclusion dermoid cyst following trauma or surgery. Procidentia can be confused with a large cervical or endometrial polyp or chronic uterine inversion.

INVESTIGATION

A midstream specimen of urine should be sent for culture and sensitivity testing before any treatment is undertaken. When urinary symptoms are present, cystometry and uroflowmetry are advisable. If frequency is particularly dominant, fluid balance charts, tests of early morning urine for acid-fast bacilli, and cystoscopy are necessary. If there is a procidentia, an intravenous urogram and blood urea test are indicated.

TREATMENT

It is important to ensure that the woman's symptoms are caused by prolapse and not by other pelvic or spinal conditions. The patient should be told that, provided there is no urinary tract obstruction or infection, prolapse carries no risk to life. If surgery is chosen, the patient should be carefully assessed beforehand to minimize the risks of postoperative morbidity. It is preferable for the patient to have completed childbearing because a successful pelvic floor repair can be disrupted by a further vaginal delivery. Coital function must be taken into account and narrowing of the vagina carefully avoided. Obese patients should be referred to a dietician for dietary control and chronic cough and constipation corrected as far as possible. Ulceration of the cervix (after first excluding any neoplastic lesion) may be managed by reducing the uterine prolapse and applying estrogen cream, if not contraindicated. The ulcer will usually heal within 7 days.

Prevention

Shortening the first and particularly second stage of delivery with an increase in operative intervention and a decline in parity are likely to decrease the incidence of prolapse. The role here of episiotomy is uncertain and controversial. Postnatal exercises have little scientific evidence to support their benefit here but are advised traditionally.

Medical treatment

Before safe anesthesia and surgery, prolapse was managed by a variety of ingenious pessaries of differing shapes and sizes. Today the role of the pessary is more restricted and is indicated below:
1. During pregnancy
2. After pregnancy (awaiting involution of tissues)
3. When the patient is medically unfit for surgery
4. As a therapeutic test to confirm that surgery might help
5. When the patient refuses surgery and prefers conservative management
6. For relief of symptoms while the patient is awaiting surgery

Older pessaries were made of vulcanized rubber and had to be changed every 3 months. Today the modern pessary is made of inert plastic and can be left in place for up to a year provided there are no adverse symptoms or signs. The most common pessary is ring shaped and is available in a variety of sizes (Figure 26.9). The two main complications are vaginal ulceration (if the pessary is too large or there is loss of vaginal sensation) and incarceration with vaginal discharge and bleeding (when the pessary has been forgotten and not changed for several years).

When prolapse occurs during pregnancy, reposition of the prolapse and insertion of a ring pessary, with additional vaginal packing if necessary and bed rest, may be sufficient.

Physiotherapy and electrical stimulation of the pelvic floor muscles have a minor role in the management of established prolapse.

Surgical treatment

The surgical repair of prolapse is one of the oldest gynecological procedures, dating back to the

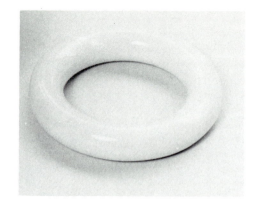

Figure 26.9 Ring pessary.

end of the nineteenth century. The majority of operations are performed through the vagina, and the abdominal route is reserved for recurrence or failure. The aims of surgery are to correct the prolapse, to maintain continence, and to preserve coital function of the vagina. These are achieved by reducing the prolapse, coapting disrupted fascia and pelvic floor musculature, and excising surplus vaginal wall skin.

Anterior colporrhaphy. When a cystocele or cystourethrocele is present, an anterior colporrhaphy, or repair, is performed. Traditionally this has also been used to cure stress incontinence. The essential features of this procedure are an anterior vaginal wall incision and dissection and display of the inferior aspect of the proximal two thirds of the urethra, the urethrovesical junction, and part of the bladder base. The urethrovesical junction is repositioned higher in the pelvis using one or two Kelly sutures. The bladder may be imbricated by a row of interrupted sutures placed either in the bladder muscle or, as I prefer, in the overlying pubocervical fascia, which remains attached to the vaginal mucosa. Any surplus skin is excised and the wound closed with an interrupted or continuous suture.

There are variations on this procedure. Pacey (1949) has emphasized the importance of locating the edge of the pubococcygeal muscle and coapting this in the midline. Ingelman-Sundberg (1946) has advocated cutting the pubococcygeal muscle behind the midpoint and uniting the anterior portion and the midline to form a further support for the bladder neck, while laterally fixing the posterior portion of the muscle.

Approximately 50% of patients will encounter

urinary retention following an anterior repair, so many gynecologists will use a catheter postoperatively. I prefer a suprapubic catheter such as a Bonanno, which has the advantage of allowing spontaneous voiding to occur before it is finally removed. It is more comfortable and less prone to urinary tract infection than a urethral catheter. The catheter is clamped the day following surgery and removed when the patient is voiding amounts greater than 200 ml and the residual urine volume is less than 100 ml.

Vaginal hysterectomy. When uterine prolapse is present, either a Manchester repair (for a first- or second-degree prolapse) or a vaginal hysterectomy may be performed. The Manchester repair consists of amputation of the cervix with an anterior and posterior colporrhaphy. After excision of the cervix, the lateral cervical (cardinal) ligaments are reunited and sutured to the remainder of the cervix. The pubocervical fascia is reconstituted and the cervical stump then covered by vaginal skin.

Modern preference is for a vaginal hysterectomy partly because it is believed to give a more satisfactory cure of prolapse and also because many seemingly healthy uteri conserved by Manchester repair are later found to contain unsuspected disease. Bonnar, Kraszewski, and Davis (1970) have found unsuspected lesions in 26% of uteri removed at vaginal hysterectomy for prolapse.

Instances in which a vaginal hysterectomy is indicated include:

1. Uterine prolapse and a uterus smaller than 14 weeks in size. (A larger uterus may be removed by morcellation.)
2. Recurrent uterine prolapse following a Manchester repair. An enterocele is more effectively repaired at the same time as a vaginal hysterectomy than with a Manchester repair.
3. An obese patient. Pitkin (1976) has shown that abdominal wound complications with abdominal hysterectomy are seven times more common in women weighing more than 200 lb (90 kg). Using a vaginal hysterectomy, no difference in morbidity or length of hospital stay was found when obese and normal-sized women were compared (Pitkin, 1977).
4. Where a painful abdominal wound is undesirable (for example, pulmonary disease) and early ambulation is advantageous.
5. Where there is vaginal prolapse and additional uterine disease such as menorrhagia.

The principles of vaginal hysterectomy are careful upward displacement of the bladder and ureters, ligation of each main pedicle, and identification of any enterocele, which is then repaired. The ovaries are inspected, and, after closure of pelvic peritoneum, the pedicles are then approximated to each other in pairs so as to reform the roof of the vault. The vaginal skin is then closed. If a vaginal hysterectomy alone is performed, bladder drainage is unnecessary.

Posterior colporrhaphy. Some clinicians maintain that pelvic floor repair or correction of incontinence by anterior colporrhaphy is incomplete without a posterior colporrhaphy or colpoperineorrhaphy. Jeffcoate (1959) has shown that in a group of women who had had an anterior and posterior colporrhaphy, 30% had apareunia or severe dyspareunia, and in a later paper (Francis and Jeffcoate, 1961) the posterior colporrhaphy was incriminated as the main cause for this. Francis and Jeffcoate were able to show that omission of the posterior colporrhaphy did not prejudice the result of prolapse repair. It would be reasonable to restrict the operation for only those patients with symptomatic and demonstrable rectocele.

The technique of posterior colporrhaphy involves dissection of the levator ani muscles and rectum via a posterior vaginal wall incision. The levator muscles and then the superficial perineal muscles are sutured together; any excess vaginal skin is cautiously excised and the vaginal wound closed.

Bladder drainage is not normally required, but in elderly persons it is a wise precaution because they often take longer to resume spontaneous micturition following pelvic surgery.

To minimize the risk of postoperative infection by anaerobic organisms, metronidazole, 500 mg, may be given as an intravenous infusion during the operation or as a 5-day course of 200 mg t.d.s. postoperatively. A simple chemotherapeutic agent (for example, nitrofurantoin [Furadantin] or nalidixic acid) can be used postoperatively while a catheter is in situ. Prophylactic heparin therapy against deep vein thrombosis should be employed, especially if the patient is obese, is a heavy smoker, or has had a past history of deep vein thrombosis.

One of the most important complications that can occur following anterior colporrhaphy is the development of incontinence in a patient who was previously continent. This has been said to be caused by correction of a previous cystocele and

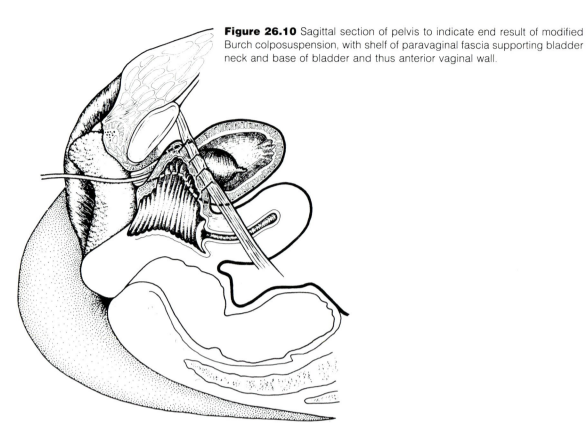

Figure 26.10 Sagittal section of pelvis to indicate end result of modified Burch colposuspension, with shelf of paravaginal fascia supporting bladder neck and base of bladder and thus anterior vaginal wall.

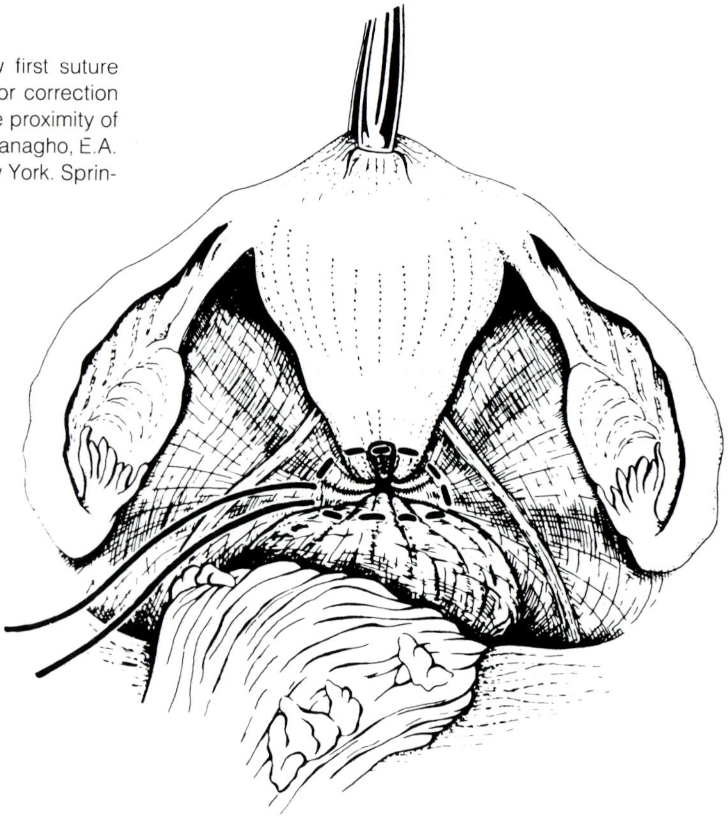

Figure 26.11 Interior of pelvis to show first suture placed in pouch of Douglas peritoneum for correction of enterocele (Moschowitz operation). Note proximity of ureters to suture. (From Stanton, S.L., and Tanagho, E.A. 1980. Surgery of female incontinence. New York. Springer-Verlag.)

removal of the valvular mechanism present at the bladder neck. I believe that this is unlikely and that incontinence is more likely to be caused by interference of the sphincter mechanism during the course of dissection with suturing, leading to inadequate support and elevation of that area.

Although most gynecologists would agree that the surgical approach to vaginal prolapse should be primarily vaginal, abdominal operations may be necessary when incontinence and prolapse coexist or when prolapse is recurrent.

Colposuspension operation. The Burch colposuspension (Burch, 1961) is used for correction of stress incontinence caused by urethral sphincter incompetence and anterior vaginal wall prolapse (Figure 26.10). The lateral fornices are approximated and sutured to the ipsilateral ileopectineal ligaments, producing elevation of the bladder neck and reduction of any cystourethrocele (Stanton, Williams, and Ritchie, 1976; Stanton and Cardozo, 1979). Enterocele formation is a complication of this procedure, and preemptive correction of an enterocele by a Moschowitz operation at the same time as a colposuspension is necessary.

Enterocele repair. Most enteroceles are repaired at the time of vaginal surgery for prolapse. Sometimes an enterocele coexists with a condition being treated by abdominal surgery, and a Moschowitz operation is the simplest method of correction. It may be conveniently performed in the course of an abdominal hysterectomy or colposuspension. It entails purse-string closure of the pouch of Douglas and is an intraperitoneal approach. Successive purse-string sutures of linen or Dexon are inserted into the pouch of Douglas peritoneum so as to obliterate it (Figures 26.11 and 26.12). Care should be taken to avoid the ureters.

A more formal repair for recurrent enterocele is that advocated by Zacharin and Hamilton (1972), which embodies a synchronous abdominal and vaginal approach. The enterocele sac is dissected and excised from above, and then from below the levator hiatus is closed by a series of sutures, guided by the abdominal surgeon. The pouch of Douglas is closed from above with successive purse-string sutures, and the vaginal skin is closed from below.

Sacral colpopexy. Recurrent vault prolapse following vaginal or abdominal hysterectomy is a difficult condition to treat. Vaginal surgery is likely to result in scarring and narrowing of the vagina, and the more effective approach is to secure the vaginal vault to the anterior sacral ligament using an abdominal incision (Birnbaum, 1973). Surgical grade plastic mesh (for example, Teflon or Ivalon) is sutured using nonabsorbable sutures to the vaginal vault and to the anterior sacral ligament, which is exposed by a small vertical incision over the second and third sacral vertebrae. Although originally no attempt was made to extraperitonealize the mesh, Cowan and Morgan (1980) have described how this may be achieved. Strict attention must be paid to asepsis because of the risk of infection of this foreign body material.

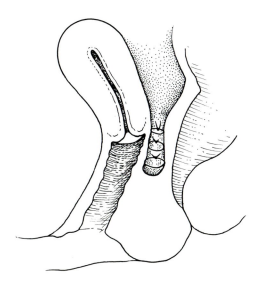

Figure 26.12 Sagittal section of pelvis showing three successive sutures inserted in pouch of Douglas peritoneum for correction of enterocele (Moschowitz operation). (From Stanton, S.L., and Tanagho, E.A. 1980. Surgery of female incontinence. New York. Springer-Verlag.)

CONCLUSION

Prolapse (and its surgical correction) is a common gynecological entity. The number of neighboring structures that can be involved in vaginal prolapse render it a complicated condition to assess and adequately treat. The clinician must be aware of the important association of urological symptoms and should carefully investigate them and decide whether abdominal or vaginal surgery is the more appropriate procedure.

REFERENCES

Birnbaum, S.J. 1973. Rational therapy for the prolapsed vagina. Am. J. Obstet. Gynecol. **115:**411-419.

Bonnar, J., Kraszewski, A., and Davis, W. 1970. Incidental pathology at vaginal hysterectomy for genital prolapse. Br. J. Obstet. Gynaecol. **77:**1137-1139.

Burch, J.C. 1961. Urethro-vaginal fixation to Cooper's ligament for correction of stress incontinence. Am. J. Obstet. Gynecol. **100:**768-774.

Cowan, W., and Morgan, H.R., 1980. Abdominal sacral colpopexy. Am. J. Obstet. Gynecol. **138:**348-349.

Francis, W., and Jeffcoate, T.N.A. 1961. Dysparenuia following vaginal operations. Br. J. Obstet. Gyneacol. **68:**1-10.

Gosling, J. 1981. Why are women continent? Proceedings of symposium ''The incontinent woman.'' London. Royal College of Obstetricians and Gynecologists.

Hawksworth, W., and Roux, J. 1958. Vaginal hysterectomy. Br. J. Obstet. Gynaecol. **65:**214-228.

Howkins, J., editor. 1971. Shaw's textbook of gynaecology. ed. 9. Edinburgh. Churchill-Livingstone.

Ingelman-Sundberg, A. 1946. Operative technique in stress incontinence of urine in the female. Nord. Med. **32:**2297-2299.

Jeffcoate, T.N.A. 1959. Posterior colpoperineorrhaphy. Am. J. Obstet. Gynecol. **773:**490-502.

Jeffcoate, T.N.A. 1967. Principles of gynaecology. ed. 3. London. Butterworths.

Keettel, W.C. 1941. Prolapse of the uterus during pregnancy. Am. J. Obstet. Gynecol. **42:**121-126.

Lewis, A.C. 1968. Major gynaecological surgery in the elderly. J. Int. Fed. Gynaecol. Obstet. **6:**244-258.

Pacey, K. 1949. Pathology and repair of genital prolapse. J. Obstet. Gynaec. Br. Emp. **56:**1-15.

Pitkin, R.M. 1976. Abdominal hysterectomy in obese women. Surg. Gynecol. Obstet. **142:**532-536.

Pitkin, R.M. 1977. Vaginal hysterectomy in obese women. Obstet. Gynecol. **49**(5):567-569.

Stallworthy, J.A. 1971. Prolapse. I. Aetiology and diagnosis. Br. Med. J.**1:**499-500.

Stallworthy, J.A. 1971. Prolapse. II. Treatment. Br. Med. J. **1:**539-540.

Stanton, S.L., Williams, J.E., and Ritchie, D. 1976. Colposuspension operation for urinary incontinence. Br. J. Obstet. Gynaecol. **83:**890-895.

Stanton, S.L., and Cardozo, L.D. 1979. Results of colposuspension operation for incontinence and prolapse. Br. J. Obstet. Gynaecol. **86:**693-697.

Zacharin, R., and Hamilton, N. 1972. The problem of the large enterocele. Aust. N.Z. J. Obstet. Gynaecol. **12:**105-109.

chapter 27

The menopause

PAUL HILTON and T. RASHMI VARMA

Young (1971) estimated that in the seventeenth century only 28% of women survived long enough to experience the menopause; currently, in developed countries, 95% of women may reach this phase of life (Studd, Chakravarti, and Oram, 1977). Ovarian failure may begin as much as 10 years before the menopause, and this prolonged period of failure of ovulation and declining estrogen production—the climacteric—represents a chronic endocrinopathy that may be associated with a variety of symptomatic and degenerative changes. With the exception of early childhood, women are more subject to urinary symptoms than men at all stages of life (Thomas et al., 1980). The different characteristics of the lower urinary tract between the sexes, particularly the relatively short urethra and less substantial pelvic floor muscle in the female, may be relevant to the development of symptoms. It is not surprising then that a significant group of women first have urinary symptoms at or about the menopause. While estrogen deficiency may undoubtedly have effects on the female lower urinary tract, the mere presentation of urinary symptoms in the climacteric should not be taken to imply a causal relationship. In considering urinary symptoms in menopausal women, it is thus

343

important that one consider the following factors:

1. The process of aging on the lower urinary tract
2. Coexistent bladder and urethral dysfunction from other causes occurring in the perimenopausal period
3. The patient's psychological reaction to the menopause and her life situation at the climacteric
4. The effects of estrogen deficiency on the lower urinary tract

PROCESS OF AGING ON THE LOWER URINARY TRACT

The effects of aging on urinary tract function and the presentation of symptoms in older patients are considered in Chapter 28.

COEXISTENT BLADDER AND URETHRAL DYSFUNCTION FROM OTHER CAUSES OCCURRING IN THE PERIMENOPAUSAL PERIOD

Many causes of urinary symptoms in women are considered in the other chapters of Part Three. All these conditions commonly appear during the climacteric. Of 750 consecutive female referrals to a specialist urodynamic unit over a 20-month period, 40% of the patients were between the ages of 40 and 60 years when symptoms began (Hilton, 1981) (Figure 27.1). The average age was 50.9 years, as compared with the average age of the menopause being 51 years (Studd, Chakravarti, and Oram, 1977). Many patients had long-standing symptoms.

PSYCHOLOGICAL REACTION TO THE MENOPAUSE

Estrogen deficiency at the climacteric may be associated with symptoms in four distinct areas: vasomotor, sexual, musculoskeletal, and emotional. The last-mentioned area particularly may have profound effects on the development of urinary symptoms. Parkes (1971) employed the term *psychosocial transition* to describe changes that are lasting in their effects, even though they occur over a short period of time, and that affect large areas of an individual's life-style. The menopause falls clearly within this definition; often it coincides with the increasing independence of children, their departure from home and marriage, and the return to a one-to-one relationship with one's spouse. At the same time, the individual's own parents may

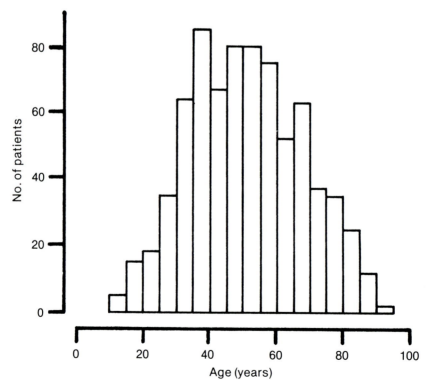

Figure 27.1 Age distribution of 750 consecutive female referrals to specialist urodynamic unit.

be approaching old age and perhaps death or geriatric dependence. These are, of course, all factors that may promote stress within the marital relationship and precipitate emotional and psychosomatic symptoms. Jeffcoate and Francis (1966) and more recently Frewen (1972) have suggested a frequent psychosomatic component to detrusor instability; thus the presentation of this condition may be anticipated with increased frequency at times of emotional stress, such as the menopause.

EFFECTS OF ESTROGEN DEFICIENCY ON THE LOWER URINARY TRACT

While aging, coexistent bladder and urethral dysfunction, and psychological factors are undoubtedly of relevance to the common presentation of urinary symptoms in the perimenopausal period, in this chapter we are mainly concerned with estrogen deficiency as it affects the lower urinary tract.

Mucosa

The vagina and distal urethra have a common embryological origin in the urogenital sinus, and this is evidenced by the similarity of their epithelial linings. In neonates the proximal urethra usually is lined by transitional epithelium continuous with that of the bladder, and the distal quarter has a nonkeratinized squamous epithelium similar to that of the vagina. In fertile and postmenopausal women the extent of the squamous epithelium increases (Huisman, 1979) and indeed may line the whole urethra and trigone (Packham, 1971).

The presence of estrogen-sensitive tissues outside the female genital tract was first demonstrated by the animal studies of Parkes and Zuckerman (1931). They found the most sensitive tissues to be the squamous epithelium of the distal urethra. Del Castillo, Argonz, and Galli Mainini (1948)

showed that urinary sediment collected at various phases of the female reproductive cycle paralleled the changes seen in vaginal smears obtained simultaneously. Subsequently, McCallin, Stewart Taylor, and Whitehead (1950) and Soloman, Panagotopolous, and Oppenheim (1958) documented the changes occurring in urinary cytology during the menstrual cycle, during pregnancy, and in the postmenopausal woman. Further cytohormonal studies by Smith (1972) have shown similar correlation between the results of distal urethral and vaginal wall smears in different phases of life. Data from our own clinic (Varma, 1982) suggest that the only 27% of menopausal women show complete estrogen deficiency in the vaginal cytology with smears showing only parabasal cells; 53% show declining estrogen stimulation, and 20% show normal smears. While estrogen dependency is certainly demonstrable in the urothelium, acute changes at the menopause are not at all obvious. It is interesting to note that women with urinary symptoms in the climacteric show a spectrum of urogenital estrogen activity similar to women with other complaints (Table 27.1).

Submucosal vascular supply

Huisman (1979) studied the structure of the female urethra in different age groups. He identified two prominent venous plexuses present in the submucosa: a distal one directly above the external urethral meatus, whose structure varied little with age, and a proximal one beneath the bladder neck, where marked age-related changes were seen. In the fertile age group the vessels were highly folded and thin walled, giving a cavernous appearance to the submucosa; in postmenopausal women these vessels became wider and lost their degree of folding (Figure 27.2). These findings, according to Huisman, lead to reduction of urethral closure.

TABLE 27.1   Karyopyknotic indices from vaginal smears in 450 women with menopausal symptoms and 150 patients with urinary symptoms in the climacteric

Karyopyknotic index	450 Menopausal patients (%)	150 Patients with urinary symptoms in the climacteric (%)
0 (atrophic)	27	30
1 to 10 (reduced activity)	53	50
>10 (normal)	20	20

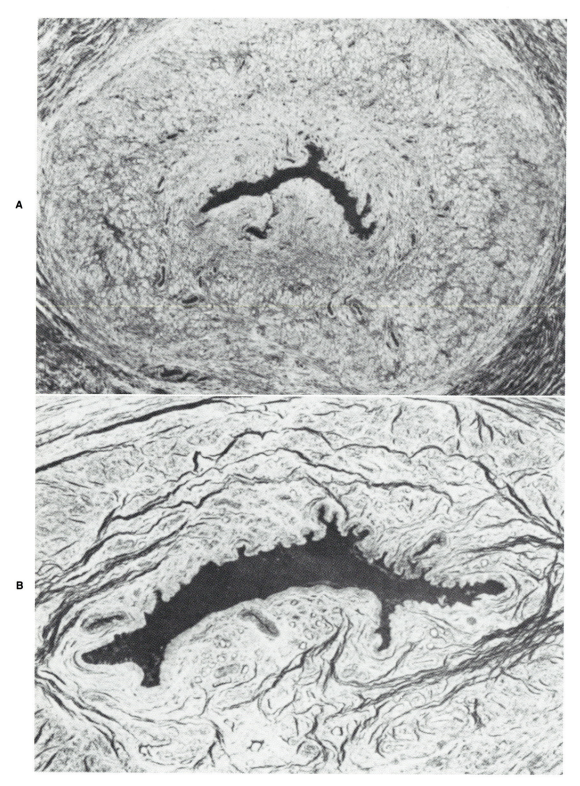

Figure 27.2 Transverse sections through human urethra just distal to bladder neck. **A,** Neonatal period. (×25.) **B,** Fertile period. (×25.) (From Huisman, A.B. 1979. Morphologie van de vrouwelijke Urethra, MD thesis, Groningen, The Netherlands.)

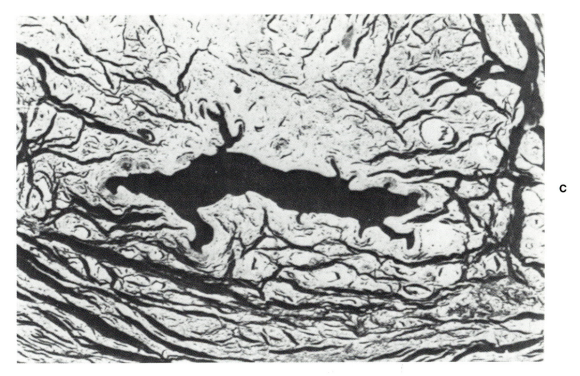

C

Figure 27.2, cont'd. C, Postmenopausal period. (×25.)

Smooth and striated muscle

The process of aging in skeletal muscle is associated with reduction in volume and replacement by adipose connective tissue. It is unlikely that such changes are hormonally determined, although by virtue of nutritional or genetic factors they are more marked in women than in men, and the overall effect is to lead to a reduction in the speed, strength, and duration of muscle contraction (Carlson, 1949). Concerning the intrinsic striated muscle of the urethra, Huisman (1979) confirmed this reduced bulk, particularly in relation to the posterior wall, where striated muscle fibers are totally deficient in postmenopausal women. Csapo (1948) established an important relationship between the contractile proteins or uterine muscle and estrogen status; it remains unclear whether other smooth muscle fibers, particularly the urethral smooth muscle, are similarly estrogen sensitive.

Connective tissues

A variety of biochemical changes have been identified within connective tissues in response to estrogen stimulation. An increase in the water and hyaluronic acid content of dermal connective tissue (Grossman, Hvidberg, and Schou, 1971) and a re-

duction in collagen breakdown and hydroxyproline excretion (Katz and Kappas, 1968) have been shown following estrogen administration. The effects of estrogen withdrawal on the connective tissue condensations of the pelvis, particularly the transverse cervical and uterosacral ligaments, might be anticipated to contribute to the development of postmenopausal uterovaginal prolapse (Brown, 1977). Similar effects on the pubovesical and pubourethral ligaments may be implicated in postmenopausal genuine stress incontinence.

URINARY SYMPTOM COMPLEXES IN POSTMENOPAUSAL WOMEN

As described previously, estrogen withdrawal at the climacteric may be associated with profound changes in the lower urinary tract; as a consequence, a number of symptom complexes may be identified. Three will be considered here: recurrent frequency and/or dysuria syndrome, voiding difficulties, and genuine stress incontinence.

Recurrent frequency and/or dysuria syndrome

Recurrent episodes of frequent painful micturition are extremely common in the female popula-

TABLE 27.2   Major areas of complaint in 450 referrals to a hormone replacement clinic

Major areas of complaint in 450 new referrals	(%)	Specific symptoms in 150 patients with urinary complaints	(%)
Vasomotor symptoms	73	Frequency	60
Dyspareunia	47	Nocturia	52
Loss of libido	40	Dysuria	40
Urinary symptoms	33	Urgency	40
Mood change	27	Urge incontinence	32
Lack of concentration	27	Stress incontinence	32
Musculoskeletal pain	25	Urge and stress incontinence	20

tion. Smith (1972) reported 719 women with these complaints from a group of 928 female referrals to a urology department over a 2-year period. In our own hormone replacement clinic at St. George's Hospital, 450 new patients have been seen in the last 4½ years. One third of these women have had significant urinary complaints, frequency and dysuria being the most common symptoms found in 60% and 40%, respectively (Varma, 1982) (Table 27.2).

Brocklehurst et al., (1972) studied the incidence of urinary symptoms in 454 women aged 45 to 64 years from a single general practice. He found a history of painful micturition in 47% of the women, with 14% having the symptom at the time of the interview. The incidence of proven urinary infection, however, was only 3.2%. Sussman et al. (1969) found a similarly low incidence of infection, 3.5%, which was independent of age in the 20- to 64-year age range. The incidence of significant bacteriuria in women with symptoms of recurrent cystitis has been found to be only 50% (Gallagher, Montgomerie, and North, 1965), and our own data would confirm this. The syndrome of recurrent episodes of frequency with dysuria in the absence of urinary tract infection has been termed *urethral syndrome*. Smith (1981) has drawn attention to the fact that women with recurring cystitis may have potential bacteriological and urethral or mechanical problems. The relationship of the onset of sexual activity to the development of such symptoms in young women is well recognized, and inadequate voiding as a result of periurethral muscle spasm or dyssynergia may also be relevant. The effect of estrogen withdrawal on the distal urethral squamous epithelium has been referred to earlier in this chapter and may also be important in the etiology of the urethral syndrome.

Voiding difficulties

The symptoms usually associated with voiding difficulty—hesitancy of micturition, slow or intermittent urinary stream, straining to void, incomplete bladder emptying, and postmicturition dribble—are too often considered to be of relevance only in the middle-aged man with prostatic enlargement. They have been shown to be common complaints in women too. Stanton, Hilton, and Oszoy (1983) reviewed the symptoms and urodynamic data of 600 consecutive female referrals to a urodynamic clinic. One hundred ninety-five patients had symptoms suggestive of voiding difficulties, and the incidence of such complaints was shown to increase with age; 99 patients had objective evidence of impaired voiding.

The presence of uterovaginal prolapse may be associated with these symptoms in a number of women, and prolapse repair has been shown to produce relief (Stanton et al., 1981). It has been suggested that previous vaginal surgery may in itself be an etiological factor in some cases, although in a prospective study of the urodynamic effects of vaginal repair, Stanton et al. (1981) found no suppport for this hypothesis. Roberts and Smith (1968) considered estrogen deficiency to be a contributory factor in the development of distal urethral obstruction in the postmenopausal woman and advocated the use of diethylstilbestrol in conjunction with urethral dilatation in the management of this condition.

Genuine stress incontinence

In a questionnaire study of urinary symptoms in women aged 35 to 60 years, Osborne (1976) reported a prevalence of troublesome stress incontinence of 26%; Brocklehurst et al. (1972) reported an incidence of 57% in women aged 45 to 64 years,

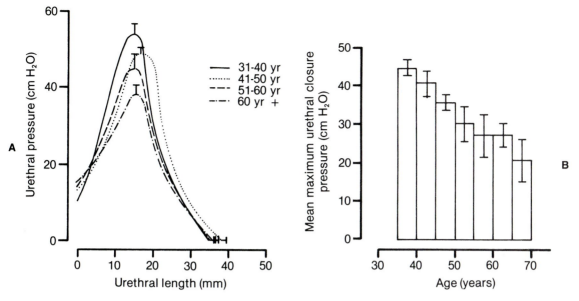

Figure 27.3 Effect of age on urethral pressure profile at rest in 120 women with genuine stress incontinence. **A,** Average urethral pressure profiles. **B,** Relationship between maximum urethral closure pressure and age, pressures plotted as mean ±1 standard error.

and others have suggested that 50% of young nullipara may experience the symptoms on occasion. Thomas et al. (1980), in a postal survey involving 22,430 people, found stress incontinence to be reported most frequently in the age group 45 to 54 years, with a slight reduction in older women; Brocklehurst et al. (1972) made a similar observation. Whether this represents a genuine reduction in the incidence of the symptom or simply an increased acceptance of symptoms by the elderly remains unproved. Nevertheless, it would seem that there is certainly no great increase in the incidence of symptom of stress incontinence at the menopause.

Several studies have shown that the urethral pressure in postmenopausal women is lower than in premenopausal women. This is undoubtedly true, although the difference appears to be age related rather than menopause related. Rud (1980) studied the effects of age on the urethral pressure profile in continent women; he found a continuous fall in maximum urethral closure pressure with increasing age but demonstrated no specific fall in relation to the menopause. Hilton (1981) described a similar age-related trend in urethral pressure in women with genuine stress incontinence (Figure 27.3).

While no definite increase in the incidence of symptoms of stress incontinence or impairment of urethral function has been demonstrated specifically in association with the menopause, several studies have attested to the efficacy of hormone replacement in the management of postmenopausal patients with genuine stress incontinence.

ASSESSMENT OF POSTMENOPAUSAL URINARY SYMPTOMS

The investigation of urinary symptoms in the menopause may be considered as follows:
1. Standard clinical data
2. Endocrine studies
3. Cytology
4. Urostatic tests
5. Urodynamic tests

Standard clinical data

The place of the clinical history and examination in the assessment of urinary symptoms is discussed in Chapter 7. In postmenopausal women a detailed urinary history is, of course, essential in addition to the history of other menopausal symptoms. The temporal relationship of urinary symptoms to the menopause should be established; estrogen deficiency symptoms may occur as much as 10 years before the menopause, although van Keep and Lauritzen (1973) found that postmenopausal urinary symptoms most commonly become manifest rather later than other climacteric symptoms, particularly the vaginal and cutaneous atrophic changes.

The limitations of physical examination in the

assessment of urinary symptoms have been stressed previously. Nevertheless, a thorough medical and neurological examination should always be carried out. Pelvic examination may reveal atrophic mucosal changes, and occasionally meatal narrowing as a result of chronic atrophic urethritis may also be evident. The efficiency of the pelvic floor may be determined by asking the patient to strain and squeeze during vaginal examination, and the extent of uterovaginal prolapse should similarly be assessed.

Endocrine studies

In postmenopausal women estrogen deficiency is evidenced by low estradiol and estrone levels and elevated gonadotropin levels (Chakravarti et al., 1976); indeed, these changes are so characteristic that they do not need to be measured in postmenopausal women. There is, however, a significant group of women with characteristic estrogen deficiency symptoms before the cessation of menstruation; in these endocrinological investigation is certainly warranted. Chakravarti et al. (1979) have shown that in such women elevation of the plasma follicle stimulating hormone level is the most reliable criterion of estrogen deficiency on which to base selection for hormone replacement therapy.

Cytology

The correlation between lateral vaginal wall cytology and urinary sediment or urethral smears has been discussed earlier in this chapter. We have also, however, pointed out our results from vaginal cytology in climacteric patients with and without urinary symptoms. The poor correlation between cytological evidence of mucosal atrophy and symptoms limits the diagnostic value of such investigations in individual patients.

Urostatic tests

Bacteriological tests. The bacteriological assessment of a midstream urine specimen is important in all patients with urinary complaints. First, their symptoms may be a direct consequence of infection in the absence of any urodynamic abnormality. Where this is a possibility, it is important to assess the response to appropriate antibiotic therapy before embarking on further investigation. Second, the repeated urethral catheterization and bladder filling required during urodynamic investigations may be uncomfortable in the presence of urinary tract infection and could theoretically lead

to an exacerbation of symptoms and perhaps to septicemia. Third, the results of urodynamic investigations themselves may be unreliable in the presence of urinary tract infection. The discomfort involved may induce extrinsic striated urethral sphincter spasm, leading to anomalous results during urethral pressure profile measurements. The increased mucosal sensitivity may give a falsely low functional bladder capacity and predispose the patient to apparently uninhibited detrusor contractions during cystometry. Finally, urodynamic investigations themselves, by virtue of their invasive nature, carry a small risk of inducing urinary tract infection. This risk has been estimated to be as low as 2% (Walter and Vejlsgaard, 1978).

In patients with intractable urinary frequency or with a sterile pyuria on standard urine culture, microscopy and culture for mycobacteria should be performed on a series of three early-morning urine specimens.

Endoscopy. Endoscopy is equally important in all patients with significant urinary sypmtoms. However, while the procedure may allow the exclusion of organic mucosal disease, vesical or urethral fistulae, or calculi, conclusions regarding the function of the lower urinary tract based solely on endoscopic findings are frequently fallacious.

Urodynamic tests

The techniques of urodynamic investigation of the lower urinary tract are described in Chapters 8 through 11 and will not be considered further here.

HORMONE REPLACEMENT THERAPY

Methods of management of defined urodynamic abnormalities are considered in Part Three under the particular pathological states and also in Part Five. We will consider here only the place of hormone replacement therapy in the clinical conditions described previously where estrogen deficiency has been considered to have at least a partial etiological role.

Urethral syndrome and other sensory abnormalities

The benefits of estrogen in the urethral syndrome have been reported by Roberts and Smith (1968). Walter et al. (1978) noted significant improvements in the symptoms of sensory urge incontinence following the use of oral estrogens in a double-blind crossover study, and Hilton (1981) showed significant subjective improvements in urinary frequency

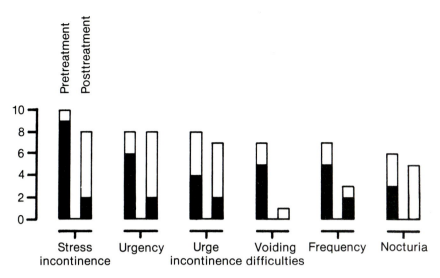

Figure 27.4 Effect of intravaginal estrogen cream on urinary symptoms of 10 postmenopausal women with genuine stress incontinence (solid bars show incidence of severe symptoms and open bars, mild symptoms).

and urgency in a group of women with detrusor-stable incontinence treated with intravaginal estrogen cream (Figure 27.4).

Voiding difficulties

Roberts and Smith (1968) advocated the use of urethral dilatation in postmenopausal women with the urethral syndrome who in addition showed endoscopic evidence of obstruction (which they inferred from the appearance of trabeculation). Eighty-three percent of the patients improved with this form of therapy, and the more refractory cases had a prolonged remission when oral estrogen replacement was given in the form of diethylstilbestrol. More recently, Smith (1981) has suggested that while the initial symptoms of atrophic urethritis may be estrogen responsive, where symptoms have been present for more than 12 months, dilatation or urethrotomy may be required to relieve the subsequent fibrosis and stricture formation. Hilton (1981), in the study referred to previously, found a highly significant reduction in the incidence of symptoms of voiding difficulty (although objective evidence in terms of improved flow rate was lacking) and found no correlation between the duration of symptoms and time since the menopause.

Urinary incontinence

Caine and Raz (1973) reported that 50% of a group of stress-incontinent women were cured or improved by estrogen replacement, and they noted a corresponding improvement in urethral pressure measurements. Walter et al. (1978) found that urge incontinence was relieved by oral estrogens, although stress incontinence was not; no urethral pressure changes were found. Both Rud (1980), using oral estrogens, and Hilton (1981), using intravaginal estrogen cream, found subjective improvement in the symptoms of genuine stress incontinence in 70% to 80% of patients.

The exact mode of action of estrogen in relieving urinary incontinence is uncertain. Urothelial proliferation certainly occurs, and it is possible that this aids the hermetic closure of the urethra. The importance of the urethral vascular supply in the maintenance of continence has been a subject of considerable debate. While Rud (1980) considered that up to one third of the urethral closure pressure was caused by a vascular contribution, Tulloch (1974) held the vascular contribution to be much less significant. Gosling, Dixon, and Lendon (1977), from their anatomical studies, found the urethral vascular supply to be unremarkable, although Huisman (1979) considered submucosal arteriovenous anastomoses to play an important role in urethral closure. Caine and Raz (1973) reported an apparent increase in the vascular component of urethral pressure following estrogen replacement therapy, although more recent studies by Walter et al. (1978), Rud (1980), and Hilton (1981) have failed to demonstrate any changes in the urethral pressure at rest following estrogen treatment. The latter two studies have both demonstrated improve-

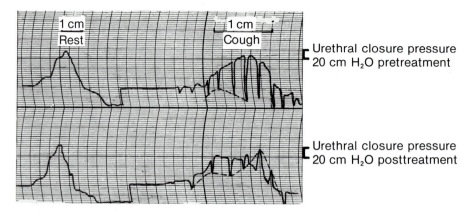

Figure 27.5 Example of resting and stress urethral closure pressure profiles before *(above)* and after *(below)* estrogen therapy.

ments in the urethral response to stress (Figure 27.5). It seems likely therefore that much of the efficacy of estrogen replacement in urinary incontinence lies in improved transmission of intraabdominal pressure rises to the urethra resulting from increased efficiency of the urethral ligamentous and muscular support.

Estrogen replacement may be given either orally, intravaginally, or by subcutaneous implantation. The symptomatic and urodynamic improvements obtained by Hilton (1981), using an intravaginal dose of estrogen equivalent to 1.25 mg conjugated estrogen daily, were similar to those obtained by Rud (1980), using 4 mg estradiol or 8 mg estriol orally). Whitehead et al. (1978) have shown that the plasma levels of estrone are of the same order, whereas those of estradiol are approximately three times higher following intravaginal administration than they are by the oral route. Certainly, then, the argument for using the intravaginal route for estrogen replacement to avoid systemic side effects is illogical; however, the choice of the latter route may mean that smaller doses may be used for the same therapeutic benefit because of the differences in metabolism of estrogen within the vaginal mucosa as opposed to the gastrointestinal tract.

CONCLUSION

Large numbers of women first have urinary symptoms during the climacteric, and while many factors may influence their presentation, estrogen deficiency may be of relevance in a significant proportion. Particularly with the symptoms of recurrent frequency and/or dysuria, sensory urgency, voiding difficulties, and urinary incontinence, es-

trogen withdrawal may be an important etiological factor. Women with these symptoms at or around the menopause justify as full an investigation as those in other age groups, and therapy for any specific urodynamic abnormality identified should be employed. Where estrogen deficiency is demonstrated, however, replacement should be considered as an important adjunct to other modes of treatment.

REFERENCES

Brocklehurst, J.C., et al. 1972. Urinary infection and symptoms of dysuria in women aged 45-64 years: their relevance to similar findings in the elderly. Age Ageing **1**:41-47.

Brown, A.D.G. 1977. Postmenopausal urinary problems. Clin. Obstet. Gynaecol. **4**(1):181-206.

Caine, M., and Raz, S. 1973. The role of female hormones in stress incontinence. Communication to the sixteenth Congress of the International Society of Urologists. Amsterdam.

Carlson, A.J. 1949. Physiologic changes in normal ageing. In Stieglitz, E.J., editor. Geriatric medicine. ed. 2. Philadelphia. W.B. Saunders Co.

Chakravarti, S., et al. 1976. Hormone profiles after the menopause. Br. Med. J. **2**:784-787.

Chakravarti, S., et al. 1979. Relation between plasma hormone profiles, symptoms, and response to estrogen therapy in women approaching the menopause. Br. Med. J. **1**:983-985.

Csapo, A. 1948. Actomyosin content in uterus. Nature **162**:218-219.

Del Castillo, E.B., Argonz, J., and Galli Mainini, C.G. 1948. Cytological cycle of the urinary sediment and its parallelism with the vaginal cycle. J. Clin. Endocrinol. Metab. **8**:76-87.

Frewen, W.K. 1972. Urgency incontinence. Br. J. Obstet. Gynaecol. **79**:77-79.

Gallagher, D.J.A., Montgomerie, J.Z., and North, J.D.K. 1965. Acute infection of the urinary tract and urethral syndrome in general practice. Br. Med. J. **1**:622-626.

Gosling, J.A., Dixon, J.S., and Lendon, R.G. 1977. The autonomic innervation of the human male and female bladder neck and proximal urethra. J. Urol. **118**:302-304.

Grosman, N., Hvidberg, H., and Schou, J. 1971. The effect of estrogenic treatment on the acid mucopolysaccharide pattern in the skin of mice. Acta Pharmacol. Toxicol. **30**:458.

Hilton, P. 1981. Urethral pressure measurement by microtransducer: observations on methodology, the pathophysiology of genuine stress incontinence, and the effects of its treatment in the female. MD thesis. Newcastle upon Tyne, England.

Huisman, A.B. 1979. Morphologie van de vrouwelijke Urethra. MD thesis. Groningen, The Netherlands.

Jeffcoate, T.N.A., and Francis, W.J.A. 1966. Urgency incontinence in the female. Am. J. Obstet. Gynecol. **94**:604-618.

Katz, F.H., and Kappas, A. 1968. Influence of estradiol and estriol on urinary excretion of hydroxyproline in man. J. Lab. Clin. Med. **71**:65.

McCallin, P.F., Stewart Taylor, E., and Whitehead, R.W. 1950. A study of the changes in the cytology of urinary sediment during the menstrual cycle and pregnancy. Am. J. Obstet. Gynecol. **60**:64-74.

Osborne, J.L. 1976. Postmenopausal changes in micturition habits and in urine flow and urethral pressure studies. In Campbell, S., editor. The management of the menopause and postmenopausal years. Lancaster, England. MTP Press, Ltd.

Packham, D.A. 1971. The epithelial lining of the female trigone and urethra. Br. J. Urol. **43**:201-205.

Parkes, A.S. and Zuckerman, S. 1931. The menstrual cycle of the primate. II. Some effect of oestrin on baboons and macaques. J. Anat. **65**:272-276.

Parkes, C.M. 1971. Psychosocial transitions—a field for study. Soc. Sci. Med. **5**:101.

Roberts, M., and Smith, P. 1968. Non-malignant obstruction of the female urethra. Br. J. Urol. **40**:694-702.

Rud, T. 1980. The effects of estrogens and gestogens on the urethral pressure profile in urinary continent and stress incontinent women. Acta Obstet. Gynecol. Scand. **59**:265-270.

Rud, T., et al. 1980. Intra-urethral pressure in women. Invest. Urol. **17**:343-347.

Smith, P. 1972. Age changes in the female urethra. Br. J. Urol. **44**:667-676.

Smith, P. 1981. Recurring cystitis in the female. Matern. Child Health **6**:353-358.

Soloman, S., Panagotopolous, P., and Oppenheim, A. 1958. Urinary cytology studies as an aid to diagnosis. Am. J. Obstet. Gynecol. **76**:57-62.

Stanton, S.L., Hilton, P., Norton, C., and Cardozo, L. 1982. Clinical and urodynamic effects of anterior colporrhaphy and vaginal hysterectomy with and without incontinence. Br. J. Obstet. Gynaecol. **89**:459-463.

Stanton, S.L., Oszoy, C., and Hilton, P. 1983. Voiding difficulties in the female: prevalence, clinical and urodynamic review. Obstet. Gynecol. **61**:144-147.

Studd, J., Chakravarti, S., and Oram, D. 1977. The climacteric. Clin. Obstet. Gynaecol. **4**(1):3-29.

Sussman, M., et al. 1969. Asymptomatic significant bacteriuria in the nonpregnant women. Br. Med. J. **1**:799-803.

Thomas, T.M., et al. 1980. Prevalence of urinary incontinence. Br. Med. J. **281**:1243-1245.

Tulloch, A.G.S. 1974. The vascular contribution to the intra-urethral pressure. Br. J. Urol. **46**:659-664.

van Keep, P., and Lauritzen, C. 1973. Ageing and oestrogens. Basel. S. Karger.

Varma, T.R. 1982. Unpublished Observations.

Walter, S., and Vejlsgaard, R. 1978. Diagnostic catheterization and bacteriuria in women with urinary incontinence. Br. J. Urol. **50**:106-108.

Walter, S., et al. 1978. Urinary incontinence in post-menopausal women treated with estrogens: a double blind clinical trial. Urol. Int. **33**:135-143.

Whitehead, M.I., et al. 1978. Systemic absorption of estrogen from "Premarin" vaginal cream. In Cooke, I.D., editor. The role of estrogen/progesterone in the management of the menopause. Lancaster, England. MTP Press, Ltd.

Young, J.Z. 1971. An introduction to the study of man. Oxford. Clarendon Press.

chapter 28

The elderly

PAUL HILTON and PETER HENRY MILLARD

URINARY TRACT CHANGES AND SYMPTOMS

With advancing age many symptoms of urinary abnormalities occur with greater frequency. Some of these symptoms are inevitable, whereas others result from the increased number of pathological findings that occur with aging. Although age changes occur at different rates in different persons, they are universal, intrinsic, progressive, and eventually deleterious.

The major change that occurs in the urinary tract with age is a gradual loss of the ability to concentrate and dilute urine, and, as in renal failure, the urine specific gravity gradually comes closer to 1.010. This is probably because of the loss of long, looped juxtamedullary nephrons, which are thought to be responsible for most of the urine concentrating power. By the age of 70 years, it is estimated that 50% of the glomeruli are lost and renal function is about half that of the young adult. This decreased function probably results from changes in the microvasculature, although hyper-trophy of tubular endothelial cells has been shown to progress to luminal occlusion and disappearance of the nephron in experimental animals. Such changes can be accelerated by high-protein diets. Decreased tubular function is associated with a re-duced ability to conserve sodium and concentrate urine and may have important consequences for the drug management of elderly patients.

In addition to being reduced in number, some nephrons hypertrophy, and in others diverticula may develop. Infections in these diverticula may lead to local inflammatory reactions, thus causing the interstitial fibrosis seen in the medulla of the aging kidney. In general, aging kidneys are shrunk-en and reduced in weight, showing changes similar to but less severe than those seen in hypertension. The net result of these changes is that the aging bladder suffers an excessive excretory load.

In a postmortem study of the bladder in elderly women, Brocklehurst (1972) showed that trabec-ulation and diverticulum formation were extremely common, and tended to be associated with reflex or uninhibited neuropathic bladders. From a functional viewpoint there are undoubtedly profound age-related effects; Brocklehurst and Dillane (1966) examined the cystometric results in non-incontinent elderly women and demonstrated a high incidence of what one would consider "abnormal results" in younger patients: 43% had bladder capacities of less than 250 ml, 50% had residual volumes over 50 ml, 38% frequently had detrusor contractions associated with leakage, and in the majority the sensation of bladder filling was delayed until bladder capacity.

The age-related cytological changes in the female urethra have been studied by Smith (1972). He showed that there is an estrogen-related aging effect in the urethral mucosa, although abrupt changes do not necessarily follow the menopause.

Urgency and frequency

Urgency and frequency are extremely common symptoms in the elderly and may be particularly distressing when mobility is restricted. In a random community sample Milne et al. (1972) found the incidence of increased diurnal frequency in elderly women to be 23% and of nocturia (two or more episodes of micturition each night) to be 25.8%. In a study of 100 incontinent elderly women Hilton and Stanton (1981) found the symptom of urgency to be a significant problem for 76%. Diurnal frequency (exceeding two voidings per hour or seven times during waking hours) and nocturia were found in up to two thirds of patients, regardless of their underlying urodynamic condition. These symptoms in general are discussed further in Chapter 23.

Voiding difficulties

The main symptoms of voiding difficulties are hesitancy, poor urinary stream, straining to void, the sensation of incomplete bladder emptying, and postmicturition dribble. Although these symptoms are undoubtedly common in elderly men, in whom prostatic hypertrophy compromises the outflow tract as an accompaniment of aging, there is as yet little information as to the incidence of these symptoms in women. Stanton, Oszoy, and Hilton (1983), in a review of 600 consecutive referrals to a specialist urodynamic unit, found evidence of significant voiding difficulty in 13.6% of younger patients as opposed to 25.5% of those over 65 years of age. In incontinent elderly women symptoms suggestive of voiding difficulty are present in up

to a third of patients (Hilton and Stanton, 1981).

Neurological disease affecting the control of micturition is probably the most common cause of these problems in the elderly woman. Lower motor neuron lesions affecting the bladder may give rise to underactivity, but more commonly upper motor neuron lesions resulting from cerebrovascular disease are found. Despite the fact that the bladder usually demonstrates uninhibited detrusor behavior, emptying may be incomplete because of intermittent spasm of the extrinsic striated sphincter. Urethral stricture is not a common problem in women, although postmenopausal atrophic changes (Roberts and Smith, 1968) and the presence of uterovaginal prolapse may be associated with voiding difficulties.

Urinary tract infection

The most obvious factor predisposing to urinary tract infection in the elderly is urinary obstruction. The increased residual volume, which seems to occur as a natural result of aging, and the frequency of discoordinate voiding patterns also predispose the elderly to urinary infection. In addition, the increased incidence of trabeculation and diverticulum formation in the aging bladder may be of relevance. Impairment of sanitary habits associated with dementia and the occasional coexistence of fecal incontinence obviously increase the risks of ascending infection even further. The increased incidence and severity of infection in elderly patients may also be exacerbated by lowered antibody response and a weakened resistance to infection. In elderly women in the community the incidence of urinary infection increases with age (Milne et al., 1972) and may be as high as 33% (Sourander, 1966). In the elderly person who is chronically ill, significant bacteriuria has been reported with twice this frequency (Mou, Siroty, and Ventry, 1962). Brocklehurst et al. (1968) showed a significant association between infected urine and the symptoms of urgency and hesitancy, although frequency of micturition, dysuria, stress incontinence, and urge incontinence showed no such relationship. The question of urinary tract infection is reviewed in detail in Chapter 24.

Urinary incontinence

Several studies in the literature relate to the prevalence of urinary incontinence in the population, although differences in interview techniques and definitions used have undoubtedly contributed to disparities in their results (Chapter 5). In a 1976 review, Milne cited the results of seven incidence studies of urinary incontinence in elderly women with results ranging from 1.6% to 42%. Yarnell and St. Leger (1979) reported that 17% of a random sample of elderly women had experienced urinary leakage in the 12 months before assessment. In a much larger survey, Thomas et al. (1980) found an incidence of 11.6% of women aged 65 years or over who experienced urinary incontinence twice or more each month. In approximately one in five of those affected, the problem was sufficient to warrant the designation "moderate" or "severe," thereby fitting the International Continence Society definition of incontinence as "urinary leakage which is objectively demonstrable and presents a social or hygienic problem" (Appendix II).

In institutions the incidence of incontinence may be considerably higher. Milne (1976) quotes figures of between 21.9% and 47% in hospitalized women. However, there is some evidence that these figures may exaggerate the problem. Willington (1969) has shown that the incidence may fall considerably in the weeks following admission to a department of geriatric medicine: on admission 33.6% of patients were incontinent of urine, but the incidence subsequently fell to 14.2% "established" cases; others have confirmed this transient nature of incontinence following hospital admission.

In purely financial terms Willington (1976) estimated that some 120,000,000 underpads were used annually in the United Kingdom at a cost of around £4,000,000 ($6,480,000). More recently a market research company (Frost and Sullivan, 1979) calculated that the current market for incontinence pads and appliances alone was on the order of £12,000,000 ($19,440,000) in the United Kingdom and £80,000,000 ($129,600,000) in Europe. However, this represents only a small proportion of the total expenditure on incontinence measures. In the early 1960s two studies of the problems of geriatric nursing (Norton, McClaren, and Exton-Smith, 1962; Adams and McIlwraith, 1963) demonstrated that about 25% of nursing time was devoted to dealing with incontinence and its sequelae. In addition, one must take into account the cost of laundry, cleaning services, and other expenditures involved in long-term inpatient care.

The costs and effects of incontinence on its elderly sufferers are no less profound. Individuals may be subjected to indignity, ridicule, ostracism, and sometimes even violence. Otherwise healthy,

active persons may become housebound and socially isolated as a result of their embarrassment. In many cases incontinence may be the breaking point that leads families to seek hospital care for their aging relatives. It has been estimated that urinary incontinence alone is the cause of more than 20% of admissions to geriatric wards (Shuttleworth, 1970).

However, urinary incontinence is not a necessary accompaniment of the aging process. Young children are disciplined by praise to excrete only in acceptable places, and this higher control of excretion is not easily lost. Many of the conditions that give rise to urinary incontinence (Chapters 15 to 21) (particularly incomplete bladder emptying, detrusor instability, and urethral sphincter weakness) are commonly found in the elderly, but not all elderly are incontinent. What then tips the balance between the individual who is predisposed to incontinence by virtue of her impaired urinary function and the patient whose impaired control can no longer be maintained? Frequently one can identify a precipitating factor that impairs control even further or robs the person of mobility or independence. A number of the more common predisposing and precipitating factors are shown on p. 357.

The relationship between urinary infection and incontinence is questionable, although in a patient already predisposed, the additional mucosal irritation caused by an acute infection may be sufficient to precipitate incontinence. Acute illness of any type, particularly infections and congestive cardiac failure, may be associated with mental confusion, and impairment of urinary control is not an uncommon manifestation of this.

Because of the multiple systems failure associated with aging, large numbers of drugs are frequently prescribed for elderly patients. Many of these may have adverse effects either on continence or voiding efficiency by virtue of their actions on adrenergic and cholinergic effector mechanisms. Other medications, particularly tranquilizers and hypnotics because they impair the individual's level of consciousness or diuretics because they increase the load on aging bladder, may be sufficient to cause loss of urinary control; this is especially true with the fast-acting diuretics.

Affective disorders in the elderly are frequently associated with apathy and inertia. Since patients may lack the motivation to perform toiletry functions regularly, incontinence frequently results.

Predisposing and precipitating factors relevant to the development of urinary incontinence in the elderly

PREDISPOSING FACTORS	PRECIPITATING FACTORS
Neurological	**Urinary infection**
Cerebral degeneration	**Acute illness**
Cerebrovascular disease	Particularly infection and congestive cardiac failure
Cerebral tumor	
Multiple sclerosis	**Drugs**
Cervical spondylosis	Effects on continence
Intervertebral disk prolapse	α-Adrenergic blockers
	Phenytoin
Renal	Reserpine
Chronic pyelonephritis	Phenothiazines
Chronic renal failure	Effects on voiding
Renal aging	Tricyclic antidepressants
Gynecological	Antihistamines
Pelvic tumor	Anticholinergic agents
Uterovaginal prolapse	Sympathomimetics
	MAO inhibitors
Rectal	Indirect effects
Tumor	Tranquilizers
Fecal impaction	Hypnotics
	Diuretics
Urethral	
Urethral sphincter weakness	**Affective disorders**
Urethral obstruction	**Hospitalization**
Vesical	**Immobilization from any cause**
Idiopathic detrusor instability	High beds, cot sides
Tumor	Chairs with fixed tables
Stone	
Pelvic surgery	

Hospitalization may have detrimental effects on continence. The access to toilet facilities is invariably more difficult in a hospital than in a patient's home; the use of high beds with cot sides and chairs of the wrong shape and size hampers mobility further, and the lack of signs in hospital wards may add to the disorientation often experienced by hospitalized elderly persons. The attitudes and expectations of hospital staff members may exacerbate the problem: the elderly are expected to be wet, so they are dressed in hospital clothes, often without underclothing, to reduce laundry problems and are seated on incontinence pads with their skirts lifted throughout the day to protect the furniture. They are therefore provided with exactly the situation in which they were stimulated as children to void, and true to staff expectations they become incontinent.

In considering incontinence in the elderly, it is helpful to differentiate between voluntary and involuntary loss of control. Involuntary loss of control can be considered to be present when there are no physical or psychological barriers preventing access to or provision of acceptable facilities but inappropriate excretion nevertheless occurs (Millard, 1979).

INVESTIGATION OF SYMPTOMS

Urodynamic investigation is considered in detail in Chapters 6 to 14. Here we discuss only procedures of relevance to the elderly and consider in particular the extent of any necessary modifications.

History and examination

A history from the patient and relatives is essential to help differentiate between voluntary and involuntary incontinence. Communication difficulties are common in the elderly, and where problems arise confirmatory information obtained from relatives, home wardens, and ward or community nursing staff may be invaluable. A Linco speech trainer is a useful aid in speaking to the very deaf.

The frequency with which urinary symptoms are found in the elderly inevitably restricts their diagnostic reliability. In a study of 100 elderly incontinent women with a variety of urodynamic diagnoses, Hilton and Stanton (1981) emphasized this point (Table 28.1). Although the symptom of stress incontinence was common in women subsequently shown to have urethral sphincter incompetence (genuine stress incontinence), it was also found in half of all elderly incontinent women and was even more common in those with voiding difficulties. Urge incontinence was common in all categories and consequently less reliable as a diagnostic aid; urination frequency exceeding two episodes per hour occurred in approximately two thirds of patients regardless of underlying urodynamic pathological condition. So, although we would advocate a complete history of all incontinent patients, the urological aspects of that history are in many respects the least helpful in the elderly. Often of more value is a thorough inquiry into the

TABLE 28.1 Incidence (percentage) of a variety of urinary symptoms related to urodynamic diagnoses in 100 elderly incontinent women

Diagnosis	Stress incontinence	Urgency	Urge incontinence	Enuresis	Frequency	Nocturia	Strain to void	Poor stream	Incomplete empyting
Detrusor instability (N = 29)	33	84	80	46	68	52	0	9	4
Detrusor instability + urethral sphincter incompetence (N = 10)	43	100	71	60	67	67	0	38	38
Urethral sphincter incompetence (N = 30)	63	70	57	30	67	50	10	30	33
Voiding difficulty (N = 14)	77	58	58	62	62	38	43	72	33
No abnormality detected (N = 12)	20	90	90	0	70	50	10	20	20
Miscellaneous (N = 5)	33	33	33	50	40	60	0	25	0
All patients (N = 100)	49	76	68	39	65	51	10	30	23

From Hilton, P., and Stanton, S.L. 1981. Br. Med. J. **282:**940-942.

general medical, neurological, psychiatric, iatrogenic, and environmental aspects of the case. A simple assessment of the mental state such as the Northwick Park Abbreviated Mental Test* should be performed:

Ability to answer each question correctly scores one mark

1. Age
2. Time (to nearest hour)
3. Address for recall at end of test—this should be repeated by the patient to ensure it has been heard correctly: "42 West Street"
4. Year
5. Name of hospital
6. Recognition of two persons (doctor, nurse, etc.)
7. Date of birth
8. Year of First World War
9. Name of present Monarch
10. Count backwards 20 - 1

Similarly the clinical examination must not be restricted to the urological features. A full assessment of the patient's general health and mobility must be performed. The patient's cardiovascular state may be relevant not only as a cause of her incontinence but also in determining the most appropriate therapy.

Palpable bladder enlargement discovered during abdominal examination is a sign of a significant voiding difficulty. During pelvic examination the extent of any uterovaginal prolapse should be assessed, and the state of estrogenization of the tissues observed. The symptom of stress incontinence is unreliable, but the demonstration of the physical sign when the patient is standing with a full bladder is a much more useful indicator of urethral sphincter incompetence. However, this sign is also frequently found in patients with voiding difficulties, in association with a chronic residual volume (Hilton and Stanton, 1981). Rectal examination should be performed to exclude fecal impaction and to assess the anal sphincter and pelvic floor tone.

Under ideal circumstances one might expect to achieve assessment and investigation of incontinent patients thus far at a primary care level. Indeed by these methods alone it has been shown that considerable diagnostic success can be achieved. Hilton and Stanton (1981) were able to reliably diagnose 60% of cases so that further urodynamic testing of patients could be restricted without loss of diagnostic accuracy (Figure 28.1).

*From Hodkinson, H.M. 1972. Age Ageing **1**:233-238.

Uroflow studies

The value of urine flow measurement in the elderly is questionable. It is generally recognized that little can be inferred from flow rates obtained from a voided volume of less than 200 ml. Since the functional bladder capacity in elderly patients is frequently reduced, voided volumes are often low and flow traces unreliable. Even with volumes exceeding 200 ml the lower acceptable limits decrease with age (Abrams and Torrens, 1979), and therefore even more caution must be used in their interpretation.

Cystometry and radiology

Much of the literature relating to bladder dysfunction in the elderly has been based on the results of single-channel cystometry (Brocklehurst and Dillane, 1966; Eastwood, 1979). Excessive respiratory and abdominal straining efforts (frequently seen during assessment of elderly patients) makes interpretation of results difficult. These may be avoided by using a dual-channel subtracted cystometry technique. Simultaneous radiological screening with cystometry in the form of videocystourethrography (Bates and Corney, 1971) is the mainstay of urodynamic investigation in most specialist centers. However, this procedure requires a degree of physical fitness on the part of the patient. By virtue of the irradiation involved and the availability of radiological facilities, it must be carried out quickly and therefore is not as applicable to elderly as to younger patients. It is our experience that the longer one takes to assess and investigate the condition of elderly patients, the more reliable the results are likely to be. Chapter 8 deals with the techniques of cystometric assessment.

Urethral pressure measurement

Although several studies on incontinence in the elderly have included data from urethral pressure profile measurements, it has been clearly shown that even in continent women the urethral closure pressure falls with increasing age (Rud, 1980). The reliability of the measurement also decreases with age (Edwards and Malvern, 1974). Therefore it would seem that the technique has very limited clinical value in the elderly.

MANAGEMENT OF URINARY INCONTINENCE

The management of urinary incontinence in the elderly may be considered in terms of (1) measures

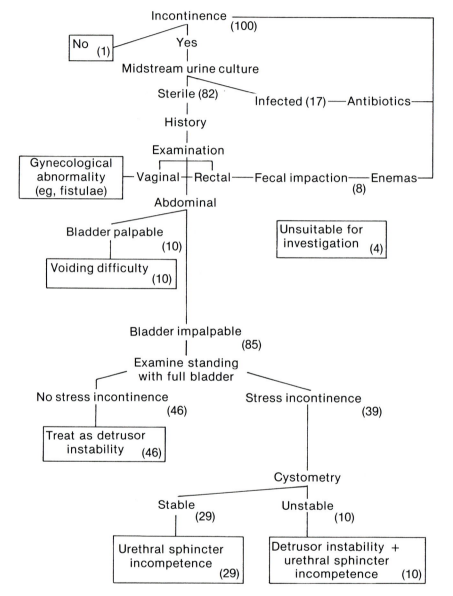

Figure 28.1 Algorithm for assessing urinary incontinence in elderly women. *Figures in parentheses,* Numbers of patients who followed each route when algorithm was applied to 100 patients retrospectively. (From Hilton, P., and Stanton, S.L. 1981. Br. Med. J. **282:**940-942.)

aimed at reducing the patient's level of incontinence, directed toward both the specific urodynamic abnormality and general rehabilitation of the patient, and (2) measures that enable the patient to cope better with whatever residual symptoms she may have.

Treatment of specific urodynamic abnormalities

Urethral sphincter incompetence (genuine stress incontinence)

Conservative treatment. The major conservative approaches to the management of urethral sphincter incontinence—physiotherapy and electrical therapy—are discussed in Chapters 41 and 36 respectively. Both techniques obviously require considerable patient compliance but are of value in the management of cooperative patients. Phenylpropanolamine is an α-adrenergic stimulant that has been found to be of some benefit in stress incontinence. Hypertension and ischemic heart disease contraindicate the use of such therapy, and adrenergic side effects including shivering and scalp tingling may occasionally be troublesome. Nevertheless, this compound has the advantage over other sympathomimetic agents of a longer period of activity. Although most reports give subjective improvement rates of close to 50%, objective evidence of the effects of phenylpropanolamine on urethral function is conflicting. Although Montague and Stewart (1979) demonstrated significant improvements in urethral pressure (using Ornade, 1 capsule b.d.), Obrink and Bunne (1978) failed to do so.

The estrogen sensitivity of the female urethra is well established (Smith, 1972), and symptomatic benefits from estrogens in postmenopausal stress incontinence have been reported (Slunsky, 1973). Although slight increases in urethral pressure and functional urethral length have been shown, it seems likely that the most significant change induced by estrogens administered either orally (Rud, 1980) or in the form of intravaginal cream (Hilton, 1981) is an improvement in the transmission of abdominal pressure rises to the urethra. In view of the frequently associated finding of atrophic vaginitis in elderly incontinent women, the use of estrogen cream is often beneficial, since, even if the degree of urinary leakage is not improved, the accompanying discomfort is often relieved.

Surgical treatment. In younger patients, surgery is the most commonly employed treatment for ure-thral sphincter incontinence. Although the operability rate is obviously lower in the elderly than in younger patients, age per se is not a contraindication to surgical treatment. Stanton and Cardozo (1980), using the Burch colposuspension in elderly women, reported an objective cure rate of 74%, comparing favorably with their cure rate of 86% in all ages (Stanton and Cardozo, 1979).

Detrusor instability. In the elderly, detrusor instability is usually managed by pharmacotherapy using the same drugs as those employed in younger patients (Chapter 17). If anticholinergic preparations are to be prescribed, visual symptoms should be investigated, since these drugs are contraindicated in glaucoma. Emepronium bromide has been reported to cause oral and esophageal ulceration, and patients should be advised to take these tablets with fluids. The use of behavior modification techniques such as biofeedback is limited; however, habit retraining (Clay, 1978) may be successfully employed in this age group for inpatients or outpatients (Chapter 39).

Voiding difficulties. The management of retention and voiding difficulties may be divided broadly into pharmacotherapy, aimed either at increasing detrusor activity or reducing urethral resistance, and surgery in the form of urethral dilatation, internal urethrotomy, or bladder neck incision. The most rational decision as to which to employ in any individual case depends on complete urodynamic assessment, including pressure flow studies. However, because of the potential cardiovascular side effects from cholinergic and sympatholytic agents in the elderly, urethrotomy has often been the preferred treatment. The management of voiding difficulties in general is considered in Chapter 21.

General rehabilitation

All staff members must be educated to realize that anyone would suffer incontinence if she or he were unable to get to a lavatory or were not given facilities when needed. Patients should be dressed in proper clothes, with pants and proper shoes. The beds should be low, with no cot sides or restraints. These conditions offer patients of any age a chance to become continent (Millard, 1979).

Toilets should be at the right height. A simple raised seat may help if the lavatory is too low. Grab rails can be affixed if necessary. Toilet paper should be provided in a single-sheet dispenser for the hemiplegic patient. At home a visit by an occupational therapist is a useful way of ensuring that the correct advice is given. Attention should be given to the height of the bed and chairs, loose carpets should be tacked down, and trailing electric cables or leads should be moved to ensure a quick, safe route to the lavatory. If nocturia is a problem, late night drinks, especially those containing weak diuretics and stimulants such as tea or coffee, should be avoided; it must be remembered that long-acting diuretics act at night as well. Many an elderly person has had incontinence precipitated by the use of a fast-acting diuretic such as furosemide (Frusemide, Lasix) or ethacrynic acid. These drugs cause diuresis over a 3- to 4-hour period, and the implication is that the patient must remain close to a lavatory. If the patient has nocturia, the light in the hall and on the stairs should be bright (at least 60 watts), and a bedside light should be provided.

As a general rule, night sedation should not be used in the elderly: the problems it causes outweigh any advantages. The elderly should be counseled instead as to the reasons why one needs less sleep with age. If necessary, a small amount of alcohol is the best night sedative.

The provision of a bedside commode can "cure" incontinence. Commodes that are less embarrassing to empty are helpful in the home. The Hassa commode, or a chemical toilet, particularly one with a flushing mechanism as used in recreational vehicles and boats, can make life much more pleasant for the elderly person and the family.

If it is determined that incontinence arises because of the inability to identify the right place, or to get to it, management should be directed at instituting a process of retraining, with reinforcement of staff and family expectations that the patient will regain control. Praise is the method of discipline and reinforcement of the elderly person's pleasure at gaining control. The act of being incontinent in an environment that expects continence is punishing enough without embarrassment by an unthinking staff. A simple record of bladder and bowel function must be kept. A 2-hour or hourly routine should be adopted in the management of incontinence, the patient being reminded to toilet after each interval. When control is regained, the provision of facilities should be adjusted to the needs of the individual.

Coping with residual symptoms

When all forms of active management of urinary incontinence have been attempted, there will inevitably be a group of patients with residual symptoms. Much can be achieved for them in the home situation to allow them to cope better. Modifications to the home environment, the provision of aids and equipment, and the use of incontinence pads and garments all fall within the role of the incontinence adviser and are considered in Chapters 40 and Appendix I.

CONCLUSION

Incontinence is not an inevitable outcome of the aging process. Urinary dysfunction symptoms are more common in the elderly, but, whatever their age, all patients who suffer urinary incontinence should have a thorough investigation and trial of treatments before being condemned to continue living under this burden.

REFERENCES

Abrams, P., and Torrens, M. 1979. Urine flow studies. Urol. Clin. North Am. **6:**71-79.

Adams, G.F., and McIlwraith, P.M. 1963. Geriatric nursing. Oxford, England. Oxford University Press.

Bates, C.P. and Corney, C.E. 1971. Simultaneous cine pressure flow cystourethrography: method of routine urodynamic investigation. Br. J. Radiol. **44:**44-50.

Brocklehurst, J.C. 1972. Bladder outlet obstruction in elderly women. Mod. Geriatr. **2:**108-113.

Brocklehurst, J.C., and Dillane, J.B. 1966. Studies on the female bladder in old age. I. Cystometrograms in non-incontinent women. Gerontol. Clin. **8:**285-305.

Brocklehurst, J.B., et al. 1968. The prevalence and symptomatology of urinary infection in an aged population. Gerontol. Clin. **10:**242-253.

Clay, E. 1978. Incontinence of urine. Part 2. Nurs. Mirror **146:**36-38.

Eastwood, D.H. 1979. Urodynamic studies in the management of urinary incontinence in the elderly. Age Ageing **8:**41-48.

Edwards, L., and Malvern, J. 1974. The urethral pressure profiles: theoretical considerations and clinical applications. Br. J. Urol. **46:**325-329.

Frost and Sullivan. 1979. Urinary incontinence in Europe: Incidence, treatment and demand for containment products. New York. Frost & Sullivan.

Hilton, P. 1981. Urethral pressure measurement by microtransducer: observations on the methodology, the pathophysiology of genuine stress incontinence and the effects of its treatment in the female. Doctoral thesis. University of Newcastle-upon-Tyne.

Hilton, P., and Stanton, S.L. 1981. Algorithmic method for assessing urinary incontinence in elderly women. Br. Med. J. **282:**940-942.

Hodkinson, H.M. 1972. Evaluation of a mental test score for assessment of mental impairment in the elderly. Age Ageing **1:**233-238.

Millard, P.H. 1979. The promotion of continence. Health Trends **11:**27-28.

Milne, J.S. 1976. Prevalence of incontinence in the elderly age groups. In Willington, F.L., editor. Incontinence in the elderly. London. Academic Press, Inc. (London), Ltd.

Milne, J.S., et al. 1972. Urinary symptoms in older people. Mod. Geriatr. **2:**198-212.

Montague, D.K., and Stewart, B.H. 1979. Urethral pressure profiles before and after Ornade administration in patients with stress incontinence of urine. J. Urol. **122:**198-199.

Mou, T.W., Siroty, R., and Ventry, P. 1962. Bacteriuria in elderly, chronically ill patients. J. Am. Geriatr. Soc. **10:**170-178.

Norton, D., McClaren, R., and Exton-Smith, A.N. 1962. Geriatric nursing problems in hospital. London. National Corporation for the Care of Old People.

Obrink, A., and Bunne, G. 1978. The effect of alpha-adrenergic stimulation in stress incontinence. Scand. J. Urol. Nephrol. **12:**205-208.

Roberts, M., and Smith, P. 1968. Non-malignant obstruction of the female urethra. Br. J. Urol. **40:**694-702.

Rud, T. 1980. Urethral pressure profile in continent women from childhood to old age. Acta Obstet. Gynecol. Scand. **59:**331-335.

Shuttleworth, K.E.D. 1970. Urinary tract diseases: incontinence. Br. Med. J. **4:**727-729.

Slunsky, R. 1973. Complex, conservative therapy of urinary incontinence in elderly women with Ubretid, oestriol and gymnastic exercises. Wien. Klin. Wochenschr. **85:**759-762. (German.)

Smith, P. 1972. Age changes in the female urethra. Br. J. Urol. **44:**667-676.

Sourander, L.B. 1966. Urinary tract infection in the aged. Ann. Med. Intern. Fenn. **55**(suppl. 45):1-55.

Stanton, S.L., and Cardozo, L.D. 1979. Results of colposuspension operation for incontinence and prolapse. Br. J. Obstet. Gynecol. **86:**693-697.

Stanton, S.L., and Cardozo, L.D. 1980. Surgical treatment of incontinence in elderly women. Surg. Gynecol. Obstet. **150:**555-557.

Stanton, S.L., Oszoy, C., and Hilton, P. 1983. Voiding difficulties in the female: prevalence, clinical and urodynamic review. Obstet. Gynecol. **61:**144-147.

Thomas, T.M., et al. Prevalence of urinary incontinence. Br. Med. J. **281:**1243-1245.

Yarnell, J.W.G., and St. Ledger, A.S. 1979. The prevalence, severity and factors associated with urinary incontinence in a random sample of the elderly. Age Ageing **8:**81-85.

Willington, F.L. 1969. Problems of urinary incontinence in the aged. Gerontol. Clin. **11:**330-356.

Willington, F.L. 1976. Hygienic methods in the management of incontinence. In Willington, F.L., editor. Incontinence in the elderly. London Academic Press, Inc. (London), Ltd.

chapter 29

Gynecological urology in the Third World

RICHARD R. TRUSSELL

It is only comparatively recently that valid statistics have become available that allow for a useful comparison of the incidence of urological symptoms between one part of the developed world and another. Most of the attempts to provide epidemiological data come from India. Pal (1980) surveyed the incidence of urinary incontinence and described 107 patients attending a urological clinic between 1977 and 1978. There were 38 cases of urinary incontinence of which 25 were described as being true stress incontinence and 14 were stress incontinence associated with prolapse. Detrusor instability was found in 10 cases.

Chakravarty and Chowdhury (1980) surveyed 100 parous nonpregnant patients and found that 50 had urinary symptoms suggesting infection, of whom 7% were found to have significant bacteriuria. The remainder of this group, together with the 50 who were asymptomatic, had sterile urine.

In less developed areas, such information is almost entirely lacking. There are many reasons for this. Most publications are hospital based and relate only sparingly to the community, and even within one country regional differences may be profound. For cultural, biological, economical, and marital reasons, a woman in the developing world is denied access to medical expertise unless her problem is disabling. Travel is often difficult and expensive. Many studies have clearly shown that maternal mortality is directly related to the distance a woman lives from a maternity center or hospital. It is true that the maternal and child health services are often the most active of the health services in the investigation and prevention of disease, and antenatal care may well be the single most effective means of reducing maternal morbidity and mortality.

These difficulties contribute to a stoicism among the women of developing countries that is only slowly changing with their changing world. When the worst happens and a tragedy such as a fistula leads to socially unacceptable urinary incontinence, it is only too common for a woman to be turned out of her home by her husband, and her search for relief becomes even more difficult. The Hamlins working in Ethiopia have found it necessary to institute a "village" to house such unfortunate women while they are waiting for surgery.

Women are embroiled in a pattern of traditional practices, some of which are harmless and some injurious. Among the Hausa tribe in Nigeria, older women make a "girishi cut" in the vagina using a razor blade (Harrison, 1979). This is carried out for a variety of complaints, both obstetrical and gynecological, and may lead to vesicovaginal fistula and death from hemorrhage. The use of caustic substances after childbirth to narrow the vagina produces vaginal ulceration and fibrosis.

Thus hard facts are difficult to come by, and data tend to be anecdotal. Notwithstanding this paucity it is clear to me that uterovaginal prolapse is less common in Africa than in Europe or the United States, and that, when it does occur, it is less liable to be accompanied by stress incontinence. This is difficult to explain in a community where laboring women are often encouraged by the traditional birth attendant to bear down from very early labor and where obstruction and prolonged labor are common and a ruptured uterus and vesicovaginal fistula may be accompanied by extensive tissue necrosis. It is tempting to conclude that there must be a factor involving pelvic connective tissue and smooth muscle that is more resilient among certain races than others, but this has never been clearly delineated.

The trauma associated with childbirth looms large in the etiology of urological problems among women in the developing world and is a major importance in the well-being of the family, on which national life ultimately depends.

To this must be added a variety of diseases that have predilection for the urogenital tract. These include syphilis, tuberculosis, schistosomiasis, lymphogranuloma venereum, amebiasis, and bladder stones.

OBSTETRICS

In most of the developing world, less than 30% of the population receives any skilled attention during labor, which will be in the hands of traditional birth attendants. Under these circumstances the maternal mortality may be as high as 300 per 100,000 live births and the perinatal mortality 80 per 1000 or more.

Although traditional birth attendants are coming increasingly under the control of the governments and many receive basic training, many remain ignorant and illiterate and have no formal contact with the health service.

Some of the social, biological, and economic determinants contributing to disorders of the urogenital tract have already been mentioned. Where adverse factors are absent and the women of a developing country are well nourished and cared for, they fare as well as those of any other region. Fiji is such an example, and Gebbie (1979) has described a perinatal mortality of about 20 per 1000 live births in New Guinea, a correspondingly low maternal mortality, and a cesarean section rate of 3%.

When, however, the dice are loaded against parturient women, obstetrical outcome will be compromised by maternal disease, cephalopelvic disproportion, long, neglected labor (Figure 29.1), infection, hemorrhage, and fetal death. Tissue necrosis will be inevitable, and when the woman survives, she will be liable to rupture of her uterus, with or without involvement of the bladder, vesicovaginal and rectovaginal fistulae, third-degree perineal tears, and trauma to the lumbosacral nerve roots.

Obstructed labor

Further difficulty follows necessary efforts to deliver the baby in obstructed labor. Tissue debility makes any form of delivery hazardous, whether by cesarean section, forceps, or *ventouse* (vacuum extraction). Even when the baby is alive, cesarean section in the presence of a severe uterine infection is not to be taken lightly, particularly because the patient may be reluctant or unable to attend the hospital for subsequent deliveries and may run the risk of trauma to the scar. The production of a uterine scar when the baby is already dead is doubly unfortunate. Indeed, dragging the molded head of a long-dead fetus up from a contracted pelvis to allow abdominal extraction may itself cause damage to tissues. In these circumstances some way to reduce the size of the dead baby is valuable. Although the day of crushing instruments such as the cephalotribe is past, trauma to the maternal tissues may be spared by perforation of the fetal head after the application of obstetrical forceps and by the

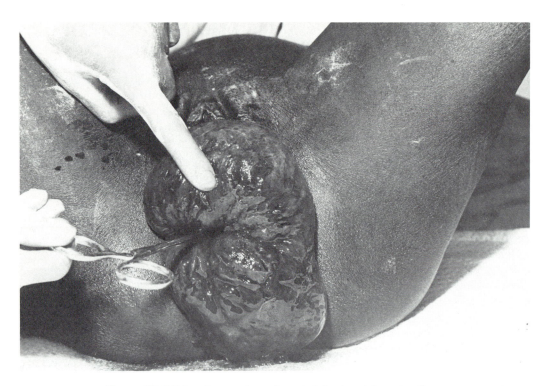

Figure 29.1 Edematous prolapsed cervix following delivery in village.

judicious use of cleidotomy and decapitation. These limited destructive procedures are not without risk, and Greenhill (1951) has commented on the morbidity resulting from ignorance and a lack of technical ability on the part of the physician. Writing in Uganda on ''Management of the dead baby'' in 1962, I reported the vaginal delivery of 151 babies following emergency admissions with neglected labor and fetal death. I recorded 8 maternal deaths, 13 ruptured uteri, 18 vesicovaginal fistulae, 3 rectovaginal fistulae, 6 severe vaginal lacerations, and 2 cases of trauma to the lumbosacral nerve roots. It is not to be concluded that these tragedies, occurring in a teaching hospital, were solely the result of unskilled obstetrical practice, but rather they resulted from the degree of devitalization to which maternal tissues had already been subjected by hours of obstructed labor.

In these circumstances the most carefully conducted forceps delivery may be followed by damage to the vagina, bladder, and rectum. Rotation with Keilland's forceps may be particularly hazardous. Even when damage to the bladder has not occurred, there may be hematuria following delivery, and an indwelling catheter will avoid overdistension of the bladder so easily missed in the puerperium.

If in spite of every effort a vesicovaginal fistula does occur, it may not be obvious until the third or fourth day, when a telltale trickle of urine will reveal the condition. It is never possible to effect repair immediately, and 3 months must elapse before a formal operation is attempted. Unfortunately, even if infection is treated vigorously, scarring may take place during this waiting period, making the subsequent operation more difficult.

Symphysiotomy

In Mulago Hospital, Uganda, from 1966 to 1969, I witnessed a swing from forceps delivery to vacuum extraction coincident with a fall in perinatal mortality and a fall in the incidence of cesarean section. At about the same time, the operation of symphysiotomy was introduced. If suitable cases are selected, this technique makes possible the delivery of a live child that could only be otherwise safely effected by cesarean section. Not only is delivery achieved vaginally, but the transverse diameter of the pelvis is permanently enlarged. The two complications reported most commonly from this operation are stress incontinence and instability of the bony pelvis. Among women in whom stress incontinence is rare, it is not surprising that symphisiotomy does not lead to this disorder if the operation is properly carried out; neither backache nor pelvic instability was recorded in this series of patients. Selection of suitable cases is all-important, and should, I believe, be restricted to failed trials of labor, where the cervix is fully dilated or almost so.

It is preferred, after the administration of local anesthesic, to apply the medium-sized cup used in vacuum extraction and to try gentle traction. If this fails, but the obstruction to vaginal delivery seems minimal, symphisiotomy may be employed. The patient's legs must be supported by assistants, whose responsibility is to prevent undue separation of the two pelvic halves at the symphysial joint. The symphysial joint is divided by a solid-bladed knife using a small incision over the middle of the joint, deflecting the urethra from the midline by a finger in the vagina acting through a urethral catheter. If the case has been well selected, subsequent delivery of the head is easy. A wide episiotomy is essential to relieve the strain on the anterior vaginal wall and the attached urethra.

Where uterine rupture is so common, digital exploration of the uterus after these procedures is mandatory. The indwelling catheter is left in place for 3 days, during which time the patient remains in bed. She then increases her mobility and usually starts walking with a frame or walking stick and is confident and stable by the tenth day. Lifting and heavy work should be avoided for a month. The symphysis heals by fibrous union, resulting in a permanent increase in the transverse diameter of the pelvis at all levels.

Bladder trauma

The close relationships between the urinary bladder on the one hand and the lower segment of uterus and the cervix on the other, mean that the bladder is frequently distorted in cases of obstructed labor, rising with the thinning lower uterine segment as high as the umbilicus. This makes it vulnerable to accidental incision when the abdomen is opened at cesarean section and liable to severe damage if the uterus ruptures.

The most common site of spontaneous rupture of the uterus is transversely in the lower uterine segment, occasionally minimizing the lower segment operation to a surprising extent. Extension distally may involve the bladder. This condition is of course primarily one arising in multigravidae who respond to obstructive labor by even stronger contractions, whereas primigravidae respond by disordered uterine action. Rupture may be spontaneous and occur at the site of a previous scar or may follow intrauterine manipulations, such as attempts at correction of an abnormal fetal lie. Although spontaneous rupture may well be a dramatic event associated with a tearing pain followed by collapse, dehiscence of the scar may take place silently and may indeed be associated occasionally with the spontaneous delivery of a live child. Every uterus that is the site of a scar must be regarded at risk of rupture during pregnancy and labor. Any deviation from the course of normal progress in the labor of such a patient demands abdominal exploration and delivery.

Damage to the bladder may also occur when the lower segment tears, and a search for this must always be made. Unlike the established vesicovaginal fistula—provided the damage is recognized immediately—repair at the time of operation in two layers is usually successful and is often easier when hysterectomy has been performed and the remaining cervix can be incorporated in the repair. Even when the tissues have been handled with the greatest care, vesicouterine, vesicocervical, or vesicovaginal fistulae may still be a sequel.

To prevent the morbidity and mortality associated with these abnormal deliveries, it is necessary to look beyond the walls of the hospital. A plan of maternal and child heath care that will accept responsibility for every mother at risk, a training scheme for traditional birth attendants, and the development of maternity centers with adequate transport to district hospitals will all play their part, but perhaps most important of all is the education of both sexes.

GYNECOLOGY
Donovanosis (granuloma inguinale)

Donovanosis, or granuloma inguinale, is fairly common throughout the tropics. It accounts for 5% of visits to venereal disease clinics in India and is more common in West Africa than in East Africa.

The disease is found much more frequently in men than women, and, with 25% of conjugal contents infected, spread is presumed to be venereal. The earliest lesion, a painless flat papule, is rarely identified. The next stage is ulceration, and itching is common. Curiously it is only as a result of the secondary infection associated with this stage that lymphadenopathy is found. Much later extensive tissue destruction may occur associated with loss of urethral tissues and elephantiasis of the vulva.

Identification depends on the examination of a small tissue snip or biopsy. Stained with Giemsa stain, intracellular Donovan bodies may be recognized. These gram-negative rods are believed to represent infection with *Calymmatobacterium granulomatis,* which are related to *Klebsiella* organisms.

Treatment is tetracycline, 2 g a day for 2 weeks, with ampicillin or chloramphenicol as an alternative. Corrective surgery must always be preceded by a full course of antibiotics.

Lymphogranuloma venereum

Lymphogranuloma venereum is caused by *Chlamydia trachomatis,* an obligate intracellular parasite which, although having many features of a true bacteria, is nevertheless a virus allied to the *C. psittaci* group.

The true incidence is unknown, but the condition is widespread in the tropics, affects both sexes, and is probably venereally transmitted. Asymptomatic female carriers may act as a reservoir. Like donovanosis, the initial painless lesion, probably a vesicle or ulcer, is rarely seen.

Early in the disease inguinal adenitis, commonly referred to as buboes (Figure 29.2), is found, sometimes unilaterally, and this stage of the disease is often associated with signs of a systemic illness, fever, and malaise. The lymph gland enlargement may go on to bubo formation both above and below the inguinal ligament and, if not treated, may break down and form multiple sinuses. When the buboes eventually heal, they leave characteristic scarring.

The local vulval condition spreads, and extensive destruction of urethra and fenestration of the labia may take place (Figures 29.3 and 29.4). At

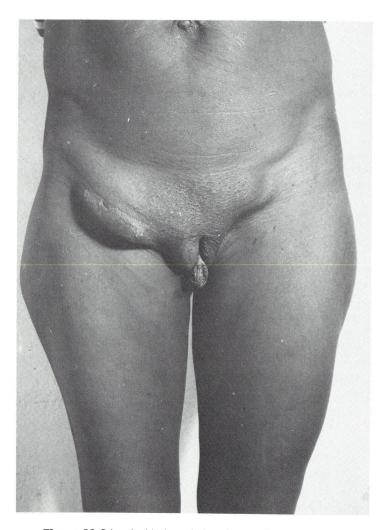

Figure 29.2 Inguinal buboes in lymphogranuloma venereum.

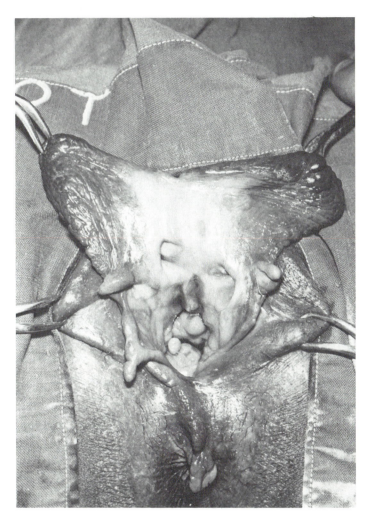

Figure 29.3 Vulva in lymphogranuloma venereum.

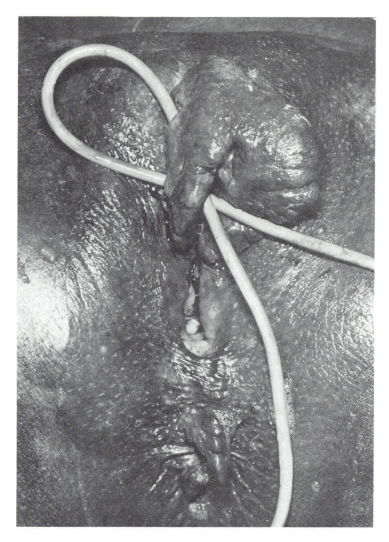

Figure 29.4 Fenestration of vulva in lymphogranuloma venereum.

this time, in about a quarter of cases, rectal symptoms occur. There is first bleeding and discharge and later perirectal cellulitis, leading to stricture formation and rectovaginal fistulae. Elephantiasis of the vulva may follow the lymphatic fibrosis (Figures 29.5 and 29.6), and prolapse may be a sequel to the straining necessary to overcome the rectal stricture. Vigorous dilatation of the anal stricture may cause a fissure, and the resulting inflammation may lead to complete bowel obstruction.

Diagnosis may be complemented by biopsy, although the tissue changes tend to be nonspecific, mainly caused by gross secondary infection (Haines and Taylor, 1962). The Frei cutaneous hypersensitivity test is of little use and, once positive, remains so for many years if not for life. Unfortunately, the complement fixation test is not specific enough to be of much assistance.

Treatment is with a 10-day course of tetracycline that may have to be repeated, but early lesions respond to sulfamethazine (sulphadimidine).

Schistosomiasis (bilharziasis)

Rivers, lakes, and canals in both the tropics and subtropics are common sources of *Schistosoma* organisms and the freshwater snails that act as intermediate hosts to these dioecious trematodes.

Of the three varieties, *S. haematobium, S. mansoni,* and *S. japonicum,* it is *S. haematobium* with its terminally spined ova that gives the most trouble in the female urinary system. Entry to the body is usually through the skin and less commonly the mouth; spread to bladder, ureters, and rectum is by the bloodstream.

After an initial hyperemia, infiltration by round cells and fibroblasts takes place, and granulations

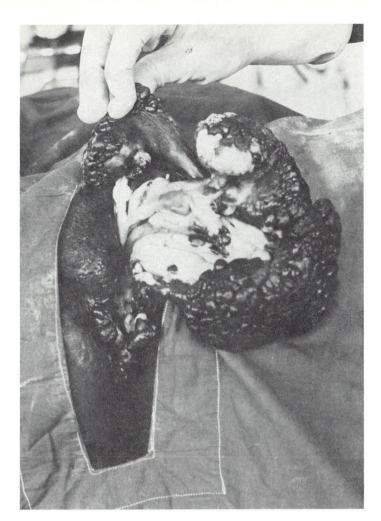

Figure 29.5 Elephantiasis of vulva in lymphogranuloma venereum.

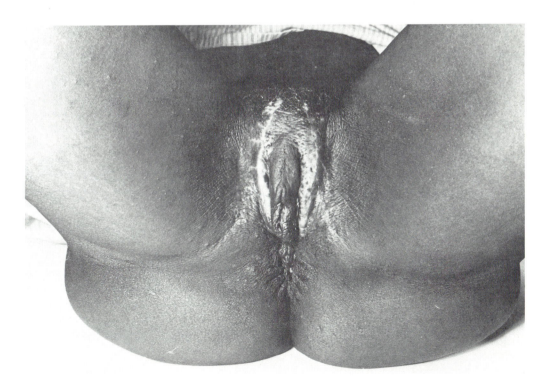

Figure 29.6 The same patient (Figure 29.5) after local vulvectomy.

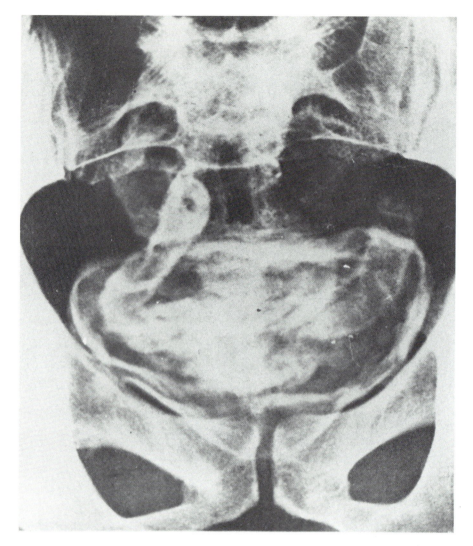

Figure 29.7 Calcification in bladder caused by schistosomiasis. (From Wallace, D.M. 1979, Ann. R. Coll. Surg. Engl. **61**:265-270.)

form. A toxin produced by live ova results in an obliterative endarteritis, and sloughing follows. Lesions in the bladder and the urethra frequently cause dense fibrosis, with calcification in long-standing cases and with great reduction of bladder capacity and scarring of the vulva and urethra. Recurrent infection is frequent and carcinoma of the bladder not uncommon. Vesicovaginal fistulae do not occur.

Diagnosis may be made by the indentification of ova from urine, feces, vaginal discharge, tissue scraping, or biopsy. Cystoscopy may show a variety of changes in the bladder mucosa ranging from hyperemia through granulation to papillomata, which may slough and ulcerate. The papillo-

mata may occasionally be seen occurring at the urethral orifice. Even if ova cannot be found in the urine after repeated examination, flat, sandy patches may be seen long afterward in the bladder. Calcification may sometimes be seen on radiographs of the lower segment of the ureter and the bladder (Figure 29.7).

Patients are often in poor general health, and this must be dealt with before the admittedly toxic drugs necessary for treatment are given. Two main groups of drugs are given, the organic trivalent antimonials parenterally and the thioxanthones orally. Intravenous antimony sodium tartrate is the established therapy, 1.5 g given in divided doses over alternate days and interrupted if side effects supervene. Other more complex antimonial compounds are available that are less toxic but more expensive.

Several countries have attempted to screen and treat the vulnerable members of their community.

Bladder calculi

Bladder calculi, or nephrolithiasis, are common in India and Africa, and some attempts have been made to determine frequency rates, but for most diseases there are few statistics dealing with the extent of the problem they present to the women who are exposed. Although calculi are considered primary in children, in adults they are usually caused by an obstructive lesion in the lower urinary tract or by a lesion leading to the accumulation of residual urine. These lesions may be found, for example, to be associated with the urethral scarring associated with vulval disease and with fistulae and are probably caused by a combination of urinary stasis and infection.

Amebiasis

Amebiasis (caused by *Entamoeba histolytica*) may occasionally cause cervical vaginal ulceration, and rectal fistula may occur. The diagnosis may sometimes be made by exfoliative vaginal cytology.

Lesions in the bladder are rare. Treatment is a combination of a tissue amebicide (metronidazole, niridazole) followed by a luminal amebicide (halogenated hydroxyquinolines, tetracycline).

Elephantiasis

Elephantiasis, with attendant difficulties of micturition and occasionally with accompanying squamous carcinoma of the vulva, will occasionally be seen by the gynecological urologist.

Acquired elephantiasis of the vulva is the end result of recurrent lymphangitis. Although *Wuchereria bancrofti* and *Brugia malayi* are probably the most common causes in the tropics (Figure 29.8), other important agents include tuberculosis (Figure 29.9), chronic pyogenic infection, malignant infiltration of regional malignant nodes, and granuloma inguinale and venereum. The retention of fluid with a high protein content stimulates the production of fibrous tissue, and the edema is of a solid nonpitting character. In the absence of malignant change, local vulvectomy is all that is required.

Urinary fistulae

Urinary fistulae occur from a variety of causes, which include obstetrical factors, local tradition, operative causes, malignancy, radiotherapy, and lymphogranuloma venereum.

Urinary fistulae associated with irregular obstetrical procedures are discussed in the section "Obstetrics."

Radiotherapy is available in all continents, although many patients in the developing world will be still denied access for years to come. Even where available, however, cases referred will tend to be those of advanced malignancy. The success rate will therefore tend to be low, and the incidence of fistulae following radiotherapy for, for example, carcinoma of the cervix, will be high.

Gynecological surgery will occasionally have to be carried out by practitioners who have little operative skill or experience. In 1980 the *Journal of Obstetrics and Gynaecology* of India (Gupta and Van Shylla) published a case that illustrates this point. A total hysterectomy for uncomplicated uterine fibromyomata was described, in the course of which both ureters were transected and two large transverse lacerations were made in the bladder, which later failed to heal.

Urethral destruction

The most difficult problems that face the gynecological urologist in the tropics include treatment of the patient who has urethral destruction to a greater or lesser extent (Figure 29.10).

Avulsion can take place during childbirth, leaving a normal urethra, usually closed at the proximal end, which may be fairly easy to reunite with the bladder, although continence may be impaired.

Lymphogranuloma, on the other hand, may in its later stages cause a smooth anterior vaginal wall leading to the internal urethral opening with no trace whatever of the original urethra, or there may be degrees of tissue loss with profound fibrosis. The creation of a new urethra will be thwarted by the aforementioned tissue destruction and the avascular nature of the remaining epithelium. In these cases it may be more beneficial to go to the bladder for neourethral tissue.

In all patients it is necessary to ensure that active disease has been adequately treated and that the patient's general condition will support the necessary surgery.

It is necessary that medical assistants be aware that a few hours' retention of urine may destroy

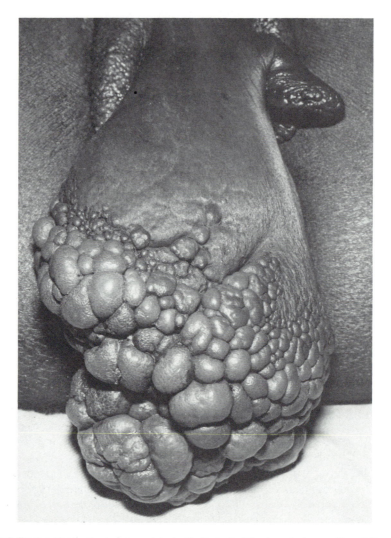

Figure 29.8 Elephantiasis of vulva associated with filariasis (*Wuchereria bancrofti* and *Brugia malayi*).

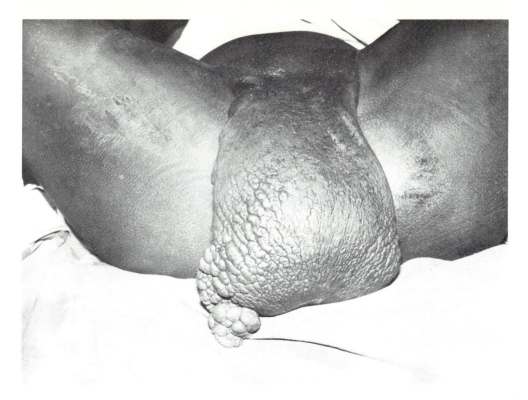

Figure 29.9 Elephantiasis of vulva associated with tuberculosis.

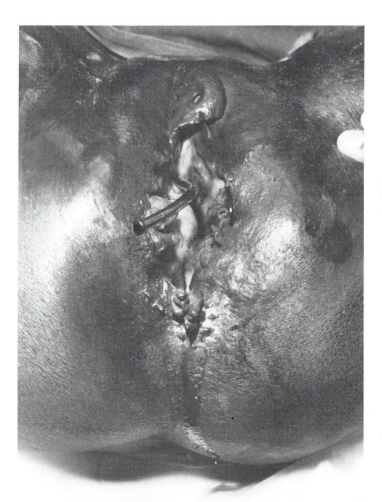

Figure 29.10 Urethral destruction associated with lymphogranuloma venereum.

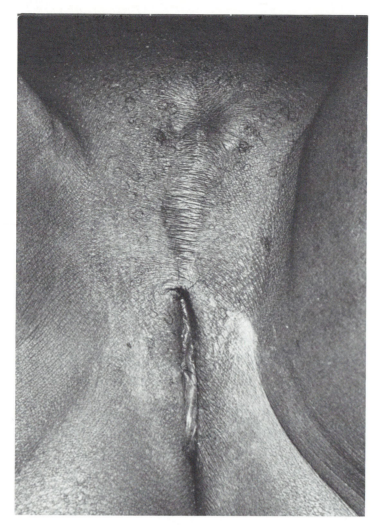

Figure 29.11 Long-term results of infantile circumcision in adult female.

what may well be the only chance of successful repair. The first attempt is always the most hopeful. The safest way to supervise the postoperative care is to insist on an hourly written record of successful urinary drainage over the full 24 hours.

Female circumcision

Female circumcision is still common in parts of Africa, and Aziz (1980), writing from Khartoum, has stated that the majority of Sudanese girls are circumcised before the age of 6 years, and that, although the procedure is multilating and sometimes results in death, it is practiced at the same rate as in the past (Figure 29.11).

Although the extent of the operation varies, the majority of patients in the Sudan had a full, or Pharaonic, circumcision, which removes the labia minora, the mons veneris, and sometimes the clitoris, usually with a sharp knife and, in the rural areas, without anesthesia. Immediate complications are hemorrhage, shock, and infection, and it is sometimes fatal. Later, there may be urinary retention, keloid formation, infertility, and marital difficulty. If pregnancy occurs, incision of the scar is often necessary before delivery can take place. The incision is then stitched again and the process repeated for each subsequent delivery.

THE FUTURE

Throughout the world, the more florid aspects of genitourinary diseases in women are seen less frequently than in the past. However, improvements in obstetrical care with a corresponding decrease in the incidence of maternal damage are taking longer to occur. Further progress will depend both on women's assumption of more responsible places in the family councils, the community, and the nation and the availability of a basic maternal and child health service, however inadequate, to replace the present care, which is available to only a fortunate few.

REFERENCES

Aziz, F.A. 1980. Gynaecologic and obstetric complications of female circumcision. Int. J. Gynaecol. Obstet. **17**(6):560-563.

Chakravarty, B.N., and Chowdhury, N. 1980. Urinary tract infection in parous women. J. Obstet. Gynaecol. **1**:140-145.

Gebbie, D.A.M. 1979. Maternity services in the developing world. Proceedings of the seventh study group of the Royal College of Obstetricians and Gynaecologists. London.

Greenhill, J.P. 1951. Principles and practice of obstetrics. Philadelphia. W.B. Saunders Co.

Gupta, H.D., and Van Shylla, S. 1980. Multiple urinary tract injuries during abdominal hysterectomy: a case report. J. Obstet. Gynaecol. **30**:825-826.

Haines, M., and Taylor, C.W. 1962. Gynaecological pathology. London. J. & A. Churchill Ltd.

Harrison, K.A. 1979. Maternity services in the developing world. Proceedings of the seventh study group of the Royal College of Obstetricians and Gynaecologists. London.

Pal, M.N. 1980. Urinary incontinence in bynecological urology. J. Obstet. Gynecol. **6**:77-78.

Trussell, R.R. 1962. Management of the dead baby. Clin. Obstet. Gynecol. **5**:1076-1088.

Psychiatric aspects

KINGSLEY R.W. NORTON

Patients seen at a gynecological urology clinic may have psychiatric as well as urological symptoms. Psychiatrists, urologists, and gynecologists in general know little about the others' specialities. The result is that little is known about areas of potential mutual interest. The aims of this chapter are to sketch in some of what is already known while highlighting areas of ignorance and to provide the reader with a psychiatric viewpoint from which it is hoped improved patient management will follow. The final section considers management and the allied question of who should manage the individual patient.

Only the psychiatric symptoms that are most commonly seen in nonhospitalized populations will be discussed in depth. No detailed accounts will be given of the symptoms of frank psychoses, such as hallucinations, delusions, and disorders of motility, or of some of the rarer neurotic symptoms (for example, obsessive-compulsive disorder). There are three reasons for this. In nonpsychiatric hospital outpatient clinics these symptoms are rarely encountered. When present, they are often though not always very obvious. They often require management in their own right largely irrespective of the urological needs. As will be seen, however, any psychiatric and any urological symptom may coexist in a patient, and management ultimately is an individual matter based on an appraisal of both physical and psychological factors.

PHYSICAL OR PSYCHOLOGICAL SYMPTOMS

There is usually agreement about whether a given symptom is physical or psychological. Sometimes, however, there may be difficulty in assigning the symptom to one or the other type. The categorization often reflects the clinician's personal conceptualization of the case and/or his or her views on the cause of the symptoms. To this extent, to contend that a given symptom is either physical or psychological is arbitrary.

A conceptual model of a hypothetical physical illness is represented diagrammatically in Figure 30.1. It emphasizes not only the presence of psychological and physiological aspects but also their continuous interaction throughout the entire length of the illness. A simple example will illustrate this point.

A woman complains to her family physician that she is going to the lavatory to pass urine more frequently than usual. She describes no other symptoms.

She has communicated information about two basic aspects of herself. First, there has been the observation of change in her usual habit. Second, she has indicated by visiting the physician that she has had some distress, which motivated her to seek help or advice. Her symptom has both physical and psychological components. The physician's knowledge of her circumstances (for example, her forthcoming marriage or final examination), of her as a person (for example, she may be rather a nervous individual), and of any relevant medical history (for example, diabetes mellitus) enables him to conceptualize her individual case and to label the symptom as predominantly physical or psychological.

Perhaps this example need not have been given. It does exemplify, however, the fact that as clinicians we acknowledge psychological distress tacitly when it is entirely appropriate, in our view, with the severity of the disorder that has been observed or reported. It is only when we perceive the distress as being inappropriately great that it acquires a distinct label.

It is unfortunate that once the inappropriateness is noted, it is often immediately afforded etiological status: the physical symptom is said to have been caused by the psychological symptom. This supposition is frequently erroneous and betrays an overly simplistic view of illness in general and of symptom production in particular. Symptom A may have precipitated symptom B, but the opposite may equally well be the case, and a third factor, C, may underlie both symptoms A and B.

In conclusion the appropriate distress that accompanies a complaint of increased urinary frequency or any other urological symptom is rightly called psychological as opposed to psychiatric. In the vast majority of cases management aimed at the urological problem, when it is successful, effects cure in both the soma and the psyche. No special management is required in these instances for the psychological aspects.

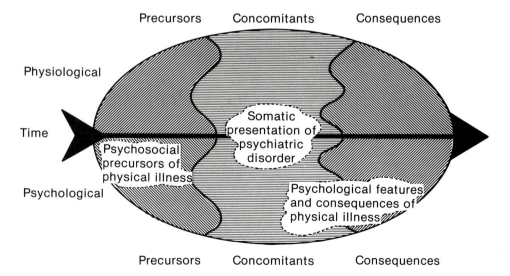

Figure 30.1 Schematic representation of interrelationship of physiological and psychological factors throughout course of hypothetical illness. (Modified and reproduced with permission from Conolly, J. 1979. Psychiatry in a general hospital. In Hill, P., Murray, R., and Thorley, A., editors. Essentials of postgraduate psychiatry. London Academic Press, Inc., Ltd. Copyright: Academic Press, Inc. Ltd. (London), Ltd.)

PSYCHOLOGICAL OR PSYCHIATRIC SYMPTOMS

Anxiety and *depression* are words that denote emotions with which everybody is familiar. When they are used in a psychiatric context, however, they refer specifically to increased frequency or intensity of the emotion and/or to its inappropriateness to the events in the patient's inner or outer worlds. Characteristically the anxious or depressed patient's state of mind or mood no longer closely mirrors what happens to her in terms of her relationships with her family and friends or with other events (internal as well as external) in her life, and her mood therefore has what can be described as an autonomy of its own. The distinction proposed between the use of the terms *psychological* and *psychiatric* therefore hinges on the notion of severity with regard to the frequency and/or intensity of the emotion as well as its degree of appropriateness to the patient's circumstances.

SEVERITY OF PSYCHIATRIC SYMPTOMS

To assess the severity of these psychiatric symptoms, it is important to know how frequently they are experienced, how intense they are, and how appropriate or understandable they appear to be in the light of the patient's experiences (including her urological problems). *Frequency* is easily evaluated. *Intensity* is a more difficult matter. One guide to this is the occurrence of changes in the patient's physical and/or social functioning. These changes, when a result of the psychiatric symptom, may be used as indices of severity (Figure 30.2). The more of these features there are, the greater the severity of the anxiety or depressive syndrome.

The fact that a certain intensity of anxiety or depression is inappropriate (for example, in response to a urological disorder) enables the clinician to identify pathological levels of anxiety and depression. In this sense, the concept of appropri-

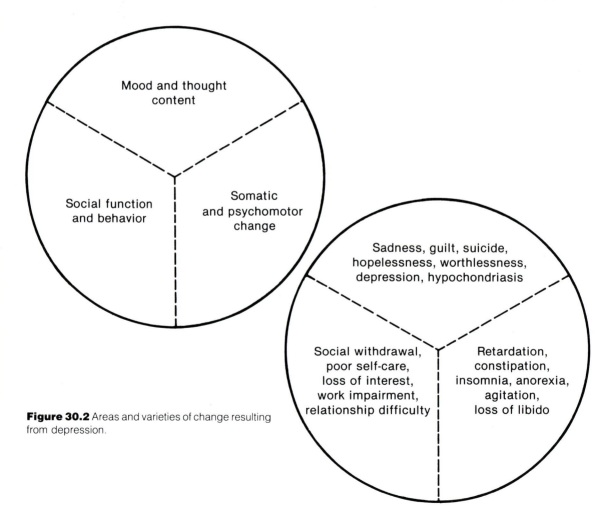

Figure 30.2 Areas and varieties of change resulting from depression.

ateness or understandability of the psychiatric symptom is a useful one and not only facilitates an assessment of the severity of the symptoms but also provides a guide to the need for treatment. Thus the disparity that is perceived on the basis of the clinician's experience as to how people feel and react to given levels of physical disease is useful.

The concept, however, is not useful in the following situation. High levels of anxiety or depression may accompany serious urological disease. The fact that such a psychological response is understandable, appropriate, or even characteristic (of such patients as a group) cannot be taken on its own as a guide to response to treatment and to treatability. Many such patients have treatable psychiatric conditions in addition to their (perhaps) untreatable urological disorders. In such a situation, history taking must involve questions about physical and social functioning if a complete picture is to be obtained and if treatable psychiatric symptoms are not to be missed.

Evaluation of the need for psychiatric treatment is thus based on the severity of the anxiety or depression in terms of its frequency, intensity, and appropriateness and also on the presence of secondary physical and social impairment.

CASUAL OR CAUSAL RELATIONSHIPS

When two symptoms or two medical conditions are common in a population, as are urological and psychiatric symptoms, there will always be an unfortunate few who by chance exhibit both types of symptoms. Within this group it would be folly to say that the psychiatric symptom caused, promoted, or precipitated the urological one, or vice versa. When such a patient is seen at an outpatient clinic, however, it is often unclear as to whether or not she comes from this group. It is also likely that with the passage of time and with the complexity of human existence, there has indeed been an interplay between the different symptoms, so that each has in fact affected the expression of the other. The same level of incontinence may be described as greater, for instance, when the patient copes less well with it because of her depression, which may have been worsened by the incontinence.

In other patients it is much clearer that one set of symptoms owes its existence, in part at least, to another set. There is, of course, again an interplay. It can be said of clinical practice that often

there is an association between psychiatric and urological symptoms, but it must be added that the nature of the association is unknown. The reason for this is that the basic scientific work has not been done to test even the hypothesis that urological and psychiatric conditions occur together with greater frequency than would be expected by chance.

UROLOGICAL SYMPTOMS ASSOCIATED WITH PSYCHOLOGICAL AND PSYCHIATRIC STATES

Common urological symptoms will now be described as they appear, according to the literature, to have associations with psychological and psychiatric states. After this, mention will be made of possible ways in which an undiagnosed psychiatric condition may be manifested by a urological symptom representing an integral part of the psychiatric disturbance. Necessarily, these two groups of symptoms will be discussed separately, but the continuing interplay between them in the individual patient must be borne in mind throughout.

Frequency

Most readers will have experienced increased urinary frequency at times of stress, such as during a visit to the dentist or on the morning of final examination. It is a common concomitant symptom of anxiety. Its severity in terms of objective change and also in terms of the amount of distress caused by it is subject to great individual variation.

Straub, Ripley, and Wolf (1949) elegantly demonstrated that there were two differing populations of people with respect to their bladder function as measured by simple cystometry. They found that talking to a mixed group of urological patients about topics known to be painful emotionally as the patients were simultaneously undergoing cystometry yielded one population whose bladders were hypermotile and another whose bladders were hypomotile. Psychological testing demonstrated that these two populations also differed in terms of their personalities.

Gynecologists (Smith, 1962; Zufall, 1963) working with patients who have the urethral syndrome, which includes urinary frequency as well as other variably present symptoms, have often concluded, usually on the basis of negative physical findings, that many cases are functional in origin. The evidence is anecdotal and clearly deserves further evaluation.

Psychoanalysts (Menninger, 1941; Yazmajian, 1966) have described abnormalities of micturition in their patients undergoing analysis. In some urinary frequency has been seen as symbolically expressing emotions such as anger or sadness. In the course of their analyses the patients, on becoming upset, would visit the lavatory instead of expressing their anger or sadness. Hypotheses concerning the psychological meaning of micturition are difficult to test. Meaning is highly personal, and such individual variation is often lost when large groups of individuals are studied.

Incontinence

Urinary incontinence is a symptom of many medical conditions. In cases of stress incontinence, the cause appears to be entirely local and, for example, repair of a genital prolapse may cure the symptom of incontinence. In other cases of incontinence, however, there may be no local pathological condition to account for the symptom, such as in patients with various neurological disorders (for example, multiple sclerosis). Many of these patients, as well as many of those who have no gross demonstrable neurological deficit, have an abnormality of bladder function—bladder instability—that shows up on investigation. In a population of patients with bladder instability, some 50% to 80% have no physical cause, and this negative finding, coupled with a history of emotional trauma antedating the onset of the symptom, has led some to the conclusion that the cause of incontinence associated with bladder instability is functional (Green, 1975). This view of causation is shared by others (Jeffcoate and Francis, 1966; Frewen, 1972). Additional evidence that they provide for this assertion stems from a high success rate in treating these patients using a psychomedical approach. This, broadly speaking, means that both physical and psychological aspects of the patient are acknowledged in an intensive inpatient treatment package. Unfortunately, scientific objectivity is again lacking, so that proper evaluation of the role played by psychological factors does not take place. The evidence that incontinence associated with bladder instability is caused by psychological factors has not been demonstrated.

One of the few studies in which there has been close collaboration between urologists and psychiatrists revealed that of 18 women with bladder instability for whom conventional treatment had failed, all 18 had severe situational problems, 17 had chronic depression, and 10 had hysterical personality traits. These patients were all offered psychiatric treatment, and in those who improved psychiatrically there was concomitant relief of urinary incontinence (Stone and Judd, 1978). The findings are striking in terms of the high psychiatric morbidity, although it is not known how typical a population this was, and there are many methodological criticisms that can be made (for example, the lack of a control group and the nonrandom selection of patients).

A group of women has been described in whom incontinence is a conscious, willful act (Green, 1975). This is probably an extreme minority of incontinent women, and they almost undoubtedly have severe personality problems.

Retention

Retention is a rare symptom in women. It is of great interest, since in a surprisingly high proportion of cases marked psychiatric disorder is seen. In one study of 37 women, 8 were found to be psychotic and there were 12 in whom the symptom was seen to be a conversion symptom as part of a hysterical neurosis (Larson et al., 1963). Such high incidences of clear psychiatric morbidity cannot be ignored, although, again, biased population sampling might falsely elevate the figures. In addition, it should be noted that the severity of the psychiatric disorder present in these patients is not closely related to the severity of the urological symptom (Barrett, 1976).

Psychoanalysts have successfully treated some of these patients (those at the neurotic end of the spectrum of disorder), and in them the symbolic meaning of the symptom centers on the control of emotions that are perceived by the patients as being dangerous (for example, angry or sexual impulses). Catheterization, it is claimed, can come to be an important avenue of eroticization, and there can be much secondary gain from the symptom through the manipulation of friends and relatives by the patient (Wahl and Golden, 1963). There is an undeniable association between psychiatric and urological morbidity, which is deserving of further study.

PSYCHIATRIC DISORDERS WITH UROLOGICAL SYMPTOMS

In theory, any psychiatric disorder may be manifested by any urological symptom. In practice, few do so. Those that most commonly do so are dis-

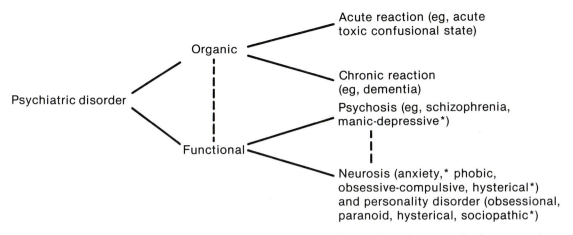

Figure 30.3 Classification of psychiatric disorders. Interrupted lines indicate that separation into groups is not always clear-cut. Asterisk indicates psychiatric disorder manifested by urological symptom.

cussed below and are marked with an asterisk in Figure 30.3.

Psychiatric disorders are divided broadly into two main groups: *organic,* where a physical lesion is known to exist and thought to account for the disorder, and *functional,* where no such lesion is known. The separation, however, is simplistic, and the disorders probably exist along a continuum, physical factors being extremely important at the organic end and psychological factors equally so at the functional end.

Anxiety neurosis

Since anxiety is a normal and universal emotion essential for human life, pathological anxiety can be defined only in relative terms. Thus complaints of anxiety are made only when it is experienced as more intense, more frequent, or more persistent than the patient is used to or can tolerate, or if it is inappropriate to her experiences. Its symptoms include weakness, dizziness, malaise, irritability, dread, panic, palpitations, dyspnea, chest pain, paresthesia, headache, tremor, sweating, flushes, dry mouth, and urinary frequency.

One study of women attending an outpatient department for problems of *recurrent cystitis,* a term that included a mixture of syndromes, found that the subjects had significantly higher numbers of psychiatric symptoms, especially anxiety, than the general population (Rees and Farhoumand, 1977).

This is not to say that the anxiety was the primary diagnosis and that the urological condition was secondary, but it is conceivable that in a number of the patients the psychiatric disorder antedated the urological symptom present. The reason for the presentation of the urological symptom may be more conscious or less conscious. Fear of stigma may be more conscious or less conscious. Fear of stigma or shame associated with psychiatric referral may prevent a patient from complaining of a psychiatric disorder but allow her to admit to a somatic one. On the other hand, she may be unaware that her urinary frequency is in part a reflection of her mental state, and she may then be caught up in a vicious circle of increased anxiety worsening the "symptom," which then causes her to become more anxious still.

Phobic neurosis

Phobic neurotic disorders typically show that the sufferer experiences pathological anxiety in specific situations only and that this usually leads to avoidance of those situations. In the literature there is an account of successful treatment of a patient who experienced urinary retention associated with the phobia of urination in public lavatories (Lamontagne and Marks, 1973). However, urological presentations of phobic disorders are probably extremely rare.

Hysterical neurosis

Hysteria is a term that has been much abused in its application to multitudes of patients who as a group have had little in common, so that its meaning is difficult if not impossible to ascertain in many instances. The label is still used, however, and here it is reserved for a neurotic disorder in which one or both of two characteristic groups of symptoms may be seen. Symptoms may be of the dissociative type, of which hysterical amnesia, hysterical fugue, and multiple personality are representative, or they may be of the conversion type, where classically neurological symptoms (but here mainly urinary retention) express symbolically unbearable unconscious emotional conflict. Anxiety provoked by the conflict threatens to overwhelm the individual's peace of mind, and this is prevented from happening (according to psychological theory) by the unconscious operation of dissociation as a mechanism of defense against the threatened disturbance. The anxiety, then, is not experienced consciously (this is called the primary gain), but the somatic symptom is the price that is paid for this emotional calm. Urinary retention is the urological symptom most often associated with hysterical neurosis. However, any other urological symptom may be associated with it.

A discussion of hysteria often leads to consideration of malingering. This is natural, since in both conversion hysteria and malingering there are complaints of symptoms for which no objective (organic) evidence can be found. The fundamental difference between these two groups of patients lies in the extent to which the person is conscious of this "deceit." In the classical case the hysterical neurotic is totally unaware that the symptom is a product of her mind, whereas the malingerer has deliberately fabricated the symptom (for example, a case of factitious urinary tract infection, hematuria, or renal calculi) (Atkinson and Earll, 1974).

The situation is often difficult to evaluate clinically. Neither hysterical patients nor malingerers may be entirely unconscious or conscious, respectively, of their motivation. There can be much emotional gain (secondary gain) from becoming sick (for example, privileged status in the family or time off from work or school). Even in those who consciously produce a physical symptom, this may be because of unwillingness or inability to seek help for real psychological distress. It is appropriate therefore that a medical rather than a legal framework take responsibility for such cases (Blackwell, 1968).

Depression

Depression (for example, following bereavement) is part of a normal human reaction to loss. It is experienced as a transient change in mood accompanying unhappy or stressful events in life. Where it becomes persistent or autonomous and no longer reflects these changes, a patient has a depressive illness. Usually there are, in addition to a lowered mood, changes in her sleep pattern (usually insomnia), appetite (usually anorexia), and libido (usually diminished). There may also be impairment of concentration and memory. Characteristically the patient feels worse first thing in the morning. She feels worthless, hopeless, helpless, and perhaps inappropriately guilty. She may become increasingly introspective, and often this focuses on her body and its functioning, which she feels has become abnormal. Hypochondriacal worries are common in depressive illness, and it is possible for urological symptoms to dominate the clinical picture. When the depression is particularly severe, the patient may believe against all contrary evidence that she has a physical illness.

Sometimes, of course, patients do have a physical disorder (for example, urinary incontinence) that has been in existence for some time and that they seek treatment for only when they fail to cope with it because of the depression. This in turn may have been precipitated by the physical symptom. The interplay of the psyche affecting the soma and vice versa is therefore very important. The patient might equally well, of course, have a third condition, such as a carcinoma, that accounts for both the depression and the urological symptom. In some cases the stigma of psychiatric illness may foster the patient's seeking treatment for the physical symptom. In other cases the physical symptom may in fact be the most troublesome to the patient, who may not recognize in herself what a clinician would call depression (Paykel and Norton, 1981).

One study of patients attending an outpatient urology clinic found that depression was associated with lower urinary tract disease but not with upper urinary tract disease (Dunlop, 1979).

It is very rare for the remaining functional psychiatric disorders to be manifested by urological symptoms. A urological disorder may, of course, be present, but this is seldom prominent, and with the following exceptions the psychiatric disorder dominates the picture. The schizophrenic patient may describe delusional beliefs regarding any part of the urinary tract; similarly she may experience somatic hallucinations (sensations perceived in the absence of external stimuli) in any part of her body, and the vulval area is not exempt from this.

Organic psychiatric syndromes

The other important disorders associated with urological symptoms are the organic psychoses. It is rare, however, for them to be manifested by a urological symptom. In the elderly any infection (for example, urinary tract infection) may precipitate an acute confusional episode, as may acute urinary retention from whatever cause. Usually the psychological symptoms and behavioral changes dominate the picture, but it is conceivable that urinary symptoms could do so. Often in this kind of situation the patient is then passed off as being ''demented,'' and the true diagnosis is not arrived at until the confusional state is reversed with the appropriate treatment.

Incontinence is a feature of advanced dementia, and if present early on in the course of this disorder, it should alert the clinician to investigate the cause of the incontinence, which is seldom caused by the brain failure itself. The only exception to this rule is in cases of normal-pressure hydrocephalus (where the patient also appears demented), when incontinence is an early symptom although not usually one that is complained of by the patient. This condition is rare but often treatable.

GUIDELINES FOR THE MANAGEMENT OF PATIENTS WITH SUSPECTED PSYCHIATRIC DISORDERS
General considerations

There are three main clinical situations in which a gynecologist may suspect a psychiatric disorder. The first is the direct observation of psychiatric symptoms. The second concerns patients whose physical symptoms persist when there is no adequate physical cause to account for them. The third concerns those patients who, according to somatic symptomatology and investigative findings, have been expected to have been helped or cured by the prescribed treatments and who have not been (Norton, 1981).

Once the suspicion of a psychiatric disorder has been raised, it is necessary to confirm or refute it. This involves gathering more historical information from the patient, especially concerning her psychosocial functioning.

The type of information needed about the patient includes simple facts about, for example, time off from work, unemployment, financial problems, marital or sexual problems, problem children, and problem parents. Short, sympathetic questions such as ''Are there any problems in the marriage?'' or later, ''Is the physical side of the relationship all right between the two of you?'' seldom offend. These inquiries can lead into direct questions about how the patient feels in her mood: ''How have

your spirits been recently?'' If there is a disturbance of mood (anxiety or depression), then it is important to find out if the areas of physical and social functioning have also been impaired. As discussed earlier, these factors provide a guide to determining both the severity of the psychiatric disorder and which type of treatment is indicated. In terms of depression, it may also be necessary to ask questions about suicidal intention. Physicians' fears about ''putting the idea into her head'' are groundless. Poor fluid or food intake and strong suicidal ideation are indicators that urgent psychiatric treatment should be sought.

In all three of these clinical situations, after psychiatric symptoms have been detected, it is appropriate to discuss with the patient both the fact of the suspected psychiatric disorder and what the approaches are to its treatment. A referral at this stage to a psychiatrist who might see the patient only on one occasion is desirable, assuming, of course, that the patient is agreeable to this course of action and that there is no more pressing need for psychiatric treatment, which might then have to be carried out against the patient's will (compulsory hospital admission).

After this step, however, management is necessarily an individual matter and must be dictated by the details of the particular clinical picture. It is important therefore to evaluate, for example, which symptom might be seen as primary and which as secondary and whether the urological or the psychiatric symptom is causing more distress. It is usually possible to get a fairly clear impression of this. As a guideline, if urological symptoms persist despite initial treatment by the gynecologist or urologist and the psychiatric symptoms are felt by the psychiatrist to be mild, then management (according to the consensus of views in the literature) is best if it is carried out by the primary care physician, namely the gynecological urologist. The approach obviously must contain an understanding of and recognition of the psychological aspect of the patient.

The following discussion concerns treatment of individual urological symptoms.

Frequency

Most authors agree that the gynecologist or urologist should manage patients with complaints of frequency, assuming that there is no major psychiatric disorder. The treatment should be aimed at both psychological and physical aspects, and it is important to explain to the patient how her symptoms were produced and to assure her, when appropriate, that the condition is benign (Smith, 1962; Zufall, 1963; Rees and Farhoumand, 1977; Frewen, 1978; Smith, 1979; Stone, 1980).

Incontinence

Treatment of urinary incontinence thought to be caused by bladder instability should be aimed at both the bladder and the psyche. Biofeedback (Cardozo et al., 1978), bladder discipline (Jeffcoate and Fracis, 1966), and psychomedical treatment (Frewen, 1978) are all claimed to be successful therapeutic approaches. Success is claimed to be a result of the conjunction of education about the condition with a psychologically supportive atmosphere in which the treatment is carried out. Treatment of incontinence from other causes is still conventional, although associated psychiatric symptoms may benefit from psychiatric treatment.

Retention

Because of the severity of the underlying psychopathological condition often seen in women with retention, there is agreement in the literature that a psychiatric consultation is advisable in most if not all cases (Barrett, 1976; Stone 1980). Various forms of psychological techniques (from interpretive psychotherapy to behavioral techniques) have proved successful in the small numbers of cases reported in the literature.

Treatment of the psychiatric symptoms will be undertaken by the psychiatrist or else by the gynecologist or urologist under the psychiatrist's guidance. The most important step is the identification of the psychiatric symptoms, since failure to recognize and correctly treat these will, apart from anything else, result in higher apparent failure rates for conventional urological treatment. This may result from poor patient compliance or from exacerbation of the urological symptoms by psychiatric disorders.

CONCLUSION

There is no substitute for an awareness of the importance of psychological factors in patients seeking treatment for "physical" disorders. A useful adjunct, although not an alternative to such awareness, may be the use of a short questionnaire such as the General Health Questionnaire (Goldberg, 1972), which is a self-administered questionnaire containing 30 questions that the patient

can easily fill in before her outpatient appointment. The originator of this questionnaire states that "a patient's score on the GHQ is in many ways analogous to the ESR in general medicine." A high score (above 4) indicates that there is probably a psychiatric disorder, but the diagnosis is not revealed. The instrument is thus a screening device detecting likely psychiatric patients who should then undergo a diagnostic interview with a psychiatrist as described earlier.

REFERENCES

Atkinson, R.L., and Earll, J.M. 1974. Munchausen syndrome with renal stones. J.A.M.A. **230**(1):89.

Barrett, D.M. 1976. Psychogenic urinary retention in women. Mayo Clin. Proc. **51**:351-356.

Blackwell, B. 1968. The Munchausen syndrome. Br. J. Hosp. Med. **1**:98-102.

Cardozo, L.D., et al. 1978. Idiopathic bladder instability treated by biofeedback. Br. J. Urol. **50**:521-523.

Conolly, J. 1979. Psychiatry in a general hospital. In Hill, P., Murray, R., and Thorley, A., editors. Essentials of postgraduate psychiatry. London. Academic Press Inc., Ltd.

Dunlop, J.L. 1979. Psychiatric aspects of urology. Br. J. Med. Psychol. **134**:436-438.

Frewen, W.K. 1972. Urgency incontinence: review of 100 cases. Br. J. Obstet. Gynaecol. **79**:77-79.

Frewen, W.K. 1978. An objective assessment of the unstable bladder of psychosomatic origin. Br. J. Urol. **50**:246-249.

Goldberg, D. 1972. The assessment of psychiatric illness by questionnaire. Maudsley Monograph. No. 21. Oxford. Oxford University Press.

Green, T.H. 1975. Urinary stress incontinence: differential diagnosis, pathophysiology and management. Am .J. Obstet. Gynecol. **122**:368-400.

Jeffcoate, T.N.A., and Francis, W. 1966. Urgency incontinence in the female. Am. J. Obstet. Gynecol. **94**:604-618.

Lamontagne, Y., and Marks, I.M. 1973. Psychogenic urinary retention: treatment by prolonged exposure. Behav. Res. Ther. **4**:581-585.

Larson, H.W., et al. 1963. Psychogenic urinary retention in women, J.A.M.A. **184**(9):697-700.

Menninger, K.A. 1941. Some observations on the psychological factors in urination and genitourinary affections. Psychoanal. Rev. **28**:117-127.

Norton, K.R.W. 1981. Could it be my nerves? A psychiatric viewpoint. Clin. Obstet. Gynaecol. **8**(1): 133-148.

Paykel, E.S., and Norton, K.R.W. 1981. Masked depression. Br. J. Hosp. Med. (In press.)

Rees, D.L.P., and Farhoumand, N. 1977. Psychiatric aspects of recurrent cystitis in women. Br. J. Urol. **49**:651-658.

Smith, D.R. 1962. Psychosomatic "cystitis." J. Urol. **87**:359-362.

Smith, P.J.B. 1979. The management of the urethral syndrome. Br. J. Hosp. Med. **22**:578-583.

Stone, C.B. 1980. Psychiatric aspects of lower urinary tract dysfunction. In Ostergard, D., editor. Gynecologic urology and urodynamics: theory and practice. Baltimore. The Williams & Wilkins Co.

Stone, C.B., and Judd, G.E. 1978. Psychogenic aspects of urinary incontinence in women. Clin. Obstet. Gynaecol. **21:**807-815.

Straub, L.R., Ripley, H.S., and Wolf, S. 1949. Disturbances of bladder function associated with emotional states. J.A.M.A. **141:**1139-1143.

Wahl, C.W., and Golden, J.S. 1963. Psychogenic urinary retention: report of 6 cases. Psychosom. Med. **25**(6):543-555.

Yazmarjian, R.V. 1966. Pathological urination and weeping. Psychoanal. Q. **35:**40-45.

Zufall, R. 1963. Treatment of the urethral syndrome in women. J.A.M.A. **184**(11):894-895.

chapter 31

Nocturnal enuresis

JOHN R. HINDMARSH

Bladder control is self-learned and normally attained by the age of 4½ years. There are two primary factors necessary for this to occur: first, there must be a mature central nervous system capable of interpreting the afferent input from the bladder and of reacting to it; and second, the bladder must be capable of holding a night's output of urine. Daytime bladder control occurs in the second year of life when postponement of micturition is learned, the process being accelerated by the child's desire to remain dry. By the age of 3, most children are reliably dry by day and usually by night. If a child has not acquired this skill by 4½ years, the attainment of reliable control becomes more difficult. Children beyond this age who are referred to a pediatrician because of incontinence of urine are termed enuretic.

Persistence of enuresis through to adult life is most frequently associated with the diurnal symptoms of frequency, urgency, and urge incontinence. Unfortunately, those patients in whom symptoms do remit are often left with the diurnal symptoms and nocturia. Under stressful stimuli the nocturnal incontinence may recur.

DEFINITION

In medical terminology enuresis has become synonymous with bed-wetting; however, the term fails to distinguish between those who never attained bladder control and those who did but at a later stage reverted back to incontinence. *Primary nocturnal enuresis* is best defined as a reflex act of micturition occurring at night in an individual who has failed to gain bladder control at the normal age in the absence of organic disease (Table 31.1). *Secondary,* or *late-onset, enuresis* refers to loss of control in an individual who formerly had gained control at the normal age. The differentiation is

TABLE 31.1   Classification of enuresis

Type	Duration
Primary with no diurnal symptoms	Lifelong
Primary with diurnal symptoms	Lifelong
Recurrent enuresis	Enuresis persists beyond age 5; control is gained but later lost
Secondary enuresis	Individual attains bladder control at normal age but later becomes enuretic

important, since the pathophysiological processes are probably different.

The use of the term *enuresis* to describe patients in an older age group with nocturnal incontinence as a result of a known disorder causes confusion and should be discouraged.

FACTORS PREVENTING THE GAINING OF BLADDER CONTROL

Enuresis is a symptom of poor nervous system control of bladder function and as such has many causes. There are also many external factors, often interrelated, that delay bladder control. At present there has been no work done to identify the neurophysiological causes of enuresis; however, it is known that the critical period of learning bladder control occurs between 2 and 4½ years of age, when the bladder capacity doubles in size (Mueller, 1960). This is achieved partially by the growth of the bladder and partially by suppression of the infantile reflexes.

For voluntary control to occur, bladder sensation must be intact to convey the impulses to the brain and the brain must be mature enough to respond correctly. The so-called maturational delay of the neural pathways results in a failure of the child to inhibit the infantile voiding reflex. This prevents the child from postponing micturition during the day, so that the functional bladder capacity remains small. *Micturition delay* does not necessarily imply that the rate of myelination of the nerves is slow but is used as a general term for slow learning of bladder control.

Some factors that adversely affect the gaining of bladder control have been identified. Bakwin

(1971) has shown that monozygotic twins are concordant for enuresis twice as frequently as dizygotic twins and has suggested that the frequency in other members of the family is directly related to the closeness of the genetic relationship. It is difficult to separate the environmental factors from the genetic influence, however. A recent study (Essen and Peckham, 1976) found overcrowding, sharing a bedroom, and being children of semiskilled and unskilled workers to be significantly related to the incidence of enuresis. Positive associations have also been found with young mothers, low birth weight, second children, and low IQs (Miller et al., 1974).

Deep sleep has been frequently quoted as being a major factor in the genesis of enuresis, but the evidence is not strong. Recent electroencephalographic studies have suggested that enuretic episodes are primarily related to bladder fullness triggering reflex activity rather than to any specific sleep stage (Kales et al., 1977).

The incidence of obstructive uropathy and enuresis has been claimed to be in the order of 1% to 3% (Forsythe and Redmond, 1974), although some authorities with a urologically based practice have reported a higher incidence.

It has been shown that there is a relationship between emotional disturbance and enuresis at all ages, with this relationship holding more strongly for girls than for boys and for those who have both diurnal and nocturnal incontinence (Rutter, Yule, and Graham, 1973).

The recorded rate of spontaneous remission is approximately 16% per annum (Forsyth and Redmond, 1974), so that by the age of 15 the incidence of nocturnal enuresis is approximately 1% of the population (Figure 31.1). The individuals who do reach adulthood yet remain enuretic have a high incidence of diurnal symptoms and a high incidence of cystometric abnormality, which takes the form of a small-capacity, unstable bladder (Hindmarsh and Byrne, 1980).

PRESENTATION
Nocturnal enuresis

Hospital referrals are unpleasant for all patients but more so for enuretic ones, who are ashamed of their symptoms and who often will not admit to incontinence until specifically asked about it. Teenagers and young adults are best seen on their own, since their parents will not only dominate the answers but inhibit good physician-patient relation-

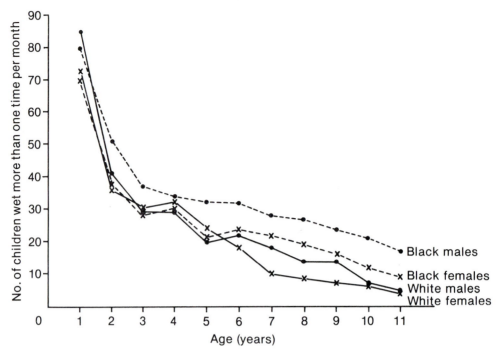

Figure 31.1 Age of attaining bladder control. (From Oppel, W.C., Harper, P.A., and Rider, R.V. 1968. Pediatrics **42**:614. Copyright American Academy of Pediatrics 1968.)

ships. Clearly, pediatric referrals rely on parental answers.

It is important to record whether the enuresis is lifelong or of recent onset. It is valuable to inquire about the longest dry period the patient has experienced. In most cases of primary enuresis the answer will be only 1 to 2 weeks. Other notable answers involve the pattern of enuresis (that is, the days of the week when wetting occurs; the time of night incontinence occurs; whether the incontinence is stable, getting worse, or improving; and if stress situations such as anxiety, tiredness, menstrual periods, or drinking bouts exacerbate the incontinence). The answers will help the physician decide whether or not the patient's enuresis is spontaneously remitting.

Diurnal symptoms

The diurnal symptoms of frequency, urgency, and urge incontinence are present in a high percentage of adults with enuresis. The incidence in childhood is less. It is sometimes difficult to decide on direct questioning whether an individual's frequency and urgency are abnormal; however, if a supplementary question about the effect of imbibing fluids is asked, it will often reveal quite a severe history of urgency. In female patients, urgency can be induced by the sound of running water, anxiety, or, peculiarly, on reaching their own doorstep.

A relationship between frequency and urgency and bladder instability has been demonstrated in enuretic adults (Hindmarsh and Byrne, 1980): in half the women with diurnal symptoms bladder instability could be demonstrated. In the others it is possible that urethral instability was the cause of the symptoms.

The presence of diurnal symptoms adversely affects the patient's chances of gaining reliable nocturnal control. Similarly, the absence of diurnal symptoms is a good prognostic sign.

Associated factors

Urinary stream. The stream is classically short and fast in enuretic patients; thus a history of hesitancy or thin stream should alert the clinician to a urethral disorder. Female patients with large floppy bladders and enuresis void by abdominal strain alone.

Family and social history. There is usually a strong family history of enuresis obtained from patients with primary enuresis; the social background and relationship of the patient to other children in the family will help determine whether a patient has primary or late-onset enuresis.

Factors exacerbating and reducing enuresis. Simply withholding or reducing the factors exacerbating enuresis may improve the patient's incontinence, particularly in those individuals with recurrent enuresis. Tiredness, anxiety, premenstrual tension, and excessive fluid consumption have all been noted to exacerbate incontinence, whereas fluid restriction, staying away from home, and relaxing weekends may be associated with less frequent episodes of incontinence. Pregnancy is not reliably associated with improvement in enuresis.

Neurological symptoms. Careful inquiry into any recent alteration in sensation or weakness of limbs is essential, since enuresis may be an early symptom of multiple sclerosis.

INVESTIGATION

The decision to whether a patient is classified as having primary enuresis or late-onset enuresis will rest with the history alone.

Children with primary nocturnal enuresis do not require detailed investigation, but a careful examination is mandatory. The lower lumbar spine is examined to exclude evidence of spina bifida; the suprapubic area is examined to exclude evidence of a chronically distended bladder; and the external genitalia are examined for abnormality. A midstream sample of urine should always be taken. Cystoscopy is of little value in the female patient.

Teenagers and young adults with enuresis should be fully investigated from age 15 onward. A careful clinical examination of the lower limbs, perianal sensation, anal tone, and bulbocavernosus reflex must be made to exclude neurological dysfunction. The number of enuretic patients who have sensory and/or motor damage of the bladder alone, without other stigmata of neurological disease, is about 3%.

Urinalysis

A routine midstream urine sample urinalysis for pus cells, glucose, and specific gravity is performed to exclude diabetes mellitus and insipidus. In patients with a tendency to nocturnal incontinence, the addition of a urinary tract infection will precipitate nocturnal incontinence.

Radiology

Radiology of the upper urinary tract is unrewarding unless the patient has a proven urinary tract infection.

In children cystography is also of limited value but will identify an abnormality in about 9% of cases, such as ureteric reflux (5%), residual urine, sacculated bladder, or urethral valve (Forsyth and Redmond, 1974). In adults studied by voiding cystography, a thickened bladder wall, prominent bladder neck, and ballooning of the posterior urethra are occasionally noted. Whiteside and Arnold (1975) studied 50 enuretic patients by cystography and deemed them normal; thus the value of voiding cystography in enuresis is doubtful.

Uroflowmetry

A free flow rate with a flowmeter is of great value in all urogynecological clinics. The majority of enuretic patients void with peak flow rates higher than normal; some are supervoiders, passing small volumes at rates above 50 ml/sec. A small number of patients will have evidence of urethral strictures, and others will have evidence of voiding by abdominal strain. The volume voided will usually be smaller than expected.

Urethral pressure measurements

The urethral closure pressure measurements (Brown and Wickham method) are of value in adult enuretic patients, since they will identify the small number of women with congenitally low urethral pressures. Supine closure pressures of less than 30 cm H_2O are incompatible with nocturnal continence. The female closure pressures demonstrate two populations: some with low and others with high values (Hindmarsh, 1980).

Cystometry

Fluid cystometry, either alone or in combination with videocystography, is probably the single most useful investigation of bladder function (see outline below).

Cystometric findings (typical enuretic adult)

I. Filling phase
   A. Normal desire to void
   B. Reduced capacity
   C. Low compliance
   D. "Unstable" bladder
II. Voiding phase
   A. Higher than normal flow rate
   B. Low volume
   C. High detrusor pressure
   D. High isometric pressure

Most studies have shown a high incidence of bladder instability in both children (Ellisan-Nash, 1949; Pompeius, 1970) and adults (Torrens and

Collins, 1975; Whiteside and Arnold, 1975; Hindmarsh and Byrne, 1980). In addition to the simple presence or absence of bladder instability, information is gained about the sensory aspect of bladder filling, residual urine, bladder capacity, and bladder compliance. During the voiding phase the flow rate, detrusor pressure, and isometric pressure can be assessed.

Residual urine is not a feature of enuretic patients. A small percentage (5%) have delay in the sensory end points, but the compliance of the bladder is usually normal in these cases, differentiating them from diabetic patients.

The conscious bladder capacity is found to be lower than normal in most enuretic patients, more so in those with unstable activity. The bladder compliance is similarly reduced.

During the voiding phase only a small number of enuretic patients show evidence of outflow obstruction. However, anxiety may result in failure of adequate pelvic floor relaxation, giving false evidence of obstruction. In enuretic patients the potential power of the detrusor muscle is high as assessed by the isometric pressure rise on the "stop" test midstream (Griffiths, 1973). It has been postulated this is caused by muscular hypertrophy.

Electromyography

In children the results of electromyography of the pelvic floor have demonstrated an irregular relaxation of the pelvic floor musculature during voiding. The significance of these findings is uncertain, and further work is awaited.

Cystoscopy

Cystoscopy should be performed after other investigations have been completed. True urethral stenosis is rare in these patients, but an increase in inflammation of the bladder neck and proximal urethra is more common, the significance being unclear. The bladder capacity has been found to be normal in children when measured at 40 cm H_2O pressure with the patient under anesthesia; in adults, however, the bladder capacity has been found to be reduced at a pressure of 10 cm of H_2O (Hindmarsh, 1980). After bladder filling, the finding of submucosal punctate hemorrhages throughout the bladder is typical, as if the functional bladder capacity has been fixed at a certain volume throughout life and the vessels have never been stretched. Trabeculation of the bladder is a feature of enuretic

patients with proven bladder instability, particularly in men, but it may also occur in women. In a few individuals cystoscopy alone induces remission, but whether this occurs by simple dilatation of the urethra or alteration of the urethral sensitivity is unknown.

TREATMENT (Figure 31.2)
Conservative treatment

Bladder training. The aim of bladder training is to increase the bladder capacity and decrease diurnal frequency with the addition of night control. The rationale is based on the finding that enuretic patients have smaller bladder capacities than normal. The proponents of this form of therapy state that the active participation of the child is essential. The child fills in a star chart, denoting dry versus wet nights, is encouraged to hold onto the urine for longer and longer periods of time, and is encouraged to record voided volumes. In pediatric studies there is conflicting evidence as to the efficacy of this form of management. In a controlled trial Harris and Purohit (1977) were unable to influence the number of episodes of nocturnal incontinence that occurred. In adults Frewen (1980) used similar techniques in women with diurnal symptoms and nocturia. He aimed at voluntary suppression of the abnormal micturition habit rather than directing treatment toward the detrusor itself. To this end he encouraged patients to prolong the period between voids. Nocturia was the first symptom to disappear. The symptomatic results were good, but the objective cystometric evidence was less convincing. Pengelly and Booth (1980) found enuresis persisting after the age of 10 to be associated with a poor result of bladder training.

Behavioral therapy. The aim of behavioral therapy is to awaken the child as he or she urinates, using a detector mechanism or enuretic alarm (Figure 31.3). The effectiveness of this therapy is thought to be related to the increased awareness of afferent input from the bladder. The results obtained rely heavily on the enthusiasm of the physician and adherence to detail concerning the use of the apparatus. After careful explanation by the physician or nurse, weekly visits by the parent and child are necessary to ensure that the device is being used correctly. The major points of importance are that the child must be aroused after each episode and changed, a record must be kept of the number of wet versus dry nights, and the apparatus must be used on consecutive nights. The problems are

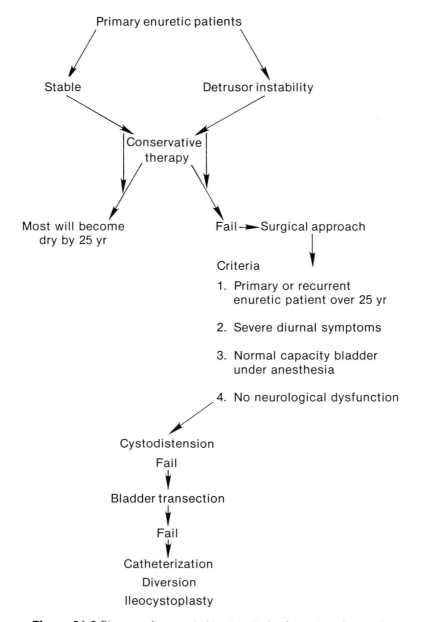

Figure 31.2 Diagram of suggested treatment plan for nocturnal enuresis.

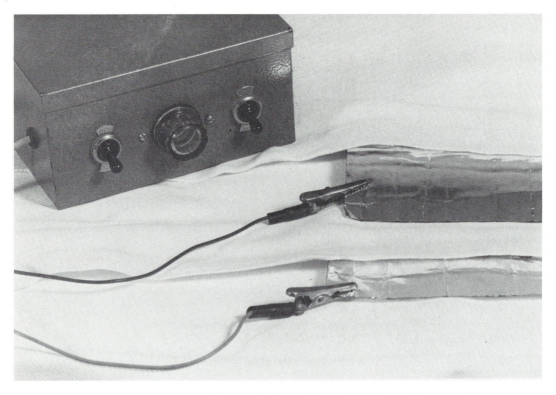

Figure 31.3 Eastleigh automatic enuresis alarm device and foils inserted between sheets.

those of family compliance, difficulty in child arousal, and malfunction or misunderstanding concerning the use of the device.

The overall results are initially good after a 10- to 16-week period, two thirds of the children being dry after completion of the course; however, relapse rates are in the order of 20%. It has been suggested that older children do less well, but a small series of enuretic adults treated by conditioning therapy does suggest an effect.

Psychotherapy. Psychotherapy may be of value in patients with late-onset enuresis, who have a stronger association with emotional and behavioral disturbance than patients with primary enuresis. Its effect, however, is mainly on improving the child's behavior and emotions rather than on reducing the number of episodes of incontinence (Shaffer, 1973). There is no evidence that psychotherapy has a place in the management of adult enuresis.

Pharmacotherapy. There are no drugs capable of ''curing'' an enuretic child at present; however, there are some capable of reducing the time it takes for spontaneous remission to occur (Table 31.2).

Imipramine has been shown to be significantly better than a placebo in a number of trials on chil-

dren. Extensive studies have shown that its effect on enuretic patients occurs within a week, and it probably works by increasing bladder capacity during the first and second parts of the night (Kales et al., 1977). Total remission is restricted to 10% to 20% at 3 months after cessation of therapy. There has been no evidence demonstrating similar effects in enuretic adults, although a recent small study of elderly patients with incontinence has suggested that it is symptomatically effective (Castleden et al., 1981).

Anticholinergic drugs such as propantheline bromide have been singularly unsuccessful when tested against a placebo (Wallace and Forsyth, 1969; Rapaport et al., 1980).

Antispasmodic treatment with flavoxate and oxybutynin has fared little better. It thus appears as if the anticholinergic effect of imipramine is not the operant. Shaffer, Hedge, and Stephenson (1978) used a competitive α-blocking agent, indoramin (Baratol), in enuretic children with negative results. These results led Stephenson (1979) to suggest that the effectiveness of imipramine in enuretic patients was primarily of central nervous system origin.

TABLE 31.2 Controlled trials of drugs used in enuresis

Drugs	Authors	Results
Imipramine	Many studies	Effective in children
Desmopressin	Ramsden et al. (1979)	Effective in adults
Amphetamines	McConaghy (1969)	Ineffective
Ephedrine	G.P. research group (1970)	Ineffective
Propantheline	Wallace and Forsyth (1969)	Ineffective
Scopolamine butylbromide	Korczyn and Kish (1979)	Ineffective
Indoramin	Shaffer, Hedge, and Stephenson (1978)	Ineffective
Phenylpropanolamine	Reece and Ransley (1980)	3 out of 5 children improved

---

Central nervous system stimulants (amphetamines) were popular in the 1960s; however, a double-blind study (McConaghy, 1969) found them to be inferior to imipramine.

The use of the antidiuretic hormone desmopressin (DDAVP) has been advocated over the years in children, although controlled studies are not available. In adults a controlled trial has shown its efficacy in reducing the number of episodes of incontinence (Ramsden et al., 1979). The major value of this drug is in adults who are only occasionally incontinent at night but who wish to be reliably dry when away from home.

All in all, the role of pharmacotherapy in enuresis can at best be regarded as being of symptomatic benefit only and will remain so until the neuropharmacological basis of this condition is elucidated.

Surgical treatment

Surgical treatment for enuresis alone is contraindicated, since remission will occur spontaneously by the age of 25; however, enuretic patients with associated diurnal symptoms resistant to all medical therapy may have symptoms of such severity that their life is miserable, demanding further treatment. It is rare that any one surgeon will see many of these patients in a lifetime; thus a detailed summary follows. The indication for these options are patients beyond the age of 20 who have severe frequency, urgency, nocturia, and incontinence resistant to current medical therapy. Only those with overactive bladders, defined by cystometric instability, should be considered, since the aim of all these modalities of treatment is to reduce the detrusor motor overactivity. Women with diurnal symptoms and a cystometrically stable bladder should not be considered.

Cystodistension. The suggestion was made that bladder instability could be caused by a sensory abnormality in the bladder wall and that bladder distension may mechanically or ischemically damage the submucosal afferent nerve plexus or stretch receptors (Dunn, Smith, and Ardran, 1974). Hydrostatic distension of the bladder with a balloon inflated to systolic blood pressure for 2 hours, with the patient under epidural anesthesia, was advocated by this group. The early results in adults were encouraging: 9 of 12 enuretic patients became completely dry at night. Of 16 children with enuresis treated by a similar method, 4 were symptom free at 1 year (Johnstone, Ardran, and Ramsden, 1977). A full 2-year follow-up showed that all the enuretic patients were dry, although some diurnal symptoms persisted (Smith and Higson, 1980).

In another study of cystodistension, Pengelly et al. (1978) were unable to repeat these findings and reported 13 enuretic patients of whom only 1 was deemed cured.

These differing results may reflect the enthusiasm of the first group, and it is indeed enthusiasm that has been shown to be of such importance in the management of enuresis in children.

Bladder transection. Bladder transection has been advocated for detrusor motor activity with or without enuresis by several authors (Essenhigh and Yeates, 1973; Gibbon et al., 1973). However, despite some experimental work, the mechanism of action of this procedure remains unknown, although either denervation or division of the detrusor muscle must play a significant role.

The indications are failed medical therapy for severe diurnal and nocturnal symptoms in adults. Most patients are initially treated by some form of hydrostatic distension. Better results are obtained in patients over the age of 25 (Hindmarsh, Essenhigh, and Yeates, 1977). The operation is not a minor procedure, but severe complications are rare.

The effect of the operation is to shift the cystometric curve to the right so that patients are able to hold onto their urine for longer periods of time and thus remain dry at night.

The longer term results from two series (Hindmarsh et al., 1977; Parsons, Boyle, and Gibbon, 1977) are similar. In the former series 44 adults with enuresis and diurnal symptoms had bladder transection performed and were followed-up for periods of 6 months to 7 years. Symptomatic relief was produced in 24 patients (16 men and 8 women). There is no evidence that the effect of the operation deteriorated after the 6-month period. In the second series 17 enuretic patients had transections performed, and 11 remained continent after a 3-month to 4-year follow-up. The postoperative cystometric findings revealed a shift to the right in 60% of cases, although cystometric patterns remained similar to those found preoperatively.

A recent report on women with enuresis (Mundy, 1980) showed that all but 3 of 11 cases transected had symptomatic relief for 8 to 25 months.

The evidence suggests that this procedure does have a place in the management of severe enuretic patients with incapacitating diurnal symptoms and should be seriously considered before diversion or ileocystoplasty procedures are performed.

Denervation procedures. Many surgeons have reported a few cases of nerve sections for the control of uninhibited bladder contractions with varying results. It is known that uninhibited contractions can be abolished by caudal anesthesia; thus the activity must be neuronally mediated. Torrens and Griffith (1974) performed selective sacral neurectomy on 17 enuretic patients and demonstrated postoperatively that the cystometrogram was markedly shifted to the right with delay in the sensory end points. The initial results were encouraging, but the long-term results have been less certain (Torrens and Hald, 1979). It appears that rerouting of the nervous channels to the bladder occurs.

Diversion and bladder-enlarging procedures. After failure of cystodistension or bladder transection, the options open are either definitive diversion or an attempt to increase the size of the bladder by cystoplasty using bowel. Sporadic papers on this subject in the past have reported good results; however, it must be said that these are major surgical procedures for a relatively benign condition and should be contemplated only under extreme circumstances.

CONCLUSION

A clear division must be made between enuretic patients with stable bladders and those with unstable bladders, since most drugs and surgical procedures are directly aimed at reducing detrusor motor activity. Only patients with mild symptoms will benefit from intensive bladder drill, a conditioning apparatus, and pharmacotherapy. Those resistant to this therapy who have severe symptoms and bladder instability may respond to cystodistension or bladder transection. It is only under extreme circumstances that diversion or ileocystoplasty should be considered.

Female patients with severe diurnal symptoms and bladder stability on cystometry are presumed to have the so-called unstable urethra, for which the only therapy available at present is intensive bladder training.

REFERENCES

Bakwin, H. 1971. Enuresis in twins. Am. J. Dis. Child. **121**:222-228.

Castleden, C.M., et al. 1981. Imipramine—possible alternative therapy for urinary incontinence in elderly. J. Urol. **125**:318-320.

Dunn, M., Smith, J.C., and Ardran, G.M. 1974. Prolonged bladder distension as a treatment of urgency and urge incontinence of urine. Br. J. Urol. **46**:645-652.

Ellisan-Nash, D.E.F. 1949. The development of micturition control with special reference to enuresis. Ann. R. Coll. Surg. **5**:318-344.

Essen, J., and Peckham, C. 1976. Nocturnal enuresis in childhood. Dev. Med. Child Neurol. **18**:577-589.

Essenhigh, D.M., and Yeates, W.K. 1973. Transection of the bladder with particular reference to enuresis. Br. J. Urol. **45**:299-305.

Forsythe, W.I., and Redmond, A. 1974. Enuresis and spontaneous cure rate. Arch. Dis. Child. **49**:259-263.

Frewen, W.K. 1980. The management of urgency and frequency of micturition. Br. J. Urol. **52**:367-369.

Gibbon, N.O.K., et al. 1973. Transection of the bladder for adult enuresis and allied conditions. Br. J. Urol. **45**:306-309.

G.P. Research Group. 1970. Sedatives and stimulants compared in enuresis. Practitioner **204**:584-586.

Griffiths, D.J. 1973. The mechanics of the urethra and of micturition. Br. J. Urol. **45**:497-507.

Harris, L.S., and Purohit, A.P. 1977. Bladder training and enuresis. Behav. Res. Ther. **15**:485-490.

Hindmarsh, J.R. 1980. Adult enuresis. M.D. thesis, England. Newcastle-upon-Tyne University.

Hindmarsh, J.R., and Byrne, P.O. 1980. Adult enuresis: a symptomatic and urodynamic study. Br. J. Urol. **52**:88-91.

Hindmarsh, J.R., Essenhigh, D., and Yeates, W.H. 1977. Bladder transection for adult enuresis. Br. J. Urol. **6**:515-521.

Johnstone, J.M.S., Ardran, G.M., and Ramsden, P.D. 1977. A preliminary assessment of bladder distension in the treatment of enuretic children. Br. J. Urol. **49**:43-49.

Kales, A., et al. 1977. Effects of imipramine on enuretic frequency and sleep stages. Pediatrics **60:**431-436.

Korczyn, A.D., and Kish, I. 1979. The mechanism of imipramine in nocturnal enuresis. Clin. Exp. Pharmacol. Physiol. **6:**31-35.

McConaghy, N. 1969. A controlled trial of imipramine, amphetamine, pad and bell conditioning and random awakening in the treatment of nocturnal enuresis. Med. J. Aust. **2:**237.

Miller, F.J.W., et al. 1974. The school years in Newcastle on Tyne. Oxford. Oxford University Press.

Mueller, S.R. 1960. Development in urinary control in children. J.A.M.A. **172:**1256-1261.

Mundy, A.R. 1980. Bladder transection for urge incontinence associated with detrusor instability. Br. J. Urol. **52:**480-483.

Parsons, K.F., Boyle, P.J., and Gibbon, N.O.K. 1977. A further assessment of bladder transection in the management of adult enuresis and allied conditions. Br. J. Urol. **49:**509-514.

Pengelly, A.W., and Booth, C.M. 1980. A prospective trial of bladder training as treatment for detrusor instability. Br. J. Urol. **52:**463-466.

Pengelly, A.W., et al. 1978. Results of prolonged bladder distension as treatment for detrusor instability. Br. J. Urol. **50:**243-245.

Pompeius, R. 1971. Cystometry in paediatric enuresis. Scand. J. Urol. Nephrol. **5:**222-228.

Ramsden, P.D., et al. 1979. D.D.A.V.P. for adult enuresis. Proceedings of the ninth International Continence Society meeting. Rome. October 4-6.

Rapaport, J.L., et al. 1980. Childhood enuresis. Arch. Gen. Psychiatry **37:**1146-1152.

Reece, D.L.P., and Ransley, P.G. 1980. Eskornade in the treatment of diurnal incontinence in children. Br. J. Urol. **52:**476-479.

Rutter, M., Yule, W., and Graham, P. 1973. Enuresis and behavioural deviance. In Kolvin, I., et al., editors. Bladder control and enuresis: clinics in developmental medicine. London. William Heinemann Medical Books, Ltd.

Shaffer, D. 1973. The association between enuresis and emotional disorders. In Kolvin, I., et al., editors. Bladder control and enuresis: clinics in developmental medicine. London. William Heinemann Medical Books, Ltd.

Shaffer, D., Hedge, B., and Stephenson, J.D. 1978. Trial of alpha adrenolytic drug (indoramin) for nocturnal enuresis. Dev. Med. Child Neurol. **20:**183-188.

Smith, J.C., and Higson, R.H. 1980. Cystodistension. In Stanton, S.L., and Tanagho, E.A., editors. Surgery of female incontinence. Vienna. Springer-Verlag KG.

Stephenson, J.D. 1979. Physiology and pharmacological basis for the chemotherapy of enuresis. Psychol. Med. **9:**249-263.

Torrens, M.J., and Collins, C.D. 1975. The urodynamic assessment of adult enuresis. Br. J. Urol. **47:**433-440.

Torrens, M.J., and Griffith, H.B. 1974. The control of the uninhibited bladder by selective sacral neurectomy. Br. J. Urol. **46:**639-644.

Torrens, M.J., and Hald, T., 1979. Bladder denervation procedures. Urol. Clin. North Am. **6:**283-293.

Wallace, R., and Forsyth, W.I. 1969. Treatment of enuresis. Br. J. Clin. Pract. **23:**207.

Whiteside, C.G., and Arnold, E.P. 1975. Persistent primary enuresis. I. Urodynamic assessment, Br. Med. J. **1:**364-367.

chapter 32

Sexual problems and urological symptoms

ELIZABETH MARGARET GORDON STANLEY and
MARGARET PATRICIA RAMAGE

Urological symptoms can be associated with sexual problems in three main ways:

1. They may be the direct cause of sexual difficulties where none previously existed.
2. They may be the *apparent* cause of a sexual problem; in this case the development of an organically based bladder problem may be conveniently used, consciously or unconsciously, to avoid further sexual contact when there is a preexisting but unacknowledged sexual problem.
3. They may be the presenting symptom of underlying sexual conflict and the emotional stress that this can create.

Sexual problems may include reduction in the frequency of sexual relationships, progressive loss of libido, and inability to reach orgasm on the part of the woman. These in turn may affect the man's sexual responsiveness, resulting in symptoms such as premature ejaculation, ejaculatory incompetence, and partial or even complete impotence.

INCIDENCE

In one study by Sutherst (1979), it was found that of 103 patients attending an incontinence clinic, 48 patients admitted that their urinary symptoms adversely affected their sexual life. In 36 patients intercourse took place less frequently than before, and in 12 patients it had ceased altogether. Reasons given for this were dysparenuia, leakage of urine during intercourse, decreased libido, depression, or simply embarrassment. In general, however, the incidence of such problems is likely to be underestimated. Many patients may be too embarrassed or ashamed to disclose problems of such an intimate nature spontaneously, or they may feel reluctant to bother the busy physician with such a "trivial" concern. This highlights the need for inclusion of questions relating to the patient's sexuality in routine history taking, especially since information concerning the presence of a sexual problem and the more detailed information subsequently elicited may influence the direction of treatment for any given urological symptom.

HISTORY TAKING

Before considering more detailed aspects of history taking, it is important to acknowledge that sex can be a highly emotive subject, as much so for physicians as for patients. Unfortunately, patients are highly sensitive to any signs of embarrassment or discomfort displayed by the physician when sexual matters are raised, and this can inhibit disclosure of a sexual problem or prevent its more detailed discussion. Therefore if the physician experiences such feelings when talking explicitly about sexual issues, it would seem preferable that this person make only the most superficial of inquiries and then, with close collaboration, refer the patient to a sexual therapist for more detailed history taking and assessment.

Initial denial of a problem should not always be accepted at face value. Observation of body language, the tone of voice, and slight hesitations in speech may provide valuable clues to suggest that the patient is being somewhat less than truthful, in which case this line of questioning should be resumed later, perhaps in a different way and when greater rapport has been established. Then, if a sexual problem is still denied, this would either indicate that these clues have been misread or that the patient is simply not yet emotionally ready to face up to it. If the latter situation is suspected, this should be noted so that the subject can again be raised at a subsequent appointment if it is thought to be appropriate. If, however, the patient does acknowledge a sexual problem and the physician feels sufficiently comfortable with more detailed sexual history taking and discussion, the following guidelines may be followed:

1. Questions asked in an open-ended manner encourage the patient to give fuller explanations, rather than having to answer yes or no.

2. The physician should not be judgmental, either explicitly or implicitly, about any aspect of the patient's behavior, values, or beliefs, no matter how odd they may seem in the light of personal experience or previous knowledge.

3. When a detailed description of the sexual problem is being obtained, the use of simple language avoids misunderstandings that commonly arise over more sophisticated terminology.

4. It is as important to elicit the patient's feelings about the facts as it is to obtain the facts themselves, and any feelings expressed should be accepted without reservation.

5. The patient's attitude toward the topics discussed should be noted (for example, the patient may be open minded, inhibited, or embarrassed).

6. It is important to understand the patient's beliefs about the normality of certain sexual practices, since misunderstandings of this kind can be the cause of much confusion and unnecessary distress. For example, a woman may say that she has never reached orgasm, but closer questioning may reveal that she is in fact orgasmic through masturbation but not during intercourse. Guilt about masturbation and a mistaken belief that the only "proper" orgasms are those achieved through intercourse may initially prevent her from volunteering this important information and could well be an important factor contributing toward her sexual difficulties.

History taking should also include specific questions about the following:

1. Onset of the sexual problem, especially in relation to that of the urological symptoms

2. Incidence of incontinence during intercourse or orgasm

3. Quality of the general relationship, previous levels of enjoyment of sexual intercourse with the current partner, and extent of disharmony caused by the sexual problem

4. Religious and family background, especially parental attitudes toward sex, nudity, and open discussion about sexual matters

5. Feelings about the onset of menstruation and adolescent sexuality

6. Early coital experiences (for example, pleasant or unpleasant, associated with guilt or anxiety)

7. Age at which the patient first masturbated and its frequency over subsequent years (With regard to questions about masturbation, it is best to assume that the patient has masturbated, thereby implying an acceptance of the normality of this practice, which in turn makes it easier for the patient to answer these questions honestly.)

8. Patient's self-image and level of acceptance of her own sexuality

9. Homosexual experiences or inclinations

This history should enable an initial assessment to be made of the relevance of the sexual problem to the urological symptoms and should indicate the most appropriate lines of management for both the urological and the sexual problems.

UROLOGICAL SYMPTOMS CAUSING SEXUAL PROBLEMS
Incontinence

The main urological symptom likely to cause sexual problems is incontinence occurring during intercourse or on orgasm, although other symptoms such as urgency, frequency, or dysuria may also be contributory. When these symptoms are caused by sphincter incompetence, neuropathic bladder disorders (including neuropathic instability), or nonneuropathic instability and when medical or surgical intervention has proved unsuccessful or the underlying lesion is untreatable, it is more likely that the urological symptoms will be found to be the major cause, rather than the effect, of any sexual problem.

Cystitis

Symptoms caused by infection, bruising, or trauma are likely to occur 24 to 36 hours after coitus and may include burning on micturition, frequency, abdominal pain, and distension. Albuminuria may be present, but frequently results of investigation for pathogenesis are negative. If untreated, this type of cystitis leads to sexual avoidance by the woman because of fear of pain and illness and by the man because of fear of contaminating or damaging his partner.

Enuresis

Enuresis is frequently associated with other personality disorders, notably difficulty in open expression of emotions. Since treatment for enuresis usually includes training in the control of body functions, this in itself can interfere detrimentally with sexual expressions. The woman is afraid to "let go" and give up control in the way that is needed for the experience of full sexual arousal and orgasm. She may also find her vulval area to be a source of embarrassment and disgust to her and may be very reluctant to share her bed with a partner. In helping enuretic women with sexual problems, much patience is called for, since the concomitant personality difficulties can make treatment slow and at times discouraging. Vaginismus may also be present, and specialist referral is usually necessary in such a case (Stanley, 1981d).

Prolapse

Severe prolapse may lead to sexual difficulties or avoidance of intercourse. The appearance of the cervix at the introitus can be somewhat daunting for the man as well as embarrassing for the woman. Prolapse may cause incontinence and make penetration difficult, and it is important that the couple understand the nature of the anatomical changes that have occurred. After surgery or other treatment some counseling of the couple may be appropriate, but it is always indicated both preoperatively and postoperatively when hysterectomy is performed. Occasionally dyspareunia occurs as a result of surgical scarring or as a result of the woman's psychological response to her altered body. In any case, at treatment follow-up some general inquiry into the quality of the patient's sexual life is indicated, with possible counseling about forms of sexual expression other than coitus (for example, masturbation or orogenital sex).

Management

Management consists largely of helping the couple come to terms with their disability and learn how to improve the quality of their sexual life despite it.

The single most important measure that can be taken to deal with such a problem is to ensure that the patient and her partner talk openly and honestly with each other about it and share the emotional feelings engendered in them by their unfortunate situation. It is surprising how many couples have never actually discussed this aspect of their lives, partly out of embarrassment or shame and partly out of a vain and irrational hope that if the problem is not talked about, perhaps it will go away. The therapeutic effectiveness of this measure alone can sometimes be quite remarkable. It may, however, be insufficient just to tell the patient to go home and talk about it with her partner, and it is always preferable to see the couple together whenever possible. Once discussion has been initiated with this outside help, it is more likely to be continued at home in a way that will enable the couple to come to terms with the problem most readily. Often in the joint interview it becomes apparent that many misunderstandings have arisen between the couple, a common one being that the woman thinks that her partner is far more disturbed by her incontinence during lovemaking than he actually is. Indeed, some men even find this to be erotically stimulating but have previously been hesitant to acknowledge this fact.

Discussion of practical measures that could be taken to minimize the intrusion of the woman's symptoms into lovemaking is also of great importance. It may seem that, for example, using a waterproof sheet on the bed is such an obvious step to take that it should not need stating, but often this is not the case, and all similar measures that could be adopted to diminish the physical discomforts of the situation should be fully discussed. Such commonsense counseling need not be unduly time consuming and may well be all that is necessary to bring about a substantial improvement in the quality of the patient's sexual life. If desired, this task can effectively be delegated to a member of the nursing staff provided this person is comfortable talking explicitly about sexual matters.

In some cases, however, the sexual problem may need to be dealt with more fully, using all the therapeutic strategies (described later) underlying the management of sexual problems. Although one does not always require specialized training to offer help along these lines, it may well seem more appropriate to refer the patient for specific sexual therapy if such additional intervention is indicated.

UROLOGICAL SYMPTOMS APPARENTLY CAUSING SEXUAL PROBLEMS

Sometimes careful history taking reveals that the sexual problem complained of clearly existed before the onset of an organically based urological problem. In this case the urinary symptoms are likely to increase the severity of the sexual problem and may well be used, consciously or unconsciously, as a convenient excuse for avoiding further sexual contact, with all the obvious implications for marital disharmony.

Management

Although some long-standing sexual problems can be resolved with minimal intervention, most are better referred to a therapist skilled in the management of sexual problems.

UROLOGICAL SYMPTOMS RESULTING FROM SEXUAL PROBLEMS

Sexual problems can undoubtedly create considerable emotional stress, and the relationship between emotional stress and idiopathic detrusor instability has been well documented (Straub, Ripley, and Wolf, 1949; Frewen, 1978). When this is the only demonstrable abnormality of bladder function, the relationship between the two problems is more clear-cut, but cause and effect may be more difficult to disentangle when detrusor instability is found in addition to other abnormalities such as sphincter incompetence or defects in the mechanism of bladder emptying.

Management

In addition to the implementation of an appropriate bladder retraining program (see Chapter 39), full discussion of the patient's sexual difficulties should take place. Sometimes the simple counseling measures described earlier can bring about dramatic improvement in the patient's urological symptoms and help clarify the cause-or-effect dilemma, as the following case history illustrates.

CASE HISTORY

Mrs. A., aged 43, had congenital deformities of the thoracic spine and ribs, a right-sided Sprengel's shoulder, and lumbosacral spina bifida. Two years before this referral she had been complaining of weakness of the right leg, and a laminectomy had been performed, at which time a cutaneous and subcutaneous developmental anomaly and a cholesteatoma were removed from the base of her spine. She was initially referred to the Urodynamic Department because of increasing urgency and urge incontinence, a variable urinary stream, and a sensation of incomplete bladder emptying, all of which followed her laminectomy. At that time, no other symptoms were declared or elicited. Videocystourethrography demonstrated a marked residual urine and detrusor instability. The urethral pressure profile was normal. Urethrotomy brought about only marginal improvement in her symptoms.

At a subsequent outpatient appointment the patient was specifically asked whether she had any particular problems with the sexual side of her life; she then volunteered that she did indeed have a complaint that was causing her great distress. She had been divorced several years previously and had recently entered into a sexual relationship with a man considerably younger than herself. For the first time in her life she had become orgasmic but only through direct manipulation of her clitoris by her partner. She also became able to masturbate herself to orgasm, but in both situations she experienced urinary incontinence. Intercourse had therefore ceased to take place, and the general quality of their relationship was deteriorating. Discussion quickly revealed that she had the mistaken belief that to reach orgasm in this way was abnormal and perverted. She was immensely relieved and reassured to be told that this was not so and that 70% of women achieved orgasm with their partner in this way only (Hite, 1976). She was also grateful to be able to unburden herself of many of her anxieties and misgivings about the age gap between herself and her partner.

Six weeks later she reported that she was no longer experiencing loss of urine on reaching orgasm, although there was no further improvement in her other urological symptoms.

In all, this patient was seen for just over 1 hour, which is admittedly more time than is usually allotted for an outpatient appointment, but it was indeed time well spent. This case also demonstrates the complexity of assessing cause and effect, especially when, as in this patient's case, a coexistent organic disorder might indicate that the detrusor instability is neuropathic rather than idiopathic and that it is therefore unlikely that the symptoms would be improved by a psychotherapeutic approach.

Sometimes, however, longer term treatment by a trained sexual therapist is indicated, as illustrated by this second case history.

CASE HISTORY

Mrs. B., aged 23, had been involved in an automobile accident 3 years before being seen in the Urodynamic Department. In this accident she had sustained a fractured pelvis in three places and a perforated bowel. Following her discharge from the hospital, she complained of weakness of the right leg and frequency, urgency, urgency incontinence, and incontinence on orgasm. She also gave a history of enuresis during childhood, and on careful questioning it became apparent that her current urinary symptoms did in fact predate the accident although to a much milder extent. Videocystourethrography demonstrated detrusor instability, but this was thought to be unrelated to her accident.

She was first seen just before becoming married, and she seemed to have many anxieties about this; in general, she appeared to be a highly anxious person. Once married, her loss of urine on reaching orgasm caused her great distress, and she found it increasingly difficult to become sexually aroused, constantly finding excuses to avoid sexual contact with her husband. In turn, this was beginning to have a detrimental effect on the quality of their general relationship.

Urethrotomy and bladder retraining through biofeedback brought about some improvement in her frequency, urgency, and urge incontinence but not in her incontinence on orgasm. She and her husband were then seen by a sexual therapist for four 2-hour sessions, in which the approach used was the same as that for any, nonspecific loss of libido. This involved education, "permission giving," and increasing the couple's communication skills (Stanley, 1981b). A vicious circle of sexual failure causing fear of failure leading to still further failure, which had developed as a result of her loss of libido, was identified and broken into by use of the "ladder concept" and a modification of Masters and Johnson's "sensate focus" (Stanley, 1981b).

The quality of their general relationship improved markedly as a result of therapy, her libido returned, and within the first 3 weeks she reached orgasm on a number of occasions without loss of urine. She continued in individual psychotherapy for a further few sessions, which focused on other problem areas, particularly her feelings of insecurity and low self-esteem and the chronic anxiety state that these engendered. Subsequently, all her urological symptoms improved still further, as did the quality of all aspects of her relationship with her husband.

GENERAL PRINCIPLES OF TREATMENT

The main causes and basic strategies underlying the management of sexual problems are shown in Figure 32.1. Whatever the relationship of the urological problem to the sexual problem, it will be found that ignorance, acceptance of cultural taboos, and failure of effective communication between the couple (Stanley, 1981a) have all played their part, either as a major cause of the problem or by acting to perpetuate it. Therefore use of the broad therapeutic strategies of education, permission giving, and teaching communication skills, common to the management of all sexual problems (Stanley, 1981b), is indicated. In addition, once sexual failure has been experienced, for whatever reason, the vicious circle of failure and fear of failure leading to further failure usually becomes established. This can be dealt with by use of the ladder concept and a modification of Masters and Johnson's sensate focus (Stanley, 1981c), which help the couple develop a more realistic concept of "success" in their sexual relationship and enable them to view sex more in terms of sharing pleasure than as a testing "performance" in which attainment of mutual orgasm is always the ultimate goal. Although these therapeutic strategies are described in more detail elsewhere (Stanley, 1981b,c), they are summarized here.

Education

Ignorance about the basic anatomy and physiology of sexual response (Master and Johnson,

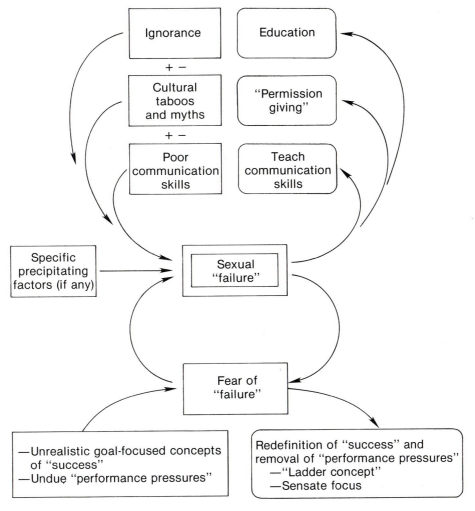

Figure 32.1 Main causes *(left)* and basic strategies underlying management *(right)* of sexual problems.

1966) and misconceptions about the normality of certain sexual practices are so widespread that some degree of education should be offered routinely once the couple's particular areas of ignorance have been identified. This can play a major role in improving the quality of the couple's sexual relationship. Many couples feel that they are unique and isolated in their difficulties, and this, coupled with ignorance of the anatomy and physiology of sexual response, gives rise to totally irrational, but greatly inhibiting, fears and fantasies. Straightforward information using models or pictures can do much to reduce anxieties and facilitate communication. An in vivo anatomy lesson cannot only be highly educational but also contains a strong element of permission giving and certainly facilitates communication between the couple (Stanley, 1981b). Useful books for their further

guidance are *The Book of Love* by David Delvin and *The Joy of Sex* by Alex Comfort.

Permission giving

Whatever other reasons can be found for a couple's experiencing a sexual problem, the cultural taboos surrounding the topic of sex and its open discussion are nearly always a contributing factor, and "permission" from an authority figure to break these taboos can prove to be highly therapeutic. Although permission giving may seem to be a somewhat abstract concept, it is in fact occurring throughout every minute of the consultation spent discussing sexual matters, simply by virtue of the fact that the physician is listening and talking about this subject in a frank and open way, with no more discomfort than would be shown during discussion of any other medical topic.

TABLE 32.1   Ladder concept

	Feelings	Genital changes
Ground level	No interest or pleasure in physical contact of any kind	None
Rung 1	Physical and emotional pleasure while cuddling without genital sensation	None
Rung 2	Feelings above heightened and early genital awareness	None or minimal
Rung 3	Moderate sexual arousal	Partial erection or lubrication
Rung 4	Strong sexual arousal but orgasm not felt to be essential	Full erection or lubrication
Rung 5	Intense sexual arousal with physical and emotional discomfort if orgasm does not occur	As above
Rung 6	Orgasm	As occur with orgasm

Teaching communication skills

At its simplest, teaching communication skills means no more than telling patients that, contrary to popular myth, they do need to let each other know what they like during lovemaking. This alone can go a long way toward helping some couples resolve their sexual problems.

A slightly more complex aspect of communication that is central to the development of both emotional and physical closeness is the ability to share emotional feelings, particularly the more negative ones, in an honest and constructive way. Poor communication can be summed up thus: ''Say what you don't mean and mean what you don't say!'' A summary of good communication can quite simply be expressed in this way: ''Mean what you say and say what you mean!'' which requires that the words spoken be consistent with the feelings experienced about the particular issue. When the tone of voice and body language (which reflect the underlying emotions) appear to be inconsistent with the statement made, communication immediately breaks down. A common example of this is the response to the question ''What is the matter?'' being ''Nothing is the matter''—but expressed in an angry or belligerent tone of voice. Clearly there *is* something the matter, but such a response leaves the receiver of such a message at best confused and negates any possibility of dealing effectively with the situation. If similar miscommunications occur repeatedly over a long period of time, no matter how trivial in itself each incident may seem, the frustration and resentment that can accumulate from these double or mixed messages can ultimately diminish sexual responsiveness.

Identifying such problems in a relationship and stressing the importance of ''saying what you mean and meaning what you say'' can do much toward helping a couple resolve their sexual difficulties; specific but more time-consuming therapeutic tools are also available (Stanley, 1981b) for couples with this kind of problem.

Redefining success

One aspect of treatment involves helping couples redefine for themselves a broader and more realistic concept of ''normal,'' ''successful'' sex. A specific therapeutic measure that may help this process is the ladder concept (Table 32.1).

A ladder with six rungs is used as the basis for discussion. The ground and each rung of the ladder are defined in terms of the intensity of physical pleasure experienced and the changes occurring in the genital region with increasing sexual arousal. By using the ladder as a framework for discussion, the couple can begin to review their ideas of what for them could constitute sexual ''success.'' It is suggested that if they so choose, they can consider that (1) the pleasure they experience on any given rung of the ladder can be valued in its own right and shared with their partner, without necessarily progressing to higher rungs every time; (2) a mutually satisfying sexual experience need not demand that both partners progress up the ladder at the same pace, always arriving at the top together; and (3) orgasm is not necessarily essential for individual satisfaction until rung five is reached. It does appear, however, that the drive for orgasmic release is greater in men than in women, possibly as a result of both cultural factors and intrinsic male-female differences. This may but need not be perceived as a problem by the couple.

Removing performance pressures

A common fantasy exists that to have good sex an erect penis must penetrate a lubricated vagina and that this should result in mutual orgasm. It can be seen now that the ladder concept can go some way toward removing such pressure to "perform." A modification of Masters and Johnson's sensate focus can also be used toward these ends. A complete ban on intercourse is imposed throughout this procedure, which for the time being removes any possibility of sexual failure, which is usually perceived only in relation to intercourse. Thus a situation is created in which the couple are more readily able to appreciate the quiet, gentle, sensual, and emotional feelings experienced at rungs one and two of the ladder, which were previously excluded from their awareness by overriding fears of failure. It is out of these less intense feelings that stronger ones grow, leading to mounting sexual arousal and orgasm, given the continuity of appropriate stimulation.

In the first stage the couple is asked to set aside 3 evenings or other periods of time in which they can be alone together for at least 2 hours. One partner is asked to lie down, as relaxed as possible and with a passive frame of mind. Using a body lotion (oils or talcum powder can be used if preferred), the other partner then begins to explore all the parts of the first partner's body, *excluding* the genital area, breasts and nipples, and the anal region. (Many couples do not appreciate the potential for pleasure of the anal region, and not all those who do may choose to use this potential.) They are asked not to view this exploration simply as a massage, since this implies only heavier forms of touch; it is often the lighter ones that the couple have failed to recognize and enjoy.

It is explained that this is primarily an exercise in sensory awareness in which the partners need to focus this awareness just on what they are experiencing at a tactile level at any given moment. They need to become aware of the differing textures of every part of their partner's body while making a conscious effort to exclude any extraneous and intrusive thoughts from their minds. As long as they are both in an appropriate mood, they will find that by keeping pleasurable sensual feelings central to their awareness, pleasure will build progressively on pleasure.

The second stage is precisely the same as the first, with the important difference that the breasts, nipples, genitals, and, if wished, the anal region are no longer out of bounds. It is stressed that these more erogenous areas should receive only intermittent attention and that the rest of the body should continue to be included in the exploration. It can also be useful to "ban" erection, high levels of sexual arousal, and orgasm for the duration of the second stage of the homework. This often proves to be invaluable paradoxical intention!

CONCLUSION

Specific questions concerning the patient's sexuality should be asked routinely of any patient seeking treatment for urological symptoms. If sexual problems are disclosed, they may be found to be either a cause or effect (or sometimes a combination of both) of the urological disorder. Regardless of the nature of this relationship, additional help for the sexual problem needs to be offered, whether by a member of the clinic staff or by referral to a trained sexual therapist.

As physicians, we have no universal sexual techniques that we can teach our patients to improve their sexual lives. We can, however, educate and give permission, and help them break into the vicious circle of fear of failure. In particular, we can help open up channels of communication between couples who experience sexual problems whereby each can teach the other how to become a good lover so that emotional feelings can be shared in a way that enhances all aspects of a close and loving relationship with another human being.

REFERENCES

Comfort, A. 1974. The joy of sex. London. Quartet Books, Ltd.

Delvin, D. 1974. The book of love. London. The New English Library, Ltd.

Frewen, W.K. 1978. An objective assessment of the unstable bladder of psychosomatic origin. Br. J. Urol. **50:**246-249.

Hite, S. 1976. The Hite report. New York. Dell Publishing Co., Inc.

Masters, W.J., and Johnson, V.E. 1966. Human sexual response. London. J. & A. Churchill.

Stanley, E.M.G. 1981a. Nonorganic causes of sexual problems. Br. Med. J. **282:**1042-1044.

Stanley, E.M.G. 1981b. Principles of managing sexual problems. Br. Med. J. **282:**1200-1202.

Stanley, E.M.G. 1981c. Dealing with fear and failure. Br. Med. J. **282:**1281-1283.

Stanley, E.M.G. 1981d. Vaginismus. Br. Med. J. **282:**1435-1437.

Straub, L.R., Ripley, H.S., and Wolf, S. 1949. Disturbances of bladder function associated with emotional states. J.A.M.A. **141:**1139-1143.

Sutherst, J.R. 1979. Sexual dysfunction and urinary incontinence. Br. J. Obstet. Gynecol. **86:**387-388.

part FOUR

URINARY TRACT IN PREGNANCY

chapter 33

Clinical aspects of the upper urinary tract in pregnancy

JOHN MALCOLM DAVISON

The changes occurring in the urinary tract during pregnancy are so extensive that nonpregnant norms are inappropriate for the management of antenatal patients. The problem becomes even more complicated as pregnancy progresses because the normal baseline alters. Cognizance of these changes is essential if early signs of renal dysfunction are to be detected or if sound advice is to be given to those women with renal problems who seek guidance on the advisability of conceiving or continuing a pregnancy already in progress.

ANATOMICAL CHANGES
Kidneys

The kidneys almost certainly enlarge during pregnancy because both vascular volume and interstitial space increase. Evidence from excretory urography performed immediately after delivery reveals that renal size is consistently greater than that predicted by standard height/weight nomograms, and repeat investigation 6 months later indicates a decrease in renal length by approximately 1 cm (Bailey and Rolleston, 1971; Kauppilla, Satuli, and Vuorinen, 1972).

A retrospective analysis of autopsy material has shown that the average weight of two normal kidneys in 137 women dying during or shortly after pregnancy was 307 g, compared with an average nonpregnant value of 250 g, and histological assessment indicated that glomerular size, but not cell number, was increased in pregnancy (Sheehan and Lynch, 1973). Examination of renal biopsy material obtained at cesarean section has been interpreted as showing that the microscopic structure of the kidney is similar in pregnant and nonpregnant women (Pollak and Nettles, 1960). Animal work seems to confirm that renal enlargement is caused by increased water content and that there is no accelerated growth during pregnancy; this is similar to the compensatory hypertrophy that occurs after unilateral nephrectomy (Davison and Lindheimer, 1980).

Ureters

The most striking anatomical change in the urinary tract is dilatation of the calyces, renal pelvis, and ureter (Figure 33.1). These changes, invariably more prominent on the right side, can be seen as early as the end of the first trimester and by the third trimester are present in 90% of women (Dure-Smith, 1970; Kauppilla, Satuli, and Vuorinen, 1972; Roberts, 1976).

The cause of the dilatation is disputed; some advocate a hormonal effect, and others obstruction (Feinstat, 1963; Roberts, 1976; Lindheimer and Katz, 1981). There is no doubt that as pregnancy progresses a supine or upright posture may cause partial ureteric obstruction as the enlarged uterus compresses the ureter at the pelvic brim. Some proponents of the obstructive theory attribute a major role to pressure from a dilated ovarian venous plexus (Bellina, Bougherty, and Mickal, 1970) (especially on the right side), the uterine veins (Kauppilla, Satuli, and Vuorinen, 1972), or the iliac vessels (Dure-Smith, 1970). Ureteric dilatation terminates at the pelvic brim where the ureter crosses the iliac artery, and at this point a filling defect termed the *iliac sign* can be seen in an excretory urogram (Figure 33.1). Failure to see dilatation below the level of the pelvic brim is not necessarily evidence in favor of an obstruction at that level, because the connective tissue sheath (Waldeyer's sheath), which surrounds the ureters as they enter the true pelvis, hypertrophies during pregnancy and could prevent hormonally induced dilatation at this level.

Dilatation of the collecting system has been assumed to be accompanied by hypotonicity and hypomotility of the ureteric muscle as well as reduced urine flow. Modern urometry, however, has demonstrated that there is increased tonicity in the upper ureter and no decrease in the frequency and amplitude of the ureteric contraction complex in pregnancy (Rubi and Sala, 1968; Mattingly and Borkowf, 1978). Furthermore, there is hypertrophy of the ureteric smooth muscle and hyperplasia of its connective tissue so that the concept of toneless, floppy ureters, their smooth muscle paralyzed by the hormonal milieu of pregnancy, is erroneous.

Vesicoureteric reflux

Since vesicoureteric reflux occurs sporadically and intermittently, it has not been possible to accurately assess its frequency. Vesicoureteric reflux occurs in approximately 3% of pregnant patients at or near term, but it is probably far more frequent (Heidrick, Mattingly, and Amberg, 1967; Mattingly and Borkowf, 1978).

The mechanism of vesicoureteric reflux remains obscure but centers around changes that occur in the intravesical ureter. With advancing pregnancy, the enlarging uterus displaces the ureters laterally and the intravesical portions are shortened, becom-

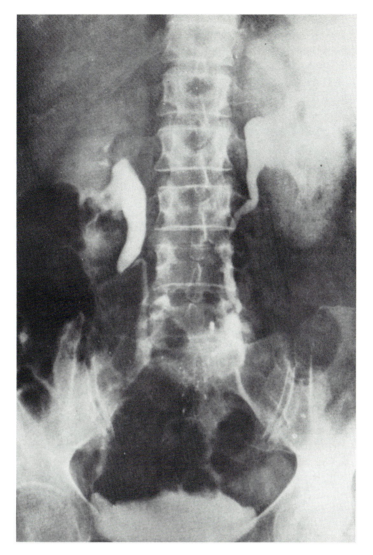

Figure 33.1 Intravenous excretory urogram taken immediately after delivery showing ureteral dilatation. Right ureter is cut off abruptly at pelvic brim where is crosses iliac artery (so-called iliac sign).

ing perpendicular rather than oblique, rendering the junction functionally less competent. Probably this is evident only when there is increased intravesical pressure such as during voiding, and it has been suggested that a minimal intramural segment length of 10 mm may be critical in the prevention of vesicoureteric reflux. Technical difficulties preclude the measurement of pressure differences between the bladder and the lower 5 cm of ureter; therefore it has been difficult to document the loss of ureteric tone that would facilitate vesicoureteric reflux. Whatever the mechanism and consequence of vesicoureteric reflux, the situation appears to be totally reversible with involution of the uterus.

Clinical implications

Urine collection. Dilatation of the urinary tract may lead to collection errors in tests based on timed urine volume, for example, 24-hour creatinine, estriol, and protein excretion. Such errors may be minimized if the pregnant woman is sufficiently hydrated to give a high urine flow and if she is positioned in lateral recumbency for an hour before and at the end of the collection. These precautions standardize the procedure and minimize dead space errors.

Radiology. Acceptable norms of kidney size should be increased by 1 cm if estimated during pregnancy or immediately after delivery. Dilatation of the ureters may persist until the sixteenth post-partum week, and elective intravenous excretory urography during this period should be deferred. Ureteric dilatation may persist in up to 11% of parous women with no history of urinary tract infection (Spiro and Fry, 1970), and whether this is a harmless sequel of normal pregnancy or represents the residuum of missed infection is not certain.

Vesicoureteric reflux. Vesicoureteric reflux may contribute to ascending infection resulting in pyelonephritis. In one series of nine patients with pyelonephritis reflux was demonstrable in three of them either in the last trimester or the postpartum period (Heidrick, Mattingly, and Amberg, 1967). Nevertheless, it was still concluded that it remains to be confirmed that vesicoureteric reflux encourages ascending infection.

Acute hydronephrosis and hydroureter. Occasionally pregnancy can precipitate acute hydronephrosis or hydroureter. Obstruction may occur at varying levels at or above the pelvic brim. When this complication develops, there may be an underlying compensated pelviureteric junction obstruction, which becomes decompensated and hence symptomatic because of the physiological changes of pregnancy (Meares, 1978). Typically, acute right loin or lower abdominal pain radiating to the groin can be relieved by ureteric catheterization, and the urine can be sterile or infected (Schloss and Solomkin, 1952). The condition should be suspected when there are recurrent episodes of pain and repeat midstream urine specimens are sterile. Diagnosis can be confirmed by using excretory urography or sonar scanning. If positioning the patient on the unaffected side (in combination with antibiotic therapy if appropriate) fails to relieve the situation, ureteric catheterization or nephrostomy may be required. Corrective surgery should be delayed, however, until the postpartum period (Meares, 1978).

PHYSIOLOGICAL CHANGES
Renal hemodynamics

Glomerular filtration rate (GFR) and effective renal plasma flow (ERPF) increase to levels about 50% to 60% above nonpregnant values (Figures 33.2 and 33.3). These increases occur shortly after conception (Davison and Noble, 1981), and all increments are present in the second trimester (Davison and Hytten, 1974; Dunlop, 1981). Why GFR increases in pregnancy is difficult to explain. The

early rise would be consistent with hormonally induced intravascular volume expansion, but the change in GFR is established long before the greatest increments have occurred, and subsequently there is no further rise in GFR as plasma volume increases.

Since GFR increases without substantial alterations in the production of creatinine and urea, plasma levels of these solutes decrease. Creatinine levels fall from a nonpregnant level of 73 μmol/L to 65 μmol/L in the first trimester, 51 μmol/L in the second trimester, and 47 μmol/L in the third trimester (Kuhlback and Widholm, 1966). The fall in plasma urea may in part be caused by reduced protein degradation as well as increased clearance of this solute. Average plasma urea levels of 3.5, 3.3, and 3.1 mmol/L in successive trimesters, rising to 4.3 mmol/L 6 weeks postpartum, have been described (Robertson and Cheyne, 1972).

Awareness of these physiological changes is important because values considered normal in nonpregnant women may reflect decreased renal function during pregnancy. Plasma levels of creatinine and urea exceeding 75μmol/L and 4.5 mmol/L, respectively, should alert the clinician to investigate renal function further.

Toward the end of pregnancy there is a fall in ERPF; this has been ascribed to the effect of posture (Chesley and Sloan, 1964), and it has been suggested that no such decrease would occur if subjects were studied serially in the left lateral position (Pippig, 1969). This interpretation has not been universally accepted, however, and the issue remains controversial (Sims and Krantz, 1958; Dunlop, 1976). Recently it has been shown that in women in lateral recumbency studied at the twenty-ninth and thirty-ninth weeks of gestation there was a significant reduction in ERPF, which suggests that the late pregnancy decrease cannot be attributed solely to the effect of posture (Ezimokhai, Davison, and Philips, 1981).

Less controversy surrounds the changes in GFR. During the last 3 weeks of pregnancy, creatinine clearance decreases (Davison, Dunlop, and Ezimokhai, 1980); this is of considerable importance when the test is used in assessment of high-risk pregnancies and when estrogen output is "corrected" for creatinine excretion (Figure 33.4).

Volume homeostasis

The average weight gain in normal pregnancy is 12.5 kg. Much of this increment consists of fluid,

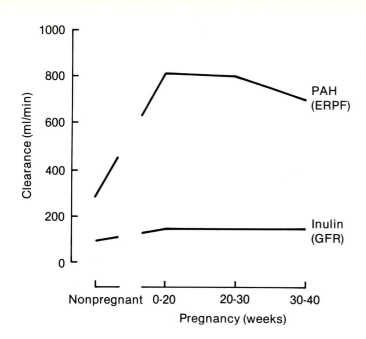

Figure 33.2 Absolute changes in ERPF and GFR measurements serially during pregnancy. (Modified from Dunlop, W. 1981. Br. J. Gynaecol. **88**:1-9.)

Figure 33.3 Weekly 24-hour creatinine clearances (GFR) over conception and in early pregnancy in nine healthy women. Solid line represents mean; stippled area represents range. *MP,* Menstrual period; *LMP,* last menstrual period.

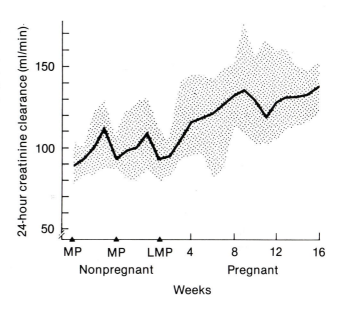

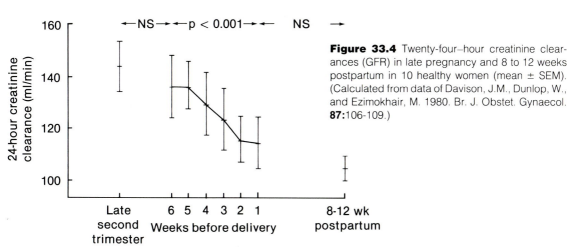

Figure 33.4 Twenty-four-hour creatinine clearances (GFR) in late pregnancy and 8 to 12 weeks postpartum in 10 healthy women (mean ± SEM). (Calculated from data of Davison, J.M., Dunlop, W., and Ezimokhair, M. 1980. Br. J. Obstet. Gynaecol. **87**:106-109.)

since total body water increases by 6 to 8 L, 4 to 6 L of which are extracellular. There are also increases in plasma volume (maximum during the second trimester and approaching 50%) and in fluid within the fetal and maternal interstitial spaces, which are greatest in late pregnancy. During normal pregnancy, there is a gradual cumulative retention of about 900 mmol of sodium, distributed between the products of conception and maternal extracellular space. The alterations in maternal intravascular and interstitial spaces produce so-called physiological hypervolemia, but maternal volume receptors sense these changes as normal. Consequently, when salt restriction or diuretic therapy limits this physiological expansion, the maternal response resembles that of salt-depleted nonpregnant subjects.

The influence of humoral changes during normal pregnancy on renal sodium handling and volume regulation is incompletely understood. Aldosterone secretion and excretion and levels of plasma cortisol, deoxycorticosterone, estrogen, and prolactin all increase during normal pregnancy. These and other factors that may influence renal sodium handling during pregnancy have been discussed in detail elsewhere (Nolten and Ehrlich, 1980; Lindheimer and Katz, 1981a).

Osmoregulation

Very early in pregnancy, plasma osmolality decreases to a level about 10 mosm/kg below the nonpregnant norm, and this can be accounted for by a concomitant fall in plasma sodium and associated anions (Figure 33.5). In view of this it might be expected that a pregnant woman would stop secreting antidiuretic hormone and arginine vasopressin and would be in a state of continuous diuresis. This does not happen, because the osmoreceptor system becomes reset in its own right and accepts and preserves the new low level of osmolality. Furthermore, there is no lag in the adjustment of the osmostat, so that polyuria is not a feature of early pregnancy (Davison, Vallotton, and Lindheimer, 1981).

Renal tubular function

Renal handling of glucose. Excretion of glucose increases soon after conception and may exceed nonpregnant values by a factor of 10 (Davison and Hytten, 1975). The glycosuria varies markedly, both from day to day and within 24 hours, but the intermittency is related neither to blood sugar concentrations nor to the stage of pregnancy.

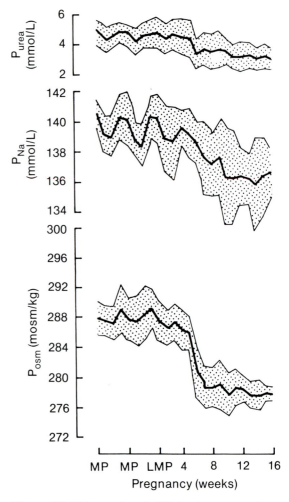

Figure 33.5 Mean values (±SD) for plasma urea (P_urea), sodium (P_Na), and osmolality (P_osm) measured at weekly intervals from before conception to first trimester in nine healthy women. *MP*, Menstrual period; *LMP*, last menstrual period.

Normal nonpregnant values are reestablished within a week of delivery (Davison and Lovedale, 1974).

Serial studies of the renal handling of glucose under infusion conditions in women with varying degrees of glycosuria have shown that glucose reabsorption is less complete during pregnancy than it is 8 to 12 weeks after delivery (Davison and Hytten, 1975). Reabsorption is always less complete in pregnant women with obvious glycosuria, and these women, although no longer clinically glycosuric following pregnancy, still show less complete reabsorption under infusion conditions when nonpregnant (Figure 33.6). Even though reabsorptive ability is less effective in pregnancy, it might be argued that the precipitating cause of glycosuria remains the striking increment in GFR.

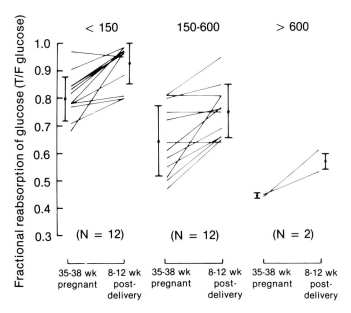

Figure 33.6 Fractional reabsorption of glucose under infusion conditions (individual values and means ± SD) in 26 women studied during late pregnancy and after puerperium. Women were divided into three groups according to their 24-hour glucose excretion (mg) during pregnancy. The within-groups significance (paired Student's *t* test) for <150 mg/day was p < 0.001; for 150 to 600 mg/day, it was p < 0.001. (Calculated from data of Davison, J.M., and Hytten, F.E. 1975. Br. J. Obstet. Gynaecol. **82**:374-381.)

Two major physiological adaptations in pregnancy have the potential to affect glucose reabsorption in opposite ways: volume expansion may inhibit the reabsorption of sodium and hence glucose, whereas increased GFR may stimulate glucose reabsorption. To further complicate the picture, work in animals has revealed that the distal parts of the nephron have a capacity to reabsorb glucose (Wenn and Stoll, 1979) and that this is much reduced in pregnancy (Bishop and Green, 1978).

It has been suggested that women with more than usual glycosuria in pregnancy may have sustained renal tubular damage from earlier untreated urinary tract infection, although they were no longer bacteriuric when pregnant (Davison and Dunlop, 1980). There can be little doubt that the phenomenon of glycosuria in pregnancy reflects an alteration of renal function rather than of carbohydrate metabolism and that testing random urine samples in pregnancy is both unhelpful in the diagnosis and control of diabetes and unrepresentative of the degree of glycosuria present.

Renal handling of uric acid. Uric acid is an end point of purine metabolism and is freely filterable at the glomerulus. It is cleared by the kidney at about 10% of the rate of insulin, implying that during its passage through the kidney most of the filtered uric acid is reabsorbed (Holmes and Kelley, 1975). The kidney's handling of uric acid is, however, more complex than simple tubular reabsorption. It appears that although a substantial proportion of filtered uric acid is reabsorbed in the proximal tubule subsequent to this, a balance between active secretion (Gutman, Yu, and Berger, 1959) and further reabsorption (Diamond and Miesel, 1975) regulates final excretion (Rieselbach and Steele, 1974).

Plasma uric acid concentration falls by at least 25% during early pregnancy. It has been suggested that this change reflects alterations in the fractional clearance of uric acid (uric acid clearance ÷ GFR), with a decrease in net tubular reabsorption (Dunlop and Davison, 1977). As pregnancy advances, the kidney appears to excrete a smaller proportion of the filtered uric acid load, and this increase in net reabsorption is associated with an increase in plasma uric acid concentration.

Uric acid concentration and renal reabsorption are significantly higher in pregnancies complicated by preeclampsia or intrauterine growth retardation (Dunlop, Furness, and Hill, 1978; Dunlop et al., 1978). Above a critical level of 350 μmol/L there is significant perinatal mortality in hypertensive patients (Redman, Beilin, and Bonnar, 1976). However, physiological variability is such that serum concentrations of uric acid below this value are of little prognostic significance (Dunlop and Davison, 1978), and a single random measurement of serum level (Hill, Furness, and Dunlop, 1977), clearance (Chesley and Valenti, 1958), or net reabsorption (Dunlop et al., 1978) is of no value. Serial measurements may be of some value in monitoring progress in preeclampsia (Beilin et al., 1974).

Other changes. Excretion of most amino acids and several water-soluble vitamins increases during pregnancy (Davison, 1975), and these increments may be yet another factor in the enhanced susceptibility to urinary tract infections in pregnancy. Urinary protein excretion is increased such that proteinuria should not be considered abnormal until it exceeds 300 mg in 24 hours, and increased protein excretion in women with known renal disease does not necessarily signify progression of the disease. Renal bicarbonate reabsorption and protein excretion appear unchanged by pregnancy (Lim, Katz, and Lindheimer, 1977).

CHRONIC RENAL DISEASE
Pathophysiology of renal dysfunction

To assess pregnancy and its altered homeostasis in the context of coexisting renal disease, it is essential to understand some of the events that occur when nephron mass has been lost. Figure 33.7 demonstrates the relationship between plasma creatinine, creatinine clearance, and nephron population. An individual may lose approximately 50% of function and yet maintain a plasma creatinine level of less than 130 μmol/L. If renal function is more severely compromised, however, then small decreases in GFR cause plasma creatinine to increase markedly. Nevertheless, a patient who has lost 75% of her nephrons may have lost only 50% of function and may have a deceptively normal plasma creatinine level. Thus evaluation of renal function should be based on the clearance of creatinine rather than on its plasma concentration.

In patients with renal disease, pathological conditions may be both chemically and clinically silent. Most individuals remain symptom free until their GFR falls to less than 25% of its original level, and many plasma constituents are frequently normal until a late stage of the disease. As renal function declines, the ability to conceive and to sustain a viable pregnancy decreases. Degrees of functional impairment that do not cause symptoms or appear to disrupt homeostasis in nonpregnant individuals do jeopardize pregnancy, and normal pregnancy is rare when renal function decreases to

a degree that nonpregnant plasma creatinine and urea levels exceed 275 μmol/L and 10 mmol/L, respectively. These increments above normal nonpregnant levels appear trivial, but they represent decrements in function of more than 50%.

Effect of renal disease on pregnancy

There are conflicting views concerning the course of pregnancy in women with renal disease, reflecting the variability of populations studied and the lack of large prospective series in which diagnosis was established by biopsy and the disease correlated with observations of fetal outcome. To some extent this situation has recently been remedied by a collaborative study in women with a variety of renal disorders, all diagnosed by renal biopsy (Katz et al., 1980, 1981).

Hypertension. Hypertension, usually of a mild degree, occurs in about 25% of pregnancies, but in half of these blood pressure is elevated before conception. Hypertension tends to be more common and more severe in women with diffuse glo-

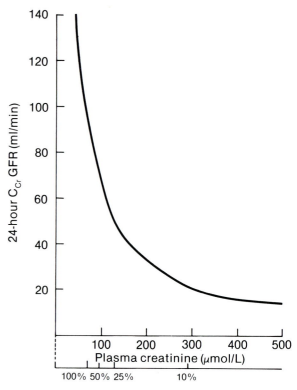

Figure 33.7 Relation of 24-hour creatinine clearance (ml/min) to plasma creatinine concentration (μmol/L) and nephron population (%), assuming a constant creatinine excretion of approximately 11.5 mmol/24 hours.

merulonephritis but it also prominent in women with focal glomerulonephritis and arteriolar nephrosclerosis.

Renal function. GFR in women with renal disease is usually lower than that of normal pregnant women, but pregnancy still evokes an increment (Figure 33.8). Toward term GFR tends to fall, but in some instances (most often in women with diffuse glomerulonephritis) renal function can decrease earlier than this. The decrement is usually mild to moderate and reverses after delivery.

Increased proteinuria is the most common renal effect of pregnancy, reflecting in part the tendency toward increased protein excretion seen in normal pregnancy. Substantially increased proteinuria occurs in about 50% of pregnancies, associated with nearly all types of renal disease, although it tends to be less common in women with chronic interstitial nephritis (predominantly of infective origin). Massive protein excretion, exceeding 3 g/24 hr, complicates 30% of pregnancies and frequently leads to nephrotic edema.

Preeclampsia. There is controversy about the incidence of preeclampsia in women with preexisting renal disease largely because the diagnosis cannot be made with certainty on clinical grounds alone, because hypertension and proteinuria may be manifestations of the underlying disease. This is clearly demonstrated by the study of Katz et al. (1980, 1981), where superimposed preeclampsia was diagnosed on clinical grounds in 13 women and eclampsia in 1 (out of 121 pregnancies in 83 women), even though 10 of these women were hypertensive and proteinuric before conception. Postpartum renal biopsy was performed in 13 of these women, and the characteristic glomerular changes of preeclampsia were evident in only 7, including the woman with eclampsia (Lindheimer, Spargo, and Katz, 1975).

Obstetrical outcome. Perinatal mortality and the incidence of preterm deliveries and small-for-dates infants are slightly higher than in healthy pregnancies. It is probable that further reductions in perinatal mortality are possible with improvements in methods of fetal surveillance and further advances in perinatal care.

Effect of pregnancy on renal disease

The studies of Katz et al. (1980, 1981) endorse the majority view that, with the exception of an increased frequency of exacerbation of pyelonephritis, pregnancy has no adverse effect on the

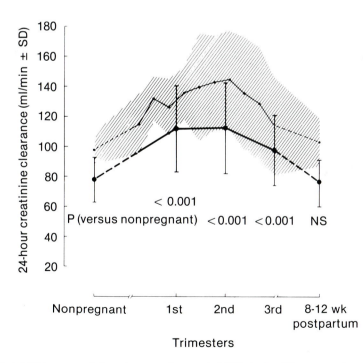

Figure 33.8 Serial 24-hour creatinine clearance (mean ± 1 SD) during 33 pregnancies of 26 women with renal disease who were studied before conception, in each trimester, and 8 to 12 weeks after delivery (solid line). Measurements from 10 healthy women (mean ± 1 SD) are shown in crosshatched area. (From Katz, A.I., et al. 1980. Reprinted from Kidney International [Vol. **18**:192-206, 1980 with permission].)

natural history of established renal parenchymal disease provided that renal function is preserved or only moderately compromised and hypertension is absent (Werko and Bucht, 1956; Kaplan, Smith, and Tillman, 1962; Felding, 1969; Strauch and Hayslett, 1974; Bear, 1976; Klockars et al., 1980). There is, however, another view that pregnancy frequently results in progression of the renal lesions and further deterioration of renal function (Tenny and Dandrow, 1961; Kincaid-Smith, Fairley, and Byllen, 1967; 1967; Fairley, Whitworth, and Kincaid-Smith, 1973). It appears, however, that in certain instances the decline in renal function in women with preexisting renal disease may have resulted from dehydration and reduced renal perfusion as a result of stringent sodium restriction and/or inadvertent diuretic therapy.

In summary, in the absence of significant hypertension or overt renal insufficiency before conception most women with mild to moderate renal disease tolerate pregnancy well. There is no evidence that pregnancy specifically accelerates the progress of their disease (Figure 33.8). The key to success is close scrutiny of the antenatal course with cooperation between obstetrician, nephrologist, and eventually pediatrician.

ASSESSMENT OF RENAL FUNCTION DURING PREGNANCY

Serial data on renal function are needed to supplement routine antenatal observations. Specialized tests involving infusion procedures are usually not available, and their use is primarily for clinical research. Tests that are available for use in routine clinical practice include the estimation of plasma urea and electrolytes, creatinine and urea clearance determination, and concentration and dilution procedures. The clinical tests are usually influenced by multiple mechanisms; for example, urea and creatinine level clearances do not measure absolute GFR, since urea is reabsorbed and creatinine is secreted by the renal tubules, so that the clearance of either gives only an approximation of the true GFR. Nevertheless, these tests have generated a great deal of empirical information and provide adequate, if not precise, assessments of renal function in numerous clinical situations.

When reporting renal function values, one should remember that correction of data to a standard body surface area of 1.73 m^2 (and thus, by implication, to a standard kidney size) is not applicable in pregnancy (Chesley and Williams,

1945). To investigate any individual's renal function, serial tests should be performed and where possible compared with the patient's nonpregnant values.

In the last analysis the assessment of renal function requires serial surveillance of creatinine clearance. If renal function deteriorates during any stage of pregnancy, reversible causes such as urinary tract infection or obstruction, subtle dehydration, or electrolyte imbalance (perhaps secondary to inadvertent diuretic therapy) should be sought. Near term, a 15% decrement in function (which affects plasma creatinine minimally) is permissible (Davison, Dunlop, and Ezimokhai, 1980) (Figures 33.4 and 33.8). If hypertension accompanies any observed decrease in renal function, the outlook is usually more serious. Immediate decisions and action may be required, and the patient should be hospitalized.

THE KIDNEY IN PREECLAMPSIA
Perspective

Preeclampsia, a hypertensive disorder peculiar to pregnancy, usually occurs after the twentieth week of pregnancy and most frequently near term; it is characterized by proteinuria, edema, and at times coagulation abnormalities. The literature is confusing and controversial, largely because it is often difficult to distinguish clinically between preeclampsia, essential hypertension, chronic renal disease, and combinations of these separate entities. For example, certain women with undiagnosed essential hypertension show a decrement in blood pressure early in pregnancy and normal levels if first examined near midpregnancy. When frankly elevated pressures are recorded near term, they are then erroneously labeled preeclamptic. Furthermore, an accelerated phase of essential hypertension (albeit a rare event during pregnancy), certain forms of renal disease (glomerulonephritis and systemic lupus erythematosus), and pheochromocytoma may all mimic preeclampsia.

These diagnostic dilemmas are best illustrated when renal biopsy has been performed immediately after pregnancies complicated by hypertension (Chesley, 1978; Lindheimer and Katz, 1981a). Table 33.1 shows the pathological diagnosis on postpartum renal biopsy of 176 patients biopsied because pregnancy was complicated by hypertension, proteinuria, and edema. In most instances the clinical diagnosis had been preeclampsia (Fisher, Luger, and Spargo, 1981). This diagnosis was

TABLE 33.1 Renal disease in 176 hypertensive pregnant women			
Diagnosis	**No. patients**	**Primigravidae**	**Multigravidae**
Preeclampsia	96	79	17
With renal disease	3	1	2
With nephrosclerosis	13	6	7
With both	2	1	1
Nephrosclerosis	19	3	16
With renal disease	4	2	2
Renal disease	31	12	19
Normal histology	8	0	8

From Fisher, K.A., et al. 1981. Medicine **60**:267-287. Copyright © 1981 The Williams & Wilkins Co., Baltimore.

wrong in 25% of primiparas and was wrong more often than not in multiparas. In addition, a surprisingly large number of patients had unsuspected parenchymal renal disease. Such information emphasizes the pitfalls inherent in interpreting reports where the diagnosis is based on clinical criteria alone. Most suspect are the series in which many of the patients labeled preeclamptic, or "toxemic," were multiparous.

Anatomical considerations

In preeclampsia the characteristic morphological lesion is glomeruloendotheliosis (Fisher, Luger, and Spargo, 1981). The glomeruli are large and swollen but not hypercellular, because of swelling of the intracapillary cells (mainly endothelial, but mesangial as well) that encroaches on the capillary lumina, giving the appearance of a bloodless glomerulus. The lesion is considered by most, but not all, investigators to be virtually pathognomonic of the disease (Lindheimer and Katz, 1981a).

Physiological considerations

Both GFR and RPF decrease in preeclampsia. The decrement in GFR is approximately 25% to 35% in mild cases, whereas the normal increase in pregnancy ranges between 40% and 50% above postpartum values. Thus despite morphological evidence of glomerular cell swelling, ischemia, and obliteration of the urinary space, GFR in preeclamptic women often remains above prepregnancy values, and the decrement may not be appreciated if one is not aware of norms of pregnancy. It should be emphasized that although functional decrements in preeclampsia are usually mild or moderate and reverse rapidly after delivery, an occasional patient may progress to acute tubular necrosis, especially when treatment or intervention is neglected.

Uric acid clearance decreases and renal reabsorption increases in preeclampsia (Dunlop et al., 1978). These changes may occur earlier (sometimes weeks before any other signs or symptoms of the disease) and be more profound than the change in GFR. The increase in renal uric acid reabsorption is accompanied by increased plasma levels of this solute, and the level of hyperuricemia correlates directly with the decrement in plasma volume that occurs in preeclampsia and indirectly with the plasma renin activity (Beaufils et al., 1981). High urate levels (≥ 350 μmol/L) correlate with the severity of the preeclamptic lesion (Pollak and Nettles, 1960), as well as with poor fetal outcome (Redman et al., 1976; Lindheimer and Katz, 1981b).

Abnormal proteinuria almost always accompanies preeclampsia, and the diagnosis is suspect without this sign, even though glomerular endotheliosis has sometimes been described in the absence of increased protein excretion. Proteinuria may be minimal, moderate, or severe (that is, in the nephrotic range). The occurrence of nephrotic syndrome deserves emphasis because in the past heavy proteinuria was believed to be uncommon in preeclampsia, and when it occurred it was considered indicative of a severe form of the disease. It is now apparent that preeclampsia is the most common cause of nephrotic syndrome in pregnancy. The severity of maternal disease is similar in preeclamptic women with heavy proteinuria and those excreting less than 3.5 g/day, although small but significant increases in fetal loss occur in women with severe proteinuria (Fisher et al., 1981). On the other hand, First et al. (1978) studied preeclamptic women with nephrotic syndrome and noted a dismal fetal outcome; however, in contrast to the study by Fisher et al. (1981), most of their patients were multiparas.

Proteinuria in preeclampsia is nonselective, although the lesion is completely reversible (Lindheimer and Katz, 1981a,b). The increased protein excretion has been attributed to vasospasm as well as to the glomerular lesion that accompanies the disease. The latter is supported by the observation that the magnitude of the proteinuria correlates with the severity of the morphologic lesion (Pollak and Nettles, 1960).

RENAL TRANSPLANTATION AND PREGNANCY

Reproductive function is abnormal in women with end-stage renal failure who experience a variety of menstrual irregularities, often fail to ovulate, and have difficulty conceiving (Lim et al., 1980; Emmanouel et al., 1981). Renal transplantation usually reverses these problems, and the resumption of regular menstrual cycles and ovulation correlates closely with the level of function achieved by the graft (Merkatz et al., 1971). It has been estimated that 1 of every 50 women of childbearing age who have a functional renal transplant will someday become pregnant (Br. Med. J., 1976), and recent review of this topic has analyzed the experience of 697 such pregnancies (Davison and Lindheimer, 1981). Inevitably it is difficult to assess the exact incidence of the various problems because some of the information in the literature is incomplete and many more pregnancies than those reported must have occurred. Excluding the large series from Denver (United States) (Penn et al., 1980), where 75% of patients had received kidneys from living related donors, only 20% of births occurred in recipients of living donor grafts. Despite the publication of case reports, series, and registry data from North America and Europe, little has been done to establish guidelines on standards of care for the transplant recipient who conceives. In some instances pregnancy was not diagnosed until the third trimester, and many patients were under the impression that they could not conceive.

Antenatal care

Management requires attention to blood pressure control, anemia, urinary tract infection, bone dis-ease, and monitoring renal function. Meticulous assessment of fetal growth is needed, and this is best performed by serial ultrasound assessment. Measurement of maternal urinary estriol excretion is of no value because the administration of steroids suppresses the synthesis of fetal adrenal steroid precursors, and in any case the transplanted kidney may not excrete estriol normally. Where there is evidence of intrauterine growth retardation, the possibility of congenital cytomegalovirus infection should be considered (Evans et al., 1975). Maternal complications include serious infection, septicemia, allograft rejection, steroid-induced hypoglycemia, and uterine rupture.

Renal function during pregnancy

Even though a transplanted kidney is ectopic, denervated, potentially damaged by previous ischemia, and immunologically foreign, the augmentation of GFR characteristic of early pregnancy in healthy women is invariably evident (Davison, 1978) (Figure 33.9). The better the renal function before pregnancy, the more satisfactory the obstetrical outcome. Even in patients with satisfactory renal function before pregnancy there may be some deterioration during the third trimester, with or without proteinuria, but this is usually transient, with normal function returning in the postpartum period. Permanent impairment of renal function may occasionally be seen, especially when it is already compromised before conception.

Allograft rejection during pregnancy

It has been reported that serious rejection episodes occur in 9% of women with pregnancies lasting into the third trimester (Rudolph et al., 1979). Although this incidence is no greater than that expected for nonpregnant transplant patients, it must be considered unusual because it has always been assumed that the privileged immunological state of pregnancy would benefit the transplant. Furthermore, there are reports of reduction or cessation of immunosuppressive therapy during pregnancy without rejection (Kaufman et al., 1967; Rifle and Traeger, 1975). Rejection occasionally occurs in the puerperium, probably caused by a return to a normal immune state (despite immunosuppression) or possibly a rebound effect from the altered immunoresponsiveness associated with pregnancy.

Even in the nonpregnant patient rejection can be a difficult diagnostic problem, and in the absence of a renal biopsy it cannot be distinguished from acute pyelonephritis and recurrent glomerulopathy.

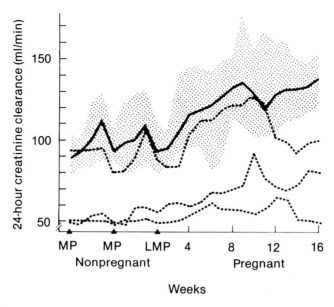

Figure 33.9 Weekly 24-hour creatinine clearance (GFR) over conception and in early pregnancy in three renal transplant patients. Solid line represents mean; stippled area represents range for nine healthy women at same period of time. *MP,* Menstrual period; *LMP,* last menstrual period.

Its clinical hallmarks are fever, decreasing urinary output, and deteriorating renal function often associated with renal enlargement and tenderness. In pregnancy the differential diagnosis must also include severe preeclampsia.

Management of delivery

Augmentation of steroids is necessary to cover the stress of delivery. Usually the transplanted kidney does not produce any mechanical dystocia in labor, and during vaginal delivery there is no apparent injury. Cesarean section is usually necessary only for purely obstetrical reasons.

Neonatal problems

There is substantial hazard to the neonate. Preterm delivery occurs in 50% and intrauterine growth retardation in 15%. One or more complications occur in about 35%, including respiratory distress syndrome, leukopenia, thrombocytopenia, adrenocortical insufficiency, and infection. There are no predominant or frequent developmental abnormalities, but any child exposed to immunosuppressive therapy in utero must have careful evaluation of the immune system and long-term follow-up.

Pregnancy counseling

Couples who want a child should discuss all the implications of pregnancy and long-term prospects.

Patients should be assessed on the basis of the following general guidelines (Davison et al., 1976):

1. Good general health for 2 years after transplantation.
2. Stature compatible with good obstetrical outcome.
3. No proteinuria.
4. No significant hypertension.
5. No evidence of graft rejection.
6. No evidence of pelvicalyceal distension on a recent excretory urogram.
7. Plasma creatinine of 180 μmol/L or less.
8. Drug therapy of prednisone, 15 mg/kg or less, and azathioprine, 2 mg/kg/day or less.

After full prepregnancy assessment has been undertaken, advice can then be given, but it can only be advice, since patients must ultimately decide for themselves what degree of risk is acceptable. Major concern is that the mother may not survive or remain well enough to raise the child she bears. Average survival figures of large numbers of patients from all over the world indicate that between 60% to 80% of recipients of kidneys from related living donors are alive 5 years after transplantation, and with cadaver kidneys the figure is 40% to 50% (Advisory Committee to Renal Transplant Registry, 1977; U.K. Transplant Service Annual Report, 1980). Functional survival of the allograft at 5 years is 45% to 65% in recipients of living donor kidneys and 30% to 35% in recipients of cadaver kidneys. Nevertheless, many patients choose parenthood in an effort to reestablish a normal life and possibly in defiance of the sometimes negative attitude of the medical establishment.

ACUTE RENAL FAILURE

Acute renal failure is a clinical syndrome characterized by a sudden and marked decrease in glomerular filtration, rising plasma urea and creatinine levels, and usually a decrease in urine output to below 400 ml in 24 hours. As a clinical diagnosis the term only describes the functional state of the kidneys without distinguishing between the different forms of underlying disease. For the most part, acute renal failure occurs in persons with previously healthy kidneys, but it may also complicate the course of patients with preexisting renal disease.

Twenty years ago the incidence of acute renal failure in pregnancy was around 0.02% to 0.05% (Kerr and Elliott, 1963) and represented about 20% of cases reported from large series (Kleinkrecht and Ganeval, 1965). At that time acute renal failure was a substantial cause of maternal mortality, since at least 20% of women with this complication died (Smith et al., 1968).

Recently there have been marked declines in cases of acute renal failure related to obstetrics, largely attributable to liberalization of abortion laws and improvements in perinatal care, thus avoiding such complications as sepsis, eclampsia, hypovolemia, and severe hemorrhage (Hawkins et al., 1975). The current incidence is probably less than 0.01% but still has the classical bimodal distribution corresponding to septic abortion in early pregnancy and preeclampsia and bleeding problems in the third trimester (Lindheimer et al., 1982). In contrast to the situation in developed countries, there are still parts of the world where the incidence of severe acute obstetrical renal failure remains high, and Chugh et al. (1976) have reported that 22% of 325 patients admitted to their unit in Northern India had complaints related to pregnancy, and 55% of these women died.

By far the majority of patients with acute renal failure have acute tubular necrosis, and on rare occasions glomerular or obstructive nephropathy occurs. However, in contradistinction to the etiologic breakdown in nonpregnant populations, a substantial number of cases are caused by acute cortical necrosis. Such cases are apt to occur late in pregnancy and seem to be frequently associated with preeclampsia and abruptio placentae. The reaons why pregnant women are so susceptible to acute cortical necrosis, the relationship of cortical necrosis to coagulopathy, and the management of acute renal failure are detailed elsewhere (Lindheimer et al., 1982).

Although necrosis may involve the entire renal cortex, causing irreversible anuria, it is usually the "patchy" variety that occurs more often in pregnancy. The latter is characterized by an initial episode of severe oliguria followed by a variable return of function and a stable period of moderate renal insufficiency (Grünfeld et al., 1980). Years later, for reasons still obscure renal function decreases again, often approaching terminal renal failure (Kleinknecht et al., 1973).

There are two rare forms of acute renal failure peculiar to pregnancy (Sun et al., 1975; Williams, 1977; Lindheimer et al., 1982). The first form, acute fatty liver of pregnancy (also called obstetrical pseudoacute yellow atrophy), is characterized by jaundice and severe hepatic dysfunction in late pregnancy or the early postpartum period. The renal failure appears to be caused by hemodynamic factors, as in the "hepatorenal syndrome," but some cases have been associated with intravascular coagulation. Recently, reversible urea cycle enzyme abnormalities resembling those seen in Reye's syndrome have been described (Weber et al., 1979). The mortality is high, with death resulting primarily from hepatic rather than renal failure.

The second form of renal failure peculiar to pregnancy goes by a variety of names, including idiopathic postpartum renal failure, or hemolytic-uremic syndrome. The patient usually has an uncomplicated pregnancy and delivery but 3 to 6 weeks into the puerperium develops severe hypertension and uremia, often accompanied by microangiopathic hemolytic anemia (Segonds et al., 1979). Pathophysiology and management have been discussed elsewhere (Remuzzi et al., 1979; Webster et al., 1980; Lindheimer et al., 1982), but suffice it to say that to date most women with this type of renal failure have died and those who survived had markedly reduced renal function.

FETAL UPPER URINARY TRACT

With the improved resolution of gray-scale ultrasound equipment and the availability of high-resolution real-time instrumentation, visualization of the fetal urinary tract can be undertaken. The normal fetal kidneys can be seen as oval areas of decreased echogenicity in the lumbar paraspinal regions, although care must be taken not to confuse them with the psoas muscles, especially in transverse views (Bernaschek and Kratochwil, 1980). Occasionally, fluid can be seen within the normal renal pelves. Since it can often be difficult to visualize normal fetal kidneys in routine scanning, their absence may not be detected. However, in the presence of oligohydramnios a careful search for fetal kidneys and bladder should always be made. The prenatal diagnosis of renal agenesis, or Potter's syndrome, can influence antenatal decision making (Cooperberg, 1980).

The two important abnormalities that can initially occur as abnormal cystic swellings in the fetal flank are multicystic kidney and hydronephrosis caused by pelviureteric junction obstruction (Lee and Blake, 1977). When compatible with life, multicystic kidney is a unilateral abnormality in which there is an atretic ureter and absence of a renal pelvis and calyces. Other abnormalities that can mimic unilateral cystic structures in the fetal renal area include ovarian cysts, gastrointestinal obstruction, mesenteric cysts, or duplication cysts of the gastrointestinal tract (Lee and Warren, 1977).

REFERENCES

Advisory Committee to the Renal Transplant Registry. 1977. The thirteenth report of the human renal transplant registry. Transplant Proc. **9:**9-26.

Bailey, R.R., and Rolleston, G.L. 1971. Kidney length and ureteric dilatation in the puerperium. Br. J. Obstet. Gynaecol. **78:**55-61.

Bear, R.A. 1976. Pregnancy in patients with renal disease: a study of 44 cases. Obstet. Gynecol. **48:**13-18.

Beaufils, M., et al. 1981. Metabolism of uric acid in normal and pathologic pregnancy. Contrib. Nephrol. **25:**132-136.

Beilin, L.J., Redman, C.W.G., and Bonnar, J. 1974. Hypertension in pregnancy. Adv. Med. **10:**3-20.

Bellina, J.H., Bougherty, C.M., and Mickal, A. 1970. Pyeloureteral dilatation and pregnancy. Am. J. Obstet. Gynecol. **108:**356-361.

Bernaschek, G., and Kratochwil, A. 1980. Echographische Studie über das Wachstum der fetalen Niere in der zweiten Schwangerschaftshälfte. Geburtshilfe Frauenheitkd **40:**1059-1064.

Bishop, J.H., and Green, R. 1979. Effects of pregnancy on glucose handling by distal segments of the rat nephron (proceedings). J. Physiol. **289:**74P-75P.

Chesley, L.C. 1978. Hypertension in pregnancy. New York. Appleton-Century-Crofts.

Chesley, L.C., and Sloan, D.M. 1964. The effect of posture on renal function in late pregnancy. Am. J. Obstet. Gynecol. **89:**754-759.

Chesley, L.C., and Valenti, C. 1958. The evaluation of tests to differentiate pre-eclampsia from hypertensive disease. Am. J. Obstet. Gynecol. **75:**1165-1173.

Chesley, L.C., and Williams, L.O. 1945. Renal glomerular and tubular function in relation to the hyperuricemia of pre-eclampsia and eclampsia. Am. J. Obstet. Gynecol. **50:**367-375.

Chugh, K.S., et al. 1976. Acute renal failure of obstetric origin. Obstet. Gynecol. **48:**642-646.

Cooperberg, P.L. 1980. Abnormalities of the fetal genitourinary tract. In Sander, R.C., and James, A.E., editors. The principles and practice of ultrasonography in obstetrics and gynecology. New York. Appleton-Century-Crofts.

Davison, J.M. 1975. Renal nutrient excretion. Clin. Obstet. Gynaecol. **2:**365-380.

Davison, J.M. 1978. Changes in renal function in early pregnancy in women with one kidney. Yale J. Biol. Med. **51:**347-349.

Davison, J.M., and Dunlop, W. 1980. Renal hemodynamics and tubular function in normal human pregnancy. Kidney Int. **18:**152-161.

Davison, J.M., and Hytten, F.E. 1974. Glomerular filtration during and after pregnancy. Br. J. Obstet. Gynaecol. **81:**588-595.

Davison, J.M., and Hytten, F.E. 1975. The effect of pregnancy on the renal handling of glucose. Br. J. Obstet. Gynaecol. **82:**374-381.

Davison, J.M., and Lindheimer, M.D. 1980. Changes in renal haemodynamics and kidney weight during pregnancy in the unanaesthetised rat. J. Physiol. **301:**129-136.

Davison, J.M., and Lindheimer, M.D. 1982. Gynaecological and obstetrical problems after renal transplantation. Nieren und Hochdruckkrankheiten. **11:**258-265.

Davison, J.M., and Lovedale, C. 1974. The excretion of glucose during normal pregnancy and after delivery. Br. J. Obstet. Gynaecol. **81:**30-34.

Davison, J.M., and Noble, M.C.B. 1981. Serial changes in 24-hour creatinine clearance during normal menstrual cycles and the first trimester of pregnancy. Br. J. Obstet. Gynaecol. **88:**10-17.

Davison, J.M., Dunlop, W., and Ezimokhai, M. 1980. Twenty-four hour creatinine clearance during the third trimester of normal pregnancy. Br. J. Obstet. Gynaecol. **87:**106-109.

Davison, J.M., Lind, T., and Uldall, P.R. 1976. Planned pregnancy in a renal transplant recipient. Br. J. Obstet. Gynaecol. **83:**518-527.

Davison, J.M., Vallotton, M.B., and Lindheimer, M.D. 1981. Plasma osmolality and urinary concentration and dilution during and after pregnancy: evidence that lateral recumbency inhibits maximal urinary concentrating ability. Br. J. Obstet. Gynaecol. **88:**472-479.

Diamond, H.S., and Miesel, A.D. 1975. Post-secretory reabsorption or urate in man. Arthritis Rheum. **18:**805-809.

Dunlop, W. 1976. Investigations into the influence of posture on renal plasma flow and glomerular filtration rate during late pregnancy. Br. J. Obstet. Gynaecol. **83:**17-23.

Dunlop, W. 1981. Serial changes in renal haemodynamics during normal human pregnancy. Br. J. Obstet. Gynaecol. **88:**1-9.

Dunlop, W., and Davison, J.M. 1977. The effect of pregnancy upon the renal handling of uric acid. Br. J. Obstet. Gynaecol. **84:**13-21.

Dunlop, W., and Davison, J.M. 1978. Plasma urate changes in pre-eclampsia. Br. Med. J. **1:**786.

Dunlop, W., Furness, C., and Hill, L.M. 1978. Maternal haemoglobin concentration, haematocrit and renal handling of urate in pregnancies ending in the births of small-for-dates infants. Br. J. Obstet. Gynaecol. **85:**938-940.

Dunlop, W., et al. 1978. Clinical relevance of coagulation and renal changes in pre-eclampsia. Lancet **2:**346-349.

Dure-Smith, P. 1970. Pregnancy dilatation of the urinary tract. Radiology **96:**545-550.

Emmanouel, D.S., Lindheimer, M.D., and Katz, A.I. 1980. Pathogenesis of endocrine abnormalities in uremia. Endocrine Rev. **1:**28-44.

Evans, T.J., McCollum, J.P.K., and Valdimasson, H. 1975. Congenital cytomegalovirus infection after maternal renal transplantation. Lancet **1:**1359-1360.

Ezimokhai, M., et al. 1981. Non-postural serial changes in renal function during the third trimester of normal human pregnancy. Br. J. Obstet. Gynaecol. **88:**465-471.

Fairley, K.F., Whitworth, J.A., and Kincaid-Smith, P. 1973. Glomerulonephritis and pregnancy. In Kincaid-Smith, P., et al., editors. Glomerulonephritis, New York. John Wiley & Sons, Inc.

Feinstat, T. 1963. Ureteral dilatation in pregnancy: a review. Obstet. Gynecol. Surv. **18:**845-852.

Felding, C.F. 1969. Obstetric aspects of women with histories of renal disease. Acta Obstet. Gyencol. Scand. (Suppl.) **48:**2-43.

First, M.R., et al. 1978. Pre-eclampsia with the nephrotic syndrome. Kidney Int. **13:**166-177.

Fisher, K.A., et al. 1980. A biopsy study of hypertension in pregnancy. In Bonnar, J., MacGillivray, I., and Symonds, E.M., editors. Pregnancy hypertension. England. MTP Press.

Fisher, K.A., et al. 1981. Hypertension in pregnancy: clinical-pathological correlations and late prognosis. Medicine **60:**267-287.

Grünfeld, J.P., Ganeval, D., and Bournerias, F. 1980. Acute renal failure in pregnancy. Kidney Int. **18:**179-191.

Gutman, A.B., Yu, T.F., and Berger, L. 1969. Tubular secretion of urate in man. Arthritis Rheum. **38:**1778-1781.

Hawkins, O.F., et al. 1975. Management of chemical septic abortion with renal failure: use of a conservative regimen. N. Engl. J. Med. **292:**722-725.

Heidrick, W.P., Mattingly, R.F., and Amberg, J.R. 1967. Vesicoureteral reflux in pregnancy. Obstet. Gynecol. **29:**571-576.

Hill, L.M., Furness, C., and Dunlop, W. 1977. Diurnal variation of serum urate in pregnancy. Br. Med. J. **2:**1250.

Holmes, E.W., and Kelley, W.N. 1975. An analysis of the bidirectional transport of uric acid by the human nephron. Arthritis Rheum. **18:**811-816.

Kaplan, A.L., Smith, J.P., and Tillman, A.J.B. 1962. Healed acute and chronic nephritis in pregnancy. Am. J. Obstet. Gynecol. **83:**1519-1525.

Katz, A.I., et al. 1980. Pregnancy in women with kidney disease. Kidney Int. **18:**192-206.

Katz, A.I., et al. 1981. Effect of pregnancy on the natural history of kidney disease. Contrib. Nephrol. **25:**53-60.

Kaufmann, J.J., et al. 1967. Successful normal childbirth after kidney homotransplantation. J.A.M.A. **200:**162-165.

Kauppilla, A., Satuli, R., and Vuorinen, P. 1972. Ureteric dilatation and renal cortical index after normal and pre-eclamptic pregnancies. Acta Obstet. Gynecol. Scand. **51:**147-152.

Kerr, D.N.S., and Elliott, R.W. 1963. Renal disease in pregnancy. Practitioner **190:**459-464.

Kincaid-Smith, P., Fairley, K.F., and Byllen, M. 1967. Kidney disease and pregnancy. Med. J. Aust. **2:**1155-1159.

Kleinknecht, D., et al. 1973. Diagnostic procedures and long-term prognosis in bilateral renal cortical necrosis. Kidney Int. **4:**390-400.

Kleinknecht, D., and Ganeval, D. 1965. Preventive hemodialysis in acute renal failure: its effect on mortality. In Friedman, E.A., and Eliahou, H.E., editors. Proceedings of Conference on Acute Renal Failure. Department of Health, Education and Welfare Publications (NIH) 74-608. Washington, D.C. U.S. Government Printing Office.

Klockars, M., et al. 1980. Pregnancy in patients with renal disease. Acta Med. Scand. **207:**207-214.

Kuhlback, B., and Widholm, O. 1966. Plasma creatinine in normal pregnancy. Scand. J. Clin. Lab. Invest. **18:**654-658.

Lee, T.G., and Blake, S. 1977. Prenatal fetal abdominal ultrasonography and diagnosis. Radiology **124:**475-477.

Lee, T.G., and Warren, B.H. 1977. Antenatal ultrasonic demonstration of fetal bowel. Radiology **124:**471-474.

Lim, V.S., Katz, A.I., and Lindheimer, M.D. 1977. Acid-base metabolism in pregnancy. Am. J. Physiol. **231:**1764-1769.

Lim, V.S., et al. 1980. Ovarian function in chronic renal failure: evidence suggesting hypothalaemic anovulation. Ann, Intern. Med. **57:**7-12.

Lindheimer, M.D., and Katz, A.I. 1981a. Pathophysiology of pre-eclampsia. Ann. Rev. Med. **32:**273-289.

Lindheimer, M.D., and Katz, A.I. 1981b. The renal response to pregnancy. In Brenner, B.M. and Rector, F.C., Jr., editors. The kidney. ed. 2. Philadelphia. W.B. Saunders Co.

Lindheimer, M.D., Spargo, B.H., and Katz, A.I. 1975. Renal biopsy in pregnancy-induced hypertension. J. Reprod. Med. **15:**189-194.

Lindheimer, M.D., et al. Renal failure in pregnancy. In Brenner, B.M., Lazarus, J.H., and Myers, B.D., editors. 1982. Acute renal failure. Philadelphia. W.B. Saunders Co.

Mattingly, R.F., and Borkowf, H.I. 1978. Clinical implications of ureteral reflux in pregnancy. Clin. Obstet. Gynecol. **21:**863-873.

Meares, E.M. 1978. Urologic surgery during pregnancy. Clin. Obstet. Gynecol. **21:**907-915.

Merkatz, I.R., et al. 1971. Resumption of female reproductive function following renal transplantation. J.A.M.A. **216:**1749-1754.

Nolton, W.E., and Ehrlich, E.N. 1980. Sodium and mineralocorticoids in normal pregnancy. Kidney Int. **18:**162-172.

Penn, I., Makowski, E.L., and Harris, R. 1980. Parenthood following renal transplantation. Kidney Int. **18:**221-233.

Pippig, L. 1969. Clinical aspects of renal disease during pregnancy. Med. Hygiene **27:**181-184.

Pollak, V.E., and Nettles, J.B. 1960. The kidney in toxaemia of pregnancy: a clinical and pathological study based on renal biopsies. Medicine **39:**469-477.

Pregnancy after renal transplantation (editorial). 1976. Br. Med. J. **1:**733-734.

Redman, C.W.G., et al. Plasma urate measurements in predicting fetal death in hypertensive pregnancy. Lancet **1**:1370-1373.

Remuzzi, G., et al. 1979. Treatment of haemolytic uraemic syndrome with plasma. Clin. Nephrol. **12**:279-284.

Rieselbach, R.H., and Steele, T.H. 1974. Influence of the kidney upon urate homeostasis in health and disease. Am. J. Med. **56**:665-675.

Rifle, G., and Traeger, J. 1975. Pregnancy after renaltransplantation: an international review. Transplant. Proc. **7**(Suppl. 1):723-728.

Roberts, J. 1976. Hydronephrosis of pregnancy. Urology **8**:1-5.

Robertson, E.G., and Cheyne, G.A. 1972. Plasma biochemistry in relation to oedema of pregnancy. Br. J. Obstet. Gynaecol. **79**:769-776.

Rubi, R.A., and Sala, N.L. 1968. Ureteral function in pregnant women. III. Effects of different positions and fetal delivery upon uterine tonus. Am. J. Obstet. Gynecol. **101**:230-237.

Rudolph, J.E., Scwihizir, R.T., nd Barius, S.A. 1979. Pregnancy in renal transplant patients: a review. Transplantation **27**:26-29.

Schloss, W.A., and Solomkin, M. 1952. Acute hydronephrosis of pregnancy. J. Urol. **68**:885-888.

Segonds, A., et al. 1979. Postpartum hemolytic uremic syndrome: a study of three cases with a review of the literature. Clin. Nephrol. **12**:229-242.

Sheehan, H.L., and Lynch, J.B. 1973. Pathology of toxaemias of pregnancy. Edinburgh. Churchill-Livingstone.

Sims, E.A.H., and Krantz, K.E. 1958. Studies of renal function during pregnancy and the puerperium in normal women. J. Clin. Invest. **37**:1764-1774.

Smith, K., et al. 1968. Renal failure of obstetric origin. Br. Med. Bull. **24**:49-56.

Spiro, F.I., and Fry, I.K. 1970. Ureteric dilatations in nonpregnant women. Proc. R. Soc. Med. **63**:462-464.

Strauch, B.S., and Hayslett, J.P. 1974. Kidney disease and pregnancy. Br. Med. J. **4**:578-582.

Sun, N.C., et al. 1975. Idiopathic postpartum renal failure: review and report of a successful renal transplantation. Mayo Clin. Proc. **50**:395-401.

Tenney, B., and Dandrow, R.V. 1961. Clinical study of hypertensive disease in pregnancy. Am. J. Obstet. Gynecol. **81**:8-15.

United Kingdom Transplant Service. 1980. Annual report. pp. 26-36.

Weber, F.L., et al. 1979. Abnormalities of hepatic mitochondrial urea-cycle enzyme activities and hepatic ultrastructure in acute fatty liver of pregnancy. J. Lab. Clin. Med. **94**:27-41.

Webster, J., et al. 1980. Prostacyclin deficiency in haemolytic-uraemic syndrome. Br. Med. J. **281**(6235):271.

Wenn, S.F., and Stoll, R.W. 1979. Effect of volume expansion on renal glucose transport in normal and uremic dogs. Am. J. Physiol. **236**:567-574.

Werko, L., and Bucht, H. 1956. Glomerular filtration rate and renal blood flow in patients with chronic diffuse glomerulonephritis during pregnancy. Acta Med. Scandin. **153**:177-186.

Williams, G. 1977. Renal disease in pregnancy. J. Pathol. **29** (suppl. 10):77-90.

chapter 34

Clinical aspects of the lower urinary tract in pregnancy

RICHARD H.G. KERR-WILSON

Previous reviews on the lower urinary tract in pregnancy have tended to be limited to particular aspects (Brown, 1978, 1981; Buchsbaum and Schmidt, 1978; Marchant, 1978; Davison, 1980; Waltzer, 1981). It is the aim of this chapter to take an overall look at the urinary tract from the point of view of the practicing obstetrician, with the exclusion of renal disease in pregnancy and pregnancy in renal transplant recipients, which have already been mentioned in Chapter 33. Urinary tract infections (see Chapter 24) and underlying physiological changes (see Chapter 33) have also been discussed and will not be considered in detail here.

NORMAL PREGNANCY
Urinary symptoms

Frequency is the most common urological symptom that occurs during pregnancy. Francis (1960a) defined frequency as voiding seven or more times during the day and once or more at night. Using these criteria, she found that 81% of a group of 400 normal pregnant women noted frequency at some stage of pregnancy. Using the definition given by the International Continence Society (see Appendix II), voiding seven or more times during the day and twice or more at night, Stanton, Kerr-Wilson, and Grant Harris (1980) found frequency to be more common in nulliparous women than in parous women. Parboosingh and Doig (1973) defined nocturia as emptying the bladder during sleeping hours on 3 or more nights of the week. Over half of their patients suffered from nocturia, irrespective of the stage of pregnancy. They noted that most of their patients accepted nocturia as being a normal feature of pregnancy; less than 4% were distressed by it.

The most common time of onset of frequency in pregnancy is the first trimester. The symptom usually becomes worse as pregnancy progresses (Francis, 1960a) but resolves by the time of the postnatal visit (Stanton, Kerr-Wilson, and Grant Harris, 1980). There does not appear to be any relationship between engagement of the fetal presenting part and frequency in the last 4 weeks of pregnancy (Stanton, Kerr-Wilson and Grant Harris, 1980).

Francis (1960a) discussed the various theories put forward to explain urinary frequency during pregnancy. Basing her conclusions on cystometrograms performed on 150 pregnant and nonpregnant women, she dismissed mechanical pressure of the uterus and increased bladder instability as causes of frequency in the first two trimesters. In her study, 100 normal pregnant women were asked to measure their fluid intake and output, and the findings were compared with a control series of 50 nonpregnant patients. She concluded that frequency during pregnancy is caused by an increase in fluid intake and urinary output (Table 34.1). This idea was given support by the evidence of Parboosingh and Doig. They showed that the major cause of nocturnal frequency in the first and second trimesters is a marked increase in overnight urine flow,

which they considered to be mainly the result of a raised overnight sodium excretion (Figure 34.1). Further work remains to be carried out to explain more fully the cause of the polydipsia and polyuria of early pregnancy.

Stress incontinence is still commonly thought to occur as a result of the act of childbirth itself. Francis (1960b), however, demonstrated that it is not parturition but pregnancy that predisposes a woman to stress incontinence. She found that 53% of primigravidae and 85% of multigravidae experienced stress incontinence of some kind during pregnancy; moreover, stress incontinence rarely, if ever, appeared for the first time after childbirth. Following delivery, 91% of women who had stress incontinence during pregnancy reported almost complete relief within a few days. The remaining 9% continued to suffer urethral incompetence as a permanent disability. She concluded that pregnancy rather than labor reveals an intrinsic defect in the sphincter mechanism; in few women can the onset of symptoms be attributed to childbirth itself. Her findings were supported by those of Beck and Hsu (1965) (Table 34.2). Most of their patients developed stress incontinence during pregnancy, and the delivery itself did not appear to be a major factor.

Stanton, Kerr-Wilson, and Grant Harris (1980) agreed that stress incontinence rarely appears de novo after childbirth if it has not already occurred during pregnancy. As with frequency, they also found no relationship between the prevalence of stress incontinence during the last 4 weeks of pregnancy and the degree of engagement of the fetal presenting part.

TABLE 34.1   Average daily fluid intake and urinary output

| No. of women | Pregnant women | | | | | | Nonpregnant women | |
| | First trimester | | Second trimester | | Third trimester | | | |
	Intake (ml)	Output (ml)	Intake (ml)	Output (ml)	Intake (ml)	Output (ml)	Intake (ml)	Output (ml)
40	1993	1895						
30			2065	2021				
30					1904	1765		
50							1434	1475

From Francis, W.J.A. 1960. J. Obstet. Gynaecol. Br. Emp. **67**:353-366.

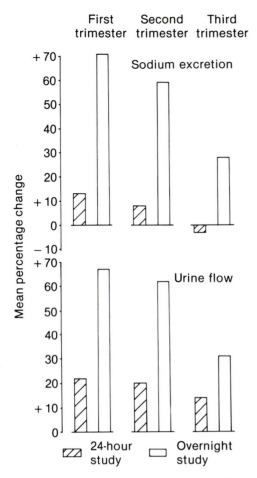

Figure 34.1 Mean sodium excretion and urine flow during 24-hour and overnight periods. Results in each trimester are expressed as percentage change relative to appropriate nonpregnant mean value. (From Parboosingh, J., and Doig A. 1973. Br. J. Obstet. Gynecol. **80**:893.)

TABLE 34.2   Time of onset of stress incontinence in 1000 random cases

	No. of cases	Stress-incontinent cases (%)
During pregnancy	202	64.5
During puerperium	44	14.1
In nulligravid state	43	13.7
After menopause	8	2.6
Miscellaneous	16	5.1
TOTALS	313	100.0

From Beck, R.P., and Hsu, N. 1965. Am. J. Obstet. Gynecol. **91**:820-823.

Stanton, Kerr-Wilson, and Grant Harris did find a slight increase in hesitancy during pregnancy. Following delivery, however, there was a marked improvement, with fewer women affected by hesitancy than before pregnancy.

Urge incontinence is the loss of urine associated with a strong desire to void; its prevalence increases during pregnancy and is not affected by descent of the presenting part. The condition is aggravated by pregnancy, so that more women suffer from it after pregnancy than before (Stanton, Kerr-Wilson, and Grant Harris, 1980).

Urodynamic studies

Results of urodynamic investigations during pregnancy have not always been consistent. This may well be a result of variations in the degree of sophistication of equipment used and of differences in the conditions under which measurements were performed. Early studies indicated an increase in bladder capacity and a decrease in intravesical pressure as pregnancy progressed. More recent experience has suggested the opposite.

Youssef (1956) carried out single intravesical pressure recordings on 10 pregnant women using a glass catheter as a simple manometer. From the early months of pregnancy, he found that the intravesical pressure was lower than normal, the first desire to void was felt between 250 and 400 ml, and the "maximum urinary urge" was not reached until the bladder contained 1000 to 1200 ml. These changes persisted into the first week of the puerperium. Francis (1960a), however, performed cystometrograms on 50 women in each trimester. She found that the average bladder capacity and the intravesical pressure remained unchanged until late in the third trimester, when there was a reduction in bladder capacity. Clow (1975) noted an increase in resting supine intravesical pressure throughout pregnancy in 25 normal pregnant women on whom cystometry was performed. Intravesical pressure rose from a nonpregnant level of 4 to 8 cm H_2O to 15 to 20 cm H_2O at term. More recently, using a twin microtip transducer catheter, Iosif, Ingemarsson, and Ulmsten (1980) obtained similar results. Simultaneous bladder and urethral pressures were measured at 12 to 16 weeks' gestation, at 38 weeks' gestation, and again 5 to 7 days after delivery in 14 healthy nulliparous women who did not experience stress incontinence. They found that the bladder pressure increased from 9 to 20 cm

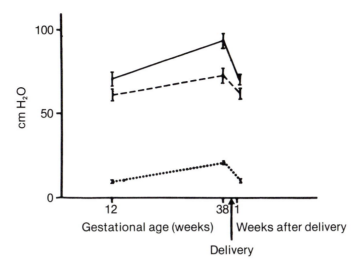

Figure 34.2 Change in maximum urethral pressure *(continuous line)*, urethral closure pressure *(dashed line)*, the bladder pressure *(dotted line)* during pregnancy and puerperium. From Iosif, S., Ingemarsson, I., and Ulmsten U. 1980. Am. J. Obstet. Gynecol. **137**:696-700. With kind permission of the authors.)

H_2O between the first and second recording and returned to its initial value after delivery (Figure 34.2). The anatomical and functional urethral length and maximum urethral pressure increased during pregnancy up until 38 weeks' gestation and after that began to decline to less than the antepartum values. As a result of changes in the urethral and bladder pressure, the urethral closure pressure increased during pregnancy up to 38 weeks' gestation and fell thereafter. The finding of a rise in bladder pressure in late pregnancy suggests a reduction in bladder capacity.

The study of urethral pressure changes was taken further by Van Geelen (1981), who investigated pressure changes in relation to mode of delivery, length of the second stage of labor, episiotomy, and serum levels of sex hormones (17 β-estradiol, progesterone, and 16 α-hydroxyprogesterone). He investigated 42 healthy nulliparous women and found that the total bladder pressure and maximum urethral pressure increased by a similar amount in both the sitting and supine positions and that the urethral closure pressure hardly varied. The rapidly increasing levels of estradiol and progesterone did not influence these parameters. In patients delivered vaginally, almost all the parameters were significantly decreased at 8 weeks postpartum, compared with early pregnancy; this decrease did not occur in women delivered by cesarean section. The postpartum change was unaffected by the length of the second stage or by the episiotomy (Figure 34.3). The anatomical urethral length gradually increased in pregnancy, whereas the functional urethral length did not change (Figure 34.4). These changes act toward maintaining continence.

The bladder and labor

Distension of the urinary bladder is often considered to be a factor in delaying the progress of labor. Kantor, Miller, and Dunlap (1949), following radiological and cystometric studies performed during labor, concluded that the distended bladder can obstruct descent early in labor until the presenting part is well below the ischial spines. According to their findings, once the presenting part is on or near the pelvic floor, the bladder usually presents no obstruction. Toppozada, Gaafar, and El-Sahwi (1967) also found the full bladder to have an inhibitory effect on uterine activity. They assessed the effect of catheterization on tocodynagraphic activity in 42 patients in the first stage of labor. Each woman had at least 300 ml of urine in her bladder, and after catheterization there was an overall increase in tocodynagraphic activity. On the other hand, in a recent study, Read et al. (1980) suggest that emptying the urinary bladder has no effect on the course of labor. They studied 68 patients in the active phase of labor for 30 minutes before and after catheterization. They found that changes in uterine activity, cervical dilatation, and descent of the fetal presenting part conformed to the normal labor pattern and were unchanged by catheterization. However, less than half of their patients had more than 300 ml of urine at cathe-

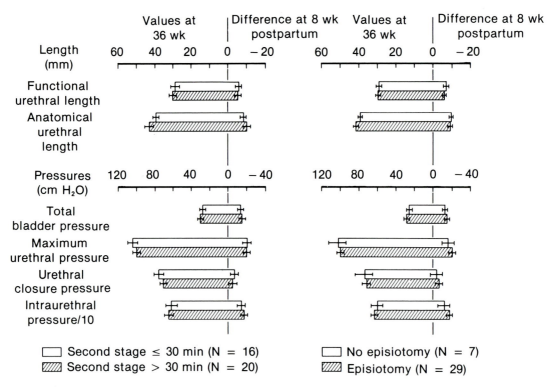

Figure 34.3 Effect of duration of second stage of labor and of presence or absence of episiotomy on functional and anatomical urethral length, total bladder pressure, maximum urethral pressure, and urethral closure pressure. (From Van Geelen, J.M. 1981. International Continence Society annual meeting. Lund.)

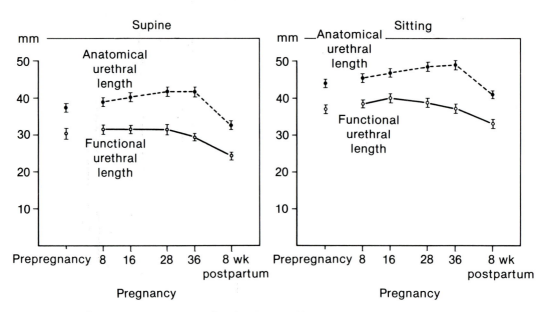

Figure 34.4 Change in anatomical and functional urethral length in supine and sitting positions. (From Van Geelen, J.M. 1981. International Continence Society annual meeting. Lund.)

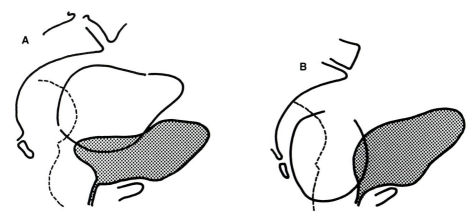

Figure 34.5 Bladder after 1 hour, **A,** and after 19 hours, **B,** of labor. Bladder base has become rotated and vesicourethral junction is funnel shaped. (Modified from Malpas, P., Jeffcoate, T.N.A., and Lister, U.M. 1949. J. Obstet. Gynaecol Br. Emp. **56:**949-960.)

terization. Their conclusions may well therefore be invalid for large volumes of urine, and until their findings are confirmed, it seems reasonable to continue to catheterize patients with distended bladders in the first stage of labor.

During the second stage of labor routine catheterization before spontaneous delivery or the application of low forceps should be abandoned. Kantor, Miller, and Dunlap (1949) concluded that routine catheterization is unnecessary in these cases, and even moderate distension of the bladder will not interfere with delivery.

The reciprocal effect of labor itself on the bladder and urethra was carefully examined by Malpas, Jeffcoate, and Lister (1949). They studied 32 women radiologically during labor and found that as labor advanced, the bladder neck became displaced forward but not upward in normal labor, and the length of the urethra remained unchanged. The vesicourethral junction became funnel shaped as a result of the bladder base being ''rolled up'' toward the lower abdomen (Figure 34.5). There was an immediate return of the bladder base and urethra to normal after delivery. They concluded that it was the rotation of the bladder base from the horizontal to the vertical that stretched the fascial investment and led to stress incontinence. Although it is difficult to confirm these findings, since such studies in labor would now be considered unethical, the conclusions have been disputed by more recent studies (Francis, 1960a; Stanton, Kerr-Wilson, and Grant Harris, 1980). These authors have shown that it is pregnancy rather than labor itself that predisposes patients to stress incontinence.

Postpartum bladder

Bennetts and Judd (1941) performed cystoscopy and intravesical measurements on 105 patients from 36 to 60 hours after vaginal delivery. Of 94 patients in whom a residual urine volume was measured, 34% had a volume greater than 250 ml, and in 6% the volume was in excess of 500 ml. At cystometry, they found hypotonic bladders with decreased bladder sensation and increased capacity in over 80% of their patients. The average bladder capacity in this group was over 865 ml, and the average detrusor pressure was less than 30 cm H_2O. These findings were independent of the type of delivery, trauma at delivery, or intrapartum analgesia. Youssef (1956), in his series of only 10 patients, had similar results, with marked hypotonia and increased bladder capacity postpartum. He pointed out that this may be an important factor in predisposing patients to postpartum retention and the formation of residual urine. These urodynamic findings were borne out by Grove (1973), who reported that loss of the desire to micturate was the most common symptom of bladder dysfunction occurring in women following delivery uncomplicated by epidural analgesia. This is most likely the result of transitory interference with the nerve supply to the bladder. Local trauma in the region of the perineum and urethra may cause inability to void but will not remove the desire to do so.

Because the pain of an overdistended bladder may not be felt during labor under epidural anesthesia, it is necessary to ensure that the bladder empties regularly and does not overdistend. If the patient cannot void normally, then intermittent catheterization should be carried out or an indwelling urethral catheter left in place; the latter can be removed within 12 hours of delivery but will need to be replaced if the patient has acute retention of urine.

PREEXISTING URINARY TRACT DISORDERS
Urinary calculi

Loin pain of indeterminate origin is a common problem in the second and third trimesters of pregnancy. The differential diagnosis includes urinary tract infection, concealed antepartum hemorrhage, and appendicitis when the pain is right sided. Calculi are often suspected but less frequently confirmed. Lattanzi and Cook (1980) have presented their results over 5 years and have summarized the data from eight previous studies, giving a total of 90 cases. They found the prevalence of urinary calculi in pregnancy to be approximately 1 per 1500, allowing for some geographical variation. The most common symptoms that they found were the acute onset of loin and iliac fossa pain, with nausea and vomiting in severe cases. Microscopic hematuria was common, but gross hematuria occurred only once. Both sides were affected equally. Symptoms occurred more often in the second and third trimesters. This may result from dilatation of the ureters allowing stones to pass further down the urinary tract, where symptoms are more likely. The only diagnostic problem was distinguishing calculi from pyelonephritis. Confirmation of the diagnosis was usually clear on radiographic examination (Cumming and Taylor, 1979).

Lattanzi and Cook recommended conservative management, since more than half of their patients passed their stones spontaneously. This was higher than that recorded in nonpregnant patients and was probably caused by the dilatation of the ureters that occurs during pregnancy. Surgical procedures when indicated usually consisted of cystoscopy with manipulation, or ureterolithotomy. There was no evidence of any harm to the fetus when such a course of management was followed, and the pregnancy itself proceeded without ill effect, apart from one case of septic shock following ureterolithotomy. Cumming and Taylor (1979) concluded that urinary calculi are readily diagnosed in pregnancy and their management is usually straightforward.

Hematuria

As in the nonpregnant patient, hematuria may be secondary to neoplasms, calculi, or inflammation anywhere in the urinary tract. In practice, hematuria during pregnancy is not common apart from when it is associated with urinary tract infection (see Chapter 24). Spontaneous rupture of a hydronephrotic kidney during pregnancy, followed by discovery of a transitional cell carcinoma of the ureteral stump in the puerperium in the same patient, has been reported (Texter et al., 1980). Another rare cause of hematuria in pregnancy is placenta percreta with invasion of the bladder.

Because of the age of patients who experience hematuria in pregnancy, an aggressive approach to evaluation had been recommended (Waltzer, 1981), although the degree of investigation will depend on the overall condition of the patient and the stage of gestation.

Other lower urinary tract disorders

Other conditions affecting the lower urinary tract not caused by the pregnancy itself are uncommon. Trauma, when it occurs, should be managed as in the nonpregnant patient (Meares, 1978). Urinary tract neoplasia is exceptionally rare in women of childbearing age. There are reports of urethral diverticula causing dystocia and urinary retention in labor (Allen et al., 1969; Brown, 1978), but these are rare.

IMAGING OF THE URINARY TRACT

An intravenous urogram may often given useful information about pregnant patients with loin pain, but obstetricians are naturally reluctant to ask for a full radiographic investigation of the urinary tract because of the risks of radiation to the fetus. It is possible, however, to gain valuable information from a single film taken 15 minutes after the injection of contrast medium. This represents the same radiation dose to the fetus as would result from a straight abdominal radiograph, such as that asked for in assessing fetal abnormality or maturity.

Postpartum intravenous urography for the detection of urinary tract disorders should be postponed for at least 6 weeks. This allows time for the physiological changes in involution to occur.

More recently, ultrasound has been used to help detect dilatation of the urinary tract during pregnancy and may result in the use of radiographs being avoided altogether. Although ureteric calculi may not be detected, hydronephrosis and hydroureter are relatively easily diagnosed.

FETAL URINARY TRACT

Some aspects of the physiology and disorders of the fetal urinary tract are beginning to be diagnosed by the use of ultrasound. The presence of urine in the fetal bladder and the fetal kidneys themselves are easily distinguished (Figure 34.6). Campbell, Wladimiroff, and Dewhurst (1973) suggested that there is cyclical voiding of the fetal bladder, with a mean cycle length of 110 minutes. They assessed the hourly fetal urine production as rising from 12 ml at 32 weeks' gestation to 28 ml at 40 weeks' gestation. More recently, Visser et al. (1981) found the cyclical emptying of the fetal bladder to be associated with changes in the fetal heart rate. They postulated that a low fetal heart rate coincides with

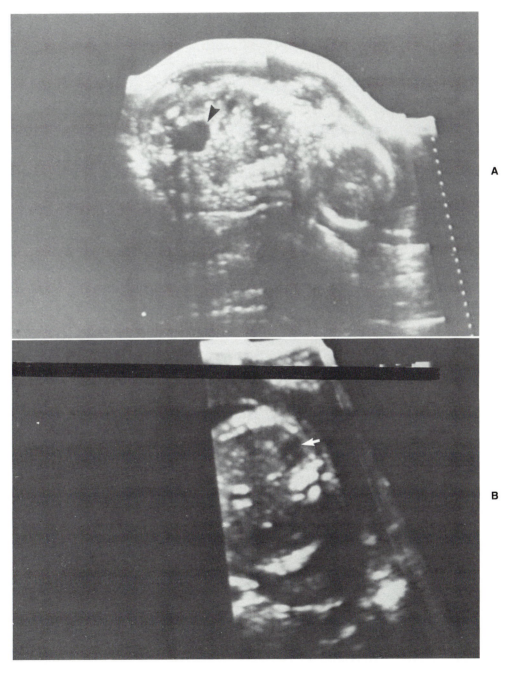

Figure 34.6 A, Ultrasonogram showing longitudinal section of fetus 27 weeks of age. Arrow designates bladder. **B,** Transverse ultrasonogram of fetus 30 weeks of age to show right kidney *(arrow).* (Courtesy of Dr. A. Duncan, Simpson Memorial Maternity Pavilion, Edinburgh, Great Britain.) *Continued.*

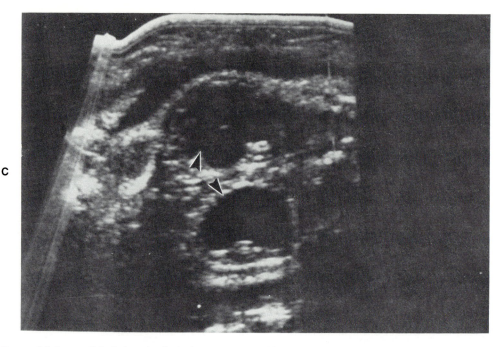

Figure 34.6, cont'd. C, Longitudinal ultrasonsogram of fetus 35 weeks of age showing congenital bilateral hydronephrosis. Fetus was later found to have trisomy 13. Arrows indicate right and left kidney.

quiet sleep and that voiding is related to a change in the sleep state.

PREGNANCY AS A CAUSE OF URINARY TRACT DISORDERS
Clinical implications of ureteral reflux

Vesicoureteral reflux is not found in nonpregnant women, or in the first and second trimesters of pregnancy (Sala and Rubi, 1972). In the last trimester, however, there is a prevalance of 3% to 4% (Heidrick, Mattingly, and Amberg, 1967; Sala and Rubi, 1972). But as Heidrick, Mattingly, and Amberg pointed out, this figure does not distinguish whether reflux occurs in 3% to 4% of all pregnant women in the last trimester, or whether it occurs in all women but only 3% to 4% of the time—a point that still remains to be clarified.

The cause of reflux in pregnancy is likewise not fully understood. Mattingly and Borkowf (1978) are of the opinion that the major factor responsible is anatomical. As pregnancy advances, there is a change in the configuration of the bladder base. The bladder and trigone are elevated into the abdomen, and the ureteral orifices are displaced laterally. This results in a shortening of the intravesical portion of the ureter, and hence a decrease in intraureteral pressure (Figure 34.7). Rubi and Sala, while not contradicting Mattingly and Borkowf, favor a more dynamic explanation. They measured

bladder and ureteral pressures before and during voiding in nonpregnant and pregnant women and found a lower rise in both ureteral and vesical pressures during voiding in pregnant women as compared with nonpregnant women. They postulated that the decreased contraction of the bladder muscles is less efficient at exerting pressure on the intravesical ureter and that the lower ureteral pressure is less effective at counterbalancing the rise in bladder pressure. Under such circumstances, diminished bladder and ureteral pressures during voiding in pregnancy might account for reflux.

The clinical significance of reflux during pregnancy is that it may provide a route for ascending infection with resulting pyelonephritis. Whether this is true cause and effect has by no means been proved. Hutch, Ayres, and Noll (1963), in a small series, found reflux to be present in 5 of 12 subjects in pregnancies complicated by pyelonephritis. Conversely, they found that just over half of a group of 23 pregnant women with proven reflux had pyelonephritis in pregnancy. Heidrick, Mattingly, and Amberg found a history of pyelonephritis occurring during pregnancy in three of nine patients in whom reflux was demonstrated either in the last trimester or immediately postpartum. This compared with 5% of patients in whom reflux was not found. They remarked on the fact that the incidence of ureterovesical reflux and pyelitis of

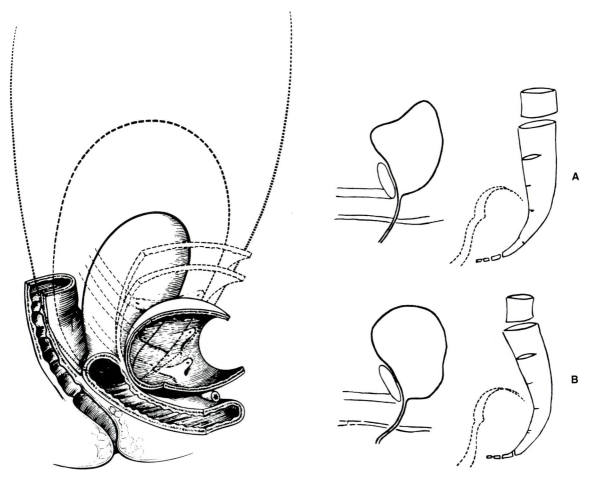

Figure 34.7 Anatomical changes of bladder base with advancing pregnancy, showing elevation of trigone and lateral displacement of ureteral orifices. (From Mattingly, R.F., and Borkowf, H.I. 1978. Clin. Obstet. Gynecol. **21**:863-873.)

Figure 34.8 Tracings of lateral urethrocystographs obtained from patient suffering from acute retention of urine caused by impaction of retroverted gravid uterus at 14 weeks' gestation. **A,** Woman is resting. **B,** Woman is attempting to void. There is no elongation or elevation of urethra. (From Francis, W.J.A. 1960. J. Obstet. Gynaecol. Br. Emp. **67**:353-366.)

pregnancy are identical at 3%. Their comment still holds true, but it remains to be confirmed that the reflux is the source of the ascending infection.

Urinary retention

The classic cause of urinary retention in early pregnancy is incarceration of the retroverted uterus at 12 to 14 weeks' gestation. This has been attributed to mechanical pressure on the neck of the bladder and elongation of the urethra (Myerscough, 1982) Since there is little difficulty in passing a catheter in the initial stages of retention in these cases, the urinary retention is unlikely to be caused by direct pressure of the uterus on the urethra. Francis (1960a) showed in addition that the theory of urethral elongation is not valid. After examining the radiographs of six women who had urethrocystography carried out at the time of retention, she illustrated that there was no elongation of the urethra and no elevation of the urethrovesical junction in these patients (Figure 34.8). She suggested that retention is caused by the retroverted uterus interfering with the normal opening mechanism of the internal urethral meatus. Once retention has been present for some time, edema of the bladder neck may make it difficult to pass a catheter as a secondary effect.

Possible complications of retention caused by a retroverted gravid uterus are abortion, urinary infection, and bladder rupture, either spontaneous or

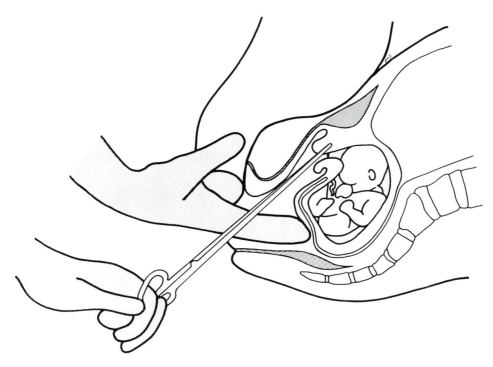

Figure 34.9 Replacement of incarcerated retroflexed uterus, with patient in knee-chest position. (Modified from Myerscough, P.R. 1982. In Munro-Kerr: Operative obstetrics. ed. 10. London. Baillière Tindall.)

as a result of attempts at rectification (Myerscough, 1982). Prophylaxis includes resting in a semiprone position and insertion of a ring pessary. Once retention has occurred, treatment should be aimed at keeping the bladder empty. If this is not successful after a few days, vaginal or rectal manipulation should be tried. If this is still not successful, it is suggested that with the patient in the knee-chest position, pressure should be exerted on the fundus while traction on the anterior lip of the cervix is carried out with vulsellum forceps (Figure 34.9).

The most common time for retention to occur in relation to pregnancy is in the puerperium. Grove (1973) found an incidence of bladder dysfunction of 14% following spontaneous delivery in patients who had not had epidural blocks during labor. Francis (1960a) concluded that retention following vaginal delivery is usually the result of spasm of the voluntary external urethral sphincter caused by pain. She explained retention following cesarean section, on the other hand, as failure of the detrusor muscle to contract. This may be the result of failure to initiate micturition by not contracting the abdominal muscles, it may be secondary to central nervous system inhibition, or it may follow local disturbance of the nerve supply at the time of operation. Postpartum retention can usually be treated

by an episode of urethral catheterization to allow the precipitating factors to resolve. If this is not successful, a cholinergic agent (for example, bethanechol) may be tried. If the patient is still unable to void sponaneously, suprapubic drainage via a Bonanno catheter is recommended while investigations for alternative causes of retention are carried out (see Chapter 21).

Other conditions

Placenta percreta with invasion of the bladder is one uncommon cause of gross hematuria in pregnancy. Two cases were reported in 1970 (Taefi et al.; Grabert et al.). One was in a gravida VIII following six cesarean sections; the other was in a gravida XIII after four cesarean sections. The diagnosis in both cases was made only at the time of laparotomy. In both cases the scars from repeated cesarean sections must have caused fixing of the placental position and weakening of the uterine wall. Complete inversion of the bladder, which usually occurs in the neonate or after the menopause, may rarely occur in labor (Armon, 1974). Replacement of the bladder may be carried out with the patient under general anaesthesia; if this is unsuccessful, injection of hyaluronidase to disperse the edema fluid or reduction by a suprapubic approach may be necessary.

CONCLUSION

Investigation of the urinary tract during pregnancy has moved from static radiographs to more complex urodynamic studies. In spite of this, myths still persist, and much of the new information remains to be verified and corroborated.

REFERENCES

Allen, L.E., et al. 1969. Pelvic dystocia secondary to urethral diverticulum and urinary retention. J. Urol. **102**:451-453.

Armon, P.J. 1974. Complete transurethral inversion of the bladder in labour. Br. J. Obstet. Gynaecol. **81**:822-824.

Beck, R.P., and Hsu, N. 1965. Pregnancy, childbirth, and the menopause related to the development of stress incontinence. Am. J. Obstet. Gynecol. **91**:820-823.

Bennetts, F.A., and Judd, G.E. 1941. Studies of the postpartum bladder. Am. J. Obstet. Gynecol. **42**:419-427.

Brown, A.D.G. 1978. The effects of pregnancy on the lower urinary tract. Clin. Obstet. Gynaecol. **5**:151-168.

Brown, A.D.G. 1981. Urinary tract problems. Hosp. Update **7**:529-536.

Buchsbaum, H.J., and Schmidt, J.D., editors. 1978. Gynecologic and obstetric urology. Philadelphia. W.B. Saunders Co.

Campbell, S., Wladimiroff, J.W., and Dewhurst, C.J. 1973. The antenatal measurement of fetal urine production. Br. J. Obstet. Gynaecol. **80**:680-686.

Chesley, L.C. 1978. Hypertensive disorders in pregnancy. New York. Appleton-Century-Crofts.

Clow, W.M. 1975. Effect of posture on bladder and urethral function in normal pregnancy. Urol. Int. **30**:9-15.

Cumming, D.C., and Taylor, P.J. 1979. Urologic and obstetric significance of urinary calculi in pregnancy. Obstet. Gynecol. **53**:505-508.

Davison, J.M. 1980. The urinary system. In Hytten, F.E., and Chamberlain, G.V.P., editors. Clinical physiology in obstetrics. London. Blackwell Scientific Publications, Ltd.

De Alvarez, R.R. 1978. Preeclampsia-eclampsia and renal diseases in pregnancy. Clin. Obstet. Gynecol. **21**:881-905.

Francis, W.J.A. 1960a. Disturbances of bladder function in relation to pregnancy. J. Obstet. Gynaecol. Br. Emp. **67**:353-366.

Francis, W.J.A. 1960b. The onset of stress incontinence. J. Obstet. Gynaecol. Br. Emp. **67**:899-903.

Grabert, H., et al. 1970. Placenta percreta with penetration of the bladder. Br. J. Obstet. Gynaecol. **77**:1142-1143.

Grove, L.H. 1973. Backache, headache and bladder dysfunction after delivery. Br. J. Anaesth. **45**:1147-1149.

Heidrick, W.P., Mattingly, R.F., and Amberg, J.R. 1967. Vesicoureteral reflux in pregnancy. Obstet. Gynecol. **29**:571-578.

Hutch, J.A., Ayres, R.D., and Noll, L.E. 1963. Vesico-ureteral reflux as cause of pyelonephritis of pregnancy. Am. J. Obstet. Gynecol. **87**:478-485.

Iosif, S., Ingemarsson, I., and Ulmsten, U. 1980. Urodynamic studies in normal pregnancy and in puerperium. Am. J. Obstet. Gynecol. **137**:696-700.

Kantor, H.I., Miller, J.E., and Dunlap, J.C. 1949. The urinary bladder during labour. Am. J. Obstet. Gynecol. **58**:354-365.

Lattanzi, D.R., and Cook, W.A. 1980. Urinary calculi in pregnancy. Obstet. Gynecol. **56**:462-466.

Malpas, P., Jeffcoate, T.N.A., and Lister, U.M. 1949. Displacement of the bladder and urethra during labour. J. Obstet. Gynaecol. Br. Emp. **56**:949-960.

Marchant, D.J. 1978. The urinary tract in pregnancy. Clin. Obstet. Gynecol. **21**:817-944.

Mattingly, R.F., and Borkowf, H.I. 1978. Clinical implications of ureteral reflux in pregnancy. Clin. Obstet. Gynecol. **21**:863-873.

Meares, E.M. 1978. Urologic surgery during pregnancy. Obstet. Gynecol. **21**:907-915.

Myerscough, P.R. 1982. Munro-Kerr's operative obstetrics. ed. 10. London. Baillière Tindall.

Parboosingh, J., and Doig, A. 1973. Studies of nocturia in normal pregnancy. Br. J. Obstet. Gynaecol. **80**:888-895.

Read, J.A., et al. 1980. Urinary bladder distention: effect on labor and uterine activity. Obstet. Gynecol. **56**:565-570.

Rubi, R.A., and Sala, N.L. 1972. Ureteral function in pregnant women. VI. Bladder and lower ureteral pressures during voiding. Am. J. Obstet. Gynecol. **113**:335-339.

Sala, N.L., and Rubi, R.A. 1972. Ureteral function in pregnant women. V. Incidence of vesicoureteral reflux and its effect upon ureteral contractility. Am. J. Obstet. Gynecol. **112**:871-876.

Stanton, S.L., Kerr-Wilson, R., and Grant Harris, V. 1980. The incidence of urological symptoms in normal pregnancy. Br. J. Obstet. Gynaecol. **87**:897-900.

Taefi, P., et al. 1970. Placenta percreta with bladder invasion nd massive haemorrhage: report of case. Obstet. Gynecol. **36**:686-687.

Texter, J.H., et al. 1980. Persistent haematuria during pregnancy. J. Urol. **123**:84-88.

Toppozada, H.K., Gaafar, A.A., and El-Sahwi, S. 1967. The urinary bladder and uterine activity. Am. J. Obstet. Gynecol. **98**:904-912.

Visser, G.H.A., et al. 1981. Micturition and the heart period cycle in the human fetus. Br. J. Obstet. Gynaecol. **88**:803-805.

Van Geelen, J. 1981. The effect of pregnancy and delivery on the urethral pressure profile (UPP) in nulliparae. Proceedings of the eleventh annual meeting of the International Continence Society. Lund. pp. 77-79.

Waltzer, W.C. 1981. The urinary tract in pregnancy. J. Urol. **125**:271-276.

Youssef, A.F. 1956. Cystometric studies in gynecology and obstetrics. Obstet. Gynecol. **8**:181-188.

part FIVE

TREATMENT

chapter 35

Applied pharmacology

ALAN J. WEIN

One of the results of the relatively recent renewed interest in the neurophysiology and neuropharmacology of the urinary bladder and its outlet has been the application of different types of pharmacological therapy to many types of voiding dysfunction. In this chapter current pharmacological treatment of voiding dysfunction within a functional scheme of therapy for disorders of micturition, specifically related to the gynecological patient, will be summarized.

SCHEMA FOR SPECIFIC TREATMENT OF LOWER URINARY TRACT DYSFUNCTION

Many recent reviews are available that describe the physiology and pharmacology of the micturition cycle (Kuru, 1965; Bradley, Timm, and Scott, 1974; Tanagho, 1978; Wein and Raezer, 1979; DeGroat and Booth, 1980; Wein, 1980). Although there are certainly differences in the manner in which each author integrates the relevant data into a theory that describes lower urinary tract function, all of these authors would doubtless agree that voiding function, and therefore voiding dysfunction, could be described in terms of two relatively discrete phases: a filling-storage phase of micturition and an emptying phase. Normal urine storage and urinary continence requires (1) the accommodation of increasing volumes of urine at a low intravesical pressure and with appropriate sensory appreciation, (2) a bladder outlet that is closed during rest and during increases in intraabdominal pressure, and (3) the absence of inappropriate bladder contraction (bladder instability or detrusor hyperreflexia). Normal emptying requires (1) a coordinated bladder contraction of significant magnitude and (2) a concomitant lowering of resistance at the level of the smooth muscle of the bladder neck and proximal urethra and at the level of the striated musculature of the external urethral sphincter.

All types of therapy for voiding dysfunction can, then, be most logically considered within a purely functional classification based on whether the primary problem seems to be one of bladder filling and urine storage or one of urine emptying (Wein, Raezer, and Benson, 1976; Wein, 1979, 1981). A further simplification of this functional classification of therapy occurs when the individual therapeutic modalities are subclassified as to whether they affect the bladder or the bladder outlet. The following outlines illustrate such a functional classification.

Supported in part by a merit review grant from the Veteran's Administration.

Therapy to facilitate bladder emptying

I. Increase intravesical pressure
  A. External compression
  B. Promotion or initiation of reflex contractions
    1. Trigger zones or maneuvers
    2. Bladder training, tidal drainage
  C. Pharmacological manipulation
    1. Parasympathomimetic agents
    2. Blockers of inhibition (?)
    3. Prostaglandins
  D. Electrical stimulation
    1. Directly to bladder
    2. To nerve root or spinal cord
II. Decrease outlet resistance
  A. At level of bladder neck
    1. Transurethral resection or incision
    2. Y-V plasty
    3. Pharmacological inhibition (α-adrenergic blockade)
  B. At level of distal mechanism*
    1. External sphincterotomy
    2. Urethral overdilatation
    3. Pudendal nerve interruption
    4. Pharmacological inhibition
      a. External sphincter/pelvic floor (striated muscle relaxant)
      b. Proximal urethra (α-adrenergic blockade)
    5. Psychotherapy, biofeedback
III. Circumvent problem
  A. Intermittent catheterization
  B. Urinary diversion

Therapy to facilitate urine storage

I. Inhibit bladder contractility
  A. Pharmacological manipulation
    1. Anticholinergic agents
    2. β-Adrenergic stimulation
    3. Musculotropic relaxants
    4. Polysynaptic inhibitors
    5. Calcium antagonists
    6. Prostaglandin inhibitors
  B. Interruption of innervation
    1. Subarachnoid block
    2. Sacral rhizotomy
    3. Bladder denervation (peripheral), cystolysis
  C. Bladder overdistension
  D. Electrical stimulation (reflex inhibition)
  E. Cystoplasty†

*Distal mechanism refers to the smooth muscle of the proximal urethra together with the external (striated muscle) urethral sphincter.
†This procedure primarily augments bladder capacity and only secondarily inhibits bladder contractility by raising the volume thresholds for sensation and distension.

II. Increase outlet resistance
  A. At level of bladder neck
    1. α-Adrenergic stimulation
    2. Vesicourethral suspension
    3. Mechanical compression
  B. At level of distal mechanism
    1. α-Adrenergic stimulation, β-adrenergic blockade (?)
    2. Mechanical compression
    3. Electrical stimulation of pelvic floor
III. Circumvent problem
  A. Intermittent catheterization
  B. Urinary diversion

My colleagues and I have found this classification to be useful from a number of standpoints. First, it is a continual reminder of the goal of the neurourological evaluation, that is, to be able to categorize the primary pathophysiology involved. Second, it serves as a constant reminder of the types of therapy available, especially in the difficult patient. Finally, it is an excellent teaching aid. Although certain modalities of therapy, such as surgical reduction of fixed anatomical obstruction and treatment of urinary tract infection, are not listed, their place within such a functional scheme of evaluation and management is quite obvious.

PRINCIPLES OF PHARMACOLOGICAL THERAPY

Most pharmacological agents produce their effects by combining with specialized functional components of cells. The cell component directly involved in the initial action of a drug is known as its receptor. The drug-receptor interaction alters the function of the cell component involved and initiates a series of biochemical and physiological changes that characterize the effects produced by that agent. Each step in neurohumoral transmission, whether peripheral or central, represents a potential point of pharmacological stimulation, inhibition, or modulation. The agents discussed here either affect a step in the initiation or transmission of neurophysiological stimuli or have a direct effect on the musculature of the bladder or the outlet.

To use a pharmacological agent intelligently, it is necessary to be familiar not only with its biochemical and physiological effects and mechanisms of action but also with all those factors that determine its concentration at its site of action. In addition, one must be thoroughly familiar with the literature surrounding the use of a particular pharmacological agent and remember that (1) agents may act at more than one site and even at several sites within a neural pathway or muscle; (2) they may have different effects in vitro and in vivo and at different concentrations; (3) they may have different effects in different species; (4) they may have different acute and long-term effects; (5) they may have multiple effects at any of the levels of action, each within a different time frame; and (6) the sensitivity, number, and type of receptors within a particular tissue can be affected by its physiological state (denervation, distension, hypertrophy, inflammation, ischemia) and by the drug itself.

Generally speaking, the simplest and least hazardous form of pharmacological therapy should be tried first. If single-agent therapy fails, a combination of therapeutic maneuvers or pharmacological agents can sometimes be used to achieve a particular effect, especially if their mechanisms of action are different and if their side effects are not synergistic. Finally, it should be noted by physician and patient alike that although great improvement often occurs with rational pharmacological therapy, a perfect result (restoration to normal status) with no side effects is seldom if ever achieved.

PHARMACOLOGICAL THERAPY TO FACILITATE BLADDER EMPTYING
Increasing intravesical pressure

Parasympathomimetic agents. Although it is likely that other excitatory neurotransmitters exist, at least a major portion of the final common pathway in physiological bladder contraction is acetylcholine-induced stimulation of the muscarinic-cholinergic receptor sites at the postganglionic parasympathetic neuromuscular junction (Wein and Raezer, 1979). Thus parasympathomimetic agents might be expected to be useful in the management of patients who exhibit a failure to empty because of inadequate bladder contractility. Acetylcholine itself cannot be used for therapeutic purposes because of its diffuse actions (central and ganglionic, as well as at the peripheral neuromuscular junction) and because of its rapid hydrolysis by acetylcholinesterase and by nonspecific cholinesterase (Koelle, 1975).

Many drugs that imitate the action of acetylcholine exist. However, only bethanechol chloride (Myotonachol, Duvoid, Urecholine) has been reported to exhibit a relatively selective action on the urinary bladder and gut with little or no action at

therapeutic doses on ganglia or on the cardiovascular system (Ursillo, 1967; Koelle, 1975). Bethanechol chloride is cholinesterase resistant and in vitro causes a contraction of the smooth muscle from all areas of the bladder (Raezer et al., 1973). A subcutaneous dose of 5 to 10 mg has been recommended for the treatment of postoperative or postpartum urinary retention. It should be used in this instance only if the patient is awake and alert and only if there is no outlet obstruction. It has been reported as being effective in the "rehabilitation" of the atonic or hypotonic bladder (Lapides, 1964, 1974; Diokno and Koppenhoeffer, 1976; Sonda et al., 1979). In this instance it is recommended that the drug initially be administered subcutaneously in a dosage of 5 to 10 mg (usually 7.5 mg) every 4 to 6 hours. The patient should be asked to try to void 20 to 30 minutes after receiving a subcutaneous dose. This regime may be initiated with indwelling catheter drainage or intermittent catheterization. When the residual urine has decreased to an acceptable level, the subcutaneous dosage is decreased by 2.5 mg and ultimately changed to an oral dosage of 50 mg q.i.d. Sometimes the drug can subsequently be discontinued completely. In cases of partial but incomplete bladder emptying, a therapeutic trial of an oral dosage of 25 to 100 mg q.i.d. can be used in conjunction with timed voidings (q. 4h.) with abdominal straining and Credé's maneuver. Bethanechol chloride has also been used to stimulate or facilitate the development of reflex bladder contraction in patients with supersacral spinal cord injury (Perkash, 1975; Diokno and Koppenhoeffer, 1976; Sonda, et al., 1979). In this instance daily divided doses similar to those employed in the rehabilitation regime or in lower dosages (2.5 to 5 mg subcutaneously or 25 to 50 mg orally) are used.

Other acetylcholine-like drugs are seldom used in the United States. Philp, Thomas, and Clarke (1980) have reported that a 4 mg oral dose of carbachol (Doryl), a cholinergic agonist that possesses some ganglionic-stimulating properties, has a much greater effect on urodynamic parameters than a 50 mg dose of bethanechol chloride, without an apparent increase in side effects. Anticholinesterase agents, which inhibit the enzymatic degradation of acetylcholine, also have the net effect of producing or enhancing cholinergic stimulation. Cameron (1966) has reported that distigmine bromide (Ubretid), a long-acting anticholinesterase, is effective in preventing postoperative urinary retention. Philp and Thomas (1980) have reported that parenteral, but not oral, distigmine improves voiding efficiency in patients with neurogenic bladder dysfunction and reflex detrusor activity. They recommend a parenteral dosage of this agent of 0.5 mg a day intramuscularly. It is also available as a 5 mg oral preparation.

The potential side effects of the cholinergic agonists and the anticholinesterase agents are similar and include flushing, nausea, vomiting, diarrhea, gastrointestinal cramps, bronchospasm, headache, salivation, sweating, and difficulty with visual accommodation. Intramuscular or intravenous administration of bethanechol chloride is contraindicated, since such use can precipitate acute and severe muscarinic side effects, resulting in acute circulatory failure and cardiac arrest. Contraindications to the use of these general categories of drugs include bronchial asthma, peptic ulcer, hyperthyroidism, enteritis, bowel obstruction, any type of bladder outlet obstruction, cardiac arrhythmia, and a history of recent gastrointestinal surgery (Koelle, 1975; Wein, 1979).

Our own efforts (mine and those of my colleagues) to facilitate bladder emptying with cholinergic stimulation have been restricted to the use of bethanechol chloride and have been disappointing (Wein, Raezer, and Benson, 1976; Wein, 1979, 1980; Wein, Raezer, and Malloy, 1980; Wein et al., 1980). We have been unimpressed with the ability of bethanechol chloride to stimulate or facilitate a physiological bladder contraction in the vast majority of patients with neuropathic or nonneuropathic disease. Gibbon (1965), Merrill and Rotta (1974), and Yalla et al. (1977) have expressed similar sentiments, at least with respect to use in neuropathic bladder dysfunction. There is no question that a subcutaneous dose of 5 mg increases the intravesical pressure at all points along the accommodation limb of the cystometrogram and also decreases the bladder capacity threshold (Lapides et al., 1963; Sonda et al., 1979; Wein, Raezer, and Malloy, 1980; Wein et al., 1980). However, the ability to stimulate a physiological bladder contraction in a patient who cannot normally initiate one is questionable, at best. What does seem to occur is an increase in tension in all areas of bladder smooth muscle, such as one would expect from in vitro studies. Some clinicians, however, believe that reflex activation is in fact an important part of the action of bethanechol (Perkash,

1975; Diokno and Koppenhoeffer, 1976; Sonda et al., 1979). This hypothesis may be at least partially supported by the recent study of Twiddy, Downie, and Awad (1980), who concluded that in cats intact pelvic reflex pathways are required for bethanechol to produce what they have described as a brisk and sustained increase in intravesical pressure during bladder filling.

Theory and in vitro experiments aside, it is difficult to find reproducible urodynamic data supporting the use of bethanechol chloride in patients who exhibit a failure to empty the bladder. Long-term studies in such patients are invariably neither prospective nor double blind and do not exclude the effects of other simultaneous maneuvers, such as treatment of urinary tract infection, bladder decompression by continuous or intermittent catheterization, timed voiding with Credé's maneuver, and other types of treatment affecting the bladder or outlet. Short-term studies in which the drug was the only variable have generally failed to demonstrate significant efficacy, at least in terms of flow and residual urine volume data (Wein, Raezer, and Malloy, 1980; Wein et al., 1980). It is generally agreed that, on an acute basis, oral doses of 50 mg or less of bethanechol chloride have little if any effect on even cystometric parameters (Diokno and Lapides, 1977; Wein et al., 1978). It is also generally agreed that, at least in a denervated bladder, an oral dose of 200 mg is required to produce the same effect as a subcutaneous dose of 5 mg (Diokno and Lapides, 1977; Philp, Thomas, and Clarke, 1980). Whether repeated doses of bethanechol or any other cholinergic agonist can achieve a clinical effect that a single dose cannot is speculative and currently under investigation. If this is not the case, the long-term response to therapy can be predicted by a urodynamic assessment before and after a single subcutaneous dose or a short oral trial has been given.

No agreement exists as to whether cholinergic stimulation produces an increase in urethral resistance (Wein, 1980; Wein et al., 1980). If such a phenomenon does occur, a logical question is whether cholinergic agonists can be combined with agents to decrease outlet resistance and thereby facilitate emptying. Khanna (1977) reported that a combination of a total daily oral dose of 50 to 100 mg of bethanechol with 20 to 30 mg or oral phenoxybenzamine (see ''Decreasing Outlet Resistance'') produced what were termed satisfactory results in a group of patients with an atonic bladder and functional outlet obstruction. Our own experience in this situation with pharmacological therapy alone has been disappointing. Certainly, most would agree that this dose of oral bethanechol rarely affects any urodynamic parameter (Lapides et al., 1963; Diokno and Lapides, 1977; Wein et al., 1978; Philp, Thomas, and Clarke, 1980).

Prostaglandins. The role of prostaglandins in lower urinary tract physiology is currently under investigation. Bultitude, Hills, and Shuttleworth (1976) hypothesized that both prostaglandins and acetylcholine were necessary for the maintenance of bladder tone and spontaneous bladder activity. This hypothesis was based on the facts that (1) prostaglandins were produced by the bladder, (2) PGE_2 and $PGF_{2\alpha}$ caused a dose-related contraction in in vitro bladder strips, and (3) inhibitors of prostaglandin synthesis caused a decrease in bladder tone and spontaneous activity. This group reported that the instillation of 0.5 mg of PGE_2 into the bladders of female patients in varying degrees of urinary retention resulted in acute emptying and improved long-term emptying in two thirds of the patients studied. Desmond et al. (1980) reported further results with this agent in patients whose bladders exhibited no contractile activity or in whom bladder contractility was relatively impaired. In their study, 1.5 mg of PGE_2 in diluent was infused into the bladder and left for 1 hour. Of 36 patients, 20 showed a strongly positive immediate response and 6 showed a weakly positive response. Fourteen patients showed prolonged beneficial effects, all but one of whom had shown a strongly positive immediate response. An intact sacral reflex arc seemed to be a prerequisite for any type of positive response. In some patients the authors noted that the effects of PGE_2 appeared to be additive to or synergistic with cholinergic stimulation. Vaidyanathan et al. (1981) reported that intravesical instillation of 7.5 mg of 15(S)–15 methylprostagladin $F_{2\alpha}$ produced reflex voiding in some patients with incomplete suprasacral spinal cord lesions. The favorable response to a single dose of the drug, where present, lasted for time periods ranging from 1 day to 2½ months.

The literature supporting the role of prostaglandins in the physiology of micturition is growing, although their exact modes of action are as yet unknown (Ghonheim et al., 1976; Andersson, Ek, and Persson, 1977; Andersson and Forman, 1978; Khanna, Barbieri, and McMichael, 1978). Although Stanton (1978) reported no success with this type of treatment, the other results described in his study are at least promising and suggest that these agents might facilitate emptying in patients with decreased bladder contractility and depressed but intact reflex function.

PGE_2 is not available in the United States in other than a rectal suppository form, and although $PGF_{2\alpha}$ is available in an injectable form, guidelines for its use do not at present include voiding dysfunction. Potential side effects with such use include bronchospasm, chills, hypotension, tachycardia, cardiac arrhythmias, convulsions, hypocalcemia, and diarrhea.

Blockers of inhibition. DeGroat and co-workers (DeGroat and Saum, 1972, 1976; DeGroat and Booth, 1980) have demonstrated a sympathetic reflex that, at least in the cat, promotes urine storage by exerting an inhibitory effect on pelvic parasympathetic ganglionic transmission. This effect, although inhibitory, is α-adrenergic in nature. Some investigators have speculated on this basis that α-adrenergic blockade, in addition to decreasing outlet resistance (discussed on the following), may in fact enhance bladder contractility by facilitating transmission through these ganglia. Guanethidine (Hartviksen, 1966) and methyldopa (Raz et al., 1977) have been used with this rationale, but subsequent reports of their efficacy have not appeared. Likewise on this basis, Raz and Smith (1976) have advocated a trial of phenoxybenzamine, an α-adrenergic blocking agent, for the treatment of nonobstructive urinary retention. Some clinicians, ourselves included, have had occasional anecdotal success using this or another exotic approach, but we would caution against the assumption, without a controlled clinical study, that improvement while a patient is taking a drug occurs solely because of it.

Decreasing outlet resistance

Inhibition of the striated sphincter. Functional obstruction can occur at the level of the striated musculature that surrounds and forms a part of the outer portion of the urethra. This entity of detrusor-striated sphincter dyssynergia is generally seen only in patients with overt neurological damage between the brainstem and the sacral spinal cord (Wein and Raezer, 1979). However, seeming striated sphincter dyssynergia, or at least a qualitatively similar disorder, can be seen in patients without an apparent structural or neurological basis (Hinman, 1974; Raz and Smith, 1976; Allen,

1977), in which case it falls into what Hinman (1980) has described as one of the syndromes of incoordination.

There is no pharmacological agent that will selectively relax the striated musculature of the pelvic floor. Various drugs do exist that are classified as centrally acting muscle relaxants (Franz, 1975). These include chlordiazepoxide (Librium), methocarbamol (Robaxin), orphenadrine (Norflex), and diazepam (Valium), the most widely used drug of this group. Effective divided daily doses of this agent are reported to range from 6 to 60 mg. The primary side effect of all the members of this group of drugs is sedation, which many believe is primarily responsible for the muscle-relaxing effect when the drugs are administered orally (Franz, 1975). Some controlled studies of the oral efficacy of these agents as muscle relaxants exist, but only a few have shown any advantage over a placebo or aspirin (Byck, 1975). In fact, oral treatment with diazepam is classified primarily as antianxiety therapy by some authorities (Byck, 1975). Potential side effects of this group of agents include drowsiness, ataxia, and fatigue. In general, we have not found the recommended oral doses to be effective in controlling striated sphincter dyssynergia caused by suprasacral spinal cord lesion. If the cause of incomplete emptying in a neurologically normal patient is obscure and the patient has what appears to be inadequate relaxation of the striated musculature of the pelvic floor, a trial of an agent such as diazepam may be worthwhile. Certainly, beneficial results do occasionally occur under these conditions. However, it should be noted that such improvement may simply be a result of the drug's antianxiety effect or a result of the intensive explanation, encouragement, and modified biofeedback therapy that usually accompany this therapy in such patients.

Dantrolene sodium (Dantrium) is a skeletal muscle relaxant that acts directly on excitation-contraction coupling (Franz, 1975). In patients with suprasacral spinal cord lesions, spasticity is often reduced and overall function improved. Although the drug has no autonomic side effects, it may induce a generalized weakness severe enough to compromise its therapeutic benefits, especially at higher doses. Adult therapy is generally begun at a dosage of 25 mg twice a day, and the dosage is increased weekly by 50 to 100 mg increments to a daily maximum of 400 mg given in divided doses. Besides the potential for generalized weakness, other potential side effects include euphoria, diz-

ziness, diarrhea, and severe hepatotoxicity, which should be checked for with frequent liver function studies. The drug has been used with success in some patients with classical detrusor-external sphincter dyssynergia (Murdock, Sax, and Krane, 1976), but Hackler et al. (1980) reported that dosages of 600 mg a day were generally required to achieve improvement in voiding function when it occurred (in approximately half of their patients). At this high-dosage range, hepatotoxicity must be carefully watched for during long-term use. We would not recommend the routine use of this agent in the patient with external sphincter dyssynergia but no other neurological findings.

Baclofen (Lioresal) is an agent that is a derivative of γ-aminobutyric acid and that causes monosynaptic and polysynaptic spinal reflex activity (Jones et al., 1970; Duncan, Shahani, and Young, 1976). In addition, it may cause a depression of the synaptic relay of primary afferent fibers in the dorsal column nuclei (Fox et al., 1978). It is useful in the treatment of skeletal spasticity from a variety of causes (Abromowicz, 1975; Roussan et al., 1975). Treatment with baclofen is started at a dosage of 5 mg t.i.d., and the dosage is doubled every 3 days until a daily dose of 60 mg is reached. Additional increases may be necessary, but the manufacturer recommends that the maximum daily dosage not exceed 20 mg q.i.d. Florante et al. (1980) reported that 73% of their patients with voiding dysfunction as a result of acute and chronic spinal cord injury showed lowered external urethral sphincter responses and a decreased residual urine volume following treatment with this agent. Their average daily oral dose, however, was 120 mg. Hachen and Krucker (1977) found a 75 mg daily oral dose to be ineffective in patients with traumatic paraplegia and external sphincter dyssynergia, whereas they found a daily intravenous dose of 20 mg to be highly effective. Potential side effects include drowsiness, insomnia, rash, pruritis, dizziness, and weakness. When usage is to be stopped, the drug should be discontinued gradually so as to prevent the hallucinations that sometimes occur after abrupt withdrawal.

β-Adrenergic agonists, especially those with β_2-characteristics (see Chapter 4 or Wein and Raezer [1979] for a complete discussion of the subclassification of β-adrenergic receptors), seem also to be able to produce relaxation of slow-twitch skeletal muscle (Olsson et al., 1979; Holmberg and Waldeck, 1980). This may account at least in part for the decrease in urethral profile parameters seen after the administration of terbutaline, a relatively specific β_2-agonist (Vaidyanathan et al., 1980). This finding may be especially significant in view of the fact that Gosling et al. (1981) have reported that the striated musculature of the external urethral sphincter, which forms a portion of the outermost urethral wall, consists exclusively of slow-twitch fibers, whereas the purely periurethral striated muscle fibers of the levator ani contain both slow-twitch and fast-twitch fibers, although the majority are also of the slow-twitch type. These observations may form the basis for further attempts to decrease outlet resistance.

Inhibition of the smooth sphincter. Regardless of the controversy surrounding the neuromorphology of the smooth muscle of the bladder neck and proximal urethra and surrounding the role of the sympathetic nervous system and the physiology of micturition, there is no question that the smooth muscle of the bladder and urethra in a variety of experimental animals and in humans contains both α- and β-adrenergic receptors. α-Receptors (producing contraction when stimulated by the sympathetic neurotransmitter) predominate in the bladder base and proximal urethra (Edvardsen and Setekliev, 1968; Donker, Ivanovici, and Noach, 1972; Raezer et al., 1973; Awad et al., 1974; Benson et al., 1976; Wein and Levin, 1979). The observation that sympatholytic drugs facilitate voiding in certain patients was first made in 1970 by Kleeman. Krane and Olsson (1973a,b) subsequently described the concept of a physiological internal sphincter, which they hypothesized as being controlled partly by a tonic stimulation, via the sympathetic nervous system, of the contractile α-receptors in the smooth muscle of the bladder neck and proximal urethra. They further hypothesized that obstructions occurring at this level during detrusor contraction were a result of inadequate opening of the bladder neck or an inadequate decrease in resistance in the area of the proximal urethra, or both. They also theorized and presented evidence to support the contention that α-adrenergic blockade could be useful and should be considered in cases of incomplete emptying despite an adequate bladder contraction in a patient without anatomical obstruction or detrusor-striated sphincter dyssynergia, an observation subsequently confirmed by others (Johnston and Farkas, 1975; Stockamp, 1975; Stockamp and Schreiter, 1975; Mobley, 1976; Whitfield et al., 1976).

A successful result, defined as an increase in flow rate and a decrease in residual urine, can often

be correlated with an objective decrease in urethral profilometry closure pressures. The phentolamine stimulation test (Olsson, Siroky, and Krane, 1977) can generally rapidly predict the effectiveness of α-adrenolytic therapy in a given situation. Urinary flow rates are measured before and after an intravenous dose of 5 mg of phentolamine (Regitine) is given, and the values are plotted on a nomogram, which relates the flow rate to the volume voided. An increase of 0.8 units on the nomogram predicts improved voiding with oral α-blocking therapy.

It has also been suggested that α-adrenergic blocking agents may decrease perineal striated muscle activity and that this action may contribute to their effect in decreasing outlet resistance (Nanninga, Kaplan, and Lal, 1977). If this is so, the mechanism must be a central one, or it must be mediated by noninnervated receptors, since histochemical examination has failed to show adrenergic nerve terminals in the striated urethral sphincter (Wein, Benson, and Jacobowitz, 1979).

There is a rationale for the addition of α-adrenolytic therapy after conventional pharmacological treatments have failed in the patient with inadequate emptying secondary to neurogenic voiding dysfunction. It has been shown that parasympathetic denervation leads to a marked increase in adrenergic innervation of the bladder, with a resultant conversion of the normal β-response of the bladder body (relaxation) to sympathetic stimulation to an α-effect (contraction) (Elmer, 1975; Norlen et al., 1976; Sundin et al., 1977). If a similar effect occurred at the level of the bladder neck and proximal urethral smooth musculature, this would produce an increase in effective α-receptor density with a resultant increase in tension that could cause a functional obstruction that should be at least partially correctable with α-adrenolytic therapy. Parsons and Turton (1980) agree with this concept of a neuropathic urethra but have ascribed the cause to decentralization supersensitivity of the urethral smooth muscle, which responds with an inappropriately high sensitivity to alterations in circulating catecholamine levels brought about as a part of cardiovascular homeostasis. They have theorized that various radical pelvic surgical procedures may result in such neurological decentralization of the urethral smooth musculature and contribute to a syndrome of functional outlet obstruction, which is especially marked with postural changes. A similar phenomenon might also be operative in certain patients with seeming obstruction at the level of the proximal urethra, but without a demonstrable neurological or anatomical lesion. If so, α-adrenolytic therapy would be expected to facilitate emptying in these subsets of patients.

Phenoxybenzamine (Dibenzyline) is the α-adrenolytic agent most commonly used by urologists and gynecologists. The initial adult dosage of this agent is 10 mg a day. An electrocardiogram and supine and standing blood pressure measurements are recommended before therapy is begun. The daily dose may be increased by 10 mg every 4 to 5 days to a recommended maximum of 60 mg. Daily doses larger than 10 mg are generally divided and given every 8 to 12 hours. The maximum effect of a particular dose usually becomes apparent 4 to 14 days after the initiation of therapy or after a change in therapy. In our experience, most patients who respond favorably to this agent do so at doses of less than 30 mg and do not respond to dose increases with incremental improvement. Some patients who respond to daily doses of 10 mg can be maintained on an even lower dose. Potential side effects include orthostatic hypotension, reflex tachycardia, nasal congestion, diarrhea, myosis, nausea and vomiting, and a generalized feeling of weakness and fatigue (Wein, 1980). In men, inhibition of seminal emission and/or retrograde ejaculation may occur.

Recently there has been a great deal of attention paid to the identification and classification of α-adrenergic receptors (for a complete discussion and bibliography see Hoffman and Lefkowitz [1980] and Weinshiebaum [1980]). At the present time it is generally accepted that α_1-receptors include typical postsynaptic α-receptors, which moderate smooth muscle contraction. α_2-Receptors include all known presynaptic autoregulatory α-receptors and also some less typical adrenergic receptors, such as those existing on human platelets. Prazosin hydrochloride (Minipress) is one of a new class of antihypertensive agents that has an affinity for postsynaptic α_1-receptors, at least in vascular smooth muscle (Atkins and Nicolosi, 1979; Graham and Pettinger; 1979). Prazosin has little affinity for α_2-receptors, in contrast to the classic α-adrenergic blocking agents, such as phentolamine and phenoxybenzamine, both of which have blocking properties at presynpatic and postsynaptic receptor sites. Prazosin has been shown to cause postsynaptic α-adrenergic blockade in the smooth muscle of the canine and human urethra (Andersson et al., 1981; MacGregor and Diokno, 1981). In addition, it has been safely and successfully used in some patients to lower outlet resistance (Andersson

et al., 1981). In this respect it may prove to be preferable to phenoxybenzamine because of its relatively selective postsynaptic action. At least with respect to equivalent hypotensive doses, phenoxybenzamine produces a greater increase in plasma norepinephrine concentration than does prazosin. Consistent with this is a greater reported incidence of tachycardia with the use of phenoxybenzamine.

Prazosin therapy is generally begun with daily divided doses of 2 to 3 mg. The dose may be titrated and very gradually increased to a maximum daily dose of 20 mg. Our subjective experience thus far is that the urodynamic effect is similar to that produced by phenoxybenzamine with fewer side effects overall. We have not used the drug in a daily dose of more than 15 mg. The major potential side effect is the occasional occurrence of the so-called first-dose phenomenon, a symptom complex of faintness, dizziness, palpitations, and, occasionally, syncope. These episodes, when they occur, generally happen within 30 to 90 minutes of the first dose and are thought to be caused by acute postural hypotension. The incidence can be minimized by restricting the initial dose of the drug to 1 mg and by administering the first dose at bedtime. Chronic side effects are generally mild and rarely necessitate drug discontinuation. Postural hypotension and tachycardia occur in a small percentage of patients, and other chronic side effects may include headaches, drowsiness, nausea, dry mouth, rash, and polyarthralgia. Sexual dysfunction in the male patient is rare.

Other agents with some α-adrenergic blocking properties at various levels of neural organization have urological side effects that may be therapeutically useful in certain circumstances. Methyldopa (Aldomet) is an antihypertensive agent that is converted to α-methylnorepinephrine, an effective neurotransmitter that functions as a presynaptic α-adrenergic receptor agonist (Weinshiebaum, 1980). α-Methylnorepinephrine interacts with these receptors at a central and perhaps peripheral nervous system level, with the end result being a decreased peripheral sympathetic effect. Raz et al. (1977) have reported improved emptying with this agent in patients with neurogenic bladder dysfunction. Clonidine (Catapres) is another antihypertensive agent that is an α-adrenergic agonist with relative specificity for presynaptic receptors at spinal and supraspinal sites (Krier, Thor, and DeGroat, 1979; Weinshiebaum, 1980). The end result, similar to that produced by methyldopa, is a decrease in peripheral sympathetic effect, reflected in the urinary tract by a decrease in the urethral closure pressure profile (Nordling, Meyhoff, and Christensen, 1979). It has been suggested that this agent may prove to produce as equivalent a reduction in outlet resistance as postsynaptic α_1-adrenergic antagonists currently in use and with fewer side effects.

β-Adrenergic stimulation has been shown experimentally to decrease the urethral closure pressure profile and, by inference, urethral resistance (Raz and Caine, 1971). The β-adrenergic receptors in the urethral smooth musculature appear to be of the β_2 type (see Chapter 4 and Wein and Raezer [1979] for a discussion of β-receptor subtypes) and, on stimulation, generally produce smooth muscle relaxation, accounting for the decrease in urethral closure pressure profile seen after the administration of terbutaline, a relatively specific β_2-agonist (Vaidyanathan et al., 1980). Whether this drug or other pharmacologically similar agents will prove to be useful in facilitating bladder emptying by decreasing outlet resistance remains to be investigated.

PHARMACOLOGICAL THERAPY TO FACILITATE URINE STORAGE
Decreasing bladder contractility

Anticholinergic agents. Atropine and agents that imitate its action produce a competitive blockade of acetylcholine receptors, primarily at postganglionic parasympathetic receptor sites. These so-called antimuscarinic agents (since they antagonize the muscarinic effect of acetylcholine) have little effect at the level of autonomic ganglia (Innes and Nickerson, 1975). Because at least a major portion of the neurohumoral stimulus for physiological bladder contraction is acetylcholine-induced stimulation of postganglionic parasympathetic cholinergic receptor sites on bladder smooth muscle (Wein and Raezer, 1979), these agents will depress true detrusor hyperreflexia of any cause (Pederson and Grynderup, 1966; Diokno et al., 1972; Innes and Nickerson, 1975; Blaivas et al., 1980). In patients with detrusor hyperreflexia and a resultant inadequacy of urine storage, the volume to the first hyperreflexic contraction will generally be increased and symptoms reduced proportionately. However, detrusor hyperreflexia, whatever its cause, can generally be only partially inhibited by antimuscarinic agents because of a phenomenon known as atropine resistance. This phenomenon refers to the fact that although atropine can completely inhibit the response of bladder smooth muscle to exogenously administered acetylcholine, it can only partially antagonize the bladder response to either pelvic nerve stimulation or direct electrical stimulation (see Chapter 2, Chapter 4, and Wein and Raezer [1979] for a complete discussion). At the present time there is no generally accepted explanation for this phenomenon. Perhaps the most attractive theory is that a major portion of the neurotransmission involved in producing bladder contraction is a result of the release of a transmitter other than acetylcholine or norepinephrine. Burnstock (1979) has proposed and supported the hypothesis that such excitatory innervation to the bladder does exist and is purinergic; that is, it liberates adenosine triphosphate. The clinical correlate of the laboratory phenomenon of atropine resistance is that it is rare to achieve a perfect result in the treatment of detrusor hyperreflexia with an antimuscarinic agent or any single type of pharmacological treatment. Often, however, significant clinical improvement is achieved that is acceptable to both patient and physician.

Propantheline bromide (Pro-Banthine) is the oral agent most commonly used to produce an antimuscarinic effect in the lower urinary tract. The adult oral dosage is 15 to 30 mg every 4 to 6 hours. Oral administration with the patient in the fasting state rather than after meals seems preferable from the standpoint of bioavailability (Gibaldi and Grundhofer, 1975). The clinical efficacy can generally be predicted by observing the effect of an intravenous or intramuscular dose on the cystometrogram (Blaivas et al., 1980). Parenteral propantheline is no longer available in many hospitals in the United States, and parenteral atropine or glycopyrrolate (Robinul) may be used instead. We generally use 0.2 mg of glycopyrrolate (available as a 1 ml single-dose vial with the usual clinical precautions) (Mirakhur, Dundee, and Jones, 1978). There seems to be little difference between the antimuscarinic effects of propantheline on bladder smooth muscle and those of other antimuscarinic agents such as glycopyrrolate, isopropamide (Darbid), hyoscyamine (Cysto-Spaz), and anisotropine methylbromide (Valpin). Some of these agents, such as glycopyrrolate, have a more convenient dosage schedule than propantheline (twice or three times a day), but their clinical effects on the lower urinary tract seem to be indistinguishable. We have recently completed a study that shows that, at least insofar as the in vitro concentration necessary to displace a muscarinic ligand is concerned, propantheline compares favorably with atropine (Table

TABLE 35.1   Displacement of 3H-quinuclidinyl benzilate by various pharmacological agents

Drug	I$_{50}$*	Relative concentrations compared with atropine
Atropine	70 ± 1.5 nmol	1
Propantheline bromide	115 ± 0.46 nmol	1.6
Glycopyrrolate	120 ± 30 nmol	1.7
Dicyclomine hydrochloride	2.65 ± 0.048 μmol	37.8
Oxybutynin chloride	3.75 ± 0.033 μmol	53.5
Imipramine	25 ± 0.4 μmol	357.1
Chlorpromazine	30 ± 0.7 μmol	428.5
Desmethylimipramine	60 ± 0.5 μmol	857.1
Phentolamine	>1 mmol	>10,000
Guanethidine	>1 mmol	>10,000
Tranylcypromine	>10 mmol	>10,000
Hexamethonium	>10 mmol	>10,000

From Levin, R.M., Staskin, D., and Wein, A.J. 1982. Neurourol. Urodynamics **1:**221-226.
*In vitro concentration necessary to displace 50% of muscarinic cholinergic receptor ligand (^{3}H-quinuclidinyl benzilate) from human urinary bladder body muscle strips.

35.1). Although there are obviously many other considerations that account for the activity of a given dose of drug at its site of action, we found no drug available orally whose direct antimuscarinic-binding potential was greater than that of the long-available and relatively inexpensive propantheline bromide.

The potential side effects of all antimuscarinic agents include dry mouth, blurred vision, mydriasis, tachycardia, drowsiness, and constipation (Innes and Nickerson, 1975). Because most of these agents possess some ganglionic blocking activity, they may also cause orthostatic hypotension at high doses. Antimuscarinic agents are contraindicated in patients with glaucoma and should be used with caution in patients with significant bladder outlet obstruction, since complete urinary retention may be precipitated.

It would seem that an agent that had a significant blocking action at the ganglionic level in addition to one at the peripheral receptor level might be more effective in suppressing bladder contractility. Methantheline (Banthine) has a higher ratio of ganglionic blocking to antimuscarinic activity than does propantheline, but propantheline, clinical dose for dose, is more potent in each respect (Innes and Nickerson, 1975). Emepronium bromide (Cetiprin) is an anticholinergic agent that has activity at both peripheral and ganglionic levels (Stanton,

1973; Ekeland and Sander, 1976; Hebjorn and Walter, 1978). It can increase bladder capacity in patients with detrusor hyperreflexia while decreasing intravesical pressure and urinary flow (Ekeland and Sander, 1976). The recommended oral dosage ranges from 100 mg t.i.d. to 200 q.i.d (Meyhoff and Nordling, 1981). However, some doubts have been raised as to its effectiveness when administered orally (Rich et al., 1977), and it seems most effective when given intramuscularly in doses of 25 to 50 mg (Rich et al., 1977; Cardozo and Stanton, 1979). Potential side effects are predominantly antimuscarinic ones, but they also include mucosal alteration, sometimes leading to oral ulcers and esophagitis.

Musculotropic relaxants (antispasmodics). Another category of drugs that inhibit bladder contractility is classified as having a musculotropic relaxant, or antispasmodic, activity. These agents fall under the general heading of direct-acting smooth muscle depressants, and their antispasmodic activity is reportedly directly on the smooth muscle at a site metabolically distal to the cholinergic receptor mechanism (Wein, 1979). In addition, all three of the agents to be discussed have been found to possess variable antimuscarinic and local anesthetic properties. Our own experience (Table 35.1) would suggest that the antimuscarinic properties (at least, of oxybutynin and dicyclomine) are considerably less than those of the classic antimuscarinic agents. However, there is still a question as to how much of their efficacy is simply a result of their atropine-like effect.

Oxybutynin chloride (Ditropan) has been described as a moderately potent anticholinergic agent with a strong, independent musculotropic relaxant activity and local anesthetic activity (Lish et al., 1965; Fredericks, Anderson, and Kruelen, 1975; Finkbeiner, Bissada, and Welch, 1977; Fredericks, Green, and Anderson, 1978). Oxybutynin has been used successfully to relieve urinary discomfort and bladder spasm following endoscopic resection (Diokno and Lapides, 1972; Paulsen, 1978). It has also been used to suppress detrusor hyperreflexia in patients with neuropathic bladder dysfunction (Thompson and Lauvetz, 1976). The recommended adult dosage is 5 mg three to four times a day. The potential side effects are the same as those of propantheline.

Dicyclomine hydrochloride (Bentyl) is another agent reported to possess a direct relaxant effect on smooth muscle, in addition to an antimuscarinic action (Johns et al., 1976; Downie, Twiddy, and Awad, 1977; Khanna et al., 1979). With an adult oral dosage of 20 mg t.i.d., dicyclomine has been reported to increase bladder capacity in patients with detrusor hyperreflexia (Fischer, Diokno, and Lapides, 1978). In our experience, to achieve a good clinical effect, the individual dose must often be raised to 30 mg. The potential side effects are similar to those of propantheline.

Flavoxate hydrochloride (Urispas) is another compound that has been reported to have a direct inhibitory action on smooth muscle in addition to local analgesic and anticholinergic properties (Kohler and Morales, 1968; Bradley and Cazort, 1970). Favorable clinical effects have been noted in patients with the symptoms of frequency, urgency, and incontinence and in patients with urodynamically documented detrusor hyperreflexia (Stanton, 1973; Delaere et al., 1977; Jonas, Petri, and Kissal, 1979). Briggs, Castleden, and Ascher (1980) reported essentially no effect of flavoxate on detrusor hyperreflexia in an elderly population, a general experience that would coincide with our own subjective impression of limited clinical efficacy (Benson et al., 1977). The drug does not generally seem to produce beneficial clinical effects in situations where other, less expensive agents have failed. However, as with all agents in this group, a short clinical trial may be worthwhile.

The recommended adult dosage of flavoxate is 100 to 200 mg three or four times a day. Reported side effects are rare and are primarily antimuscarinic in nature. If in fact any of these agents do exert an inhibitory effect on bladder muscle contractility that is independent of an antimuscarinic action, there exists a therapeutic rationale for combining their use with that of a relatively pure antimuscarinic agent. Our own philosophy has always been to cautiously try to combine pharmacological agents that have different primary mechanisms of action (and, hopefully, different side effects), with the idea of achieving an additive clinical benefit without a corresponding increase in the number or severity of side effects.

Polysynaptic inhibitors. Polysynaptic inhibitors have previously been discussed under the heading of agents that decrease outlet resistance secondary to an inhibitory effect on the striated pelvic floor musculature. Baclofen (Lioresal) has also been shown to depress detrusor hyperreflexia secondary to a spinal cord lesion (Kiesswetter and Shober, 1975; Roussan et al., 1975). A double-blind crossover study by Taylor and Bates (1979) showed that the drug could be very effective also in decreasing day and night urinary frequency and incontinence in patients with ideopathic detrusor hyperreflexia. Cystometric changes, however, were not recorded in this study, and it should be noted that considerable improvement was also obtained with a placebo.

β-Adrenergic agonists. β-Adrenergic receptors, β_2 in nature, can be demonstrated in human bladder muscle, more so in the region of the body than in the region of the base (Wein and Levin, 1979; Wein and Raezer, 1979). β-Adrenergic stimulation can cause significant increases in the capacity of animal bladders with a moderate density of β-adrenergic receptors (Larson and Mortensen, 1978). Terbutaline (Bricanyl) has been reported as having a good clinical effect in patients with urgency and urge incontinence, but no significant effect on the bladders of neurologically normal persons without voiding difficulty. Norlen, Sundin, and Waagstein (1978) have pointed out that these results are compatible with those in other organ systems, since β-adrenergic stimulation causes no acute change in total lung capacity in normal persons but does favorably affect patients with bronchial asthma.

Calcium antagonists. Calcium plays an important role in excitation-contraction coupling in striated, cardiac, and smooth muscle (Andersson, 1978). The dependence of contractile activity on the inflow of calcium from extracellular sources or on its release from intracellular stores varies from tissue to tissue, but interference with these processes, interference with intracellular calcium-using mechanisms, or acceleration of calcium extrusion from the cells are all under study as potential mechanisms for the mediation of at least vascular smooth muscle relaxation (Zelis, 1981).

This type of therapy is potentially applicable to the inhibition of bladder contractility. The calcium antagonist nifedipine has been shown to effectively inhibit contraction induced by several agents in human (Forman et al., 1978) and guinea pig (Sjogren and Andersson, 1979) bladder muscle. In addition, this agent has been shown to be capable of completely blocking the noncholinergic portion of the contractile activation produced by electrical field stimulation in rabbit bladder (Husted et al., 1980). Nimodipine, a more stable nifedipine analog, showed a maximum inhibitory action of 69% on the response of the rabbit urinary bladder to electrical field stimulation and, in combination with atropine, resulted in complete inhibition of the response of this preparation to electrical field stimulation (Husted et al., 1980). Nifedipine more effectively inhibited potassium-induced contractions than carbachol-induced ones, whereas terodiline, an agent with calcium antagonist and anticholinergic properties, had the opposite effect. However, terodiline caused complete inhibition of the electrically induced response of rabbit detrusor to field stimulation. Terodiline in low concentrations seems to have mainly an antimuscarinic action; at higher concentrations a calcium antagonistic effect becomes evident (Husted et al., 1980). In vitro experiments appear to show that these two effects are at least additive with regard to bladder contractility. Whether the calcium antagonistic properties of terodiline contribute to its clinical effectiveness and whether the drug is more effective than standard antimuscarinic agents remains to be established. However, Rud et al. (1980) reported that this agent in oral dosages of 12.5 mg two or three times a day produced a marked decrease in the number of hyperreflexic contractions produced by rapid filling of the bladder or by coughing in a group of seven women with urgency incontinence and two with nocturnal enuresis. The amplitude of the contractions was decreased, and bladder capacity was approximately doubled.

Very few anticholinergic side effects were produced.

In a double-blind crossover study of 12 women with motor urge incontinence, Ekman et al. (1980) reported an increase in bladder capacity and in the bladder volume at which urgency was experienced in all but 1 of the patients treated with terodiline, whereas placebo treatment had no effect on either objective parameters or on subjective symptoms. Palmer, Worth, and Exton-Smith (1981) reported the results of a double-blind placebo trial with a single 20 mg daily dose of flunarizine in 14 female patients with urinary frequency, incontinence, and urodynamically proved detrusor instability. In the calcium antagonist–treated group a statistically significant decrease in urgency was produced, but there was no decrease in the frequency of micturition. Although there was a trend toward improvement of cystometric parameters, this was not significant at the 0.05 level.

The side effects produced in patients who have been treated with these agents for voiding dysfunction have been extremely small, but it should be noted that the potential side effects of calcium antagonists in general can be considerable and consist of hypotension, facial flushing, headache, dizziness, abdominal discomfort, constipation, nausea, skin rash, weakness, and palpitations. Although work in this area is obviously in its infancy, this class of agents may prove to be a promising alternative or addition to existing drugs for the inhibition of bladder contractility.

Prostaglandin inhibitors. As mentioned previously, prostaglandins are one class of compounds proposed as having an important role in excitatory neurotransmission in the lower urinary tract. Thus there exists at least a theoretical mechanism whereby inhibitors of prostaglandin synthesis might decrease bladder contractility. Cardozo et al. (1980) reported such effects in a double-blind placebo study of 30 women with detrusor instability, using the prostaglandin synthetase inhibitor flurbiprofen in dosages of 50 mg t.i.d. Frequency, urgency, and urge incontinence were all significantly reduced, as was the detrusor pressure rise during bladder filling. Abnormal detrusor activity, however, was not abolished in significantly more drug-treated patients than placebo-treated ones, and actual bladder capacity likewise showed no change. It was concluded that the drug did not abolish detrusor instability but delayed the intravesical pressure rise until the level of distension was greater. Forty-three percent of the patients, unfortunately, experienced side effects while taking the drug; these consisted of nausea and vomiting, headache, indigestion, gastric distress, constipation, and rash.

Cardozo and Stanton (1980) reported symptomatic improvement in patients with detrusor instability given indomethacin, another prostaglandin synthetase inhibitor. Unfortunately, this was a short-term study with no cystometric data, and the drug was compared only with bromocriptine. The incidence of side effects attributable to indomethacin was relatively high.

Again, other agents in this category may in the future prove to be clinically useful in inhibiting bladder contractility, with a low incidence of side effects, either alone or in combination with other agents. It is unfortunate that the most common such agent, aspirin, is only a relatively weak inhibitor of prostaglandin synthesis.

Dimethyl sulfoxide. Dimethyl sulfoxide (DMSO), an industrial solvent, is now being used by many people in the United States for the treatment of arthritis and other musculoskeletal disorders. The only formulation approved for human bladder use is a 50% solution, generally used for bladder instillation in patients with interstitial cystitis (Medical Letter, 1980). Stewart and Shirley (1976) reported symptomatic improvement in 75% of patients with interstitial cystitis so treated and improvement in bladder capacity in 80% of these patients. Generally, one 50 ml instillation is carried out every other week for a total of six treatments. The unpleasant garliclike odor of DMSO is its primary side effect and makes double-blind placebo studies impossible. However, cataracts have been reported in experimental animals, and for this reason, eye evaluation is recommended with chronic therapy. As a last resort, this drug has been used by some clinicians in the ever-frustrating patient with the urgency-frequency syndrome but without objective evidence of detrusor hyperreflexia or true interstitial cystitis. Although anecdotal improvement is sometimes reported, few if any formal reports of the results of such usage exist.

Bromocriptine. Bromocriptine (Parlodel) is an ergot alkaloid that activates dopamine receptors (Parkes, 1979). It has been reported to inhibit norepinephrine release by stimulation of α_2-adrenergic receptors (presynaptic) (Ziegler et al., 1979). On this basis it might be expected to decrease outlet resistance, but it has in fact been used in the treatment of detrusor hyperreflexia. Although Farrar

and Osborne (1976) reported encouraging preliminary success in this regard, subsequent experience by others has been disappointing (Abrams and Dunn, 1979).

Increasing outlet resistance

α-Adrenergic agonists. As previously described, the bladder neck and proximal urethral smooth musculature contain α-adrenergic receptor sites that, on stimulation, produce contraction. Such stimulation increases the maximum urethral pressure and maximum urethral closure pressure (Ek et al., 1978; Obrink and Bunne, 1978). Various pharmacological agents that can be administered orally are available to produce this type of stimulation with relatively mild side effects. Ephedrine is a noncatecholamine sympathomimetic agent that directly stimulates both α- and β-adrenergic receptors (Innes and Nickerson, 1975b). It is used in an adult dosage of 25 to 50 mg q.i.d. Theoretically, at least, any β-adrenergic effect that the drug has should simultaneously depress bladder contractility, but we have not been impressed that this latter mechanism is operative in clinically used doses. Potential side effects of all agents that produce a peripheral sympathetic effect include blood pressure elevation and anxiety and insomnia caused by central nervous system stimulation. All of these agents should be used with caution in patients with hypertension, cardiovascular disease, and hyperthyroidism. Pseudoephedrine hydrochloride (Sudafed) is a stereoisomer of ephedrine that is used for similar indications with similar precautions (Wein, 1979). The adult dosage is 30 to 60 mg q.i.d. The 30 mg dose form is available in the United States without a prescription. Tachyphylaxis seems to be a problem with the long-term usage of both ephedrine and pseudoephedrine.

Phenylpropanolamine hydrochloride shares the pharmacological potencies of ephedrine and is approximately equal in peripheral potency, while causing less central stimulation (Innes and Nickerson, 1975b). In doses of 50 mg t.i.d., this agent has been shown to be effective in some cases of stress incontinence (Awad, Downie, and Kiruluta, 1978). Fifty milligrams of this substance, 8 mg of chlorpheniramine (an antihistamine), and 2.5 mg of isopropamide (an antimuscarinic agent) were combined into a sustained-release capsule called Ornade used primarily for the relief of symptoms of allergic rhinitis. Stewart, Banowsky, and Montague (1976) found this agent to be particularly effective in treating many patients with mild sphinc-teric incontinence. The adult dosage was one cap-sule b.i.d. Recently the antimuscarinic has been removed from the formulation, leaving the other agents in the same dosage.

An improvement in patients with stress urinary incontinence has been reported also with a 100 mg sustained-release capsule of norephedrine chloride given b.i.d. (Ek et al., 1978; Obrink and Bunne, 1978.

All of these agents, which produce an α-adren-ergic effect on the smooth muscle of the bladder neck and proximal urethra, have been noted to in-crease outlet resistance sufficiently to improve many cases of mild to moderate stress inconti-nence. Total cure rates of over 50% in women with stress urinary incontinence have been reported (Awad, Downie, and Kiruluta, 1978). Our own experience, however, agrees with that of Obrink and Bunne (1978) and Ek et al. (1978), who have reported that stimulation by such agents often pro-duces improvement but rarely produces total dry-ness in cases of severe or even moderate stress incontinence. A clinical trial is certainly worth-while, however, and will, at the least, assure the patient that the possibility of one type of nonsurgi-cal therapy has been explored.

β-Adrenergic antagonists. Theoretically, β-adrenergic blocking agents might be expected to "unmask" or potentiate an α-adrenergic effect, thereby increasing outlet resistance. Gleason et al. (1974) reported success in treating certain patients with stress incontinence with 10 mg of propranolol q.i.d. The beneficial effect, however, became man-ifest only after 4 to 10 weeks of treatment, a fact that is difficult to explain on a pharmacological basis. However, such treatment has been suggested as an alternative method of pharmacological ther-apy (to α-adrenergic stimulation) in patients with hypertension and stress incontinence. Recently, few if any reports have appeared to support this approach, and it should be noted that others have been unable to show significant increases in ure-thral profilometry pressures in normal women after the administration of a β-adrenergic blocking agent (Donker and van der Sluis, 1976).

Estrogen therapy. Salmon, Walter, and Geist first reported the use of estrogen in the treatment of stress urinary incontinence in 1941. In 1973 Caine and Raz reported that a daily dose of 2.5 mg of Premarin improved stress incontinence and in-creased urethral pressures in postmenopausal pa-tients—effects that they attributed to mucosal pro-liferation with a consequently improved mucosal seal effect and to enhancement of the α-adrenergic response of urethral smooth musculature to en-dogenous catecholamines. Schreiter, Fuchs, and Stockamp (1976) reported similar benefits after 10 days of treatment with daily divided doses of 6 mg of estriol. They showed also that the effects of estrogen and exogenous α-adrenergic stimulation were additive. Hodgson, et al. (1978) reported that the sensitivity of the rabbit urethra to α-adrenergic stimulation was estrogen dependent, since castra-tion caused a decrease in sensitivity and treatment with low levels of estrogen reversed this effect. Recent experiments in our laboratory (Levin, Sho-fer, and Wein, 1980; Levin, Jacobowitz, and Wein, 1981) have suggested that parenteral estrogen ad-ministration can change the α-adrenergic receptor content and the autonomic innervation of the lower urinary tract of immature female rabbits. Whether the levels achieved by commonly used oral estrogen preparations or by estrogen vaginal creams (simply providing a convenient vehicle for systemic ab-sorption) can increase the α-adrenergic receptor content of the bladder outlet or the mucosal seal effect is still a matter for speculation and is currently under study. The potential long-term effects of such treatment must be carefully con-sidered, however, in light of the current contro-versy over whether estrogen therapy predisposes the patient to the development of endometrial car-cinoma.

Tricyclic antidepressants

Some authors have found tricyclic antidepres-sants, particularly imipramine hydrochloride (Tof-ranil, Presamine) to be particularly useful agents for facilitating urinary storage (Milner and Hills, 1968; Petersen, Andersen, and Hansen, 1974; Rae-zer et al., 1977; Castleden et al., 1981). All of these drugs possess varying degrees of at least three major pharmacological actions (Hollister, 1978). They are sedatives, presumably on a central basis. They have central and peripheral anticholinergic actions at some, but not all, sites. They block the active transport system in the presynaptic nerve ending, which is responsible for the reuptake of the released amine neurotransmitters serotonin and norepinephrine. In addition, they have antihista-minic properties (Richelson, 1979), and at least desimipramine has been shown to desensitize α_2-receptors on central noradrenergic neurons (Spyraki and Fibiger, 1980). Many such compounds are available and have been categorized as to their relative potency, insofar as their effect on the reuptake of serotonin and norepinephrine is concerned and insofar as their antihistaminic and anticholinergic activity is concerned.

Imipramine inhibits the reuptake of both serotonin and norepinephrine and possesses moderate antihistaminic and anticholinergic properties (Hollister, 1978; Richelson, 1979; Rosenbaum, Maruta, and Richelson, 1979). Imipramine has prominent systemic anticholinergic effects (Byck, 1975); however, it does not appear to have a significant antimuscarinic effect on bladder smooth muscle (Diokno et al., 1972; Dhattiwalla, 1976; Tulloch and Creed, 1979; Olubadewo, 1980). Tulloch and Creed (1979) have noted the same to be true with respect to the effect of imipramine on salivary gland function. A strong, direct inhibitory effect on bladder smooth muscle does exist, however, that is neither adrenergic nor anticholinergic (Dhattiwalla, 1976; Benson et al., 1977; Fredericks, Green, and Anderson, 1978; Tulloch and Creed, 1979; Olubadewo, 1980). This may be caused by a local anesthetic–like action at the nerve terminals in the adjacent effector membrane—an effect that seems to occur also in cardiac muscle (Bigger et al., 1977)—or by inhibition of the participation of calcium in the excitation-contraction coupling process (Olubadewo, 1980).

Clinically, the drug seems to be effective in decreasing bladder contractility and in increasing outlet resistance (Mahoney, Laferte, and Mahoney, 1973; Raezer et al., 1977; Tulloch and Creed, 1979; Castleden et al., 1981). This latter effect is presumably caused by the peripheral blockade of the reuptake of norepinephrine, which would tend to produce or enhance an α-adrenergic effect in the smooth muscle of the bladder base and proximal urethra. Theoretically, at least, this latter action might also tend to stimulate the predominantly β-adrenergic receptors of the bladder body smooth musculature, an action that, if it occurred, would further facilitate urine storage by decreasing the excitability of the smooth muscle in that area. The clinical effect of imipramine on lower urinary tract function is often evident only after days to weeks of treatment, a phenomenon shared by the antidepressant effects of the drug. This may explain why the acute effects of a parenterally administered dose on detrusor hyperreflexia were not noted to be very striking (Diokno et al., 1972; Cardozo and Stanton, 1979). The usual adult dosage of imipramine when used for voiding dysfunction is 25 mg q.i.d. We have given only half that dosage in elderly patients, although Castleden et al. (1981) begin with a single 25 mg nighttime dose in elderly patients and increase this every third day by 25 mg until the patient is improved, has side effects, or reaches a dose of 150 mg.

The most frequent side effects are those attributable to the systemic anticholinergic activity: dry mouth, constipation, dizziness, blurred vision, and tachycardia. Weakness, fatigue, headache, muscle tremors, and epigastric distress may also result, as well as excessive sweating and an allergic type of obstructive jaundice (Byck, 1975; Richelson, 1979; Rosenbaum, Maruta, and Richelson, 1979). Imipramine is contraindicated in patients receiving monoamine oxidase inhibitors because of the danger of potentiating adverse side effects. Like all agents producing a sympathomimetic effect, it should be used with caution in patients with hypertension or cardiovascular disease. In our experience, its effects on the lower urinary tract are often at least additive to those of the atropine-like agents. Consequently, a combination of imipramine and propantheline is sometimes especially useful in decreasing bladder contractility (Raezer et al., 1977). If imipramine is to be used in conjunction with an atropine-like agent, it should be noted that the anticholinergic side effects of the drugs may be additive. If the drug is to be prescribed for voiding dysfunction, the patient should be thoroughly informed of the usual indications, all potential side effects, and, in the United States, of the fact that this drug is not approved by the Federal Regulatory Agency for use in the treatment of any voiding dysfunction. Recently a report of the onset of significant side effects (severe abdominal distress, nausea, vomiting, headache, lethargy, and irritability) following abrupt cessation of high-dose imipramine in children has appeared (Petti and Law, 1981). It would seem prudent therefore to discontinue the drug gradually in patients receiving high doses. Unfortunately, most, if not all, antidepressants can be shown electrophysiologically and hemodynamically to depress the myocardium (Burgess and Turner, 1980; Muller and Schulze, 1980). Whether this will prove to be a legitimate concern in patients receiving relatively small oral doses for lower urinary tract dysfunction remains to be seen and is a potential matter of concern.

TABLE 35.2   Acknowledged and potential effects of various pharmacological agents on urine storage and emptying

Agent	Facilitate emptying		Facilitate storage	
	Increase bladder contractility	Decrease outlet resistance	Inhibit bladder contractility	Increase outlet resistance
Acetylcholine-like agents	+ +			
Anticholinesterases	+ +			
Prostaglandins (E$_2$ and F$_{2\alpha}$)	+ +			
Digitalis	+			
α-Adrenergic blocking agents	+	+ +		
β-Adrenergic stimulating agents		+ +	+	
Centrally acting muscle relaxants*		+ +	+	
Polysynaptic inhibitors		+ +	+	
Direct-acting skeletal muscle relaxants		+ +	+	
Atropine-like agents			+ +	
Ganglionic blocking agents			+ +	
Musculotropic relaxants			+ +	
Calcium antagonists			+ +	
Antihistamines			+ +	
Theophylline			+ +	
Phenothiazines		+	+ +	
Phenytoin		+	+ +	
Prostaglandin inhibitors			+ +	
Narcotics*			+	
Tricyclic antidepressants			+ +	+ +
α-Adrenergic stimulating agents			+	+ +
L-Dopa				+ +
Amphetamines				+ +
β-Adrenergic blocking agents	+			+

+ +, Accepted, widely acknowledged clinical effects; +, theoretical or laboratory effects and/or effects that are not widely clinically acknowledged.
*These act primarily through central effects and may cause decreased emptying on the basis of oversedation or bladder inhibition.

EFFECTS OF VARIOUS PHARMACOLOGICAL AGENTS ON URINE STORAGE AND EMPTYING

It is obvious from the foregoing discussion that any one of a number of agents prescribed for reasons unrelated to voiding dysfunction can affect autonomic nervous system and receptor function and can thereby influence urine storage, urine emptying, or both. Agents that decrease outlet resistance may predispose a patient to stress or sphincteric incontinence or worsen an already existing condition. Agents that increase intravesical pressure by increasing bladder muscle contractility may decrease functional bladder capacity, since the threshold pressure at which the sensation of distension is perceived will be reached at a lower intravesical volume. Thus an increase in urinary frequency and perhaps a feeling of urgency may occur under these circumstances. Agents that inhibit bladder contractility may decrease the urinary flow rate and may cause relative or even complete urinary retention. If emptying is inhibited, an increase in residual urine may well occur, with an increase in urinary frequency because of a decreased functional capacity. Compounds that increase outlet resistance can cause the same end effects on voiding efficiency as those that decrease bladder contractility. It is obvious that adverse and unwanted pharmacological effects on lower urinary tract function do not occur in the great majority of patients treated with agents that can potentially do so. Such effects are usually most manifest in those patients whose pretreatment voiding status already borders on being pathological. Some of these agents and their potential effects are listed in Table 35.2.

REFERENCES

Abrams, P.H., and Dunn, M. 1979. A double blind trial of bromocriptine in the treatment of idiopathic bladder instability. Br. J. Urol. **51**:24-27.

Abromowicz, A., editor. 1975. Baclofen (Lioresal). Med. Lett. Drugs Ther. **20**:43.

Allen, T.D. 1977. The non-neurogenic neurogenic bladder. J. Urol. **117**:232-238.

Andersson, K.E. 1978. Effects of calcium and calcium antagonists on the excitation contraction coupling in striated and smooth muscle. Acta Pharmacol. Toxicol. **43**(1):5-14.

Andersson, K.E., Ek, A., and Persson, C.G.A. 1977. Effects of prostaglandins on the isolated human bladder and urethra. Acta Physiol. Scand. **100**:165-171.

Andersson, K.E., and Forman, A. 1978. Effects of prostaglandins on the smooth muscle of the urinary tract. Acta Pharmcol. Toxicol. **43** (suppl. 2):90-95.

Andersson, K.E., et al. 1981. Effects of prazosin on isolated human urethra and in patients with lower motor neuron lesions. Invest. Urol. **19**:39-42.

Atkins, F.L., and Nicolosi, G.L. 1979. Alpha adrenergic blocking activity of prazosin. Biochem. Pharmacol. **28**:1233-1237.

Awad, S.A., Downie, J.W., and Kiruluta, H.G. 1978. Alpha-adrenergic agents in urinary disorders of the proximal urethra. I. Stress incontinence. Br. J. Urol. **50**:332-335.

Awad, S.A., et al. 1974. Distribution of alpha and beta adrenoreceptors in human urinary bladder. Br. J. Pharmacol. **50**:525-529.

Benson, G.S., et al. 1976. Adrenergic and cholinergic stimulation and blockade of the human bladder base. J. Urol. **116**:174-175.

Benson, G.S., et al. 1977. Comparative effects and mechanisms of action of atropine, propantheline flavoxate, and imipramine on bladder muscle contractility. Urology **9**:31-35.

Bigger, J.T., et al. 1977. Cardiac antiarrhythmic effect of imipramine hydrochloride. N. Engl. J. Med. **296**:206-208.

Blaivas, J.G., et al. 1980. Cystometric response to propantheline in detrusor hyperreflexia: therapeutic implications. J. Urol. **124**:259-262.

Bradley, D.V., and Cazort, R. 1970. Relief of bladder spasm by flavoxate: a comparative study. J. Clin. Pharmacol. **10**:65-68.

Bradley, W.E., Timm, G.W., and Scott, F.B. 1974. Innervation of the detrusor muscle and urethra. Urol. Clin. North Am. **1**:3-28.

Briggs, R.S., Castleden, C.M., and Asher, M.J. 1980. The effect of flavoxate on uninhibited detrusor contractions and urinary incontinence in the elderly. J. Urol. **123**:665-666.

Bultitude, M.I., Hills, N.H., and Shuttleworth, K.E.D. 1976. Clinical and experimental studies on the action of prostaglandins and their synthesis inhibitors on detrusor muscle in vitro and in vivo. Br. J. Urol. **48**:631-637.

Burgess, C.D., and Turner, R. 1980. Cardiotoxicity of antidepressant drugs. Neuropharmacology **19**:1195-1199.

Burnstock, G. 1979. Past and current evidence for the purinergic nerve hypothesis. In Baer, H.P., and Drummond, G.I., editors. Physiological and regulatory functions of adenosine and adenine nucleotides. New York. Raven Press.

Byck, R. 1975. Drugs and the treatment of psychiatric disorders. In Goodman, L.S., and Gilman, A., editors. The pharmacological basis of therapeutics. ed. 5. New York. Macmillan Publishing Co., Inc.

Caine, M., and Raz, S. 1973. The role of female hormones in stress incontinence. Presented at the sixteenth Congress of Societé International d'Urologie. Amsterdam.

Cameron, M.D. 1966. Distigmine bromide (Ubretid) in the prevention of postoperative retention of urine. Br. J. Obstet. Gynaecol. **73**:847-848.

Cardozo, L.D., and Stanton, S.L. 1979. An objective comparison of the effects of parenterally administered drugs in patients suffering from detrusor instability. J. Urol. **122**:58-59.

Cardozo, L.D., and Stanton, S.L. 1980. A comparison between bromocriptine and indomethacin in the treatment of detrusor instability. J. Urol. **123**:399-401.

Cardozo, L.D., et al. 1980. Evaluation of flurbiprofen in detrusor instability. Br. Med. J. **280**:281-282.

Castleden, C.M., et al. 1981. Imipramine—a possible alternative to current therapy for urinary incontinence in the elderly. J. Urol. **125**:318-320.

DeGroat, W.C., and Booth, A.M. 1980. Physiology of the bladder and urethra. Ann. Intern. Med. **92**:312-315.

DeGroat, W.C., and Saum, W.R. 1972. Sympathetic inhibition of the urinary bladder and of pelvic ganglionic transmission in the cat. J. Physiol. **220**:297-314.

DeGroat, W.C., and Saum, W.R. 1976. Synaptic transmission in parasympathetic ganglia in the urinary bladder of the cat. J. Physiol. **256**:137-158.

Delaere, K.P., et al. 1977. Flavoxate hydrochloride in the treatment of detrusor instability. Urol. Int. **32**:337-381.

Desmond, A.D., et al. 1980. Clinical experience with intravesical prostaglandin E$_2$: a prospective study of 36 patients. Br. J. Urol. **52**:357-366.

Dhattiwalla, A.S. 1976. The effect of imipramine on isolated innervated guinea pig and rat urinary bladder preparations. J. Pharm. Pharmacol. **28**:453-454.

Diokno, A.C., and Koppenhoeffer, R. 1976. Bethanechol chloride in neurogenic bladder dysfunction. Urology **8**:455-458.

Diokno, A.C., and Lapides, J. 1972. Oxybutynin: a new drug with analgesic and anticholinergic properties. J. Urol. **108**:307-309.

Diokno, A.C., and Lapides, J. 1977. Action of oral and parenteral bethanechol on decompensated bladder. Urology **10**:23-24.

Diokno, A.C., et al. 1972. Comparison of action of imipramine (Tofranil) and propantheline (Pro-Banthine) on detrusor contractions. J. Urol. **107**:42-43.

Donker, P.J., Ivanovici, F., and Noach, E.L. 1972. Analysis of the urethra pressure profile by means of electromyography and the administration of drugs. Br. J. Urol. **44**:180-193.

Donker, P.J., and van der Sluis, C. 1976. Action of beta-adrenergic blocking agents on the urethral pressure profile. Urol. Int. **31**:6-12.

Downie, J.W., Twiddy, D.A.S., and Awad, S.A. 1977. Antimuscarinic and noncompetitive antagonist properties of dicyclomine hydrochloride in isolated human and rabbit bladder muscle. J. Pharmcol. Exp. Ther. **201**:662-668.

Doxley, J.C., and Roach, A.G. 1980. Presynaptic α-adrenoreceptors: in vitro methods and preparations utilized in the evaluation of agonists and antagonists. J. Auton. Pharmacol. **1**:73.

Duncan, G.W., Shahani, B.T., and Young, R.R. 1976. An evaluation of baclofen treatment for certain symptoms in patients with spinal cord lesions. Neurology **26**:441-446.

Edvardsen, P., and Setekleiv, J. 1968. Distribution of adrenergic receptors in the urinary bladder of cats, rabbits, and guinea pigs. Acta Pharmacol. Toxicol. **26**:437-445.

Ek, A., et al. 1978. The effects of long-term treatment with norephedrine on stress incontinence and urethral closure pressure profile. Scand. J. Urol. Nephrol. **12**:105-110.

Ekeland, A., and Sander, S. 1976. A urodynamic study of emepronium bromide in bladder dysfunction. Scand. J. Urol. Nephrol. **10**:195-199.

Ekman, G., et al. 1980. A double blind crossover study of the effects of terodiline in women with unstable bladder. Acta Pharmacol. Toxicol. **46**(1):39-43.

Elmer, M. 1975. Stimulation of adrenergic nerve fibres to the urinary bladder of the rat. Acta Physiol. Scand. **94**:517-521.

Farrar, D.J., and Osbourne, J.L. 1976. The use of bromocriptine in the treatment of the unstable bladder. Br. J. Urol. **48**:235-238.

Finkbeiner, A.E., Bissada, N.K., and Welch, L.T. 1977. Uropharmacology. IV. Parasympathetic depressants. Urology **10**:503-510.

Fischer, C.P., Diokno, A., and Lapides, J. 1978. The anticholinergic effects of dicyclomine hydrochloride in uninhibited neurogenic bladder dysfunction. J. Urol. **120**:328-329.

Florante, J., et al. 1980. Baclofen in the treatment of detrusor-sphincter dyssynergy in spinal cord injury patients. J. Urol. **124**:82-84.

Forman, A., et al. 1978. Effects of nifedipine on the smooth muscle of the human urinary tract in vitro and in vivo. Acta Pharmacol. Toxicol. **43**:111-118.

Fox, S., et al. 1978. Action of baclofen on mammalian synaptic transmission. Neuroscience **3**:495-515.

Franz, D.N. 1975. Drugs for Parkinson's disease: centrally acting muscle relaxants. In Goodman, L.S., and Gilman, A., editors. The pharmacological basis of therapeutics. ed. 5. New York. Macmillan Publishing Co., Inc.

Fredericks, C.M., Anderson, G.F., and Kreulen, D.L. 1975. A study of the anticholinergic and antispasmodic activity of oxybutynin (Ditropan) on rabbit detrusor. Invest. Urol. **12**:317-319.

Fredericks, C.M., Green, R.L., and Anderson, G.F. 1978. Comparative in-vitro effects of imipramine, oxybutynin, and flavoxate on rabbit detrusor. Urology **12**:487-491.

Ghonheim, M.A., et al. 1976. The influence of vesical distention on the urethral resistance to flow: a possible role for prostaglandins? J. Urol. **116**:739-743.

Gibaldi, M., and Grundhofer, B. 1975. Biopharmaceutic influences on the anticholinergic effects of propantheline. Clin. Pharmacol. Ther. **18**:457-461.

Gibbon, N.O. 1965. Urinary incontinence in disorders of the nervous system. Br. J. Urol. **37**:624-632.

Gleason, D.M., et al. 1974. The urethral continence zone and its relation to stress incontinence. J. Urol. *112*:81-88.

Gosling, J.A., et al. 1981. A comparative study of the human external sphincter and periurethral levator ani muscles. Br. J. Urol. **53**:35-41.

Graham, R.M., and Pettinger, W.A. 1979. Prazosin. N. Engl. J. Med. **300**:232.

Hachen, H.J., and Krucker, V. 1977. Clinical and laboratory assessment of the efficacy of baclofen on urethral sphincter spasticity in patients with traumatic paraplegia. Eur. Urol. **3**:237-240.

Hackler, R.H., et al. 1980. A clinical experience with dantrolene sodium for external urinary sphincter hypertonicity in spinal cord injured patients. J. Urol. **124**:78-81.

Hartviksen, K. 1966. Discussion. Acta Neurol. Scand. Suppl. **42**:180.

Hebjorn, S., and Walter, S. 1978. Treatment of female incontinence with emepronium bromide. Urol. Int. **33**:120.

Hinman, F. 1974. Urinary tract damage in children who wet. Pediatrics **54**:143-150.

Hinman, F., Jr. 1980. Syndromes of vesical incoordination. Urol. Clin. North Am. **7**:311-319.

Hodgson, B.J., et al. 1978. Effect of estrogen on sensitivity of rabbit bladder and urethra to phenylephrine. Invest. Urol. **16**:67-69.

Hoffman, B.B., and Lefkowitz, R.J. 1980. Alpha adrenergic receptor subtypes. N. Engl. J. Med. **302**:1390-1396.

Hollister, L.E. 1978. Tricyclic antidepressants. N. Engl. J. Med. **299**:1106-1109.

Holmberg, E., and Waldeck, B. 1980. On the possible role of potassium ions in the action of terbutaline on skeletal muscle contractions. Acta Pharmacol. Toxicol. **46**:141-149.

Husted, S., et al. 1980. Anticholinergic and calcium antagonistic effects of terodiline in rabbit urinary bladder. Acta Pharmacol. Toxicol. **46**(1):20-30.

Innes, I.R., and Nickerson, M. 1975a. Atripine, scopolamine, and related antimuscarinic drugs. In Goodman, L.S., and Gilman, A., editors. The pharmacological basis of therapeutics. ed. 5. New York. Macmillan Publishing Co., Inc.

Innes, J.R., and Nickerson, M. 1975b. Norephedrine, epinephrine, and the sympathomimetic amines. In Goodman, L.S., and Gilman, A., editors. The pharmacologic basis of therapeutics, ed. 5. New York. Macmillan Publishing Co., Inc.

Jonas, U., Petri, E., and Kissal, J. 1970. Effect of flavoxate on hyperactive detrusor muscle. Eur. Urol. **5**:106.

Jones, R.F., et al. 1970. A new agent for the control of spasticity. J. Neurol. Neurosurg. Psychiatry **33**:464-468.

Johns, A., et al. 1976. The mechanism of action of dicyclomine hydrochloride on rabbit detrusor muscle and vas deferens. Arch. Int. Pharmacodyn. Ther. **224**:109-113.

Johnston, J.H., and Farkas, A. 1975. Congenital neuropathic bladder: practicalities and possibilities of conservational management. Urology **5**:719-727.

Khanna, O.P. 1976. Disorders of micturition: neuropharmacologic basis and results of drug therapy. Urology **8**:316-328.

Khanna, O.P., Barbieri, E.J., and McMichael, R. 1978. Effects of prostaglandins on vesicourethral smooth muscle of rabbit. Urology **12**:674-681.

Khanna, O.P., et al. 1979. In-vitro study of antispasmodic effects of dicyclomine hydrochloride on vesicourethral smooth muscle of guinea pig and rabbit. Urology **13**:457-462.

Kiesswetter, H., and Schober, W. 1975. Lioresal in the treatment of neurogenic bladder dysfunction. Urol. Int. **30**:63-71.

Kleeman, F.J. 1970. The physiology of the internal urinary sphincter. J. Urol. **104**:549-554.

Koelle, G. 1975. Parasympathomimetic agents. In Goodman, L.S., and Gilamn, A., editors. The pharmacologic basis of therapeutics. ed. 5. New York. Macmillan Publishing Co., Inc.

Kohler, F.P., and Morales, P.A. 1968. Cystometric evaluation of flavoxate hydrochloride in normal and neurogenic bladder. J. Urol. **100**:729-730.

Krane, R.J., and Olsson, C.A. 1973a. Phenoxybenzamine in neurogenic bladder dysfunction. I. A theory of micturition. J. Urol. **110**:650-652.

Krane, R.J., and Olsson, C.A. 1973b. Phenoxybenzamine in neurogenic bladder dysfunction. II. Clinical considerations. J. Urol. **110**:653-656.

Krier, J., Thor, K.B., and DeGroat, W.C. 1979. Effects of clonidine on the lumbar sympathetic pathways to the large intestine and urinary bladder of the cat. Eur. J. Pharmacol. **59**:47-53.

Kuru, M. 1965. Nervous control of micturition. Physiol. Rev. **45**:425-494.

Lapides, J. 1964. Urecholine regimen for rehabilitating the atonic bladder. J. Urol. **91**:658-659.

Lapides, J. 1974. Neurogenic bladder: principles of treatment. Urol. Clin. North Am. **1**:81-97.

Lapides, J., et al. 1963. Comparison of action of oral and parenteral bethanechol chloride upon the urinary bladder. Invest. Urol. **1**:94-97.

Larsen, J., and Mortensen, S. 1978. Effect of ritodrine on the bladder capacity in unanaesthetized pigs. Acta Pharmacol. Toxicol. **43**:405-408.

Levin, R.M., Jacobowitz, D., and Wein, A.J. 1981. Autonomic innervation of the rabbit urinary bladder following estrogen administration. Urology **17**:449-453.

Levin, R.M., Shofer, F.S., and Wein, A.J. 1980. Estrogen-induced alteration in the autonomic responses of the rabbit urinary bladder. J. Pharmacol. Exp. Ther. **215**:614-618.

Levin, R.M., Staskin, D., and Wein, A.J. 1982. The muscarinic cholinergic binding kinetics of human urinary bladder. Neurourol. Urodynamics **1**:221-226.

Lish, P.M., et al. 1965. Oxybutynin: a musculotropic antispasmodic drug with moderate anticholinergic action. Arch. Int. Pharmacodyn. **156**:467.

MacGregor, R.J., and Diokno, A.C. 1981. The alpha adrenergic blocking action of prazosin hydrochloride on the canine urethra. Invest. Urol. **18**:426-429.

Mahoney, D.T., Laferte, R.O., and Mahoney, J.E. 1973. Observations on sphincter augmenting effect of imipramine in children with urinary incontinence. Urology **2**:317-323.

Medical Letter. 1980. Dimethyl sulfoxide (DMSO). Med. Lett. Drugs Ther. **22**:93.

Merrill, D.C., and Rotta, J. 1974. A clinical evaluation of detrusor denervation supersensitivity using air cystometry. J. Urol. **111**:27-30.

Meyhoff, H.H., and Nordling, J. 1981. Br. J. Urol. **53**:129-133.

Milner, G., and Hills, N.F. 1968. A double blind assessment of antidepressants in the treatment of 212 enuretic patients. Med. J. Aust. **1**:943-947.

Mirakhur, R.K., Dundee, J.W., and Jones, C.J. 1978. Evaluation of the anticholinergic actions of glycopyrronium bromide. Br. J. Clin. Pharmacol. **5**:77-84.

Mobley, D.F. 1976. Phenoxybenzamine in the management of neurogenic vesical dysfunction. J. Urol. **116**:737-738.

Muller, J., and Schulze, S. 1980. Imipramine cardiotoxicity: an electrocardiographic and hemodynamic study in rabbits. Acta Pharmacol. Toxicol. **46**:191-199.

Murdock, M.M., Sax, D., and Krane, R.J. 1976. Use of dantrolene sodium in external sphincter spasm. Urology **8**:133-137.

Nanninga, J.B., Kaplan, P., and Lal, S. 1977. Effect of phentolamine on perineal muscle EMG activity in paraplegia. Br. J. Urol. **49**:537-539.

Nordling, J., Meyhoff, H.H., and Christensen, N.J. 1979. Effects of clonidine on urethral pressure. Invest. Urol. **16**:289-291.

Norlen, L., Sundin, T., and Waagstein, F. 1978. Beta-adrenoceptor stimulation of the human urinary bladder in vivo. Acta Pharmacol. Toxicol. **43**(11):26-30.

Norlen, L., et al. 1976. The adrenergic innervation and adrenergic receptor activity of the feline urinary bladder and urethra in the normal state and after hypogastric and/or parasympathetic denervation. Scand. J. Urol. Nephrol. **10**:177-184.

Obrink, A., and Bunne, G. 1978. The effect of alpha adrenergic stimulation in stress incontinence. Scand. J. Urol. Nephrol. **12:**205-208.

Olsson, C.A., Siroky, M.B., and Krane, R.J. 1977. The phentolamine test in neurogenic bladder dysfunction. J. Urol. **117:**481-485.

Olsson, C.A., et al. 1979. Effects of β-adrenoceptor agonists on airway smooth muscle and on slow contracting skeletal muscle: in vitro and in vivo results compared. Acta Pharmacol. Toxicol. **44:**272-276.

Olubadewa, J.O. 1980. The effect of imipramine on rat detrusor muscle contractility. Arch. Int. Pharmacodyn. **245:**84-94.

Palmer, J.H., Worth, P.H.L., and Exton-Smith, A.N. 1981. Flunarizine: a once-daily therapy for urinary incontinence. Lancet **2:**279-281.

Parkes, D. 1979. Drug therapy: bromocriptine. N. Engl. J. Med. **301:**873-878.

Parsons, K.F., and Turton, M.B. 1980. Urethral supersensitivity and occult urethral neuropathy. Br. J. Urol. **52:**131-137.

Paulson, D.F. 1978. Oxybutynin chloride in control of post transurethral vesical pain and spasm. Urology **11:**237-238.

Pedersen, E., and Grynderup, V. 1966. Clinical pharmacology of the neurogenic bladder. Acta Neurol. Scand. Suppl. **42:**111.

Perkash, I. 1975. Intermittent catheterization and bladder rehabilitation in spinal cord injury patients. J. Urol. **114:**230-233.

Petersen, K.E., Anderson, O.D., and Hansen, T. 1974. Mode of action and relative value of imipramine and similar drugs in the treatment of nocturnal enuresis. Eur. J. Clin. Pharmacol. **7:**187-194.

Petti, T.A., and Law, W. 1981. Abrupt cessation of high dose imipramine therapy treatment in children. J.A.M.A. **246:**768-769.

Philp, N.H., and Thomas, D.G. 1980. The effect of distigmine bromide on voiding in male paraplegic patients with reflex micturition. Br. J. Urol. **52:**492-496.

Philp, N.H., Thomas, D.G., and Clarke, S.J. 1980. Drug effects on the voiding cystometrogram: a comparison of oral bethanechol and carbachol. Br. J. Urol. **52:**484-487.

Raezer, D.M., et al. 1973. Autonomic innervation of canine urinary bladder: cholinergic and adrenergic contributions and interaction of sympathetic and parasympathetic systems in bladder function. Urology **2:**211-221.

Raezer, D.M., et al. 1977. The functional approach to the management of the pediatric neuropathic bladder. J. Urol. **117:**649-654.

Raz, S., and Caine, M. 1971. Adrenergic receptors in the female canine urethra. Invest. Urol. **9:**319-323.

Raz, S., and Smith, R.B. 1976. External sphincter spasticity syndrome in female patients. J. Urol. **115:**443-446.

Raz, S., 1977. Methyldopa in treatment of neurogenic bladder disorders. Urology **9:**188-190.

Richelson, E. 1979. Tricyclic antidepressants and histamine H-1 receptors. Mayo Clin. Proc. **54:**669-674.

Ritch, A.E.S., et al. 1977. A second look at emepronium bromide in urinary incontinence. Lancet **1:**504-506.

Rosenbaum, A.H., Maruta, T., and Richelson, E. 1979. Drugs that alter mood. I. Tricyclic agents and monoamine oxidase inhibitors. Mayo Clin. Proc. **54:**335-344.

Roussan, M.S., et al. 1975. Bladder training: its role in evaluating the effect of an antispasticity drug on voiding in patients with neurogenic bladder. Arch. Phys. Med. Rehabil. **56:**463-468.

Rud, T., et al. 1980. Terodiline inhibition of human bladder contraction: effects in vitro and in women with unstable bladder. Acta Pharmacol. Toxicol. **46**(1):31-38.

Salmon, U.J., Walter, R.I., and Geist, S.H. 1941. The use of estrogen in the treatment of dysuria and incontinence in post menopausal women. Am. J. Obstet. Gynecol. **42:**845.

Schreiter, F., Fuchs, P., and Stockamp, K. 1976. Estrogenic sensitivity of alpha receptors in the urethral musculature. Urol. Int. **31:**13-19.

Sjögren, C., and Andersson, K.E. 1979. Effects of cholinoceptor blocking drugs, adrenoceptor stimulants and calcium antagonists on the transmurally stimulated guinea pig urinary bladder in vitro and in vivo. Acta Pharmacol. Toxicol. **44:**228-234.

Sonda, L.P., et al, 1979. Further observations on the cystometric and uroflometric effects of bethanechol chloride on the human bladder. J. Urol. **122:**775-777.

Spyraki, C., and Fibiger, H.C. 1980. Functional evidence for subsensitivity of noradrenergic α-2 receptors after chronic desipramine treatment. Life Sci. **27:**1863-1867.

Stanton, S.L. 1973. A comparison of emepronium bromide and flavoxate hydrochloride in the treatment of urinary incontinence. J. Urol. **110:**529-532.

Stanton, S.L. 1978. Diseases of the urinary system. Drugs acting on the bladder and urethra. Br. Med. J. **1:**1607-1608.

Stewart, B.H., Banowsky, L.H.W., and Montague, D.K. 1976. Stress incontinence: conservative therapy with sympathomimetic drugs. J. Urol. **115:**558-559.

Stewart, B.H., and Shirley, S.W. 1976. Further experience with intravesical DMSO in the treatment of interstitial cystitis. J. Urol. **116:**36-38.

Stockamp, K. 1975. Treatment with phenoxybenzamine of upper urinary tract complications caused by intravesical obstruction. J. Urol. **113:**128-131.

Stockamp, K., and Schreiter, F. 1975. Alpha adrenolytic treatment of the congenital neuropathic bladder. Urol. Int. **30:**33.

Sundin, T., et al. 1977. The sympathetic innervation and adrenoreceptor function of the human lower urinary tract in the normal state and after parasympathetic denervation. Invest. Urol. **14:**322-328.

Tanagho, E.A. 1978. The anatomy and physiology of micturition. Clin. Obstet. Gynecol. **5:**3-26.

Taylor, M.C., and Bates, C.P. 1979. A double blind crossover trial of baclofen—a new treatment for the unstable bladder syndrome. Br. J. Urol. **51:**504-505.

Thompson, I.M., and Lauvetz, R. 1976. Oxybutynin in bladder spasm, neurogenic bladder and enuresis. Urology **8:**452-454.

Tulloch, A.G., and Creed, K.E. 1979. A comparison between propantheline and imipramine on bladder and salivary gland function. Br. J. Urol. **51:**359-362.

Twiddy, D.A.S., Downie, J.W., and Awad, S.A. 1980. Response of the bladder to bethanechol after acute spinal cord transection in cats. J. Pharmacol. Exp. Ther. **215:**500.

Ursillo, R.C. 1967. Rationale for drug therapy in bladder dysfunction. In Boyarsky, S., editor. The neurogenic bladder. Baltimore. The Williams and Wilkins Co.

Vaidyanathan, S., et al. 1980. Beta adrenergic activity in human proximal urethra: a study of terbutaline. J. Urol. **124:**869-871.

Vaidyanathan, S., et al. 1981. Study of intravesical instillation of 15(5)-15 methyl prostaglandin F-2$_\alpha$ in patients with neurogenic bladder dysfunction. J. Urol. **126:**81-85.

Wein, A.J. 1979. Pharmacologic approaches to the management of neurogenic bladder dysfunction. J. Cont. Educ. Urol. **18**(5):17.

Wein, A.J. 1980. Pharmacology of the bladder and urethra. In Stanton, S.L., and Tanagho, E.A., editors. Surgery of female incontinence. Berlin. Springer-Verlag.

Wein, A.J. 1981. Classification of neurogenic voiding dysfunction. J. Urol. **125:**605-609.

Wein, A.J., Benson, G.S., and Jacobowitz, D. 1979. Lack of evidence for adrenergic innervation of the external urethral sphincter. J. Urol. **121:**324-326.

Wein, A.J., and Levin, R.M. 1979. Comparison of adrenergic receptor density in urinary bladder in man, dog, and rabbit. Surg. Forum **30:**576-578.

Wein, A.J., and Raezer, D.M. 1979. Physiology of micturition. In Krane, R., and Siroky, M., editors. Clinical neurourology. Boston. Little, Brown & Co.

Wein, A.J., Raezer, D.M., and Benson, G.S. 1976. Management of neurogenic bladder dysfunction in the adult. Urology **8:**432-443.

Wein, A.J., Raezer, D.M., and Malloy, T.R. 1980. Failure of the bethanechol supersensitivity test to predict improved voiding after subcutaneous bethanechol administration. J. Urol. **123:**202-203.

Wein, A.J., et al. 1978. The effect of oral bethanechol chloride on the cystometrogram of the normal adult male. J. Urol. **120:**330-331.

Wein, A.J., et al., 1980. The effects of bethanechol chloride on urodynamic parameters in normal women and in women with significant residual urine voumes. J. Urol. **124:**397-399.

Weinshiebaum, R.M. 1980. Antihypertensive drugs that alter adrenergic function. Mayo Clin. Proc. **55:**390-402.

Whitfield, H.N., et al. 1976. The effect of adrenergic blocking drugs on outflow resistance. Br. J. Urol. **47:**823-827.

Yalla, S.V., et al. 1977. Detrusor-urethral sphincter dyssynergia. J. Urol. **118:**1026-1029.

Zelis, R.F. 1981. Calcium entry blockers in cardiologic therapy. Hosp. Pract. August, pp. 49-56.

Ziegler, M.G., et al. 1979. Bromocriptine inhibits norepinephrine release. Clin. Pharmacol. Ther. **25:**137-142.

chapter 36

Electrical therapy

STANISLAV PLEVNIK

Electrical stimulation of the neuromuscular structures involved in the function of the bladder and the urethra has been the subject of research and has been in routine use for the past two decades. It is used for the correction of both urinary incontinence and retention.

This chapter reviews methods of electrical stimulation currently in use and the mechanisms by which they act and suggests future research objectives in this area. From among the rather large and varied number of methods of electrical stimulation that are available on the market or are otherwise suggested for the correction of urinary dysfunctions, primarily those that have been more or less objectively evaluated are discussed.

ELECTRICAL STIMULATION FOR URINARY INCONTINENCE

Two different methods of electrical stimulation for the correction of urinary incontinence are in use and are classified according to the time of application and the intensity of the electrical stimuli: long-term, or chronic, electrical stimulation and short-term, or maximum, electrical stimulation.

Chronic electrical stimulation

Caldwell (1963) was the first to introduce chronic electrical stimulation for the correction of urinary incontinence in humans. He used an implantable radio-linked electrical stimulator with electrodes adjacent to the urethral musculature. Many patients with urinary incontinence of varying causes were treated with this method. In about 50% of the cases treatment was successful.

The relatively low rate of success as compared with the risks of implantation speeded up the replacement of the implantable stimulators by noninvasive stimulation techniques using nonimplantable stimulators. These consist of an external generator and electrodes in the form of various designs of vaginal and anal plugs. They are used by patients continuously during their daily activities and during the night if needed. These devices usually consist of an external, miniature, battery-operated pulse generator, which is carried on the patient's clothing and is connected to the vaginal plug electrodes (Figure 36.1) or anal plug electrodes (Figure 36.2) by a cable. Different designs and sizes of electrodes are used, such as the vaginal ring pessary (Alexander and Rowan, 1968; Hill et al., 1968), the elliptical Hodge's pessary, cylindrical vaginal plug electrodes (De Soldenhoff and McDonnel, 1969), expandable vaginal electrodes (Fall et al., 1978), and the anal plug electrodes (Hopkinson and Lightwood, 1967). The electrodes are made of different materials such as stainless steel and silver- and

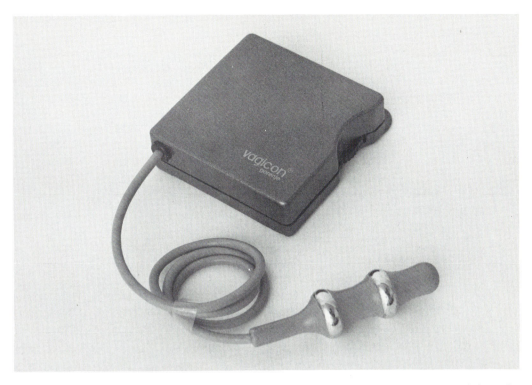

Figure 36.1 Gorenje Vagicon: box containing battery and pulse generator with vaginal cylindrical electrodes. (Courtesy of GORENJE, Velenje, Yugoslavia.)

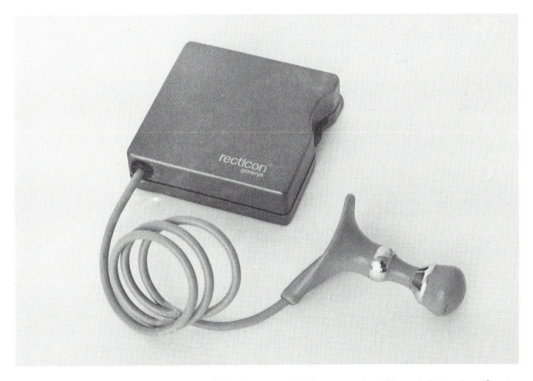

Figure 36.2 Gorenje Recticon: box containing battery and pulse generator with anal electrodes. (Courtesy of GORENJE, Velenje, Yugoslavia.)

gold-plated titanium and are incorporated into a plug consisting of materials such as polyethylene, silicon rubber, Perspex, Plexiglas, and acrylic. The shapes of these electrodes are selected with the aims of provoking a good pelvic floor contraction when stimulated and achieving maximum retention during stimulation. The materials of the electrodes are inert so as not to cause electrical corrosion, which could lead to damage of the stimulated tissue.

Both the cable leading from the electrodes to the external unit and the external unit itself are inconvenient and impractical. To avoid this an automatic integrated system in the form of a vaginal plug was developed (Figure 36.3) (Suhel, 1976; Suhel, Kralj, and Plevnik, 1978). This complete system

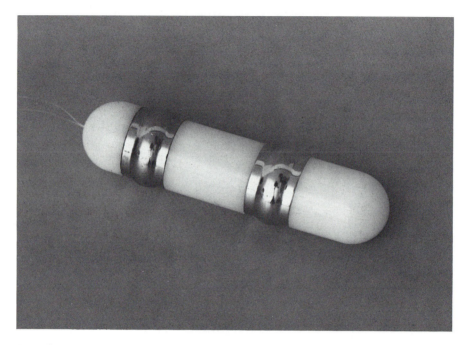

Figure 36.3 Gorenje Vagicon-X: automatic integrated vaginal stimulator. (Courtesy of GORENJE, Velenje, Yugoslavia.)

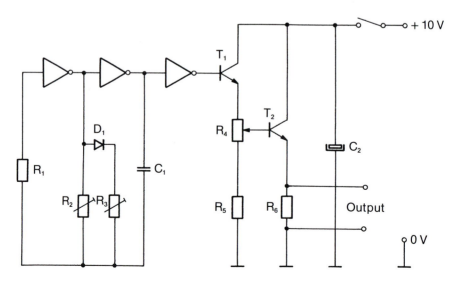

Figure 36.4 Electronic circuit of electrical stimulator.

together with the battery and electronic circuit is placed in a waterproof housing made of Plexiglas. The electrodes are made of stainless steel. The system is automatically turned on when the electrodes come in contact with the walls of the vagina and turned off when the contact is broken by their removal.

The electronic circuits of the stimulators are more or less based on the same principle (Figure 36.4). They contain a complementary multivibrator, which feeds an emitter-follower output stage from which a continuous train of monophasic rectangular pulses of different frequencies and pulse widths is delivered.

Those parameters of electrical stimuli that are considered to be optimum and that are most frequently applied (via either implanted electrodes or anal or vaginal electrodes) have a frequency of 20 Hz and a pulse width of 1 msec. The amplitude of the stimulus is in a range from 4 to 12 V (Caldwell, 1967; Riddle, Hill, and Wallace, 1969; Alexander and Rowan, 1970; Harrison and Paterson, 1970; Plevnik et al., 1977). On the other hand, some researchers use higher frequencies of up to 200 Hz and pulse widths of down to 0.2 msec (De Soldenhoff and McDonnell, 1969; Hopkinson, 1972).

The amplitude of the stimulus is adjusted by the patient up to the intensity where the stimulator can still be comfortably used. In the case of the automatic vaginal electrical stimulator, the amplitude of the stimulus cannot be adjusted and is fixed at a value of 8 V.

Short-term maximum electrical stimulation

Moore and Schofield (1967) described a qualitatively different method of electrical stimulation for the treatment of urinary incontinence, which they called maximum perineal electrical stimulation. Contrary to stimulation with chronic implantable and nonimplantable stimulators, which extends over several hours daily for prolonged periods of time, they stimulated only once. They applied faradic stimulation to the perineal body of anesthetized patients to obtain four to six maximum tetanic contractions of all the voluntary musculature. The faradic surge consisted of 1 msec pulses and lasted for 2 to 3 seconds, the pause before a subsequent faradic surge being 2 to 3 seconds. The surging stimulus was applied between a unipolar electrode placed on the perineal body and an indifferent electrode placed under the sacrum. The intensity of the stimulation was increased until all

the voluntary musculature gave maximum contraction. This method was used by different researchers, their results ranging from 30% success to complete failure. Many patients benefited but reverted to the original state after several months. This method is no longer in use.

Encouraged by the results of Moore and Schofield, Godec and Cass (1978) used the method of acute maximum electrical stimulation in patients with urinary incontinence. The method consists of a 15- to 25-minute application of electrical stimulation to unanesthetized patients. The high-intensity electrical stimuli with amplitudes from 100 to 150 mA, frequency 20 Hz, and pulse width 1 msec were applied concurrently via anal plug electrodes and needle electrodes inserted into the levator ani muscle. The applications of stimulation were repeated 4 to 10 times with 2 to 3 days between applications.

Plevnik and Janez (1979) used a modified method of maximum electrical stimulation. They stimulated via only anal or vaginal plug electrodes, using one channel unit generating constant current pulses (Figure 36.5). The current applied ranged from 15 to 100 mA in adults and from 7 to 25 mA in children. The adults adjusted the amplitude of the stimulation by themselves up to the level of tolerable discomfort (Janez, Plevnik, and Vrtacnik, 1980; Plevnik et al., 1980).

Short-term maximum electrical stimulation is intended for treatment in inpatient and outpatient clinics and exceptionally for use in the patient's home. A therapeutic effect is observed mostly after the first or second application of maximum electrical stimulation and lasts from several days to several months. Therefore the stimulation should be repeated periodically, depending on the duration of the therapeutic effects.

Indications and contraindications

Nonimplantable electrical stimulation can successfully be used in most types of urinary incontinence that are caused by urethral sphincter incompetence as well as for bladder instability. It proved to be of benefit in patients with genuine stress incontinence, idiopathic urge incontinence, urgency, frequency, enuresis, and neuropathic incontinence (De Soldenhoff and McDonnell, 1969; Alexander and Rowan, 1970; Alexander et al., 1970; Harrison and Paterson, 1970; Edwards and Malvern, 1972; Godec, Cass, and Ayala, 1976; Plevnik et al., 1977; Godec and Cass, 1978; Plevnik and Janez, 1979).

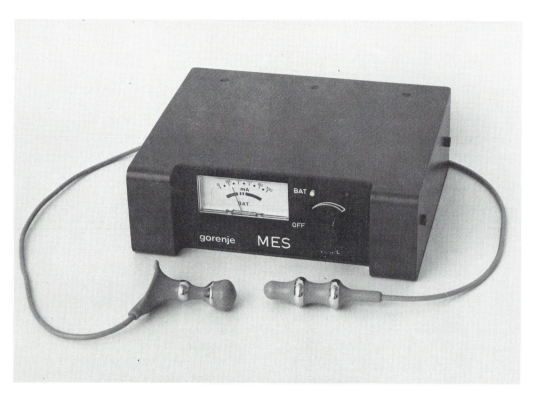

Figure 36.5 Gorenje MES: stimulator for maximum electrical stimulation with electrodes. (Courtesy of GOR-ENJE, Velenje, Yugoslavia.)

Urinary incontinence caused by urethral sphincter incompetence can be successfully treated by application of either chronic or short-term maximum electrical stimulation. In the case of incontinence caused by bladder instability, I recommend short-term maximum electrical stimulation, although chronic stimulation can also be successful in some patients. The average success rate is moderate, that is, up to 50%, although it varies from 10% to 90% among different researchers. In the case of urge incontinence caused by objectively confirmed detrusor instability, the success rate of treatment with maximum electrical stimulation is somewhat higher (Kralj et al., 1977; Janez et al., 1980). The stimulation can result in a cure but mostly will result in different degrees of improvement of the symptoms of incontinence.

Electrical stimulation is contraindicated in patients with retention of urine except when it is caused by an upper motor neuron lesion and when the patient has pronounced autonomous hyperreflexia. There is no place for electrical stimulation in patients whose incontinence is caused by urinary fistulae or ectopic ureter.

Selection of patients and methods

My experience in the use of nonimplantable electrical stimulation for the treatment of urinary incontinence suggests the following guidelines for preparing patients for electrical stimulation and for choosing it from among the methods of treatment available (Plevnik and Janez, 1979) (Figure 36.6). Before treatment the patient should undergo careful urological, urodynamic, and neurological examination to obtain a precise diagnosis of the type and degree of incontinence. Before the application of electrical stimulation, general measures have to be taken, such as treatment or urinary tract infection, reduction of body weight if necessary, and exercises for pelvic floor muscles, which can later be combined with electrical stimulation.

Many different ways of selecting patients and methods of electrical stimulation have been suggested by different authors. Most of them are based on the observation of pelvic floor contraction during electrical stimulation (Alexander et al., 1970) or on urodynamic measurement of urethral and bladder responses to electrical stimulation (Harrison and Paterson, 1970), which predict the clinical

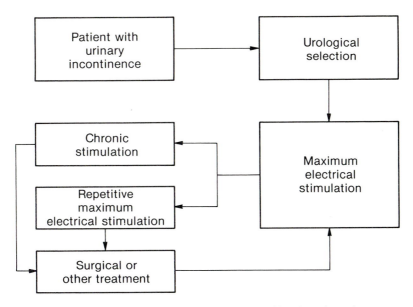

Figure 36.6 Scheme of management of patient with urinary incontinence.

effects of stimulation. Among my patients treated with electrical stimulation the only reasonably reliable prediction of the effect of electrical stimulation was obtained by observing the clinical state of the patients in the period of time after the application of maximum electrical stimulation. Regardless of the results of urodynamic and neurological examination, one to two applications of maximum electrical stimulation should be carried out. The positive temporary effect of maximum electrical stimulation can be a good, although not entirely reliable, guide for further application of either maximum electrical stimulation or chronic nonimplantable electrical stimulation. It is interesting to note that although in some patients two applications of maximum electrical stimulation produced no effect, those patients benefited later by further stimulation.

After the test application with maximum electrical stimulation, the chronic nonimplantable stimulator should be prescribed primarily for those patients in whom incontinence is caused by urethral sphincter incompetence. In cases where it does not affect the weakened urethral closing muscles because of the limited strength of the stimuli, maximum electrical stimulation should be prescribed as a further treatment. The repetitive treatment with maximum electrical stimulation could increase the excitability of the urethral closing mechanism and thus enable the continuation of treatment with chronic stimulation.

Maximum electrical stimulation should be prescribed whenever an unstable bladder appears to be the main cause of incontinence. In cases where chronic electrical stimulation usually fails to inhibit bladder activity, it is caused by the limited strength of the stimulation (Teague and Merrill, 1977).

When incontinence is caused by both urethral sphincter incompetence and bladder instability, maximum electrical stimulation applications are recommended, with chronic stimulation applied in the periods between maximum electrical stimulation applications as well as afterward if necessary. It can be expected in many of these cases that bladder instability will diminish or cease after the application of maximum electrical stimulation, whereas urethral sphincter incompetence will remain.

In appropriate patients, unsuccessful treatment with electrical stimulation is followed by surgery, sometimes with only partial success. In some of these patients in whom the anatomical changes have been corrected but incontinence still remains, further treatment with electrical stimulation can improve the remaining disability.

The place of electrical stimulation in the hierarchy of treatment methods differs among clinical institutions. Most of the researchers apply electrical stimulation as a last resort for curing urinary incontinence. This approach is understandable when implantable electrical stimulators are used; however I consider nonimplantable electrical stimulation as the next step if general measures have failed to bring relief to the patient.

Mode of action

Urethral closure. By electrical stimulation of the anogenital area using either implanted or vaginal or anal electrodes, the motor as well as sensory nerves can, in theory, be excited. Therefore there is the possibility of direct as well as reflex electrical stimulation, this being the subject of disagreement among many investigators. The prevalence of direct stimulation was suggested in many previous studies (Caldwell, Flack, and Broad, 1965; Alexander and Rowan, 1966), whereas more recent studies suggest the prevalence of reflex stimulation (Collins, 1972; Brindley, Rushton, and Craggs, 1974; Trontelj et al., 1974). The number of directly or reflexly excited motor units innervating the muscles involved in the urethral closing mechanism depend on the place and intensity of stimulation, with the frequency and duration of stimulus taken as constant.

Whereas it is more or less clear how electrical stimulation excites the pelvic floor muscles, the question of what particular pelvic floor muscles are being stimulated is much more difficult to answer. On the other hand, the mechanisms of continence as well as of incontinence are far from being elucidative. With commonly used methods of investigation, we are not able to determine precisely how and by which muscles of the pelvic floor closure of the urethra is provided. In patients with urinary incontinence caused by urethral sphincter incompetence (for example, genuine stress incontinence), the measurement of static urethral pressure as well as urethral length frequently fails to objectify incontinence or improvement or failure during electrical stimulation.

Relatively high urethral pressure response, which shows up immediately after the onset of electrical stimulation and lasts from 2 to 3 minutes, declines until it reaches a considerably lower sustained value (Harrison, 1976). It can be speculated that the fast-twitch muscle fibers of the pelvic floor are activated during the initial phase of the response; a decline of pressure follows because of their fatigue. The role of fatigue in maintaining continence is a question to be answered.

Bladder inhibition. It has been shown that in patients with urinary incontinence caused by detrusor instability, electrical stimulation produces not only reflex contraction of the urethral closure muscles but also the reflex inhibition of the antagonist, that is, the detrusor muscle (Godec, Cass, and Ayala, 1975; Rakovec, Plevnik, and Kralj, 1977). This finding was confirmed by measuring cystometric curves and bladder capacities before and during electrical stimulation. If present, the uninhibited bladder contractions were reduced or ceased completely. Bladder inhibition requires higher intensities of stimulation as compared with those needed to produce urethral closure (Teague and Merrill, 1977).

Therapeutic effects. It has been known for some time that chronic electrical stimulation of weakened urethral closing muscle as well as the weakened skeletal muscle produces not only a strengthening of the muscles during stimulation but also long-term recovery of the muscles. Theoretically, neuromuscular structures must be preserved to a certain degree if response to electrical stimulation or therapeutic effects is to be expected.

More recent research on muscle fiber and efferent nerve electrical stimulation reveals that the sustained strengthening of the weakened skeletal muscle can be caused by functional change of fast-twitch muscle fibers into slow-twitch muscle fibers as a result of training with low-frequency electrical stimulation for long periods of time (Salmons and Vrbova, 1969). Thus a qualitative change of primary structure takes place. The fast-twitch muscle fibers may take over the function of the slow ones, so that the recovered muscle is able to produce slower and less powerful but more sustained contractions with less fatigue. In the case of electrically stimulated urinary closing muscles, the proposed mechanism has to be verified.

Previous interpretation of the mechanism of muscle recovery could serve only to a certain extent as an explanation of the recovery of incontinent patients with urethral sphincter incompetence. Some of these patients benefited immediately after test stimulation examination when the suitable type of chronic electrical stimulator was determined (Plevnik et al., 1977). Therefore some so far inexplicable changes in neural activity should presumably cause recovery of urethral neuromuscular function, since achievement of the functional change of muscle structure needs much longer periods of stimulation. In most cases of recovery it is possible that an interaction of sustained changes in neural and muscular activity takes place.

Contrary to chronic electrical stimulation, short-term maximum electrical stimulation produces temporary or sustained therapeutic effects in patients with incontinence caused by urethral sphincter incompetence as well as in patients with incontinence caused by bladder instability. Some strikingly prompt temporary or sustained changes of neural origin must be involved in producing such temporary or sustained therapeutic effects on bladder and urethral function. A sustained increase in tonic activity of sphincteric motor units, as shown by methods utilizing electromyography (EMG) was observed in patients after one application of maximum electrical stimulation (Vodusek and Kralj, 1979). The mechanism that enables such prompt sustained changes in the neural function is unknown.

As seen from the results of treatment of different types of incontinence, one session of anal or vaginal maximum electrical stimulation produced complete or partial improvement of a temporary nature, whereas in a smaller percentage of cases sustained recovery was achieved. In some patients several successive monthly maximum electrical stimulation sessions revealed sustained recovery or gradual improvement after each session. This implies that temporary recovery can be converted to sustained recovery with repetitively applied maximum electrical stimulation.

Future research trends

Electrical stimulation for urinary incontinence is a rather poorly accepted method of treatment despite its beneficial effects and simplicity of use. The main reason is probably insufficient exploration of its mode of action. Therefore future research should be directed primarily toward the exploration of the mode by which electrical stimulation functions.

In several preliminary studies new, more physiological, methods of stimulation were proposed, such as on-demand stimulation and intermittent alternating electrical stimulation. On-demand stimulators provide electrical stimulation during increased activity of the pelvic floor muscles, which occurs during holding, coughing, and sneezing, and is intended for the correction of genuine stress incontinence. Either vaginal EMG (Armstrong, 1970) or anal pressure (Plevnik et al., 1977) is used as a control signal. Intermittent alternating electrical stimulation was designed to reduce the fatigue and therefore to produce sustained contraction of the pelvic floor muscles by stimulating them alternately via vaginal and anal electrodes (Plevnik and Janez, 1978).

It seems that for the moment there is no need to seek new methods of stimulation, since we do not fully understand the functioning of the existing, commercially available, electrical stimulators. Unless we know more precisely what is being stimulated, what should be stimulated, and what the mechanisms of therapeutic effects and their duration are so that we might predict them, clinician acceptance of this method of treatment is unlikely.

If we want to know what should be stimulated or otherwise corrected to provide continence, undoubtedly the mechanism of continence itself as well as the mechanisms of different types of incontinence should be further elucidated.

In most of the types of incontinence that are caused by an unstable bladder, such as motor urge incontinence and incontinence caused by reflex neurogenic bladder, the beneficial effects of electrical stimulation are caused by electrically induced inhibition of the uninhibited contractions of the detrusor, which are the cause of incontinence.

Sustained increase of urethral pressure as well as increase of the tonic EMG activity of the striated sphincter is also achieved as a consequence of stimulation in some patients (Plevnik and Janez, 1979; Vodusek and Kralj, 1979). With the aim of achieving optimum utilization of electrical stimulation and obtaining insight into the physiological mechanisms of the observed therapeutic effects, several questions that relate to the neural structures involved in these changes, to the optimum method of stimulation that produces the most prolonged therapeutic effects, and to the ability to predict these effects need to be answered. The role of inherent coordinating reflex activity between the bladder and the urethra in producing the therapeutic effects should also be explored.

In the case of incontinence caused by urethral sphincter incompetence such as genuine stress incontinence, the situation is far more complicated. The mechanisms of continence and incontinnence during rest and during stress have not been fully explored. It is intuitively understood that as long as there is positive urethral closure pressure, there should be no leakage of urine and therefore the patient should be continent. The resultant forces that originate from different passive and active bladder, urethral, and periurethral structures tend to compress or to open the urethral lumen and in the phase of continence produce the positive urethral closure pressure.

Compressing forces, which are created by elastin

and collagen fibers, vascular bed, smooth muscles of the urethra, slow-twitch striated external sphincter, and slow- and fast-twitch peri-urethral striated muscles (Gosling, 1979), are possibly low-speed developing forces and should serve mainly for the maintenance of the basal level of compression, which enables a positive urethral closure pressure during rest, bladder filling, and slow changes, that is, slow increases of intravesical pressure. The fast-twitch periurethral striated muscle fibers possibly produce high-speed developing forces that maintain positive urethral closure pressure during the fast increases of intravesical pressure, which occur during coughing for instance.

It would be important to know which particular periurethral muscles are producing the urethral compression during stress as well as whether they are aiding urethral closure during electrical stimulation. Most of the female patients with genuine stress incontinence have no significant denervation of the pelvic floor muscles as shown by EMG (Vodusek, Janko, and Kralj, 1979). On the other hand, in many patients electrical stimulation provides no benefit even though the patients have little or no peripheral denervation. Therefore even if electrical stimulation presumably produces a sufficient contraction of the urethral closing muscles, continence will not be achieved when other changes such as decrease in the compressive action of the urethral sphincter mechanism caused by postpartum anatomical change are present. By measuring the urethral and detrusor pressures during coughing and straining, the distribution of urethral and bladder pressure–transmission ratio during stress was estimated in continent and stress-incontinent women (Constantinou, Faysal, and Govan, 1980; Constantinou and Govan, 1980; Faysal et al., 1981). Surprisingly, in continent women during stress this ratio had the greatest increase in the distal half of the urethra and not at the point of the maximum resting urethral profile. This finding indicates that during stress the reflex action of the urethral, or more likely the periurethral muscles such as levator ani muscles that are located in the distal third of the urethra, produce the greatest positive urethral closure pressure. In the patients with stress incontinence the ratio of urethral and bladder pressure–transmission proved to be much lower as compared with the normal controls. One of the next steps in the investigation of the functioning of electrical stimulation would certainly be to study the effects of electrical stimulation on transmission ratio. The other approach to determining which particular muscles are stimulated would possibly involve the measurement of circular pressure distribution in the individual cross sections of the urethral lumen (Hilton and Stanton, 1981).

The concept of opening forces rather than pressures is new. In a preliminary study (1981), I estimated the bladder circumference from semilateral

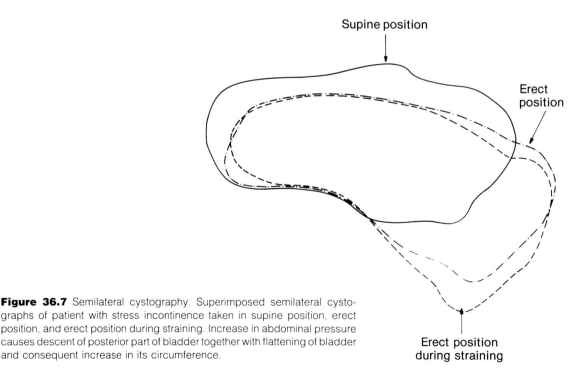

Supine position

Erect position

Erect position during straining

Figure 36.7 Semilateral cystography. Superimposed semilateral cystographs of patient with stress incontinence taken in supine position, erect position, and erect position during straining. Increase in abdominal pressure causes descent of posterior part of bladder together with flattening of bladder and consequent increase in its circumference.

cystographs taken in the supine and erect position during rest and during straining with and without electrical stimulation of the pelvic floor. The results obtained indicate an increase of bladder circumference and flattening of the bladder during the increase of abdominal pressure and decrease of circumference during electrical stimulation (Figures 36.7 and 36.8). Since the bladder geometry changes during increase of abdominal pressure, it seems that there is no hydrostatic pressure transmission to the urethra. The bladder is pressed against the pelvic floor in a way that cannot be compared with a balloon placed in a pressurized water chamber (Figure 36.9). Therefore it seems that there is no transmittable structure that would permit the abdominal forces to act radially on the urethra and thus cause its compression. Increase of the bladder circumference means an increase in the stretching of the bladder wall that is likely to produce an increase in the forces on the bladder wall that act to open the bladder neck. The decrease of the bladder circumference during electrical stimulation of the pelvic floor indicates that the pelvic floor support also has a function in reducing the flattening of the bladder and hence limiting the development of the opening forces. Studies should be further pursued in this direction. It would also be interesting to explore the relationship of this new concept to the initiation of voiding and to the detrusor contraction provoked by stress.

ELECTRICAL STIMULATION FOR URINARY RETENTION

Although extensive efforts have been made to mimic electrically the micturition reflex and thus to provide effective urinary bladder evacuation in spinal cord–injured patients, the results obtained were rather poor compared with the results of electrical stimulation in the treatment of urinary incontinence.

Numerous attempts to empty the bladder using implanted electrodes by direct bladder stimulation, pelvic nerve stimulation, sacral nerve stimulation, or spinal cord stimulation failed to provide satisfactory urinary bladder control. Failures were caused by many factors such as pain, technical and biological problems at the electrode tissue interface, and electrode wires. The main problem was electrically induced detrusor sphincter dyssynergia caused by insufficiently controlled current spread. Detailed reviews of different methods of controlled micturition through electrical stimulation are given by Bradley, Timm, and Chou (1971) and Schmidt and Tanagho (1979).

The need to provide effective electrical control of micturition remains. Brindley (1977) attempted to control micturition by stimulating ventral sacral nerve roots of neurologically intact baboons by using an implanted stimulator. Strong electrical stimuli were delivered in bursts with 2-second intervals between the bursts. Since smooth muscle relaxes much more slowly than striated muscle, the bladder contracted smoothly, but striated muscles relaxed during the intervals and allowed the urine to be expelled. Using the same stimulator, he was also able to provide effective closure of the urethra between micturitions by stimulating the roots with weak electrical stimuli that activated the striated closing muscles only, since the somatic nerve fibers are substantially larger and therefore more electri-

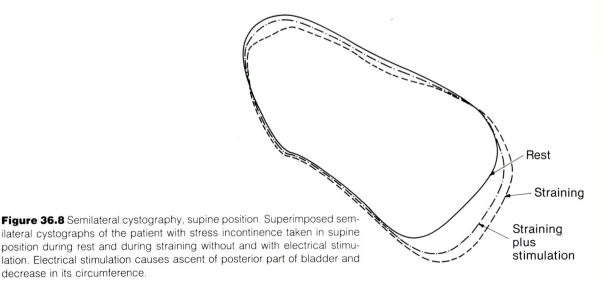

Rest

Straining

Straining plus stimulation

Figure 36.8 Semilateral cystography, supine position. Superimposed semilateral cystographs of the patient with stress incontinence taken in supine position during rest and during straining without and with electrical stimulation. Electrical stimulation causes ascent of posterior part of bladder and decrease in its circumference.

Abdominal pressure, P_1

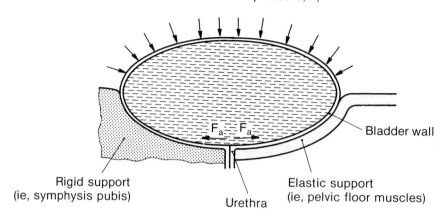

Rigid support
(ie, symphysis pubis)

Bladder wall

Urethra

Elastic support
(ie, pelvic floor muscles)

Increased abdominal pressure, P_2

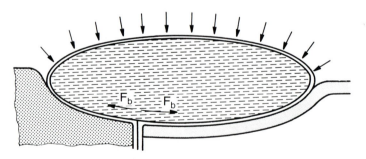

Circumference (b) > Circumference (a)

$$F_b > F_a$$

Figure 36.9 Schematic presentation of concept of opening forces. Increase of abdominal pressure causes flattening of bladder with consequent increase in bladder circumference. Circumference of ellipse under *(b)* is 19% greater than circumference under *(a)*. Areas of both ellipses are equal. Resultant stretch of the bladder wall produces increase of forces, *F*, in bladder wall, which tend to open bladder neck.

cally sensitive than parasympathetic nerves. A different approach was suggested by Schmidt, Bruschinin, and Tanagho (1978) from the studies carried out on paraplegic female dogs. By electrical stimulation of the ventral root of the sacral nerve having the greatest detrusor representation and by selected division of somatic fibers from the stimulated sacral root they were able to avoid electrically induced detrusor sphincter dyssynergia and thus provide effective voiding. The effectiveness of this proposed method will most likely be verified in humans.

It also seems of interest to mention the beneficial effects of epidural spinal cord electrical stimulation in patients with multiple sclerosis and urinary retention caused by a spastic sphincter. The use of upper thoracic epidural spinal cord stimulation caused inhibition of the tonic activity of the somatic sphincter associated with voluntary initiation and maintenance of voiding (Cook et al., 1979).

On the other hand, nonimplantable short-term maximum electrical stimulation benefited patients with upper motor neuron lesions who had urinary retention as well. In a preliminary study treatment with maximum electrical stimulation was successful in paraplegics with long-standing as well as recent lesions who had not developed reflex bladders; it was also successful in paraplegics with long-standing lesions who had well-developed reflex bladders and in whom retention occurred afterward (Plevnik, et al., 1980). Maximum electrical stimulation seems to balance favorably the integrated reflex activity involved in micturition. It produced prolonged facilitation of the bladder and also prolonged inhibition of the urinary closing muscles. Similar urodynamic responses were obtained from the study of acute bladder and urethral responses to maximum electrical stimulation (Janez, Plevnik, and Suhel, 1979). More detailed urodynamic and neurophysiological studies are necessary for a better understanding of the mechanisms of these therapeutic effects.

REFERENCES

Alexander, S., and Rowan, D. 1966. Closure of the urinary sphincter mechanism in anaesthetized dogs by means of electrical stimulation of the perineal muscles. Br. J. Surg. **52:**808-812.

Alexander, S., and Rowan, D. 1968. An electric pessary for stress incontinence. Lancet **1:**728.

Alexander, S., and Rowan, D. 1970. Electrical control of urinary incontinence: a clinical appraisal. Br. J. Surg. **57:**766-768.

Alexander, S., et al. 1970. Treatment of urinary incontinence by electric pessary: a report of 18 patients. Br. J. Urol. **42:**184-190.

Armstrong, D.R. 1970. An electronic device that provides demand stimulation of muscle. Master's thesis. Belfast. Queen's University.

Bradley, W.E., Timm, G.W., and Chou, S.N. 1971. A decade of experience with electronic stimulation of the micturition reflex. Urol. Int. **26:**283-303.

Brindley, G.S. 1977. An implant to empty the bladder or close the urethra. J. Neurol. Neurosurg. Psychiatry **40:**358-369.

Brindley, G.S., Rushton, D.N., and Craggs, M.D. 1974. The pressure exerted by the external sphincter of the urethra when its motor nerve fibers are stimulated electrically. Br. J. Urol. **46:**453-462.

Caldwell, K.P. 1963. The electrical control of sphincter incompetence. Lancet **2:**174.

Caldwell, K.P. 1967. The treatment of incontinence by electronic implants. Ann. R. Coll. Surg. Engl. **41:**447-449.

Caldwell, K.P., Flack, F.C., and Broad, A.F. 1965. Urinary incontinence following spinal injury treated by electronic implant. Lancet **1:**846-847.

Collins, C.D. 1972. Observations on the effect of electrical stimulation. Proc. R. Soc. Med. **65:**832.

Constantinou, C.E., Faysal, M.H., and Govan, D.E. 1980. The impact of bladder neck suspension on the mode of distribution of abdominal pressure along the female urethra. In Zinner, N., and Sterling, A., editors. Female incontinence. New York. Alan Liss, Inc.

Constantinou, C.E., and Govan, D.E. 1980. Contribution and timing of transmitted and generated pressure components in the female urethra. In Zinner, N., and Sterling, A., editors. Female incontinence. New York. Alan Liss, Inc.

Cook, A.W., et al. 1979. Neurogenic bladder: reversal by stimulation of thoracic spinal cord. N. Y. State J. Med. **79:**255-258.

De Soldenhoff, R., and McDonnel, H. 1969. New device for control of female urinary incontinence. Br. Med. J. **4:**230.

Edwards, L., and Malvern, J. 1972. Electronic control of incontinence: a critical review of the present situation. J. Urol. **44:**467-472.

Fall, M., et al. 1978. Long-term intravaginal electrical stimulation in urge and stress incontinence. Scand. J. Urol. Nephrol. **44:**55-63.

Faysal, M.H., et al. 1981. The impact of bladder neck suspension on the resting and stress urethral pressure profile: a prospective study comparing controls with incontinent patients preoperatively and post operatively. J. Urol. **125:**55-60.

Godec, C., and Cass, A. 1978. Acute electrical stimulation for urinary incontinence. Urology **12:**340-342.

Godec, C., Cass, A.S., and Ayala, G.F. 1975. Bladder inhibition with functional electrical stimulation. Urology **6:**663-666.

Godec, C., Cass, A.S., and Ayala, G.F. 1976. Electrical stimulation for incontinence. Urology **7:**388-397.

Gosling, J. 1979. The structure of the bladder and urethra in relation to function. Urol. Clin. North Am. **6:**31-38.

Harrison, N.W., and Paterson, P.J. 1970. Urinary incontinence in woman treated by electronic pessary. Br. J. Urol. **42:**481-485.

Harrison, N.W. 1976. The basis of electrical stimulation in urology. In Williams, D.I., and Chisholm, G.D., editors. Scientific foundations of urology. London. William Heinemann Medical Books, Ltd.

Hill, D.W., et al. 1968. Electric pessary for stress incontinence. Lancet **2:**112-113.

Hilton, P., and Stanton, S.L. 1981. Personal communication.

Hopkinson, B.R. 1972. Electrical treatment of incontinence using an external stimulator with intra-anal electrodes. Ann. R. Coll. Surg. Engl. **50:**92-111.

Hopkinson, B.R., and Lightwood, R. 1967. Electrical treatment of incontinence. Br. J. Surg. **54:**802-805.

Janez, J., Plevnik, S., and Suhel, P. 1979. Urethral and bladder responses to anal electrical stimulation. J. Urol. **122:**192-194.

Janez, J., Plevnik, S., and Vrtacnik, P. 1980. Maximal electrical stimulation for female urinary incontinence. Proceedings of the first joint meeting of the International Continence Society and Urodynamic Society. Los Angeles.

Kralj, B., et al., 1977. Urge incontinence and maximal electrical stimulation. Proc. of seventh annual meeting of the International Continence Society. Portoroz.

Moore, T., and Schofield, P.F. 1967. Treatment of stress incontinence by maximum perineal electrical stimulation. Br. Med. J. **3:**150-151.

Plevnik, S. 1981. The bladder deformation during increase of the abdominal pressure. (In press.)

Plevnik, S., Fliser, K., and Kralj, B. 1977. Anal pressure-controlled electrical stimulator. Digest of papers, first Mediterranean conference on Med. and Biol. Enging., Sorrento, **1:**21-24.

Plevnik, S., and Janez, J. 1978. Alternating intermittent electrical stimulation of urethral closing muscles. Proceedings of the tenth annual meeting of International Continence Society. Rome.

Plevnik, S., and Janez, J. 1979. Maximal electrical stimulation for urinary retention: a report on 98 cases. Urology **14:**638-646.

Plevnik, S., et al. 1977. Effects of functional electrical stimulation on the urethral closing muscles. Med. Biol. Eng. Comput. **15:**155-167.

Plevnik, S., et al. 1980. Maximal electrical stimulation for urinary dysfunctions. Proceedings of the International Conference on Reh. Engng. pp. 230-233, Toronto.

Rakovec, S., Plevnik, S., and Kralj, B. 1977. The mechanisms of the action of electrical stimulation of muscles. Urol. Int. **32:**232-237.

Riddle, P.R., Hill, D.W., and Wallace, D.M., 1969. Electronic techniques for the control of adult urinary incontinence. Br. J. Urol. **41:**205-210.

Salmons, S., and Vrbova, G. 1969. The influence of activity on some contractile characteristics of mammalian fast and slow muscles. J. Physiol. **201:**535-549.

Schmidt, R.A., Bruschini, H., and Tanagho, E.A. 1978. Feasibility of inducing micturition through chronic stimulation of sacral roots. Urology **12:**471-477.

Schmidt, R.A., and Tanagho, E.A. 1979. Feasibility of controlled micturition through electric stimulation. Urol. Int. **34:**199-230.

Suhel, P. 1976. Adjustable nonimplantable electrical stimulators for correction of urinary incontinence. Urol. Int. **31:**115-123.

Suhel, P., Kralj, B., and Plevnik, S. 1978. Advances in nonimplantable electrical stimulators for correction of urinary incontinence. J. Life Sci. **8:**11-16.

Teague, C.T., and Merrill, D.C. 1977. Electric pelvic floor stimulation: mechanisms of action. Invest. Urol. **15:**65-69.

Trontelj, J.V., et al. 1974. Electrical stimulation for urinary incontinence: a neurophysiological study. Urol. Int. **29:**213-220.

Vodusek, D., Janko, M., and Kralj, B. 1979. Electromyography of the pelvic floor muscles in incontinent female patients. Zdrav. Vestn. **48:**577-578.

Vodusek, D., and Kralj, B. 1979. Change in sphincter EMG activity after strong electrical stimulation. Proceedings of the ninth annual meeting of International Continence Society. Rome.

chapter 37

Bladder drainage

STUART L. STANTON

Catheter drainage of the bladder is a day-to-day procedure carried out by nurses and physicians and sometimes by patients. Apart from the latter, familiarity with catheterization may sometimes result in neglect of important principles of asepsis and lead to urinary tract infection. Nursing and medical staff may be unaware of the advances in catheter design and drainage that can save nursing time and enhance patient comfort.

The indications for catheter drainage are as follows:

1. Acute urinary retention (Chapter 21) from whatever cause will require catheterization, especially if incontinence (chronic retention with overflow), recurrent urinary tract infection, or deterioration of the upper urinary tract occurs.

2. Following pelvic surgery (urological, rectal, or gynecological), postoperative urinary retention caused by pain, anatomy, or local edema can result and require catheterization.

3. Injury to the bladder and urethra following trauma or surgery requires catheterization to allow free drainage of urine and promote healing without the risk of fistula formation.

4. Persistent urinary incontinence, which is a social or hygienic problem, requires catheterization.

The complications of continuous catheter drainage are discomfort, urinary tract infection, encrustation with urinary salts both on the inside and outside of the catheter, and a decrease in bladder capacity if catheter drainage is maintained for a long time.

475

The following methods of catheterization will be described:

1. Urethral, which may be a single event.
2. Intermittent, carried out by the patient.
3. Continuous indwelling.
4. Suprapubic via an open cystostomy, using a transurethral obturator, or via a stab incision.

If the catheter is to be retained, it should be attached in a sterile fashion to a closed drainage system that does not allow urine to track back from the bag and can be drained regularly without entry of organisms. There should be a urine-sampling sleeve fitted on the drainage tube to allow sampling without interruption of the closed circuit system.

URETHRAL CATHETERIZATION

Urethral bladder drainage is the oldest and simplest method of catheterization. The flexible rubber catheter was first manufactured in the nineteenth century, and in 1937 Foley described a self-retaining balloon catheter, which bears his name and is now almost synonymous with urethral catheterization. Latex (which is an irritant to the urethral mucosa) has begun to be superseded by Neoplex and Silastic materials, which are less irritant, have a limitless shelf life, can be used for 6 to 8 weeks if necessary, and evoke minimum encrustation by urinary salts. Caution should be exercised in choosing between Silastic and Silastic-coated catheters, since they will vary in their internal gauge and ability to withstand internal and external encrustation (George, Feneley, and Slade, 1978).

Types

The common urethral catheters are shown in Figure 37.1. They may be classified as non-self-retaining (for example, Nelaton) or self-retaining with an inflatable balloon (for example, Foley). The former is used when catheterization is a brief event such as immediately before pelvic surgery, for investigative purposes, or to fill the bladder before insertion of a suprapubic catheter.

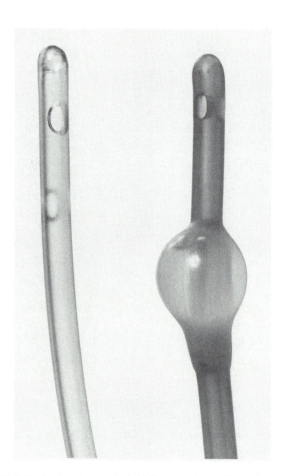

Figure 37.1 Urethral catheters: *Left*, Nelaton catheter. *Right*, Foley catheter.

Indications

The indications for urethral catheterization are as follows:

1. Trauma to the bladder and urethra with or without hematuria, when certain and dependable bladder drainage or urethral stenting is required.
2. Filling the bladder before insertion of suprapubic catheter.
3. During investigation of bladder and urethral function.

Technique

The technique of urethral catheterization varies considerably. Sadly it is often delegated to a junior nurse or physician who may be unaware of the importance of sterility and have never been shown a safe technique. While catheterization in the female is less uncomfortable than in the male, an effort should be made to make this as pain free a procedure as possible. The catheter should be well lubricated with a surface anesthetic gel. A No. 12 to 14 F gauge catheter is usually adequate for the female urethra. The catheter, sterile swabs, antiseptic solution, and a collecting vessel should be immediately at hand. A mask is not necessary, but hands should be washed and gloved. One hand parts the labia and exposes the external urethral meatus; keeping this position, the meatus is swabbed once or twice with antiseptic solution in a downward direction, and the catheter is passed directly into the meatus for about 6 cm. Then the hand separating the labia is placed suprapubically to exert pressure on the bladder and express urine (Figure 37.2). When urine flow ceases, the catheter is slowly withdrawn (never advanced, as this causes entry of organisms into the urethra). The residual urine should be measured if necessary. If the catheter is to be indwelling, the bulb should be inflated with only about 10 ml of sterile saline or water and connected to a closed drainage system. The catheter should be secured to the thigh to prevent the balloon tugging on the bladder neck.

Complications

Complications of urethral bladder drainage include urethritis, leakage, and failure of the balloon to deflate.

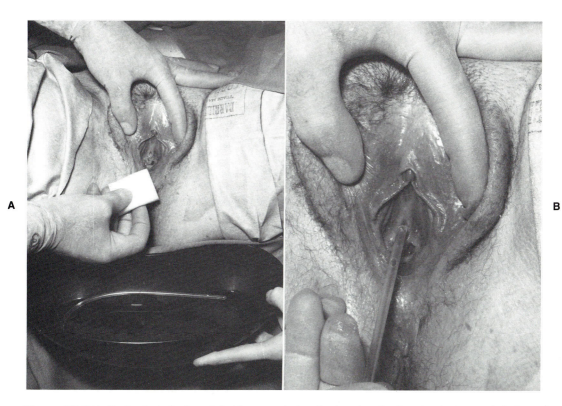

Figure 37.2 Urethral catheterization: **A,** Labia are parted and external urethral meatus is cleansed. Catheter is close at hand. **B,** Catheter introduced directly into external urethral meatus. *Continued.*

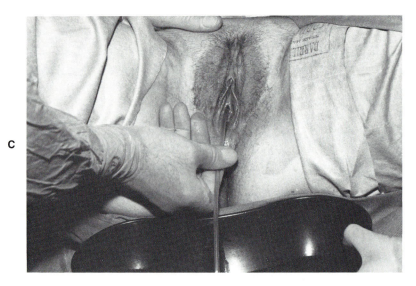

C

Figure 37.2, cont'd. C, Suprapubic pressure aids expression of urine.

Urethritis. Urethritis results from irritation by a latex catheter. If the catheter is tight fitting, it will block off the paraurethral glands, preventing their secretions from escaping and leading to paraurethral abscess formation.

Leakage. Leakage results from too much water being instilled into the balloon; 5 to 10 ml can be withdrawn, and this is usually effective. Alternatively, if too large a catheter has been used in the past, the urethra may become grossly dilated. The use of an even larger catheter only aggravates the problem, and suprapubic catheterization may be more suitable. Sometimes leakage resulting from uninhibited detrusor contractions occurs, and this may be treated by propantheline (Pro-Banthine) or a similar antispasmodic preparation.

Failure of the balloon to deflate. Old-fashioned methods to burst the balloon, such as injection of ether or water into the balloon, are to be eschewed. These only leave fragments of balloon inside the bladder to form a nidus for a calculus. Either the catheter can be cut and allowed to deflate over 24 hours or, more effectively, the balloon can be pulled firmly down to the bladder neck and a sterile stylet introduced through the anterior vaginal wall to puncture the balloon. The balloon should be checked afterward to ensure that no material remains behind, in which case endoscopic removal will be required.

Disadvantages

The disadvantages include the discomfort of a urethral catheter (including difficulty with inter-

course if the catheter is indwelling) and the uncertainty of knowing whether micturition will resume once the catheter is removed, which may necessitate further urethral catheterization. Finally, residual urine cannot be measured (as it can with a suprapubic catheter) without further catheterization or the use of ultrasound measurement.

INTERMITTENT SELF-CATHETERIZATION
Indications

Intermittent clean catheterization by the patient was first described by Lapides et al. in 1972 for patient with obstructive uropathy complicated by urinary tract infection with pyelonephritis and hydronephrosis. Its aim was to avoid overdistension of the bladder and the sequela of ischemia of the bladder wall. The feasibility of unsterile but clean catheterization was based on the concept that host resistance rather than the invading microorganisms was the most important determinant of urinary infection. Since then, reports of the practicability and benefits of this method have been published by many clinicians (Lyon, Scott, and Marshall, 1975; Whitfield and Mayo, 1976: Madersbacher and Weissteiner, 1977).

Technique

The patient must have a reasonably dextrous hand and must be able to place herself in the position for self-catheterization. She should be taught the techinque by the nursing staff, who will first instruct her in anatomy with the aid of a mirror placed between her legs while the patient lies su-

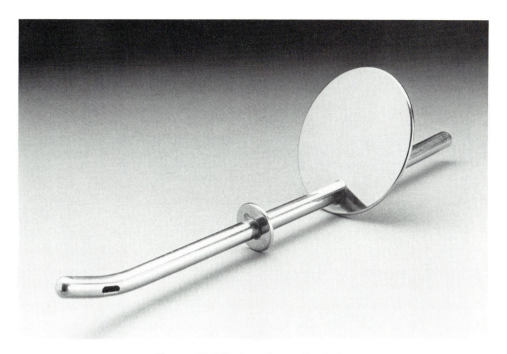

Figure 37.3 Bruijnen-Boer self-catheter.

pine. The patient then washes her hands and either stands with one leg flexed and placed on a chair or sits in bed in an upright position, flexing her knees, and abducting her thighs. A receiver is placed between her legs. Parting her labia with one hand, the patient uses the other hand to clean the external urethral meatus with antiseptic solution. She can watch this either with a mirror or use the specially designed catheter of Bruijnen-Boer (Figure 37.3), which has a mirrored surface incorporated. The catheter is carefully inserted and the urine drained into the receiver. This is carried out 1 to 3 times a day, depending on the need. Long-term antimicrobial therapy may be given, or regular midstream urine specimens may be taken and antimicrobial agents prescribed accordingly. The technique is suitable for both children and the elderly.

Complications

The major complications of self-catheterization is urinary tract infection, but most series report a coincident overall fall in infection. Lapides et al. 1976 state that no patient suffered renal deterioration as judged by intravenous urogram, blood urea nitrogen, and serum creatinine levels.

SUPRAPUBIC CATHETERIZATION

Suprapubic catheterization is intended to decrease urinary tract infection, encourage prompt return to spontaneous micturition following pelvic surgery, and avoid the need for recatheterization for urinary retention. It was described by Hodgkinson and Hodari (1966), and many authors since then have attested to its value, particularly in the care of patients after pelvic surgery (Bonanno, Landers, and Rock 1970; Mattingly, Moore, and Clark, 1972; Hilton and Stanton, 1980).

Types

There are many different catheters available.

Bonanno catheter. The Bonanno catheter (No. 6 Fr gauge, manufactured by Becton, Dickinson & Co.) can be inserted close to a suprapubic incision and is secured by two small tabs sutured to the skin. The sutures will hold the catheter in place for about 3 weeks, which is ideal for postoperative use. The gauge is adequate, provided hematuria does not occur; this may block the catheter. It can easily be inserted in the office or the ward using local anesthetic (Figure 37.4).

Cystocath. The Cystocath, (No. 8 Fr gauge, manufactured by Dow Corning Corp.) is secured to the skin by a large round adhesive flange. This limits its insertion close to a wound. The three-way tap is not as simple to operate as the clamp on the Bonanno catheter (Figure 37.5).

Stamey catheter. The Stamey percutaneous catheter (No. 10 Fr gauge, manufactured by Vance

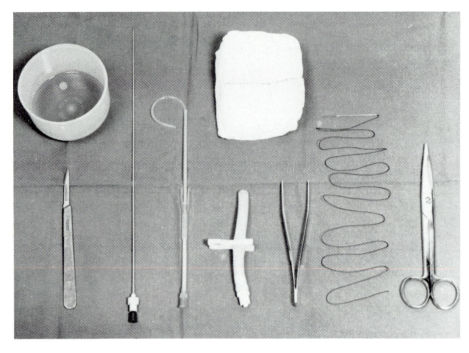

Figure 37.4 Bonanno catheter with instruments required for its insertion.

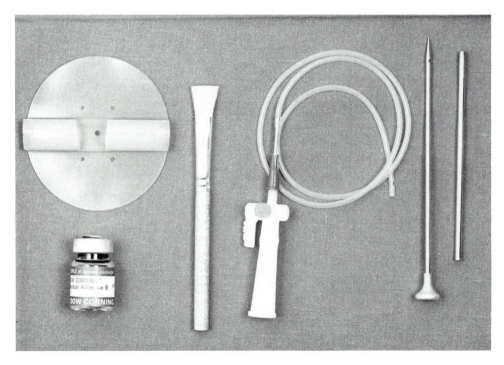

Figure 37.5 Cystocath set.

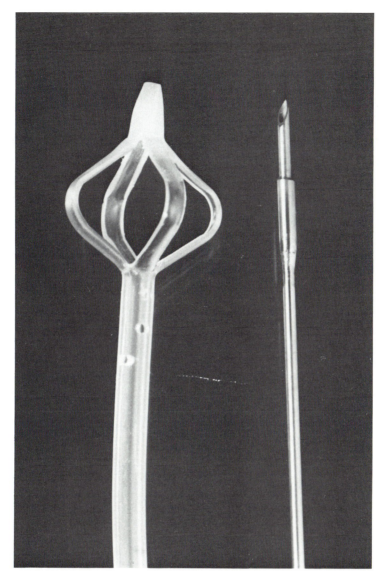

Figure 37.6 Stamey catheter. *Right*, Catheter straightened with stylet in place before insertion. *Left*, Malecot end is shown without stylet in place.

Products, Inc.) has a Malecot-designed end to retain it within the bladder and is strapped to the skin (Figure 37.6).

Argyle Ingram catheter. The Argyle Ingram trocar catheter (No. 12 or 16 Fr gauge, manufactured by Sherwood Medical Industries, Inc.) is more solid in construction and has an additional irrigation channel. It is secured by an intravesical balloon and flange sutured to the skin. It is ideal where hematuria is expected (Figure 37.7).

Foley catheter. A Foley catheter may be used suprapubically.

Indications

The indications for suprapubic catheterization are as follows:

1. Following pelvic surgery (All gynecological, urological, and rectal operations may be complicated by postoperative urinary retention. In particular, operations to correct incontinence frequently give rise to acute retention. Suprapubic catheterization allows spontaneous voiding and measurement of residual urine without further catheterization.)

2. In the management of acute retention, when

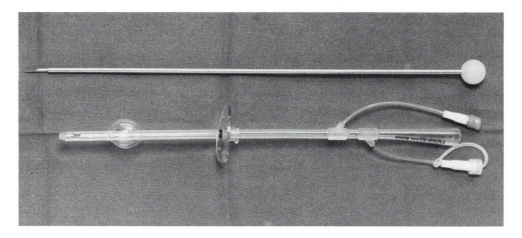

Figure 37.7 Argyle Ingram trocar catheter, 12-gauge, with stylet above.

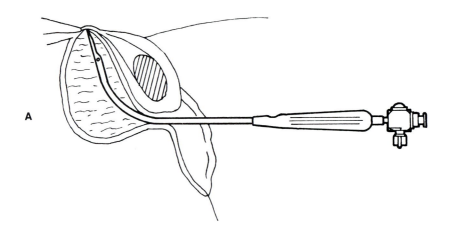

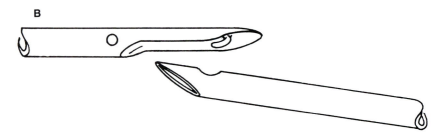

Figure 37.8 A, Robertson's cystotrocar introduced into bladder. **B**, Close-up of hook at end of trocar to connect with eye of catheter.

spontaneous voiding has not occurred despite several urethral catheterizations.

3. Urethral trauma or surgery, when urethral catheterization may be prejudicial to healing.
4. When bladder drainage is required in the presence of acute vulvovaginal irritation and when urethral catheterization may cause further discomfort.

Advantages

The advantages of suprapubic catheterization over a urethral catheter are a decreased incidence of urinary tract infections (Andersen et al., 1982), more comfort for the patient, and easier management for the nursing staff.

Disadvantages

The disadvantages of suprapubic catheterization include potential risk of bowel injury and the need for its insertion by medical rather than nursing staff.

Contraindications

The contraindications of suprapubic catheterization include inability to distend the bladder, a recent cystostomy, and gross hematuria if small-gauge catheters are used.

Technique

The suprapubic catheter may be inserted either with the help of a sound or Robertson's cystotrocar (1973) (Figure 37.8) passed transurethrally. The cystotrocar allows the bladder to be filled and has a small hook at its distal end to secure the suprapubic catheter and pull it into the bladder. The rigidity of this instrument may limit its use following certain bladder neck operations for incontinence. Alternatively, the catheter can be inserted at open cystostomy or by closed stab technique. Either a local anesthetic or a general anesthetic (when carried out at the end of an operation) may be used. The bladder is filled aseptically with between 400 and 500 ml of sterile water. A small stab incision is made in the midline about 3 cm above the symphysis pubis, and the catheter is inserted. A free flow of fluid should be obtained. If not, the catheter should be reinserted. When drainage is satisfactory, the catheter is fixed in position and connected to a drainage bag.

Complications

The immediate complications include perforations of the large or the small bowel. The catheter should be removed and a fresh catheter resited. Conservative treatment consisting of observation and metronidazole (Flagyl) or a cephalosporin will usually suffice. Hematuria may occur on the first day following insertion as a result of trauma or later as a result of cystitis or irritation of the bladder mucosa by the catheter. In the absence of urinary tract infection, hematuria usually settles spontaneously. Sometimes after working satisfactorily for 1 to 2 days, the catheter fails to drain. This is either due to blockage or to extrusion of the catheter from the bladder into the extravesical space. The catheter should be detached from the drainage tube and sterile water syringed backward and forward gently. If there is a block, it can be cleared. Aspiration will yield the equivalent amount that was injected. If the catheter is outside the bladder, this maneuver may be painful and no fluid will be reaspirated. The catheter should be resited.

Later complications include leakage around the catheter. This may be due to fracture of the catheter or to urine tracking back along its insertion. The most common place for a fracture to occur is the junction between the portion of the catheter in the bladder and the external portion. To detect a fracture, the catheter is gently pulled out 2 cm and clamped close to the skin. The catheter is disconnected from the drainage tube and 5 to 10 ml of fluid is inserted through a sterile syringe. If leakage occurs, a break is present and the new catheter should be reinserted. Finally, a portion of the indwelling catheter may become detached and remain within the bladder when the catheter is withdrawn. The catheter should always be carefully inspected when it is withdrawn; any retained portion can be removed endoscopically.

CATHETER AND DRAINAGE BAG MANAGEMENT

A closed drainage system is important in the prevention of urinary tract infection, and it should be interrupted only if the catheter is blocked or leaks. Most systems are provided with a simple clamp that will allow spontaneous voiding; this should be used rather than a spigot.

Intermittent clamping to allow the bladder to regain tone is rather unscientific, and many clinicians are skeptical of its use. However, Segal and Corlett (1979), in a controlled study of patients following bladder neck surgery for incontinence, found that intermittent clamping encouraged an early return of spontaneous voiding and removal of the catheter.

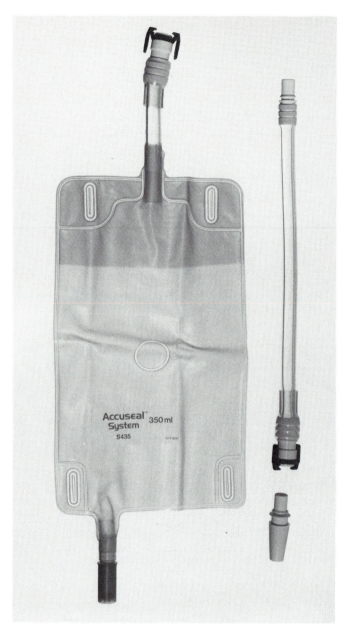

Figure 37.9 Squibb connections for drainage tube and bag.

My own routine following either vaginal or suprapubic surgery is to clamp the catheter on the second day and to release it later that day when the patient complains of discomfort or after 8 hours when the residual urine is measured. This is carried out by moving the patient onto her side and allowing the catheter to drain for 15 to 30 minutes. The catheter is then left on open drainage overnight. A strict input and output fluid chart is maintained and an input of about 2.5 L/day is encouraged. The procedure is repeated each day until the patient voids amounts up to 200 ml of urine, by which time the residual urine will usually fall below 100 ml. The catheter is then clamped overnight, and the patient is awakened once to void. If the patient is able to void, does not have retention, and has morning residual urine of less than 300 ml, the catheter can be removed.

The prevention and treatment of postoperative retention is often inadequate. Anxiety is probably

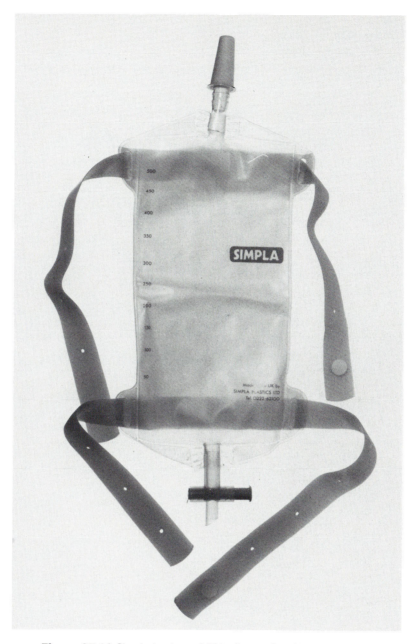

Figure 37.10 Simpla leg bag of 500 ml capacity with two leg straps.

an important factor, and both the operation and the subsequent catheter drainage should be carefully explained to the patient before and after the surgery. Drugs such as diazepam (Valium), 10 to 20 mg, as night sedation (Stanton, Cardozo, and Kerr-Williams, 1979), bethanechol (Urecholine), 25 to 100 mg t.d.s., distigmine bromide (Ubretid), 5 mg daily, or phenoxybenzamine (Dibenzyline), 10 mg daily (with a prior check on the patient's ECG and lying and standing blood pressure to detect cardiac

ischemia and avoid hypotension), can be tried. Intravesical instillation of various prostaglandins have been used with inconsistent results thus far (Stanton, Cardozo, and Kerr-Williams, 1979).

Antimicrobial therapy

Antimicrobial therapy is controversial and is discussed further in Chapter 24. Opinion is divided between therapy according to the results of regular midstream urine specimens for culture and sensitivity and the use of prophylactic drugs such as nitrofurantoin (Furadantin) or nalidixic acid (Neggram), with recourse to broader agents such as trimethoprim (Syraprim) or amoxicillin (Amoxil) when required.

Ambulation

Continuous catheter drainage after the patient is discharged from the hospital requires a suitable drainage bag. The connecting tube needs to be shorter, and the bag should have a reasonable capacity to avoid frequent emptying yet be sufficiently small to be concealed under clothing. A capacity of 350 to 500 ml is convenient.

The connection should be easy to manipulate, for example, the Squibb drainage system (Figure 37.9). The bag can be attached to a belt around the waist or, more satisfactorily, to a leg bag (Figure 37.10). This can be drained as required and need only be changed at weekly intervals or when the catheter has to be changed.

Many patients will accept and cope with the inconvenience of temporary ambulatory catheter drainage, if it appreciably reduces their hospital stay.

REFERENCES

Andersen, J., Fischer-Rasmussen, W., Molsted Pedersen, L., and Nielsen, N. 1982. Suprapubic bladder drainage reduces rates of urinary infection and of impaired voiding after colposuspension/vaginal repair. Proceedings of the twelfth annual International Continence Society Meeting, Leiden, pp. 96-98.

Bonanno, P.J., Landers, D.E., and Rock, D.E. 1970. Bladder drainage with the suprapubic catheter needle. Obstet. Gynecol. **35:**807-813.

Foley, F.E.B. 1937. A self retaining bag catheter. J. Urol. **38:**140-143.

George, N.J., Feneley, R.C., and Slade, N. 1978. Trial of long term catheterisation in the elderly: initial findings. Proceedings of the eighth International Continence Society Meeting, Manchester, pp. 19-20.

Hilton, P., and Stanton, S.L. 1980. Suprapubic catheterisation. Br. Med. J. **281:**1261-1263.

Hodgkinson, C.P., and Hodari, A.A. 1966. Trocar suprapubic cystostomy for post operative bladder drainage in the female. Am. J. Obstet. Gynecol. **96:**773-783.

Lapides, J., Diokno, A.C., Gould, F., and Lowe, B. 1976. Further observations on self-catheterisation. J. Urol. **116:**169-171.

Lapides, J., Diokno, A.C., Silber, S., and Lowe, B. 1972. Clean intermittent self-catheterization in the treatment of urinary tract disease. J. Urol. **107:**458-461.

Lyon, R.P., Scott, M.P., and Marshall, S. 1975. Intermittent catheterization rather than urinary diversion in children with meningomyelocele. J. Urol. **113:**409-417.

Madersbacher, H., and Weissteiner, G. 1977. Intermittent self catheterization as an alternative in the treatment of neurogenic urinary incontinence in women. Eur. Urol. **3:**82-84

Mattingly, R.F., Moore, D., and Clark, D. 1972. Bacteriologic study of suprapubic bladder drainage. Am. J. Obstet. Gynecol **114:**732-738.

Robertson, J.R. 1973. Suprapubic cystoscopy with endoscopy. Obstet. Gynecol. **41:**624-627.

Segal, A., and Corlett, R.C. 1979. Post operative bladder training. Am J. Obstet. Gynecol. **133:**366-370.

Stanton, S.L., Cardozo, L., and Kerr-Williams, R. 1979. Treatment of delayed onset of spontaneous voiding after surgery for incontinence. Urology **8:**494-496.

Whitfield, H., and Mayo, M. 1976. Intermittent non-sterile self catheterization. Br. J. Surg. **63:**330-332.

chapter 38

Urinary diversion

HUGH N. WHITFIELD

The diversion of urine by bypassing part of the urinary tract is a procedure full of important implications for both the patient and the surgeon; before making that decision it is essential to recognize the possible consequences of such a step. Urinary diversion is surgically straightforward, but to reverse the process and restore normal urinary drainage is fraught with ethical and moral difficulties as well as surgical problems. In this chapter the indications for urinary diversion are set out and the methods available are reviewed. The choice of the diversion procedure and the indications will vary from one surgeon to another; if my views do no more than stimulate disagreement and critical thought, they will have achieved their purpose.

INDICATIONS FOR DIVERSION
Incontinence

Severe urinary incontinence causes so much misery that major surgery is justified to relieve the distress. The prevalence of urinary incontinence in the community increases with age, and in one survey (Thomas et al., 1980), 8.5% of women between the ages of 15 and 64 and 11.6% of women over 65 admitted to urinary incontinence; in a fifth of these women the incontinence was moderate or severe. Much higher figures have also been reported. Nemir and Middleton (1954) and Wolin (1969) found that 50% of nulliparous women had some degree of stress incontinence, which is not much different from the figure reported by Brocklehurst et al. (1972) in women 45 to 64 years of age, although Osborne (1976) found an incidence of only 26% in women of similar age. This latter study highlights the difficulty of objectively assessing the severity of incontinence.

It is possible to quantitate the degree of urine loss with sophisticated devices such as the Urilos Nappy, but a very useful assessment can be made from inquiring about the type of protection that has to be worn. Any patient who wears 10 or more sanitary pads each day, or who finds she needs to use 2 at a time, or who uses paper towels torn to an appropriate size has a problem severe enough to warrant consideration of a urinary diversion.

Causes. Because urinary incontinence is a blanket diagnosis, the clinician must always identify the cause of incontinence before deciding on treatment.

Neuropathic bladder. Of all the causes of incontinence in women, neuropathic disorders are the most common indication for urinary diversion. The neuropathic lesion may be congenital, and many girls with spina bifida need a urinary diversion early in life, although intermittent nonsterile self-catheterization has been strongly advocated (Lapides

487

et al., 1974; Lyon, Scott, and Marshall, 1975). Acquired neurological diseases may result in disabling urinary incontinence, and disseminated sclerosis is the most common of such diseases. Those patients with a neuropathic bladder who harbor a large residual urine volume can be managed more satisfactorily by intermittent catheterization than those who have little or no residual urine (Whitfield and Mayo, 1976).

Sphincter weakness. It is very uncommon for women with pure sphincter weakness incontinence to need a urinary diversion, although there are a few patients who undergo multiple repair operations unsuccessfully in whom the resulting fibrosis around the urethra, bladder base, and bladder neck make further surgery impossible and in whom a urinary diversion may have to be considered. Pelvic irradiation can cause similar fibrotic problems that make the bladder neck sphincter incompetent, often with a small-capacity bladder, making a urinary diversion necessary.

Detrusor instability. There are a number of patients who have severe detrusor instability but in whom no underlying neurological disorder can be detected. These patients are labeled as having idiopathic instability. Those most severely affected, who fail to respond to any form of antispasmodic drug or to bladder overdistension (Whitfield and Mayo, 1975; Smith, 1981), will need a urinary diversion.

Congenital disorders. There are other congenital disorders that give rise to urinary incontinence and for which a urinary diversion is necessary. The most common of these is bladder exstrophy when reconstruction is not feasible.

Pelvic malignant disease

If the primary management of a pelvic malignant disease of the female genital tract includes anterior exenteration, a permanent diversion procedure is necessary, and an ileal loop urinary diversion is the procedure of choice. Whenever it is decided that radical pelvic surgery of this nature is indicated for the total removal of a pelvic malignancy, the potential for eradicating the malignancy fully justifies such major surgery.

Much more controversial is the problem of incurable pelvic malignant disease that is causing bilateral ureteric obstruction and renal failure. If the patient is in renal failure from a gynecological pelvic malignant disease that has not been treated, some form of urinary diversion of one or both sides

is mandatory. Prolonged remissions after radiotherapy may be seen even in the presence of advanced local disease, and on occasions the ureteric obstruction may resolve spontaneously after radiotherapy and/or chemotherapy. Percutaneous nephrostomy drainage of one or both kidneys (Saxton Ogg, and Cameron, 1972) provides satisfactory urinary drainage for several weeks, but if a longer period of drainage is necessary, a ring nephrostomy is more reliable (Figure 38.1). The restoration of normal urinary drainage may require ureteric reimplantation; this is not always straightforward following pelvic irradiation, and the interposition of an isolated segment of ileum between the bladder and ureter(s) may be necessary.

When bilateral ureteric obstruction occurs from recurrence of a malignant disease that is already being treated, the decision as to whether or not a urinary diversion should be performed becomes much more difficult. However, there is no need to make a hasty decision, since percutaneous drainage of the kidney can be performed to overcome the immediate crisis. If at a later stage the decision is made not to perform a more permanent diversion, a percutaneous nephrostomy tube, which is removed, will not leave behind a urinary fistula, since the small track will close quickly.

The prognosis that can be expected under these circumstances has been the subject of a retrospective study by Fallon, Olney, and Culp (1980). In a group of 15 patients with carcinoma of the cervix whose average age was 47 years at the time of nephrostomy, the mean survival time was 18 months after the relief of obstruction, and the quality of life was reasonably good in most cases.

METHODS OF DIVERSION

The urine may be diverted at any site from the kidney to the urethra, and a perurethral bladder catheter is just as much a method of urinary diversion as is a nephrostomy. Different sites of diversion are used for varying indications, but in practical terms the clinician most often has to decide initially whether he anticipates a period of urinary diversion lasting a few weeks (short term), a few months (medium term), or a few years (long term).

Short-term diversion

The technique of establishing a percutaneous nephrostomy was first described in 1955 by Goodwin, Casey, and Woolf and is now recognized as a most

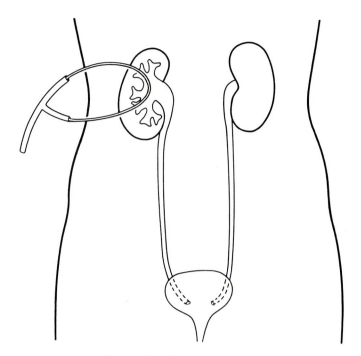

Figure 38.1 Ring nephrostomy.

satisfactory method of draining an obstructed kidney (Bartley, Chidekel, and Radberg, 1965). An advantage of the procedure is that it can be performed with the patient under a local anesthetic with radiological or ultrasound control. Patients in chronic renal failure are often poor anesthetic risks, and once satisfactory drainage has been achieved, there is a rapid improvement in the patient's condition, which allows definitive treatment to be started quickly.

The details of the technique have been fully described (Off and Saxton, 1969). A fine needle is used to locate the renal pelvis, and contrast medium is injected into the collecting system. A large needle that will accommodate a guide wire is then passed into the renal pelvis through the parenchyma to establish a watertight seal. A No. 7 French gauge pigtail catheter is passed over the guide wire, and when this catheter is in a satisfactory position, the guide wire is removed and the catheter sewn to the skin.

There is a risk that this kind of nephrostomy tube may become blocked, either with debris from an infected system or by a blood clot, but there are many cases in which very satisfactory drainage has been provided for several weeks and in some cases for several months. The disadvantage, however, is that the tube is vulnerable to being accidentally pulled out, and since, of necessity, it has been placed into the kidney through a posterior approach, it is sometimes uncomfortable for the patient.

Medium-term diversion

If drainage of an obstructed upper urinary tract is likely to be needed for a period of several months, a formal nephrostomy is required. The operation is usually performed on one side only— the side that seems to be performing better as judged on renography or excretion urography.

A ring nephrostomy (Figure 38.1) is the most satisfactory technique for establishing this type of drainage from the kidney. The operation was first described by Tressider (1957) and has several advantages over an end type of nephrostomy. The drainage tube cannot fall or be pulled out; if it becomes blocked, the tube can be easily changed by railroading another tube into place. It is possible to site the tube exits from the skin anteriorly where they cause the least discomfort and inconveninence to the patient.

After the kidney has been exposed through a standard incision, the renal pelvis is opened between stay sutures, and one end of the nephrostomy tube is attached to a malleable probe that is brought out through the parenchyma overlying a lower calix. The opposite end of the tube is similarly brought out through an upper calix, and side holes are cut in the tube where it lies in the renal pelvis. The tube is sewn to the renal capsule where it emerges, and the renal pelvis is closed. Prophylactic antibiotics are not necessary unless there is preexisting urinary tract infection, and postoperative antibiotics are best reserved for symptomatic episodes of infection.

Although this method is not designed for permanent diversion, there are patients in whom very satisfactory long-term drainage has been provided in this way and in whom renal function has remained stable.

Permanent urinary diversion

There are three techniques available that are commonly considered for permanent urinary diversion.

Ureterosigmoidostomy. A ureterosigmoidostomy (Figure 38.2) is simple to perform and spares the patient the necessity of a stoma. It depends on the integrity of the innervation of the anal sphincter for its success and is therefore contraindicated in any patient in whom a urinary diversion is being performed for incontinence as a result of a neuropathic bladder disorder. The quality of life depends very much on the ability of the patient to prevent flatus from being passed at any time, since fecally contaminated urinary leakage will inevitably occur at such a time. Control during the day may be achieved, but leakage at night is common. Those who have best control are those in whom the diversion was performed early in life, for example, for bladder exstrophy. Elderly patients often experience difficulty in gaining urinary control after a ureterosigmoidostomy, since the anal sphincter is unable to provide satisfactory continence. In my experience a ureterosigmoidostomy is not a suitable method of diversion for patients with idiopathic bladder instability, since the anal sphincter function is also often inadequate in this group.

Preoperatively an effective preparation of the large bowel is necessary so that the patient undergoes surgery with an empty colon. The ureters are divided low in the pelvis and anastomosed sepa-

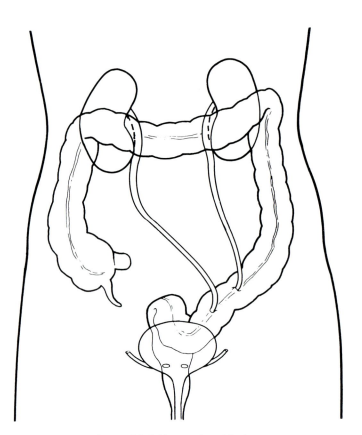

Figure 38.2 Ureterosigmoidostomy.

rately into a tenia coli of the sigmoid colon, using an antireflux technique, the most common one being that which was described by Leadbetter (1950). The use of splints across the anastomosis is optional, but a rectal tube should be used for the first 48 hours. Suitable prophylactic preoperative antibiotics, such as a combination of gentamycin and metronidazole, should be given, although prolonged courses of oral antibiotics should not be necessary. The left ureter is usually anastomosed higher up than the right one, and the sigmoid colon should be fixed so that the anastomoses lie without tension.

Ileal loop diversion. The ileal loop urinary conduit (Figure 38.3) was first described by Bricker in 1950. Over the past 20 years this operation has been regarded by many people as the method of choice for urinary diversion.

The technique requires a length of ileum to be isolated on its mesentery. The terminal 6 to 8 inches of ileum are not suitable, since the arterial supply comes from the ileocolic artery and runs parallel to the bowel; whereas more proximally arcades from the superior mesenteric artery are arranged radially and a suitable length of ileum with a good

vascular supply can be chosen. The modification of the ureteroileal anastomosis described by Wallace (1970), in which the ureters are spatulated and joined to them, has proved to greatly reduce the incidence of stenosis at the ureteroileal junction after end-to-side anastomosis as originally described by Bricker.

Fashioning a satisfactory stoma is the key to the success of the operation. Preoperatively the site for the stoma must be chosen with care so that it lies on the summit of any skin fold in the iliac fossa. The patient should be examined lying, standing, and sitting so that the best site can be identified. An adequate length of ileum is necessary so that after the distal end of the loop has been everted, a spout protrudes a minimum of 1 inch from the skin surface. Retraction and prolapse of the stoma and parastomal herniation can be avoided by suturing both the peritoneum and the external oblique aponeurosis to the ileum as it passes through the abdominal wall. The use of a T tube stent is optional. The site of the ureteroileal anastomosis should be extraperitonealized.

Colonic conduit diversion. The colonic conduit diversion operation was popularized in the United

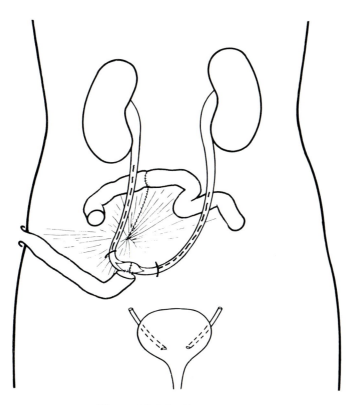

Figure 38.3 Ileal loop diversion.

Kingdom in the 1960s by Mogg (1965), who emphasized the low incidence of late complications and the opportunity to fashion an antireflux anastomosis between the bowel and the ureters to reduce the incidence of upper urinary tract infection and impairment of renal function. For these reasons the operation is still strongly advocated in some centers as being superior to an ileal conduit.

After full bowel preparation, a suitable length of colon is isolated using either the sigmoid colon or, in patients who have undergone extensive pelvic irradiation, a length of transverse colon. Whichever segment is chosen, it needs to be at least 8 inches long, since, following division of the bowel, the loop tends to shorten. In the case of the sigmoid colon conduit, the segment is mobilized with an arterial supply derived from the inferior mesenteric artery. By dividing the superior hemorrhoidal artery, adequate mobilization of the distal end of the loop can be obtained. The sigmoid mesentery does not have to be divided proximally very far away from the bowel. The proximal end of the conduit is closed and the ureters implanted by a suitable antireflux technique, such as that described by Leadbetter (1950) for a ureterosigmoidostomy. Similar care needs to be taken in siting the stoma.

Other methods. It is well recognized that no single method of urinary diversion is entirely satisfactory, and there have been many attempts to modify existing methods and to devise new ones.

A cutaneous ureterostomy sounds attractive on the surface, but although it is simple to perform, stomal stenosis is almost inevitable, even when the ureter is widely dilated. There are occasional indications for performing one of the several varieties of ureterostomy, particularly in children, but the procedure can be regarded only as a short-term method of diversion, and the precise indications are beyond the scope of this chapter.

There have been attempts to fashion a continent diversion. A leakproof vesicostomy has been described by Turner-Warwick (1976), in which a nippled ileal segment is interposed between the bladder and the skin. The patient then catheterizes the stoma intermittently. Ashken (1974) has described a continent ileocecal urinary diversion, but the results have shown that there are problems.

LONG-TERM RESULTS OF DIVERSION

Reports of the long-term follow-up of patients who have undergone one of these forms of diversion enable comparisons to be made of the incidence of complications.

Ureterosigmoidostomy has been criticized because of the potential for electrolyte imbalance and for the incidence of ureteric reflux, ascending infection, and subsequent renal impairment. Hyperchloremic acidosis is a well-recognized problem and can cause life-threatening illness, but it is now evident that other forms of diversion may be associated with metabolic disturbances, and in terms of renal function there may be little to choose from other than a ureterosigmoidostomy or a conduit.

With more experience in ileal loop diversions, it has become apparent that there is a high incidence of late complications. Stomal stenosis, upper tract dilatation, recurrent infections, and psychological disturbances are all common (Schwartz and Jeffs, 1975; Dunn et al., 1979). However, the incidence of these problems after colonic conduit diversion is similarly high. Dunn et al. (1979) reported an incidence of late complications of 82% after ileal loop diversion, and after colonic conduit there was an incidence of 61.5% for stomal stenosis, 22% for ureterocolic stenosis, and 48% for upper tract deterioration in a series of 41 children reported by Elder, Moisey, and Rees (1979).

There have been a number of reports over the past 50 years of colonic carcinoma occurring at the site of ureterocolic anastomosis after a ureterosigmoidostomy (Spence, Hoffman, and Fosmire, 1979). The combination of endogenous secondary amine in the gut, urinary nitrate, and suitable bacterial flora can lead to the formation of N-nitroso compounds, one of which is known to be carcinogenic to animals. The mean tumor latency of cases reported in the literature is 24 years, and it may be that the population at risk includes those who have colonic loops (Stewart et al., 1981). There has also been an isolated report of a patient developing an adenocarcinoma at the site of a ureteroileal anastomosis (Shousa, Scott, and Polak, 1978). Certainly, there is enough evidence to justify investigating patients who have had ureterosigmoidostomies at regular intervals by estimation of urinary carcinogens and by flexible colonoscopy.

Any method of urinary diversion carries a risk of complications, which increases with time, and the high incidence of these problems makes it all the more important to pick the right timing for a diversion and to choose the operation most suitable for a particular patient.

REFERENCES

Ashken, M.H. 1974. An appliance-free ileocaecal urinary diversion: preliminary communication. Br. J. Urol. **46:**631-638.

Bartley, O., Chidekel, N., and Radberg, C. 1965. Percutaneous drainage of the renal pelvis for uraemia due to obstructed urinary outflow. Acta Chir. Scand. **129:**443-446.

Bricker, E.M. 1950. Bladder substitution after pelvis evisceration. Surg. Clin. North Am. **30:**1511-1521.

Brocklehurst, J.C., et al. 1972. Urinary infection and symptoms of dysuria in women aged 45-65 years: their relevance to similar findings in the elderly. Age Ageing **1:**41-47.

Dunn, M., et al. 1979. The long-term results of ileal conduit urinary diversion. Br. J. Urol. **51:**458-461.

Elder, D.D., Moisey, C.U., and Rees, R.W.M. 1979. A long-term follow-up of the colonic conduit operation in children. Br. J. Urol. **51:**462-465.

Fallon, B., Olney, L., and Culp, D.A. 1980. Nephrostomy in cancer patients: to do or not to do? Br. J. Urol. **52:**237-242.

Goodwin, W.E., Casey, W.C., and Woolf, W. 1955. Percutaneous trocar (needle) nephrostomy in hydronephrosis. J.A.M.A. **157:**891-894.

Lapides, J., et al. 1974. Follow-up on unsterile, intermittent self-catheterisation. J. Urol. **111:**184-187.

Leadbetter, W.F. 1950. Trans. Am. Assoc. Gen. Surg. **42:**39-51.

Lyon, R.P., Scott, M.P., and Marshall, S. 1975. Intermittent catheterisation rather than urinary diversion in children with meningomyelocele. J. Urol. **113:**409-417.

Mogg, R.A. 1965. The treatment of neurogenic urinary incontinence using the colonic conduit. Br. J. Urol. **37:**681-686.

Nemir, A., and Middleton, R.P. 1954. Stress incontinence in young nulliparous women. Am. J. Obstet. Gynaecol. **68:**1166-1168.

Off, C.S., and Saxton, H.M. 1969. Percutaneous needle nephrostomy. Br. Med. J. **4:**657-660.

Osborne, J.L. 1976. Post-menopausal changes in micturition habits and in urine flow and urethral pressure studies. In Campbell, S., editor. The management of menopause and postmenopausal years. Lancaster, England. MTP Press, Ltd.

Saxton, H.M., Ogg, C.S., and Cameron, J.S. 1972. Needle nephrostomy. Br. Med. Bull. **28:**210-213.

Schwartz, G.R., and Jeffs, R.D. 1975. Ileal conduit urinary diversion in children: computer analysis of follow-up from 2 to 16 years. J. Urol. **114:**285-288.

Shousa, S., Scott, J., and Polak, J. 1978. Ileal loop carcinoma after cystectomy for bladder exstrophy. Br. Med. J. **2:**397-398.

Smith, J.C. 1981. The place of prolonged bladder distension in the treatment of bladder instability and other disorders: a review after 7 years. Br. J. Urol. **53:**283.

Spence, H.M., Hoffman, W.W., and Fosmire, G.P. 1979. Tumour of the colon as a late complication of ureterosigmoidostomy for exstrophy of the bladder. Br. J. Urol. **51:**466-470.

Stewart, M., et al. 1981. The role of N-nitrosamine in carcinogenesis at the ureterocolic anastomosis. Br. J. Urol. **53:**115-118.

Thomas, T.M., et al. 1980. Prevalence of urinary incontinence. Br. Med. J. **281:**1243-1245.

Tressider, G.C. 1957. Nephrostomy. Br. J. Urol. **29:**130-133.

Turner-Warwick, R. 1976. Leak-proof cystostomy. J. Urol. Nephrol. **2**(suppl. 8):405-413.

Wallace, D.M. 1970. Uretero-ileostomy. Br. J. Urol. **42:**529-534.

Whitfield, H.N., and Mayo, M.E. 1975. Prolonged bladder distension in the treatment of the unstable bladder. Br. J. Urol. **47:**635-639.

Whitfield, H.N., and Mayo, M.E. 1976. Intermittent non-sterile self-catheterisation. Br. J. Surg. **63:**330-332.

Wolin, L.H. 1969. Stress incontinence in young, healthy, nulliparous, female subjects. J. Urol. **101:**545-549.

chapter 39

Bladder retraining

CHRISTINE NORTON

The idea that the bladder is an organ susceptible to training is well known to every mother who has toilet trained a child. Yet it is only fairly recently that clinicians have recognized the therapeutic potential of this idea in treating lapses from the habit of continence learned as a toddler. The failure to recognize this potential earlier is not surprising, since it is usually the urologist or gynecologist whom adult women with symptoms of bladder dysfunction consult, rather than the psychologist. Fortunately, the boundaries between disciplines are becoming more flexible, and clinicians are increasingly willing to borrow methods more commonly used elsewhere. This is of benefit to those women with symptoms of bladder disturbance that have proved to be notoriously resistant to remedy by drugs or surgery.

DEFINITIONS

Several methods of bladder retraining (called *retraining, drill,* or *habit retraining*) have been described in the medical and nursing literature. They have been used to treat either the urgency, frequency, and urge incontinence syndrome of symptoms (with or without proved detrusor instability) or the nonspecific incontinence of institutionalized patients (especially the elderly or mentally handicapped). Although the methods differ in detail (de-

pending on the type of patient, her symptoms, and the clinician's preferences), most are based on a common presumption of the psychosomatic origin of incontinence (rather than genuine stress or overflow incontinence) and its amenability to treatment by psychotherapeutic means.

The term *bladder training* has also on occasion been used to denote management of the symptom of stress incontinence by pelvic floor reeducation (see Chapter 41) or to describe intermittent clamping of an indwelling catheter to restore bladder tone before withdrawal of the catheter. These uses will not be discussed here.

PRINCIPLES

Nearly all the retraining programs have certain common principles. A careful history of the problem must be taken, a physical examination performed, and, where facilities are available, urodynamic investigation undertaken to make a diagnosis of the cause of incontinence. Any obvious contributory factor (for example, urinary tract infection or constipation) should receive appropriate attention. Once the decision to retrain has been made, a full explanation should be given to the patient about the nature of her condition, its supposed causes, and the planned course of treatment. Some programs described are for patients already hospitalized; others include 2 weeks of hospitalization at the beginning of the treatment, and a few have been conducted on an outpatient basis. Nearly all of them emphasize the importance of careful and accurate charting as a means of defining the problem, of planning the regime, and of providing feedback to both patient and staff on progress toward continence. Some authors have used drug therapy as an additional aid. All have stressed the need for commitment and enthusiasm from the staff involved if the venture is to be successful. Three months is the average time span for retraining programs.

CLINICAL PROGRAMS
Jeffcoate and Francis' regime

While many people had probably been using various elements of bladder retraining for a number of years, Jeffcoate and Francis (1966) were the first to describe retraining as a planned, coherent regime for the management of urge incontinence in women. They postulated the cause of the symptom as being psychological conflict leading to an irritable detrusor muscle. In a series of 300 women with urge incontinence, they found a peak incidence in women between 40 and 60 years of age and an organic lesion accounting for detrusor instability in only 18% of the women. One hundred fifty women had a clear emotional upset to explain the onset of symptoms. Management was based on discipline to overcome the long-standing ''bad habit'' (48 patients had reported lifelong abnormal micturition patterns).

All patients were hospitalized and had a cystoscopy performed. The initial few also had a urethral dilatation, but this was later discontinued, since it was not found to be helpful. Careful teaching was then given as to the cause of the problem and how to break the vicious circle of urgency and fear of incontinence by toileting according to the clock rather than by desire. Most began with a program of voiding every 1 or 2 hours and were not permitted to void before the allocated time. When each time interval was achieved without discomfort, it was increased by half an hour with the objective that within 2 to 3 weeks a voiding pattern of every 3½ or 4 hours would be established. No pattern was imposed at night, but evening fluids were restricted and a mild sedative given to poor sleepers. All patients were given anticholinergic therapy while in the hospital and after discharge, and those who appeared to be tense were given tranquilizers.

Hospital admission removed the patient from the supposed causal environment and enabled firm, yet sympathetic nursing staff to ensure that the patients adhered to the program. Discharge from the hospital was consequent on the patient's lasting 3½ hours without discomfort between voidings and feeling a restored confidence in her bladder function. Perineal pressure (by sitting on a sandbag or wearing a vaginal tampon) was recommended as an aid in resisting urgency.

Among the 247 women with no organic lesion, a 67% cure rate was reported 1 year or later after treatment. Only 27 women failed entirely to respond, and of those who had initial success but later relapsed, a return to the stressful environment was cited as a reason.

Frewen's regime

In 1972 Frewen described a very similar retraining program that he has since elaborated on and developed a theory to explain (Frewen 1976, 1978, 1980). He believes that the symptoms of urge incontinence and frequency and the disorder of detrusor instability are usually psychosomatic in origin when no neurological or other organic lesion can be found. His regime, which he calls psychomedical treatment, involves hospital admission, issue of a printed sheet explaining the disorder and treatment, drug therapy (usually anticholinergics—propantheline [Pro-Banthine] for younger patients, emepronium bromide [Cetiprin] for the elderly—and a psychotropic agent such as diazepam [Valium]), and a micturition chart. The aim is to build up the individual's confidence in her own ability to overcome her problems and depends heavily on staff support and encouragement. Ten days of hospitalization are followed by close outpatient supervision for 3 months. Frewen (1978) reported an 82.5% cure rate for 40 women with detrusor instability after 3 months (*cure* being defined as symptom free with reversion to a stable cystometrogram). The seven cases of failure all involved patients with unrelieved personal stresses. Symptomatic cure predated the return to cystometric normality by 1 to 3 months. In 1980 Frewen suggested that the habit of frequency may actually be a precursor of detrusor instability and reported success in outpatient retraining of women with frequency and urgency but stable bladders. The idea that these patients would later exhibit instability if left untreated is interesting but as yet unsubstantiated. If true, it is possible that prompt early retraining of women with these symptoms could prevent instability from developing.

Frewen's regime has been tried by other authors. Jarvis and Millar (1980) reported a controlled trial of 60 women, aged 27 to 79 years, with detrusor instability. All patients were hospitalized for cystoscopy and urethral dilatation; they were then randomly allocated to either an inpatient bladder drill group of a control group of patients who were advised that they should now be able to hold their urine for 4 hours and were then discharged. Bladder drill involved a careful explanation and allocation of a time interval, initially usually 1½ hours, during which the patient had to wait out the period or be incontinent. As each interval was attained, it was then increased by a half hour each day until voiding every 4 hours was achieved. No drugs were used. The mean hospital stay was 6.25 days. After 3 months 90% of the patients in the bladder drill group were continent and 83.3% were symptom free. In the control group 23.3% of the patients were cured. All those cured had stable bladders, and those not helped remained unstable. This study has helped identify retraining rather than drug therapy as the effective element of Frewen's regime.

Pengelly and Booth (1980) reported a series of 28 women with detrusor instability in which 19 were cured or improved at 3 months with the use of a similar regime. An analysis of their results failed to identify predictors of which patients would be likely to do well, but some factors were associated with a bad result: especially, failure to show improvement during the first 2 weeks of treatment, an isometric detrusor pressure rise greater than 100 cm H_2O on interruption of micturition, and nocturnal enuresis that had persisted after 10 years of age.

Elder and Stephenson (1980) also reported success (86% cure or improvement rate) in treating urge incontinence and found that women with stable or noncompliant bladders did better on retraining programs than those exhibiting detrusor contractions. They, like Frewen, believe that this may be an earlier stage of the same complaint.

Habit retraining

Methods of bladder retraining described for use with hospital inpatients often emphasize theories of behavior modification. Newman (1962) postulated that the stress caused to elderly people by hospitalization, which is so often coincident with social degradation and a loss of human dignity,

may lead to an ultraparadoxical urination pattern (that is, a negative response to what normally is a positive conditioned stimulus), such as failing to micturate on the toilet, then immediately wetting the bed. According to Newman, a lifetime's conditioned response may break down under strain, and there may be a regression to earlier childhood habits.

Clay (1978) has outlined a habit-retraining program used with geriatric inpatients that emphasizes the importance of maintaining the individual's dignity and privacy and of recognizing what may be deterrents in the hospital environment to continence (for example, cold, unclean toilets or a lack of privacy). The principle is to discover the individual's own natural pattern of micturition during a preliminary check period of 2 to 3 days, when the patient is observed frequently (for example, every 2 hours) for evidence of incontinence and offered toilet facilities and the results are carefully charted. The regime involves keeping those micturition times when the patient was dry and voided during the check period, discontinuing times when she was dry and did not void, and bringing forward those times when she was found to be incontinent in an effort to "catch" the wetness (Figure 39.1). The regime is thus individualized and should fit the patient's own voiding pattern. The times are reveiwed every few days and adjusted as necessary, until a habit is formed. If the correct pattern is found, the patient should eventually be able to maintain it herself without nursing reminders, thus forming an important step in rehabilitation. In a 13-week trial of the program in a geriatric hospital, the following results were achieved:

	Men	Women
Number	20	11
Mean age (yr)	79	85
Success	12	8
Partial	4	1
Failed	3	2
Died	1	0

In the absence of any diagnostic aids and with the use of only the nursing resources available, such results are very encouraging. Those patients who failed to improve were those in whom no apparent pattern of micturition emerged. For such patients a rigid regime of toileting regularly by the clock is recommended.

The same habit-retraining regime has been found to be easy to use and effective with elderly outpatients, provided that the patient (or her relatives)

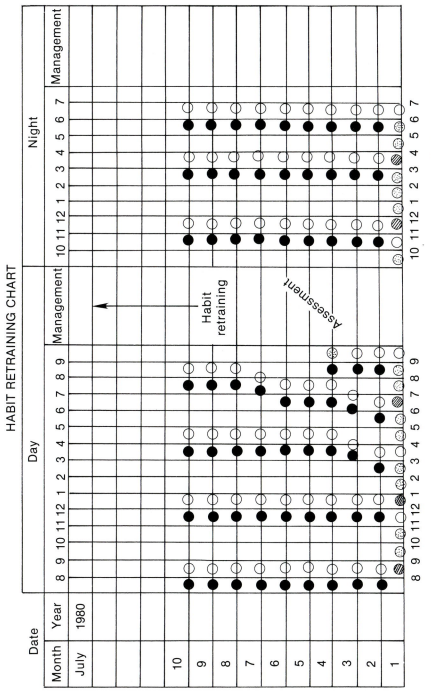

Figure 39.1 Graphic monitor showing time adjustments, time extensions, and evolving pattern of urination. ●, Continent; ○, passed urine in toilet; ⬚, incontinent; ⊙, did not pass urine in toilet. (From Clay, E.C. 1980. Geriatr. Nurs. November/December, p. 253. Copyright © 1980, American Journal of Nursing Company. Reproduced, with permission, from Geriatric Nursing, American Journal of Care for the Aging.)

498

is able to keep reasonable charts and is not too disorientated to remember the time. Timing devices can be of help for forgetful patients (Roe, 1977). I see patients on a weekly or twice-weekly basis for review of their progress and to adjust times as necessary.

Much of the literature relating to bladder retraining for institutionalized patients is on the mentally handicapped, especially children, but there seems to be no reason why the same principles of shaping behavior cannot apply to adults. Woods and Guest (1980) have pointed out the necessity of finding out what constitutes a reward or punishment for each individual when undertaking behavior modification. Tierney (1973) achieved good results with a shaping program for achieving successive approximations toward the target behavior of continence for mentally handicapped children by offering praise and personal contact for appropriate toilet behavior and giving minimal contact (but not punishment) for incontinent behavior. Barker (1979) found that in a retraining program for nocturnal enuresis in mentally handicapped adults, greater success was achieved if the patient was not only aroused at the time of peak incidence of enuresis, toileted, and reinforced for continent behavior, but also forced to deal with the consequences if inappropriate urination occurred (for example, having to change the wet bed).

Biofeedback

Biofeedback is another form of bladder retraining that has been successfully used to treat detrusor instability (Cardozo et al., 1978) and is described in more detail in Chapter 17. Hafner (1981) has described the use of biofeedback in urinary retention in teaching the patient to initiate detrusor contractions. Maizels, King, and Firlit (1979) have used biofeedback from EMG and flow rate recordings to retrain girls with vesical sphincter dyssynergia to relax the urethral sphincter. The use of biofeedback techniques as an aid in retraining deserves further attention.

CONCLUSION

Research into methods and uses of retraining for bladder dysfunction is as yet in its early stages. Even so, there is a remarkable degree of agreement as to how such programs should be run and also how successful they can be. For the symptoms of urgency, frequency, and urge incontinence with no neurological basis, retraining is the treatment of choice. Its value for women with neuropathic detrusor instability remains to be tested. Most studies to date have involved hospitalization, but a few have suggested that this may be unnecessary (for example, Frewen, 1980). Likewise, the necessity for coincident drug therapy is questionable (Jarvis and Millar, 1980). Whatever method is employed, a clear understanding by the patient of the causes of her disorder and the treatment, careful charting, and staff with enthusiasm and the ability to impart their faith in the procedure to the patient are the basis on which any retraining program should be built.

REFERENCES

Barker, P. 1979. Nocturnal enuresis: an experimental study involving two behavioural approaches. Int. J. Nurs. Stud. **16:**319-327.

Cardozo, L., et al. 1978. Biofeedback in the treatment of detrusor instability. Br. J. Urol. **50:**250-254.

Clay, E.C. 1978. Incontinence of urine. Nurs. Mirror. March 9, p. 36; March 16, p. 23.

Elder, D.D., and Stephenson, T.P. 1980. An assessment of the Frewen regime in the treatment of detrusor dysfunction in females. Br. J. Urol. **52:**467-471.

Frewen, W.K. 1972. Urgency incontinence. Br. J. Obstet. Gynaecol. **79:**77-79.

Frewen, W.K. 1976. Urgency incontinence. Br. J. Sex. Med. **3:**21-24.

Fewen, W.K. 1978. An objective assessment of the unstable bladder of psychosomatic origin. Br. J. Urol. **50:**246-249.

Frewen, W.K. 1980. The management of urgency and frequency of micturition. Br. J. Urol. **52:**367-369.

Hafner, R.J. 1981. Biofeedback treatment of urinary retention. Br. J. Urol. **53:**125-128.

Jarvis, G.J., and Millar, D.R. 1980. Controlled trial of bladder drill for detrusor instability. Br. Med. J. **281:**1322-1323.

Jeffcoate, T.N.A., and Francis, W.J.A. 1966. Urgency incontinence in the female. Am. J. Obstet. Gynecol. **94:**604-618.

Maizels, M., King, L.R., and Firlit, C.F. 1979. Urodynamic biofeedback: a new approach to treat vesical sphincter dyssynergia. J. Urol. **122:**205-209.

Newman, J.L. 1962. Old folks in wet beds. Br. Med. J. **5295:**1824-1827.

Pengelly, A.W., and Booth, C.M. 1980. A prospective trial of bladder training as treatment for detrusor instability. Br. J. Urol. **52:**463-466.

Roe, P.F. 1977. Incontinence timing device. Age Ageing **6:**238-239.

Tierney, A.J. 1973. Toilet training. Nurs. Times. **69:**1740-1745.

Woods, P.A., and Guest, E.M. 1980. Toilet training the severely retarded: the importance of evaluation. Nurs. Times. **76**(suppl. 12):53-56.

chapter 40

Pads and mechanical methods

CHRISTINE NORTON

Today there are a bewildering variety of incontinence aids on the market, and the list is growing almost daily as an increasing number of designers and manufacturers realize the huge market potential offered by incontinence. The aim of this chapter is not to provide a comprehensive catalog but rather to give an indication of the types of products available and to provide a guide to patient suitability and selection of aids. Three types of aids—pads and pants, occlusive devices, and collection devices—as well as catheterization are considered.

PADS AND PANTS

Pads and pants are a means of concealing and containing incontinence rather than curing it. As such, they should *never* (as they all too often have in the past) represent a first line of management and should seldom be the only management a patient receives. Nonetheless, they do have an important part to play, and a comprehensive service for incontinent people includes professional advice as to what is available for their individual needs (see Appendix 1). The attitude sometimes encoun-

tered that "we do not believe in pads here" is almost as dogmatic as former policies of "pads for everyone." An individual assessment will indicate which patients need a special incontinence garment and which sort is likely to suit their needs best.

Before the patient is advised on or issued pads and pants, it must first be ascertained that the patient is sufficiently incontinent to warrant their use. As soon as someone is given a special garment, there is a danger that she will start to feel in some way abnormal and that everyone else will view her as such. If a patient has only a small or occasional amount of leakage, formal incontinence garments are unlikely to be appropriate, especially since most patients will be managing adequately with either changes of underwear or panty liners and sanitary napkins.

Indications

Patients for whom pads may be useful include those in the following groups:
1. Those awaiting investigation.
2. Those on a waiting list for surgery.

499

3. Those undergoing treatment that, by its nature, takes time to be effective (for example, pelvic floor exercises, bladder retraining programs).

4. Those in whom the correct diagnosis has not yet been established or for whom initial treatment has been unsuccessful.

5. Those who have made an informed decision that they do not wish active treatment or who wish to delay it (for example, surgery). Each individual has the right to an explanation of the alternatives open to her, and some feel that they can manage their symptoms adequately with the help of a good pad. This will apply especially to those who have had multiple procedures or who are otherwise in poor health.

6. Those who have tried all available treatments without success. There is as yet no treatment with guaranteed success for all causes of incontinence, and a number of failures have to be accepted in the patient population.

7. Those for whom investigation and active treatment is inappropriate (for example, the very sick) or unavailable.

Principles

If the patient decides to try pads, then a proper assessment as to needs and suitability must be made. It is no longer acceptable merely to hand over a supply of whatever happens to be in stock, first and most important because the patient's needs vary so much and second because the pads and pants are individually very different. Shepherd and Blannin (1980) in a trial of incontinence garments found that "no one product will suit everybody" and concluded that a range of items must be provided if all needs are to be considered. An experienced advisor can assess the patient's needs and order accordingly.

When such an assessment is made, many factors need to be taken into account. The absolute *volume* of leakage will determine the size and absorbency of the pad needed. The *pattern* of urine loss (that is, constant dribble or occasional flood) will affect choice of pad and the number supplied. *Skin problems* and *sensitivities* will indicate which materials are appropriate for the pants. The patient's *personal preferences* as to the look and feel of the garments are very important; the choice must be acceptable esthetically to the individual (and her husband), and many refuse otherwise adequate garments that they feel they could not hang out on their washing line or take to the launderette. Younger women will often prefer a lighter, briefer garment to the more substantial underwear that the elderly favor. *Comfort* of a garment is important. Some people dislike any plastic in contact with the skin, and others find elastic irritates. A wet pad next to the vulva may cause irritation and discomfort. Pads and pants vary a lot in the softness of their materials. There is also a psychological component to comfort in that if the wearer feels that a garment is bulky and shows through her clothes or fears that it may rustle, she is likely to feel awkward using it.

Naturally it is important that the incontinence garment be "safe," that is, leakproof. The purpose of wearing it is to enable the incontinent person to mix socially without embarrassment or fear that her problem will be revealed to others and to protect her environment from soiling. People place varying emphasis on this quality. Some prefer comfort and will risk occasional accidents and choose a small pad that is adquate for most of the time; others go to extraordinary lengths and put up with great discomfort to ensure a watertight system at all times. Advice on the best clothing materials to disguise a wet patch (for example, some man-made fibers and darker colors) can help the patient conceal the slight leak and thus enable her to choose a more comfortable alternative.

More minor, yet still important, considerations are the *quality* and *cost* of the product. The pad must not disintegrate when wet yet should be easy to dispose of. The pants should wash well and easily, preferably by machine if for institutional use. They should dry quickly and last a reasonable length of time without the material becoming hardened or wearing out. Costs vary tremendously; and, although some of the least expensive products are a false economy because of poor quality, it does not always follow that the most expensive is best. Where possible the least expensive combination that will fulfill the individual's requirements adquately should be chosen.

All the preceding factors are of varying importance to each patient; the final choice depends on a balance between her need for comfort, safety, esthetic choices, economic resources, and washing facilities.

With all garments there is a need for accurate measuring and sizing of the pants, and an adequate supply of pads has to be ensured. Until the patient has actually tried an item, it is impossible to be certain that it is suitable; therefore it is wise to allow the patient to take samples home to try during her normal activities to ensure they work as expected. Only after such a trial period is it possible for the patient to be confident enough to order a long-term supply. Even then, needs may change over time.

Types available

Plastic pants. Fortunately the traditional approach of using a larger version of babies' plastic or rubber pants for the incontinent adult is dying out, although they are still seen in some places and are still the most widely available pant type obtainable at the pharmacy or by mail order. Most women find plastic garments unacceptable, both because of degrading associations with childhood and because of discomfort, perspiration, and skin problems. Being advised to use plastic pants is taken by many as a sign that they have no hope of recovery. However, they can be secure and dependable garments. They are especially suitable for use when the patient is sleeping away from home or attending lengthy public functions or in any situation in which the patient feels leakage would be a disaster. The pants are usually used with the length of padding cut to individual requirements.

There are, however, more acceptable alternatives for most needs.

Marsupial pants. First described by Willington (1973), marsupial pants represent a more modern approach and are one of the most popular garments available. They consist of a pant made from soft, hydrophobic material with a waterproof pouch sewn on the outside to hold the pad (Figure 40.1). When leakage occurs, urine passes through the material of the pants and is absorbed by the pad. Providing the pad is changed before it becomes soaked, the patient is separated from her excreta and has a relatively dry material next to the skin. They are available in a standard white material, in patterned materials, in a bikini version, and with a side-opening for disabled people. There are some minor restrictions as to users; for example, the patient needs reasonable manual dexterity to get the pad into the pouch, and she must maintain a good level of personal hygiene and be prepared to launder the pants properly. They are unsuitable for fecal incontinence or for people with vaginal discharges and work less well for use in bed.

Plastic-backed pads. There are a variety of pads with plastic backing available. They tend to be more expensive than ordinary padding but can work either with the patient's own close-fitting pants or with a very simple stretch garment. There

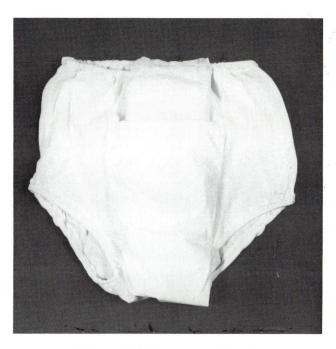

Figure 40.1 Kanga marsupial pants.

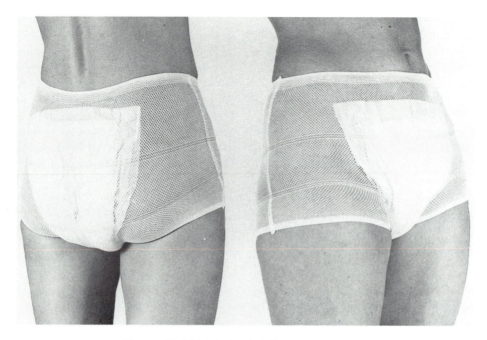

Figure 40.2 Molnlycke Maxi-Plus pants and pad.

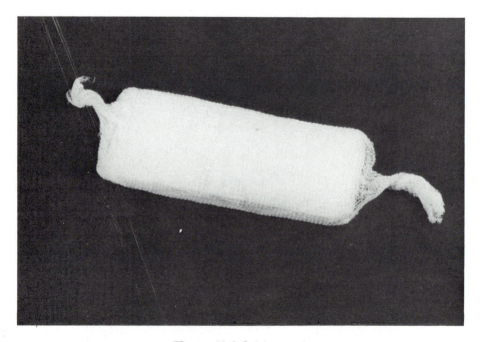

Figure 40.3 Gelulose pad.

is a range of pad sizes and absorbencies from different sources. An example of a large pad supplied with Helenca stretch pants is shown in Figure 40.2. These pads can be used for double incontinence, but the larger versions may present a disposal problem.

Protective pants with padding. Rather than being made of plastic, some pants are now made of softer waterproof material either completely or with a protective gusset. Some have interlinings of a soft material next to the skin. They are usually supplied with a roll of padding that can be cut to an appropriate length. This is an advantage because it lends flexibility; for example, more can be cut off when the patient is going out or is having a "bad day." Thus the waste of wearing a large pad all the time is avoided.

New absorbent materials. Much work is being done on the development of substances that will absorb and retain fluid, for example, the gelulose pad, which incorporates a powder that gels on contact with urine and will hold many times its own volume (Figure 40.3). At present this is an expansive option, but it is hoped, that with further research these substances will become less expensive and more widely used in the management of incontinence.

OCCLUSIVE DEVICES
Indications

It has been found that the presence of a device in the vagina may lessen or even prevent urinary leakage. As with pads, devices are seldom appropriate as a first line of management because they contain rather than treat incontinence and will work only while in situ (unlike electrical stimulation; see Chapter 36). Many of the same indications apply as for pads, for example, for those patients awaiting treatment or who wish to delay it or those who failed to respond to other therapy. Additional considerations are patient acceptability (many women object to the idea of wearing a device in the vagina), dexterity (a reasonable manipulative ability is required to insert most devices), vaginal sensation (which, if impaired, involves a risk of pressure necrosis), and the problem of finding a device that will both fit the vagina and prevent incontinence.

The exact mechanism of action of these devices is uncertain. Some may elevate the bladder neck; others raise resting urethral pressure by direct contact. They may lengthen the urethra, although the relevance of urethral length to continence is con-

troversial. There is some work to suggest that a device can improve the transmission of raised intraabdominal pressure to the midurethra (Hilton, 1981).

Principles

A device should be easy to insert, comfortable to wear, and, of course, improve continence. It should also be easy to extract and clean and involve minimum risk of pressure necrosis or infection. Most should be used only with medical recommendation and supervision. The patient must receive clear instructions on use and when to seek medical advice. Three of the more common approaches are described.

Tampon. Some women find that an ordinary tampon is helpful in controlling stress incontinence. This is a simple solution if leakage occurs only intermittently, for example, when playing a sport. However, if worn continuously, it can cause vaginal soreness and dryness (because of the absorbent nature of its material), and it may also be expensive. An alternative foam rubber tampon is now available (Figure 40.4). It has a string for extraction and is reusable after washing. Its value has yet to be tested in clinical trials.

Edward's pubovaginal spring. Edward's pubovaginal spring is a rigid plastic device with a triangular portion that lies over the pubic bone and an arm that is inserted into the vagina and "sprung" to exert gentle pressure against the anterior vaginal wall and urethra (Figure 40.5). The device is available in several sizes. Edwards and Malvern (1973) found a 70% improvement using this device but encountered one case of vaginal ulcer. It can be difficult to use in the obese patient and where there is vaginal narrowing, and special care is needed if vaginal sensation is impaired. It has to be removed before voiding.

Bonnar device. The Bonnar device is a soft, inflatable silicone rubber device (Figure 40.6). The arms of the device fit into the lateral vaginal fornices, and the balloon is inflated via a small pump to exert pressure anteriorly. The balloon can be deflated without extraction for voiding by reversing the pump. Cardozo and Stanton (1979) found problems with the device, which was too large or too small in 8 out of 20 patients, and over half of the patients found it of no help at all. Only 2 (10%) chose to keep the device after the trial. Nevertheless, it is certainly worthwhile trying for carefully selected patients.

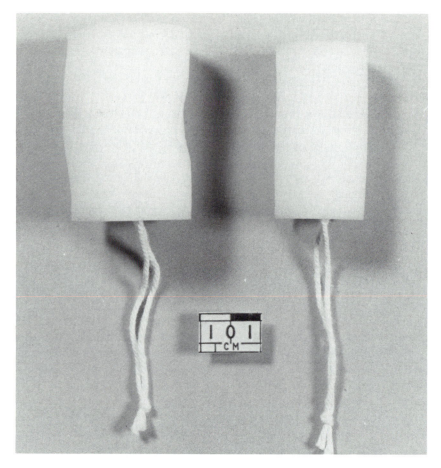

Figure 40.4 Rocket pessary.

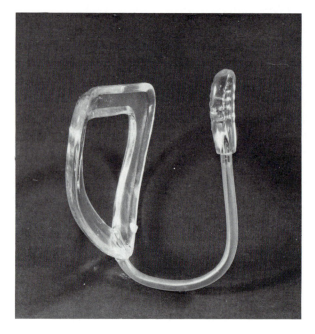

Figure 40.5 Edward's pubovaginal spring.

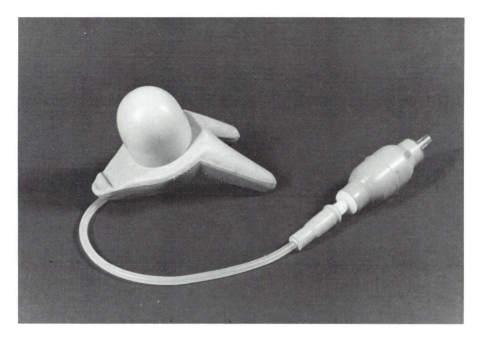

Figure 40.6 Bonnar device.

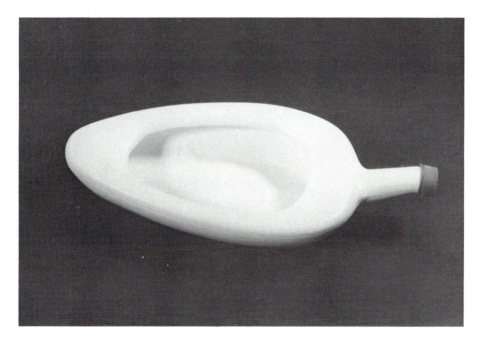

Figure 40.7 Slipper bedpan.

COLLECTION DEVICES

Female collection devices attached to the body have so far proved unsuccessful because of the obvious anatomical difficulties involved in ensuring a leakproof seal around the female genitalia. There are, however, some useful hand-held urinals for women that may enable a patient with extreme urgency to retain continence. They are most useful for those who are too immobile to transfer quickly or reliably onto a toilet or commode or on journeys with no toilet facilities.

The slipper bedpan is easily slipped under the body and is generally spillproof (Figure 40.7). The St. Peter's Boat (Figure 40.8) is useful for those

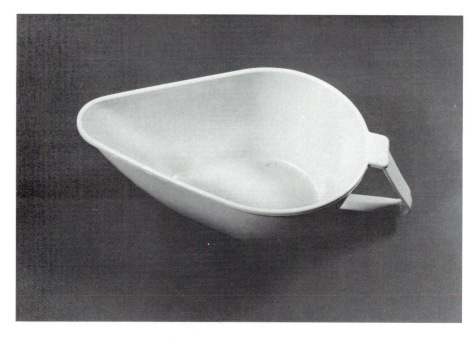

Figure 40.8 St. Peter's Boat.

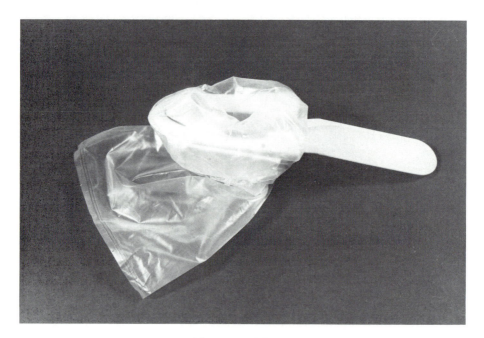

Figure 40.9 Feminal.

who can get to the edge of a chair, as is the Feminal (Figure 40.9). This is shaped to fit the female vulva closely and collects urine in a disposable plastic bag. Some women find that a simple funnel with tubing into a receptacle is adequate. Most urinals require some dexterity if they are not to be spilled and, as with all the other aids, will be of use only if the individual's needs have been correctly assessed and a product selected accordingly.

CATHETERIZATION
Intermittent self-catheterization

The technique of intermittent self-catheterization has been most widely used for patients with neuropathic bladder lesions. It has been described as aseptic and performed by nurses (Pearman, 1976) or clean and self-administered (Lapides, et al., 1972). It is the latter that has gained popularity recently and is now used for a wider group of patients (see also Chapter 37).

Indications. The use of clean, intermittent self-catheterization is indicated for female patients with significant postmicturition residual urine volumes if (1) there is evidence of progressive upper tract damage, (2) recurrent problematic urinary tract infections occur, of (3) overflow incontinence is present. Women may have residual urine for many reasons, for example, neuropathic lesions, following incontinence surgery, or decompensated bladder (MacGregor and Diokno, 1979). Idiopathically, especially in old age, the mechanism may be caused by overflow obstruction, atonic detrusor, or a detrusor-sphincter dyssynergia.

Procedure. The procedure is best taught to the patient by an experienced female nurse or doctor. Many women find the idea unpleasant at first and need to talk about their worries. The majority have never looked at the female genitalia before. An understanding teacher, together with a careful explanation of bladder anatomy, physiology, and the rationale for using self-catheterization, can reassure most patients. Explanation that it will not involve the masks and gloves they have seen used in the hospital and that with practice inserting a catheter becomes as easy as inserting a tampon will dispel much of their anxiety.

The patient should be carefully taken through the necessary steps. The equipment should be assembled—disposable female catheter (No. 12 to 14 Fr gauge), wet cotton wool ball, lubricant, mirror, and receptacle or toilet—and the patient should wash her hands. The patient should be placed in a convenient and comfortable position so that a good view of her vulva is obtained in the mirror. Some patients manage this with sitting on a toilet with an adapted shaving mirror attached to the seat. Others prefer a semirecumbent position on the floor or bed. Some patients squat or stand with one foot to a chair or on the toilet edge. The chosen position depends both on coexistent disabilities and on home circumstances. If right-handed, the patient should part the labia minora with the left hand, exposing the urethral meatus and give one downward swab with the cotton wool ball to cleanse the area. The catheter should be inserted by using a little lubricant jelly if desired until urine flows into the toilet or receptacle. The key to success is a good view in the mirror, and problems may occur if the meatus is intravaginal (for example, post-surgical), disability prevents good positioning, or there is impaired manual dexterity. In such circumstances, a relative might be taught the procedure.

If the meatus is missed and the catheter enters the vagina, it should be withdrawn and washed, and the procedure should be started again. When the urine stops flowing, gentle manual pressure may be exerted suprapubically to ensure that no residual remains. The patient should then slowly withdraw the catheter, pausing if the stream begins again. The catheter should be washed and stored in a clean, dry place to be ready for the next use. If infection is a problem, it may be advisable to leave the catheter soaking in a mild antiseptic solution between uses.

Frequency of catheterization depends on the clinician's instructions. Most women manage self-catheterization very easily and can dispense with the mirror after practice. The technique can be performed almost anywhere, and all the items required will fit into a handbag. It is important to ensure that the patient feels confident before she is sent home, and it is useful to have an information sheet for her to take home. If teaching is carried out on an outpatient basis, the patient should be told when and where to seek help, for example, if infection or bleeding occurs.

There are several types of catheters used for intermittent self-catheterization. The most suitable are round-ended plastic catheters with lateral eyes (for example, Portex Scott catheter). Each may be used for about 1 week and then discarded.

Long-term. A long-term indwelling catheter is often a realistic alternative for patients in whom all treatments, pads, and collection devices have failed to render them sufficiently continent to be socially acceptable. A catheter can enable incontinence to be kept private and may allow people who would otherwise need permanent institutional care to be managed in the community. Although catheter use almost inevitably results in urinary tract infections, there is no need to treat such infections unless symptoms occur (Brocklehurst, 1977).

There are many long-term catheters available. Most are made of pure silicone or are silicone coated. The former tend to have a larger internal bore for the same external diameter and therefore offer better drainage potential (George, Feneley, and Slade, 1978). Costs vary greatly, and the best choice will usually be the least expensive catheter

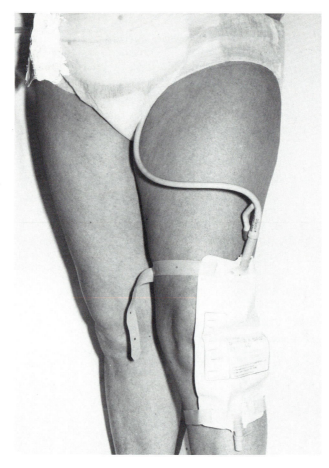

Figure 40.10 Leg bag.

that offers adequate drainage (Blannin and Hobden, 1980). The choice of size depends largely on the individual's propensity to block the catheter. Size Nos. 14, 16, or 18 Fr gauge should be adequate for most women. The temptation to replace a leaking catheter with a larger size should be resisted because most leakage is caused by either detrusor instability, a blocked catheter, or too much water in the retaining balloon. This balloon needs only enough in it to be self-retaining (usually 5 to 10 ml). Larger amounts result in a pool of undrained urine around the balloon and may even irritate an unstable bladder.

Catheters should be changed according to individual needs. Some people block their catheters much more readily than others, whatever management is used. Most catheters should last 2 to 3 months before being changed. If blockage or encrustation is a problem, regular washouts with water may prove useful, but they are not necessary as a routine in the absence of such problems. There

is no reason why a sensible patient, or relative, cannot be taught to perform the washouts.

The catheter should be attached to either a comfortable leg bag (most suitable for the nonambulant patient) (Figure 40.10) or a sporran-held bag (Figure 40.11). Daytime bags should be small enough to be discrete and light (usually 350 ml) and should be exchanged for a larger drainage bag at night. For home use the same bag can be reused for up to 1 week if it is washed in soapy water or a mild antiseptic after changing. A catheter should be allowed continuous uninterrupted drainage, except in special circumstances such as swimming or sexual intercourse, when it may be plugged for short periods. Some women find intercourse with a catheter in situ uncomfortable because it causes trauma. A change of coital position may help, but some prefer to use a short-term catheter, which is removed and replaced after intercourse.

The patient who is catheterized will need careful explanation and instruction, especially at first. She

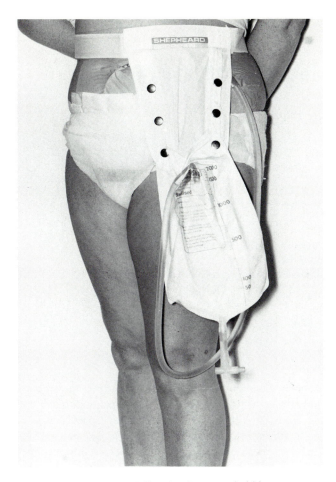

Figure 40.11 Shepherd sporran-held bag.

should know exactly when to seek help (for example, failure to drain for several hours, hematuria) and what is normal (sediment in the urine, occasional abdominal cramps). Scrupulous personal hygiene should be maintained, preferably with daily baths. If a catheter is dealt with in an experienced and matter-of-fact way by the nurse, there is no need for the patient to feel she is abnormal or have to worry about her catheter. Providing she has an adequate supply of bags and can rely on professional help and advice if needed, a catheter should be a welcome relief from the problems of incontinence.

REFERENCES

Blannin, J.P., and Hobden, J. 1980. The catheter of choice. Nurs. Times **76**:2092-2093.

Brocklehurst, J. 1977. Urinary infections: not all patients need treatment. Mod. Geriatrics **7**:33-36.

Cardozo, L.D., and Stanton, S.L. 1979. Evaluation of a female urinary incontinence device. Urology **13**(4):398-401.

Edwards, L., and Malvern, J. 1973. Long-term follow-up results with the pubo-vaginal spring device in incontinence of urine in women: comparison with electronic methods of control Br. J. Urol. **45**:103-108.

George, N.J., Feneley, R.C., and Slade, N. 1978. Trial of long-term catheterisation in the elderly—initial findings. Proceedings of the eighth annual meeting of the International Continence Society. Manchester. England.

Hilton, P. 1981. Personal communication.

Lapides, J., et al. 1972. Clean intermittent self-catheterisation in the treatment of urinary tract diseases. J. Urol. **107**:458-461.

MacGregor, R.J., and Diokno, A.C. 1979. Self-catheterisation for the decompensated bladder: a review of 100 cases. J. Urol. **122**:602-603.

Pearman, J.W. 1976. Urological follow-up of 99 spinal cord injured patients initially managed by intermittent catheterisation. Br. J. Urol. **48**:229-310.

Shepherd, A., and Blannin, J.P. 1980. A clinical trail of pads and pants used for urinary incontinence. Nurs. Times **76**:1015-1016.

Willington, F. 1973. Marsupial principle in maintenance of personal hygiene in urinary incontinence. Br. Med. J. **3**:626-628.

chapter 41

Physiotherapy

DOROTHY A. MANDELSTAM

In cases where pelvic floor dysfunction contributes to urinary incontinence, physical therapy has an important part to play. It involves the reeducation and strengthening of the muscles concerned by means of voluntary exercise, the use of electricity, or a combination of these. It is particularly applicable in the treatment of genuine stress incontinence. General lack of awareness of function and poor neuromuscular coordination of the pelvic floor muscles in women with stress incontinence was commented on by Kegel (1949), in whose opinion such poor coordination is probably phylogenetic, relating to the assumption of the erect posture by humans. It has also been recognized (Muellner, 1958) that some people manage the mechanics of micturition with skill and speed, whereas others are "slow and clumsy." As pointed out by Muellner, our ability to void at will involves a voluntary mechanism mediated through the use of intraabdominal pressure and pelvic floor muscles. Observation commonly reveals great personal variation in ability to stop and start the urinary stream.

During the last two decades our knowledge has been increased by a number of studies relating to the pelvic floor and its role in the control of micturition and defecation. While some of this knowledge is still controversial, certain new aspects need to be considered.

In general, the treatment of genuine stress incontinence is surgical, but strengthening of the pelvic muscles can alleviate symptoms in varying degrees. In the management of incontinence, the idea of muscle strengthening by electronic stimulation is in no way novel, as is illustrated by the multiplicity of devices produced for this purpose. On the other hand, treatment by voluntary exercise has been neglected because of a certain element of vagueness in its aims, in the way in which it has been carried out, and in the selection of suitable patients. Some comparative evaluation of the various methods of muscle strengthening is needed; so far, there has been a lack of controlled trials, but urodynamic techniques now make objective measurement possible.

SELECTION OF PATIENTS

Pelvic floor reeducation is desirable in postnatal women, particularly those who have had urinary incontinence throughout pregnancy. Certain postmenopausal women will benefit provided no gross anatomical distortion exists, age in itself being relatively unimportant (Kegel, 1951). Some women under consideration for surgical treatment may improve sufficiently to make surgery unnecessary. In cases where an operation has been unsuccessful or only partially effective, muscular reeducation is indicated. In cases where genuine stress incontinence is accompanied by only a minor degree of prolapse, results can also be gratifying. In cases where genuine stress incontinence is accompanied by detrusor instability, results will be less satisfactory, but if bladder training has been instituted, pelvic floor contractions can reinforce this effort. It has been shown by cystometric examination that this helps inhibit bladder activity (Wilson, 1976).

PELVIC FLOOR

The muscular component of the pelvic floor consists of an arrangement of three diaphragms: the levator ani, the urogenital diaphragm, and the superficial perineal group of muscles. Treatment is mainly directed toward activating the deepest layer, the levator ani. Concomitant action of the superficial perineal group follows. Each levator muscle arises from the posterior aspect of the os pubic adjacent to the symphysis, and most fibers pass almost horizontally backward toward the coccyx. Some fibers insert into the tendinous area of the perineum, in common with the superficial perineal group, and others mingle with the anal sphincter. The components of the levator ani muscles together form a sling with an interlevator cleft, closed by fascia but allowing the passage of the urethra, vagina, and rectum. The pubococcygeal muscle, the anterior portion of the levator ani, is the most important component in relation to the function and support of the urethra and vagina. The free medial margins of the pubococcygeus are easily felt through each lateral wall of the vagina. On contraction these margins tend to approximate and can produce voluntary interruption of micturition.

In cases where the level of the pelvic floor has descended, the muscles are less effective in supporting the region of the bladder neck. This is often caused by stretching of musculofascial tissue such as occurs in childbirth, and it can be remedied by improving muscle tone, since muscles and fascia are complementary. If there has been fascial rupture, physical therapy in itself is not sufficient and surgery is indicated.

Continence, in urodynamic terms, is dependent on the intraurethral pressure remaining higher than the intravesical pressure. The factors contributing to urethral resistance are a competent bladder neck, the intrinsic urethral mechanism together with the external sphincter musculature, and the pelvic floor, although their relative importance is uncertain. In practice, the strengthening of the pelvic muscles gives greater support to the bladder neck region, restoring the relationship of the urethra and bladder base and thus improving the urethral closure mechanism.

The second factor requiring consideration is the urethral musculature. Gosling (in Chapter 1) has shown the external sphincter to be an intrinsic part of the urethra and not, as previously thought, part of the pelvic musculature outside the urethra. It consists of specialized slow-twitching fibers capable of maintaining tone over prolonged periods of time, whereas the levator ani contains, in addition, a population of fast-twitching fibers capable of rapid action in stopping the flow of micturition. The levator ani assists the external sphincter in maintaining continence, particularly during any increase in abdominal pressure. Active exercise can improve the automatic function of the urethra. According to Jones (1950), both smooth and striated muscles are directly affected by exercise. Measurement of the urethral pressure profile before and after treatment demonstrates increased urethral resistance.

The third factor contributing to urethral resistance is the pelvic floor. Reflex activity of the pelvic floor is constant, even during sleep. Any increase in intraabdominal pressure is resisted by increased reflex muscle activity. During normal micturition or defecation, inhibition of this activity occurs, thus allowing relaxation of the pelvic floor with consequent passage of urine or feces. In elderly sedentary people these muscles may well show atrophy and affect bladder and bowel performance. Fecal incontinence can arise from a passively overstretched pelvic floor (Parks, 1975). Years of straining at stool can result in lengthened and inefficient muscle fibers and also in stretching of the nerves supplying them. The same effect may be caused by the trauma of childbirth. The implications of pelvic floor dysfunction are considerable.

TREATMENT BY EXERCISE

The aim of exercise is to counter any descent of the pelvic viscera and restore their normal anatomical relationships, thereby improving the sphincteric function.

An accurate history is necessary and should include details of the incontinence, including its onset, duration, and severity. The patient is given a very simple description of the pelvic floor and its workings, and the aims and method of treatment are then discussed (see box on p. 513). A local examination will reveal any general atony. During

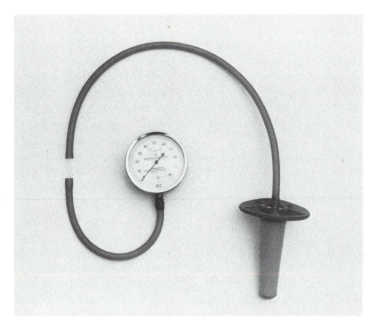

Figure 41.1 Kegel perineometer.

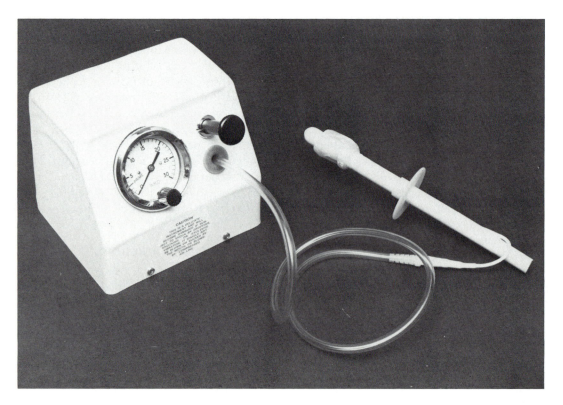

Figure 41.2 Pelvic floor "exerciser."

Instructions for the patient: exercises to strengthen the pelvic floor

The pelvic muscles cannot be seen, but they can be felt and identified in the following way:

1. Sit or stand and without tensing the muscles of the legs, seat, or abdomen, imagine that you are trying to control a bowel movement by tightening the ring of muscle around the anus. This will help you identify the **back** part of the pelvic floor.
2. When you are in the middle of passing urine, try to stop the flow and then restart it. If you do this every time you empty your bladder, you will become aware of the **front** muscles of the pelvic floor.

These muscles, back and front, are the ones to be exercised as follows. Working from the back to the front, tighten both sections while counting to four slowly and then release them. Do this four times, about once an hour. You can do these exercises anywhere—sitting or standing, while watching TV, or waiting for the bus. There is no need for them to interrupt your normal daily activity.

---

palpation of the lateral walls of the vagina, the tone of the pubococcygeal muscle can be determined by asking the patient to "tighten up." A request to cough or strain down will show the presence of any marked prolapse of the anterior wall and may inadvertently confirm any stress incontinence. If a definite cystocele or urethrocele is present, surgery is indicated. Any posterior displacement of the anal opening in relation to a horizontal line between the posterior margins of the ischial tuberosities, as well as the presence of a rectocele, indicates surgery. During palpation of the vagina, muscle awareness can be taught by asking the patient to act as though she is trying to stop a bowel movement and to interrupt a flow of urine. This is reinforced later by actually stopping and starting the flow during micturition.

A perineometer (Figure 41.1) is a useful teaching aid (Mandelstam, 1976, 1978). First devised in the United States by Kegel, this consists of a vaginal resistance chamber attached to a meter that registers an increase in pressure when the appropriate muscles contract. Care has to be taken to ensure that the abdominal, gluteal, and adductor muscles are not being used at the same time. Kegel intended it as a means of recording progress and

to be used by patients at home as an "exerciser." (Figure 41.2).

Having learned to contract the relevant muscles, the patient is asked to do so slowly four times every hour or when convenient. Practice must become habitual but need not interfere with her daily routine. The average length of treatment is 3 months, with monthly checks. Should the patient be overweight, attention to diet is encouraged.

It is frequently claimed that patients are not sufficiently motivated to continue exercising, but this has not been my experience. Any incontinent subject has a real incentive to become "dry." There is a further inducement when it becomes apparent that increased pelvic muscle tone leads to greater sexual satisfaction for both partners (Scott, 1979). Employing a similar form of treatment in Norfolk, England, Harrison (1979) reported that in a retrospective survey conducted from 1970 to 1976 of some 212 patients, 199 became symptom free.

OTHER METHODS OF TREATMENT
Faradism

The use of an electrical stimulus, together with exercises, has been an accepted treatment for many years. An alternating current of bearable but sufficient strength is produced to stimulate the levator ani. It has been shown that only the use of an internal electrode will effectively stimulate these muscles, yet approximately five external methods are in current use (Scott, Green, and Couldrey, 1969). An interferential current is now used in some centers. However, unless muscle contraction is verified by digital examination, the effectiveness of treatment cannot be assumed; thus it is hardly surprising that sometimes physical therapy is considered to be of little value.

In a controlled trial, Brown (1981) compared the different forms of physical treatment with objective assessment including urethral pressure measurements. He found that while pelvic floor exercises were effective, the addition of an electrical stimulus had no particular value and that treatment success seemed to depend on teaching muscle awareness. The perineometer was used both as a visual aid and as a means of measuring and recording any improvement.

Turner (1979) appraised a group of patients treated by maximum faradic stimulation while they were under anesthesia, along with daily exercise; two thirds of the patients showed symptomatic improvement and demonstrated a return to normal pressure profile measurement. Since this was not a controlled trial, however, it is difficult to assess the comparative importance of the two elements in this treatment.

Electronic devices

A constant, pulsed electric current delivered by a vaginal or rectal electrode can be used to stimulate the pelvic floor. These devices (see Chapter 36), though effective, are inconvenient to wear, especially during micturition and defecation, and are not acceptable to all patients. In one trial, a group of patients used a galvanic direct-current stimulator (the Vagette) and another group performed Kegel exercises using the perineometer (Scott, 1979). Muscle improvement, measured by the Kegel meter, was found to be present in both groups, as well as improvement in sexual response and function.

CONCLUSION: THE CASE FOR TREATMENT BY EXERCISE

There is ample clinical evidence to show that muscular reeducation can in many cases alleviate the symptom of stress incontinence. A technique of voluntary exercise that is effective and simple for both patients and instructor could make this treatment more acceptable, as an alternative to surgery in certain cases and as an adjunct to it in others. A device similar to the perineometer could be available in clinics and physical therapy departments to be used in a number of ways: for the assessment of muscle performance, as a visual teaching aid, and as an "exerciser." Patient motivation is important, as is an informed, convincing instructor, be it physician, nurse, or therapist. In the United Kingdom there are several incontinence clinics with specialist nurse advisors who carry out physical therapy of the pelvic floor as part of the general care of incontinent patients. It is hoped that this skill will become more widespread.

Both surgery and physical therapy have the same aim in view, namely to elevate the proximal urethra and bladder neck. Surgery by the vaginal approach "pushes" up these structures, and surgery by the suprapubic approach "pulls" them up. Physical therapy aims to restore the urethrovesical relationship by "lifting."

REFERENCES

Brown, A.D.G. 1980. Physiotherapy. Communication to the annual meeting of the International Uro-Gynaecological Association. New Orleans.

Gosling, J.A., et al. 1981. A comparative study of the human external sphincter and periurethral levator ani muscles. Br. J. Urol. **53:**35-41.

Harrison, S.M. 1979. Gynaecological conditions. In Downie, P.A., editor. Cash's textbook of physiotherapy in some surgical conditions. ed. 6. London. Faber & Faber, Ltd.

Jones, E.G. 1950. Role of active exercise in pelvic muscle physiology. West. J. Surg. Obstet. Gynecol. **58:**1-10.

Kegel, A.H. 1949. The physiologic treatment of poor tone and function of the genital muscles and of urinary stress incontinence. West. J. Surg. Obstet. Gynecol. **57:**527-535.

Kegel, A.H. 1951. Physiologic therapy for urinary stress incontinence. J.A.M.A. **146:**915-917.

Mandelstam, D.A. 1976. Re-assessment of the use of the perineometer in the treatment of stress incontinence. Communication to the annual meeting of the International Continence Society. Antwerp, Belgium.

Mandelstam, D.A. 1978. The pelvic floor. Physiotherapy **64:**236-239.

Muellner, S.R. 1958. The voluntary control of micturition in man. J. Urol. **80:**473-478.

Parks, A.G. 1975. Anorectal incontinence. Proc. R. Soc. Med. **68:**681-690.

Scott, B.O., Green, J., and Couldrey, B.M. 1969. Pelvic faradism: investigation of methods. Physiotherapy **55:**302-305.

Scott, S.R. 1979. A clinical study of the effects of galvanic vaginal muscle stimulation in urinary stress incontinence and sexual dysfunction. Am. J. Obstet. Gynecol. **135:**663-665.

Turner, A.G. 1979. An appraisal of maximal faradic stimulation of pelvic muscles in the management of female urinary incontinence. Ann. R. Coll. Surg. Engl. **61:**441-443.

Wilson, T.S. 1976. A practical approach to the treatment of incontinence of urine in the elderly. In Willington, F.L. editor. Incontinence in the elderly. Academic Press, Inc. London.

APPENDICES

Role of the incontinence advisor

CHRISTINE NORTON

There are as many different interpretations of the role of incontinence advisor as there are posts in existence. The position is new and as yet largely undefined. Few centers have, until relatively recently, recognized the need for an advisor as part of a comprehensive urodynamic or incontinence clinic. Most advisors are female registered nurses; thus this will be assumed throughout this appendix. However, this is in no way intended to undervalue the often excellent work carried out by a small number of advisors with alternative qualifications (in the field of social work, psychology, or physiotherapy, for example).

The Chief Nursing Officer for England and Wales has identified incontinence as a priority area for nursing and for improvement in standards of care, suggesting the designation of a nurse in each Health District to act as a specialist, resource person, and education focus (Friend, 1977). In 1979 Isaacs suggested that the most rational approach to tackling the huge problem of incontinence was to set up medical incontinence clinics with hospital backup and access to adequate supplies and resources. An incontinence nurse advisor was seen as a key person in such a scheme, and it is the role of the advisor as part of the team in this context that will be described here. Obviously, precise interpretation of the role will depend on local factors, the specialities of the medical team members, patient characteristics, and the interests and expertise of each advisor.

The number of advisors at present in England and Wales is uncertain. In 1981 it was estimated that there were fewer than 30 full-time incontinence advisors in the United Kingdom (Norton, 1981). The majority are based in specialist units largely funded by research grants rather than in service posts. Some work totally in hospitals, some in the community, and the majority in both. A few are in isolated clinics with no medical backup at all.

517

Many spend a large proportion of their time in educational roles, whereas a few are seen exclusively as "catheter and pad nurses." It is clear that with the trend toward appointing more advisors, there is a need for a realistic job description.

SCOPE

At every stage of the patient's contact with an incontinence clinic, the advisor has a part to play. She will (1) make an assessment of the patient's incontinence and the effect it is having, (2) contribute toward reaching a diagnosis and realistic treatment plan, (3) participate in treatment and manage those patients who fail to regain continence, (4) advise other professionals about incontinence, (5) teach, (6) participate in research, (7) liaise with manufacturers, and (8) act as a resource person serving the surrounding population.

ADVISOR'S ASSESSMENT

In some circumstances the advisor may make an assessment before a clinic visit, especially if the problem sounds relatively simple, such as constipation or a urinary tract infection, or mechanical, such as inadequate or inaccessible toilet facilities. Sorting out such problems at the referral stage enables the best use to be made of costly and time-consuming urodynamic investigations for those with genuine bladder dysfunction. If the remedies the advisor suggests fail to restore continence after a reasonable trial, then the patient can undergo a full investigation. This management by the advisor before or sometimes instead of an investigation should be emphasized.

More usually, the advisor's and the medical assessment will be made in conjunction, the former complementing the latter by illuminating many different aspects of the patient's problem. The advisor should assess the patient in a relaxed, unhurried atmosphere, giving the patient time to fully express her feelings about her condition. If the patient is elderly or disabled, it is best to conduct this initial interview in her usual environment (whether at home or in an institution), so that the patient's interaction with her surroundings and facilities for coping with problems can be observed. If relatives or friends wish to be involved, it is tactful to ensure that the patient consents to their knowledge of her condition and its treatment.

It is wise when making an assessment to employ checklists so that no topic of potential importance is left undiscussed. This should not, of course, be used as a rigid, structured questionnaire for the interview, but it does provide a useful baseline record from which to measure progress and highlights areas needing attention when a treatment plan is being formulated. An example of an assessment checklist for use with female outpatients is shown in Figure I.1 (Norton, 1980).

Record chart

When assessing the type and degree of bladder dysfunction, it is useful to have an accurately charted record of fluid balance, micturition, and incontinence, initially for 5 to 7 days. The patient's own undocumented estimate of the severity and frequency of her problem is often very inaccurate, and a chart can reveal many features, such as the pattern of incontinence, that suggest its cause (for example, polydipsia or polyuria). It also provides one parameter on which to judge the severity of the problem and the extent of treatment warranted. It is notable that the act of keeping a chart is often therapeutic in itself, the patients returning them with comments such as "This was the best week I've had in years" or "I thought it was a lot worse than this." Almost all patients are able to keep accurate charts if properly instructed, and charts can be modified, if necessary, for those with very poor eyesight or insufficient dexterity to manage measurement.

Physical signs

The patient should be observed for signs of restricted mobility, lack of manual dexterity, or failing eyesight, since these can precipitate incontinence if accompanied by urgency of micturition or inaccessible toilet facilities. Sometimes the provision of a walking aid does more to make the patient dry than control of her uninhibited detrusor contractions. If the advisor is not present during the medical examination, the skin condition and personal hygiene will need separate inspection. The skin of many incontinent patients may be excoriated, especially if plastic has been worn next to the skin or personal hygiene is less than scrupulous. The experienced nurse will also recognize senile atrophy of the genitalia, detect any sizable residual urine on bimanual examination, exclude constipation with fecal impaction as a contributing factor to incontinence, and assess pelvic floor tone and awareness.

Psychological assessment

Psychological assessment is equally as important as clinical assessment. The advisor has a real role

CONFIDENTIAL

Checklist for nursing assessment of adults incontinent of urine

Name .... Hosp no ....
Address ....
Telephone no .... Date of birth ....
Age............. Occupation (present or past)...............................
Referred by ....
GP name ....
        Address ....
        Telephone no ....
Seen in Urodynamic Unit? Yes/No Diagnosis:

Relevant past medical history:

Obstetric:
Gynaecological:
Neurological:
Psychiatric:
Other medical conditions (present):

Current medication:

Urinary Symptoms

Average daily intake:
Average daily output: ⎫ Fluid balance
Average volume voided: ⎭ chart or estimate?
Does patient restrict fluids?
Frequency day/night:
Urgency?
How long can patient 'hold on' after initial desire to void?
Pain or burning on micturition?
Sensation of bladder fullness?

Signs/symptoms of retention

Hesitancy:
Poor stream:
Incomplete emptying:
Post micturition dribble:
Is bladder palpable?
Does suprapubic pressure improve flow?
     – is this used regularly?

Incontinence

Time since onset:
Circumstances at onset:
        Change school/job/retirement:
        Hospitalized:
        Acute illness:
        Emotional crisis:
        Constipation:
        Drug therapy:
        Other:
Is incontinence worse/same/improving?
Does condition vary – How:
                    Circumstances:
Frequency of incontinence day/night:
How much urine is lost (dribble – entire contents):
        Does this vary?

Events precipitating incontinence:
        Cough/laugh/sneeze/strain: Difficulty getting to/onto toilet:
        Walking: No specific event:
        Change of position: Event not known:
        Urgency: Other:

Do these events *always* produce incontinence?
Is patient ever free from problem?

Mobility

Comments on mobility problems:

Manual dexterity

Comments on dexterity problems:

Eyesight

Problems with washing:

        dressing:
        personal hygiene:
        getting to/onto toilet:

MSSU result:

Bowels

Faecal incontinence?
Comments:
Bowel actions per week (average):
Constipation?
Rectal examination done/not done:

Vaginal examination

Skin condition: Residual urine:
Pelvic floor tone: Comments:
Atrophic changes:

Psychological factors

Attitude to problem

        Distressed:
        Apathetic:
        Denial:
        Coping:
        Comments:

Orientation

        Fully alert and orientated:
        Orientation slightly impaired:
        „   moderately impaired:
        „   severely impaired:
        Comments:

Psychiatric state

        Depressed:
        Anxious:
        Other:

Social network

Official – which services are involved

        District nurse   Laundry service
        Health visitor   Linen loan
        Social worker   Home adaptation
        Home help   Loan of equipment
        Attendance allowance   Day centre/clubs

Unofficial

        Who does patient live with?
        Who visits regularly?
        Social activities:
Are any of the above unaware of incontinence:
        – does patient wish incontinence to be secret from anyone?
        Is incontinence affecting family relations?
        Is incontinence affecting sexual activity (as relevant)

Environment

Toilet facilities

Does patient use:
Toilet: private/share   Commode
indoors/outdoors   Urinal
stairs involved   Catheter
distance from usual base   Other

Aids and equipment being used:

        Pads and pants – who supplies?
                        are they satisfactory?
        Other aids:
        What aids have been tried in the past?
        Comments:

Financial:

Is incontinence a financial burden?
        Comments:

Assessment of problems

1. Physical   a. bladder   What needs changing/aims
              b. general
2. Psychological
3. Environmental
4. Financial

Action: Toilet training   Bell and buzzer
         Pads and pants   Call in other care workers
         Aids/devices   Medical referral
         Home adaption   Other
         Pelvic floor excercises

Follow-up notes:

Figure I.1 Incontinence advisor incontinence checklist for use with female outpatient.

in providing support and encouragement to the patient and, where necessary, the family. If dementia is suspected, simple mental testing will determine the feasibility of treatment options (although if disorientation is present, it should not be assumed that it is the cause of the incontinence). Depression and anxiety are commonly expressed by incontinent women, but cause and effect are difficult to disentangle (see Chapter 30). Severe apathy or even denial of incontinence requires some time spent in conversation to gain the patient's trust and restore confidence.

Social aspects

Social problems may likewise influence or be influenced by incontinence. Fear of embarrassment in public can lead to social withdrawal and eventual isolation, which then reinforces incontinent behavior because the individual lacks motivation to make an effort to stay dry. Feelings of degradation and worthlessness can lead to a downward spiral of squalor and neglect. Those incontinent women who do not withdraw do nevertheless experience great problems in conducting a social life involving everyday contact with others in the home, at work, shopping, or at social functions. Family activities may be restricted by the patient's continual search for toilets or refusal to undertake long journeys. Caring for an elderly relative can become an unbearable strain if incontinence supervenes. Sexual relations are naturally more difficult if one partner suffers nocturnal enuresis or incontinence during intercourse (see Chapter 32).

Some patients undoubtedly do use bladder problems as a means of manipulating their social lives and the people around them. This may especially be seen in some institutional settings where incontinence can become rewarding, resulting in human contact and attention. One cannot dismiss such patients as merely seeking attention without probing for a reason for their need to act in this way.

Environment

The physical environment can determine a patient's ability to cope with any given degree of bladder dysfunction. Urgency leading to urge incontinence may cause a woman to give up her job because of inaccessible toilet facilities. Shopping may be restricted to familiar centers well supplied with public conveniences. In the home, stairs or the distance to an outside toilet may present a huge obstacle to the elderly person taking fast-acting diuretics. The environment should be assessed with a view toward suggesting improvements as to how washing and toilet facilities may be improved.

Financial considerations

Financial problems are very relevant in cases of incontinence. Some patients go to great expense to purchase aids, many of which are not available on prescription. Sometimes financial considerations may preclude an otherwise suitable treatment, piece of equipment, or home modification.

MANAGEMENT
Explanation

In some clinics the advisor will be involved in the urodynamic investigation. It is reassuring for the patient to have continuity of personnel during this procedure. The nature of the tests should be fully explained to the patient and maximum privacy and dignity preserved.

Diagnosis

The nursing assessment supplements clinical and urodynamic investigation so that a full picture of each patient's incontinence is provided. Among patients the causes of incontinence will vary from purely physical defects such as sphincter incompetence to a complex interaction of psychosocial and environmental factors. The treatment planned for each individual must be made with the diagnosis, her preferences, and all other factors considered. Physical diagnosis alone is unlikely to provide a flexible enough basis for treatment to cover all needs.

Treatment

The incontinence advisor can participate in the treatment offered by other team members and should develop her own areas of expertise. Preoperative counseling before surgery for incontinence is very important, since each patient must make an informed decision as to whether or not to undergo a procedure that is not lifesaving. The advisor may be involved in all forms of conservative treatment, including drugs, electrical devices, physiotherapy, bladder drill, or biofeedback, and may be the principal therapist for bladder retraining or pelvic floor reeducation (see Chapters 39 and 41). Continuity of care is very important for patients who are possibly likely to need several types of treatment.

The advisor must have the trust and confidence of her patients if advice on the more intimate aspects of incontinence control is to be accepted. Fear of odor is the most commonly expressed worry of incontinent women, and many regard odor as the greatest problem caused by their incontinence (Norton, 1982). Help with personal hygiene, disposal of soiled pads and clothes, adequate ventilation, and the use of suitable clothing materials and proprietary products can minimize the risk of odor. Reassurance that fresh, adequately dilute, and uninfected urine should not smell can help to restore confidence. Good skin care can relieve much of the discomfort attendant on being wet. Sexual counseling can help with the problem of incontinence during intercourse. Advice on modification of clothing style enabling one to undress quickly or to avoid obvious wet patches is important. Many patients are unaware that they can regulate fluid intake to coincide with the easiest times to cope or that certain types of drinks may make their incontinence worse (for example, tea, coffee, and red wine).

The advisor should know which pads, aids, and equipment are available locally, how to obtain them, and how much they might cost the patient (see Chapter 40). The use of catheter drainage, either with a long-term indwelling catheter or through intermittent self-catheterization can likewise be regularly reviewed to ensure that the technique is sound and up to date and that it is the best method for the individual's needs.

TEACHING

The subject of incontinence is generally poorly covered in the training of medical and paramedical personnel. Anyone with expertise in this area has an obligation to spread this knowledge among colleagues and to help change attitudes toward incontinence. It is not feasible for all incontinent patients to be seen in specialist units, so the aim of teaching must be, first, to spread principles of prevention of incontinence and, second, to teach the simple methods of treatment to all health care workers so that only the more intractable cases will need referral. Formal lectures and informal discussion groups are important, but probably most individuals can be taught by watching the advisor at work, and those already working with the patient can be involved in the assessment and treatment of the incontinence so that they can learn to manage subsequent cases themselves.

If the advisor is to teach, she must keep abreast of current literature and methods, and she will be helped in this endeavor by having contact with others working in similar situations. In the United Kingdom there is an Association of Continence Advisors, whose aim is to facilitate contact and exchange of ideas and techniques.

RESEARCH

Since the role of the incontinence advisor is a recent innovation, there has been little research into the best methods of applying knowledge in this field. The results of an ongoing study on the cost-effectiveness of advisors are being awaited (Ramsbottom, 1981).

LIAISON WITH INDUSTRY

There will always remain a sizable minority of patients for whom medical and nursing advice does little to relieve their incontinence. For such people, good aids and equipment can enable them to cope with their incontinence and lead a normal life. There is much scope for improvement in the range of items currently available, and it is hoped that through close cooperation between advisors and industry, better products can be developed to meet the needs of the patient. New products need proper testing in well-designed trials and in a variety of situations to determine their effectiveness and patient suitability.

CONCLUSION

The precise role of the incontinence advisor has not yet been crystallized, and the details of this role will probably always depend on local needs and circumstances. Often the advisor's contribution to patient care will be in the form of suggesting many minor improvements to help the patient cope with her problem and offering psychological support throughout. Sometimes she may be the principal therapist. A balance will need to be struck between having an ongoing case load and teaching other professionals. As yet, there is no form of training for this post. It is hoped that as the role of the incontinence advisor becomes established, appropriate training will follow.

REFERENCES

Friend, P. 1977. Promotion of continence and management of incontinence. Department of Health and Social Security Circular CNO (SNC) **77**:1.

Isaacs, B. 1979. Water, water everywhere. R. Soc. Health J. **4**:155-165.

Norton, C. 1980. Assessing incontinence. Nursing **18**:789-791.

Norton, C. 1981. Communication to the first meeting of the Association of Continence Advisors. London.

Norton, C. 1982. The effects of urinary incontinence in women. Rehabil. Med. **4**:9-14.

Ramsbottom, F. 1981. Personal communication.

appendix II

Definitions— International Continence Society

FIRST REPORT ON THE STANDARDISATION OF TERMINOLOGY OF LOWER URINARY TRACT FUNCTION

Produced by the International Continence Society, February, 1975*

Members: Patrick Bates, William E. Bradley, Eric Glen, Hansjörg Melchior, David Rowan, Arthur Sterling and Tage Hald (Chairman)

This report contains the first set of recommendations dealing with the terminology of lower urinary tract function. Specifically, it covers the storage of urine in the bladder, urinary incontinence and units of measurement. The recommendations were subject to discussion during the Fourth Annual Meeting of the International Continence Society in Mainz, Germany in September, 1974.

These standards are proposed to facilitate comparison of results by investigators who use urodynamic methods. It is recommended that the acknowledgement of these standards in written publications be indicated by a footnote to the section "Methods and Material" or its equivalent: "Methods, definitions, and units conform to the standards proposed by the International Continence Society except where specifically noted."

URINARY INCONTINENCE

Incontinence is a condition where involuntary loss of urine is a social or hygienic problem and is objectively demonstrable. Loss of urine through channels other than the urethra is extraurethral incontinence.

Stress incontinence denotes: 1. a symptom,
　　　　　　　　　　　　2. a sign, and
　　　　　　　　　　　　3. a condition = genuine stress incontinence.

The *symptom* "stress incontinence" indicates the patient's statement of involuntary loss of urine when exercising physically (in the broadest possible sense of the words).

The *sign* "stress incontinence" denotes the observation of involuntary loss of urine from the urethra immediately upon an increase in abdominal pressure.

The *condition* "genuine stress incontinence" is involuntary loss of urine when the intravesical pressure exceeds the maximum urethral pressure but in the absence of detrusor activity.

Urge incontinence is involuntary loss of urine associated with a strong desire to void. Urge incontinence may be subdivided into *motor urge incontinence*, which is associated with uninhibited detrusor contractions, and *sensory urge incontinence*, which is not due to uninhibited detrusor contractions.

Reflex incontinence is voluntary loss of urine due to abnormal reflex activity in the spinal cord in the absence of the sensation usually associated with the desire to micturate.

From International Continence Society. 1976. Br. J. Urol. **48**:39-42.
*Revised following discussion during the business meeting of the International Continence Society, Mainz, 1974.

Overflow incontinence is involuntary loss of urine when the intravesical pressure exceeds the maximum urethral pressure due to an elevation of intravesical pressure associated with bladder distension but in the absence of detrusor activity.

PROCEDURES RELATED TO THE EVALUATION OF URINE STORAGE
Cystometry

Cystometry is a method by which the pressure-volume relationship of the bladder is measured. Zero reference for pressure is the level of the superior edge of the symphysis pubis.

Specify: Access: 1. transurethrally,
                   2. percutaneously.
       Medium: 1. liquid,
                   2. gas.
       Temperature: state temperature in degrees Celsius.
       Position of patient: 1. supine,
                           2. sitting,
                           3. standing.
       Filling: 1. continuous,
                 2. incremental.
                 The precise filling rate should be stated.* When using incremental method, also state volume of increment.

Technique:
1. single or double lumen catheter or multiple catheters,
2. type of catheter (manufacturer),
3. size of catheter,
4. measuring equipment.

Findings: Before starting to fill, residual urine should be measured. The presence of contractions exceeding 15 cm H_2O clearly indicates an uninhibited detrusor contraction when the patient has been asked to inhibit. Pressure elevations smaller than 15 cm H_2O indicate that clinical judgement should be exercised. An indication of the volume at first desire to void should be made.

Maximum cystometric capacity is the volume at which the patient has a strong desire to void.

Effective cystometric capacity is the maximum cystometric capacity minus the residual urine.

Compliance indicates the change in volume for a change in pressure. It is defined as $C = \Delta V \Delta p$ where ΔV is the volume increment and Δp is the change in pressure associated with this volume increment. During cystometry, it is taken for granted that the patient is awake and not sedated. If otherwise, this should be specified.

Urethral closure pressure profile

Urethral closure pressure profile denotes the intraluminal pressure along the length of the urethra with the bladder at rest.

Zero reference for pressure is the level of the superior edge of the symphysis pubis.

To be meaningful, bladder pressure should be measured simultaneously.

Specify:
1. catheter type and size,
2. measurement technique,
3. rate of infusion,
4. continuous or intermittent withdrawal,
5. rate of withdrawal,
6. bladder volume,
7. position of patient: *(a)* supine,
                               (b) sitting,
                               (c) standing.

*For general discussion, the following terms for the range of filling rate may be used:
1. up to 10 ml per minute is a *slow fill cystometry;*
2. 10-100 ml per minute is a *medium fill cystometry;*
3. over 100 ml per minute is a *rapid fill cystometry.*

Findings (see Figure II.1)

Maximum urethral pressure is the maximum pressure of the measured profile.

Maximum urethral closure pressure is the difference between the maximum urethral pressure and the bladder pressure.

Functional profile length is the length of the urethra along which the urethral pressure exceeds bladder pressure.

(*Total profile length* is not generally regarded as a clinically useful parameter.)

UNITS OF MEASUREMENT

In current urodynamic literature there is no standardisation in the units of measurement. For example, intravesical pressure is sometimes measured in mm Hg and sometimes in cm H_2O. When Laplace's law is used to calculate tension in the bladder wall, it is often found that pressure is then measured in dyne cm^{-2}. This lack of uniformity in the systems used leads to confusion when other parameters, which are a function of pressure, are computed, for instance, "compliance," "urethral resistance," etc. From these few examples it is evident that standardisation is essential for meaningful communication. Many journals now require that the results be given in SI Units.

This system will be used in all future I.C.S. papers. The following report is designed to give guidance in the application of the SI system to urodynamics and defines the units involved. The principal units to be used are listed below.

Quantity	Acceptable unit	Symbol
volume	millilitre	ml
time	second	s
flowrate	millilitres/second	ml s^{-1}
pressure	centimetres of water*	cm H_2O
length	metres or submultiples	m, cm, mm
velocity	metres/second or submultiples	m s^{-1}, cm s^{-1}
temperature	degrees Celsius†	°C

A fuller explanation of the SI system follows.

LE SYSTÈM INTERNATIONAL d'UNITÉS (SI UNITS)

At the Conférence Générale des Poids et Mesures (CGPM) in Paris in 1960 it was agreed internationally that this system of units (abbreviated to SI in all languages) should be adopted for all scientific and technical work. It is an extension and refinement of the traditional metric system and is rational, coherent and comprehensive. It is therefore logical that this system should be used in all urodynamic studies.

There are 7 fundamental units; all other units are derived from these. The 3 basic mechanical quantities are mass, length and time. The complete list is given below.

Quantity	Unit	Symbol
mass	kilogramme	kg
length	metre	m
time	second	s
temperature	kelvin	K
electric current	ampere	A
luminous intensity	candela	cd
amount of substance	mole	mol

*The SI Unit is the pascal, but it is only practical at present to calibrate our instruments in cm H_2O. One centimetre of water pressure is approximately equal to 100 pascals (1 cm H_2O = 98.07 Pa). When calculating parameters that are a function of pressure, for example, "compliance", the pascal must be used to avoid confusion. Measurements reported in millimetres of mercury will not be acceptable.

†The SI Unit is the degree Kelvin. The Kelvin temperature interval is identical with the degree Celsius (centigrade) temperature interval. The Kelvin scale starts at absolute zero (-273.16°C), and this is inconvenient in medical practice. The Celsius scale will therefore be used.

As in the metric system a prefix may be added to the unit to indicate that a multiplier of the form 10^a has been applied.

Prefix	Symbol	Multiplier	Remarks
tera	T	10^{12}	
giga	G	10^9	
mega	M	10^6	
kilo	k	10^3	
hecto	h	10^2	1
deca	da	10^1	1
deci	d	10^{-1}	1,2
centi	c	10^{-2}	1,3
milli	m	10^{-3}	
micro	μ	10^{-6}	
nano	n	10^{-9}	
pico	p	10^{-12}	

REMARKS

1. An endeavour is being made to reduce unnecessarily fine division by discouraging the general use of exponent values, $a = +2, +1, -1, -2$.
2. The prefix "deci" may be used to specify a volume of $10^{-3} m^3 = 1\ dm^3$ since the litre has been redefined as 1 dm^3 exactly.
3. Although "centi" is one of the discouraged prefixes, it is too well established to be eliminated at the present time.

DERIVED SI UNITS

These units are composed of combinations of the fundamental units; some of them have been given special names.* A few examples of commonly used units are listed below.

area	= (length)^2	= m^2	= *square metre*
volume	= (length)^3	= m^3	= *cubic metre†*
flowrate	= volume per unit time	= $m^3 s^{-1}$	= *cubic metres per second‡*
density	= mass per unit volume	= $kg\ m^{-3}$	= *kilogrammes per cubic metre*
velocity	= distance in unit time	= $m\ s^{-1}$	= *metres per second*
acceleration	= velocity increase in unit time	= $m\ s^{-2}$	= *metres per second per second*
force	= mass × acceleration	= $kg\ m\ s^{-2}$	= *newton (N)**
energy	= force × displacement	= $N\ m$	= *joule (J)**
power	= energy per unit time	= $N\ m\ s^{-1}$	= *watt (W)**
pressure	= force per unit area	= $N\ m^{-2}$	= *pascal (Pa)**
stress	= force per unit area	= $N\ m^{-2}$	= *pascal (Pa)**
tension	= force per unit length	= $N\ m^{-1}$	= *newtons per metre*
momentum	= mass × velocity	= $kg\ m\ s^{-1}$	= *kilogramme metres per second*
electric charge	= electric current × time	= $A\ s$	= *coulomb (C)**
potential difference	= energy to move 1 coulomb	= joules per coulomb	= *volt (V)**
electric resistance	= potential difference for 1 ampere	= volt per ampere	= *ohm (Ω)**

USE OF SI UNITS AND THEIR MULTIPLES

The symbol of a prefix is considered to be combined with the unity symbol to which it is directly attached forming a new unit symbol which can be raised to a positive or negative power.

$$e.g.,\ 1\ cm^3 = (10^{-2}m)^3 = 10^{-6}m^3$$
$$1\ kN\ m^{-2} = 10^3 N\ m^{-2}$$

When expressing a quantity by a numerical value and a certain unit, it has been found convenient to use units resulting in numerical values between 0.1 and 1000.

$$e.g.,\ 14300\ N = 14.3\ kN$$
$$0.00564\ m = 5.64\ mm$$

†Another unit which is accepted is *litre* $= 1\ dm^3$.
‡Another unit which is accepted is *litres per sound* $= dm^3\ s^{-1}$.

SECOND REPORT ON THE STANDARDISATION OF TERMINOLOGY OF LOWER URINARY TRACT FUNCTION

Produced by the International Continence Society, August 1976*

Members: Patrick Bates, Eric Glen, Derek Griffiths, Hansjörg Melchior, David Rowan, Arthur Sterling, Norman Zinner, Tage Hald (Chairman)

INTRODUCTION

This report contains the second set of recommendations dealing with the terminology of lower urinary tract function. It covers micturition and recommendations for the use of symbols. The recommendations were subject to discussion during the Fifth Annual Meeting of the International Continence Society in Glasgow, Scotland, September 1975.

These standards are proposed to facilitate comparison of results by investigators who use urodynamic methods. It is recommended that the acknowledgement of these standards in written publications be indicated by a footnote to the section "Methods and Material" or its equivalent: "Methods, definitions, and units conform to the standards proposed by the International Continence Society except where specifically noted."

Urodynamics encompasses the morphological, physiological, biomechanical and hydrodynamic aspects of urine transport. This report deals with the urodynamics of the lower urinary tract.

PROCEDURES RELATED TO THE EVALUATION OF MICTURITION
Flow rate

Flow rate is defined as the volume of fluid expelled via the urethra per unit time. It is expressed in ml/s.

Specify: 1. Patient environment and position: (1) supine
                                                 (2) sitting
                                                 (3) standing.
        2. Filling: (1) by diuresis: (i) spontaneous
                                    (ii) forced (specify regimen)
               (2) by catheter: (i) transurethral ⎫
                                   (ii) suprapubic ⎬ state rate.
        3. Fluid—indicate temperature.
Technique: 1. Measuring equipment.
          2. Solitary procedure or combined with other measurements.
Definitions:
1. *Continuous flow* (see Figure II.2).
   Flow time is the time over which measurable flow actually occurs.
   Time to maximum flow is the elapsed time from onset of flow to maximum flow.
   Maximum flow rate is the maximum measured value of the flow rate.
   Voided volume is the total volume expelled via the urethra.
   Average flow rate is voided volume divided by flow time.
2. *Intermittent flow or continuous flow with substantial terminal dribbling* (see Figure II.3).
   The same parameters are applicable if care is exercised in measuring flow time as defined above, *i.e.* time intervals between flow episodes are disregarded, or if the duration of very low terminal flow is disregarded.

Voiding time is total duration of micturition, *i.e.* includes interruptions. In continuous flow situation, voiding time is equal to flow time.

Flow pattern
Specify pattern description. This cannot be defined at present and is best illustrated.

From International Continence Society. 1977. Br. J. Urol. **49**:207-210.
*Revised following discussion during the business meeting of the International Continence Society, Antwerp, September 1976.

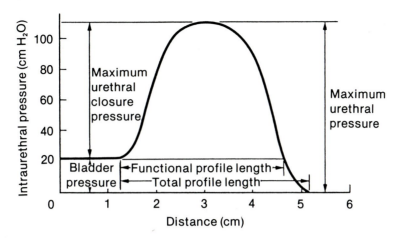

Figure II.1 A schematic representation of the urethral closure pressure profile.

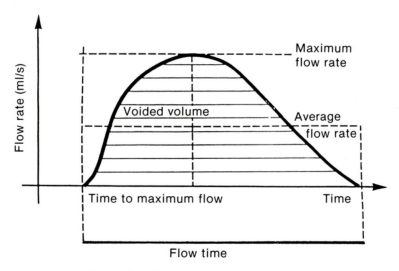

Figure II.2 Diagram of continuous flow curve.

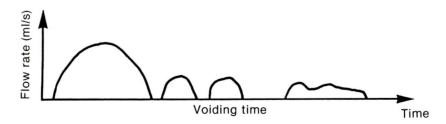

Figure II.3 Diagram of intermittent flow curve.

Comment:

Measurement of the flow rate has value

(a) as screening procedure

(b) in assessing results of treatment

(c) in assessing progression of disease.

However, as an isolated measurement it has limitations. In particular it may have to be related to bladder pressure, initial and residual volume in the bladder and of course age and sex.

Pressure measurements during micturition

Zero reference for all pressure measurements is the level of the superior edge of the symphysis pubis. Pressures are expressed in cm H_2O.

Specify: Access to intravesical pressure (1) transurethral
                                                          (2) suprapubic
                                                          (3) telemetry.
                  Access to abdominal pressure   (1) rectal
                                                          (2) gastric
                                                          (3) intraperitoneal.
              Position (1) supine
                         (2) sitting
                         (3) standing.
Technique: 1. Catheter type and size.
                 2. Measuring equipment.
Definitions (see Figure II.4):

Intravesical pressure is the pressure within the bladder.

Abdominal pressure is taken to be the pressure surrounding the bladder. In current practice it is estimated from rectal, gastric or intraperitoneal pressure.

Detrusor pressure is that component of intravesical pressure which is created by forces in the bladder wall (passive and active). It is estimated by subtracting abdominal pressure from intravesical pressure.

Opening time is the elapsed time from initial rise in detrusor pressure to onset of flow. This is the initial isovolumetric contraction period of micturition. Time lags should be taken into account.

The following parameters are applicable to measurements of each of the pressure curves: intravesical, abdominal and detrusor pressure (see Table II.1):

Premicturition pressure is the pressure recorded immediately before the initial isovolumetric contraction.

Opening pressure is the pressure recorded at the onset of measured flow.

Maximum pressure is the maximum value of the measured pressure.

Pressure at maximum flow is the pressure recorded at maximum measured flow rate.

Contraction pressure at maximum flow is the difference between pressure at maximum flow and premicturition pressure.

Postmicturition events are at present not well understood and so cannot be defined.

It is common practice to relate pressure and flow by calculation of a resistance factor. However, caution should be exercised in interpreting this number. The subject of resistance factors will be dealt with in a later report.

Symbols

It is often helpful to use symbols in a communication.

The system below has been devised to standardise a code of symbols for use in urodynamics.

The rationale of the system is to have a basic symbol representing the physical quantity with qualifying subscripts.

The list of basic symbols largely conforms to international usage. The qualifying subscripts relate the basic symbols to commonly used urodynamic parameters (Table II.2).

If all parameters were to be given standard symbols the system would be clumsy. If further qualifiers therefore are required they should follow this system and be defined.

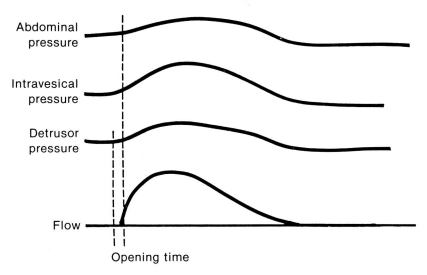

Figure II.4 Diagram of corresponding pressures and curve of flow. The order of presentation of curves as shown above is recommended.

TABLE II.1   Parameters of pressure in the micturition cycle

| | Pressure curves | | |
	Intravesical	Abdominal	Detrusor
Premicturition pressure	Intravesical premicturition pressure	Abdominal premicturition pressure	Detrusor premicturition pressure
Opening pressure	Intravesical opening pressure	Abdominal opening pressure	Detrusor opening pressure
Maximum pressure	Maximum intravesical pressure	Maximum abdominal pressure	Maximum detrusor pressure
Pressure at maximum flow	Intravesical pressure at maximum flow	Abdominal pressure at maximum flow	Detrusor pressure at maximum flow
Contraction pressure at maximum flow	Intravesical contraction pressure at maximum flow	Abdominal contraction pressure at maximum flow	Detrusor contraction pressure at maximum flow

---

TABLE II.2   List of symbols

Basic symbols		Urological qualifiers		Value	
Pressure	p	Bladder	ves	Maximum	max
Volume	V	Urethra	ura	Minimum	min
Flow rate	Q	Ureter	ure	Average	ave
Velocity	v	Detrusor	det		
Time	t	Abdomen	abd		
Temperature	T				
Length	l				
Area	A				
Diameter	d	Example:			
Force	F	$p_{ves,\,max}$ = maximum intravesical pressure			
Energy	E				
Power	P				
Compliance	C				
Work	W				

THIRD REPORT ON THE STANDARDISATION OF TERMINOLOGY OF LOWER URINARY TRACT FUNCTION

Procedures related to the evaluation of micturition: Pressure-flow relationships. Residual urine

Produced by the International Continence Society, February 1977*

Members: C.P. Bates, W.E. Bradley, E.S. Glen, D. Griffiths, H. Melchior, D. Rowan, A. Sterling and T. Hald (Chairman)

This report continues with recommendations on procedures related to the evaluation of micturition. It covers pressure-flow relationships and residual urine. These recommendations were subject to discussion during the Seventh Annual Meeting of the International Continence Society in Portoroz, Yugoslavia, September 1977.

These standards are proposed to facilitate comparison of results by investigators who use urodynamic methods. It is recommended that the acknowledgement of these standards in written publications be indicated by a footnote to the section "Methods and Material" or its equivalent: "Methods, definitions and units conform to the standards proposed by the International Continence Society except where specifically noted."

PRESSURE-FLOW RELATIONSHIPS

To accomplish micturition a driving pressure is necessary. The driving pressure for micturition is the pressure within the bladder. This pressure can be generated by detrusor contraction (p_{det}), by abdominal pressure (p_{abd}) or by both ($p_{ves} = p_{det} + p_{abd}$). The urethra is an irregular and distensible conduit whose walls and surroundings, which have active and passive elements, influence the flow of urine through it. The bladder and urethra each have their own characteristics and in combination these characteristics determine the pressure-flow relationships of micturition. The relationships vary throughout a micturition and, in one individual, from one micturition to the next. Many attempts have been made to reduce the pressure-flow relationships to "urethral resistance factors" in an attempt to distinguish between normal and pathological conditions.

The following formulae have all been used at one time or another.

(1) p_{ves}/Q

(2) p_{ves}/Q^2

(3) $\sqrt{p_{ves}}/Q$

(4) p_{det}/Q

(5) p_{det}/Q^2

(6) $(p_{ves} - E_{str})/Q$

(7) $(p_{ves} - E_{str})/Q^2$

(8) $(p_{ves} - E_{str})p_{ves}$

(9) $d_{ura,eff} = \left[\dfrac{32\rho fl Q^2}{\Delta p g \pi^2} \right]^{0.2}$

From International Continence Society. 1980. Br. J. Urol. **52**:348-350. © British Association of Urological Surgeons.

*Revised following discussion during the business meeting of the International Continence Society, Portoroz, Yugoslavia, September 1977. Reprinted from *Scand. J. Urol. Nephrol.* (1978) **12**, 191-193.

E_{str} is the kinetic energy per unit volume in the external stream, sometimes (unfortunately) called the "exit pressure", and $d_{ura.eff}$ is a calculated "effective urethral diameter".

ρ = density of fluid
f = Fanning's friction factor
l = urethral length
Δ_p = friction loss
g = acceleration due to gravity.

Ideally we should like to choose the most useful of the above formulae and recommend it for general use. However, all of them originate from rigid tube hydrodynamics. The urethra is not a rigid tube. Therefore these factors vary not only during micturition but also from one micturition to another and so cannot provide a valid comparison between patients. They may even be misleading.

However, pressure-flow studies are still valuable since some characteristic pressure-flow patterns may be identified. For example:

(a) Low flow rate accompanied by high pressure indicates obstruction.

(b) High flow rate accompanied by low pressure indicates freedom from obstruction.

(c) Intermittent flow rate associated with abdominal contractions and absence of detrusor activity indicates motor impairment of the detrusor.

(d) Intermittent interruptions of the flow in the absence of abdominal straining, with concomitant increases in the intravesical pressure, indicate intermittent contractions of the urethral and/or periurethral striated musculature.

In all cases the urodynamic findings should be assessed in conjunction with the results of routine urological investigations.

Presentation of pressure-flow relationships

It is suggested that it is more useful to present both the flow rate and the corresponding intravesical or detrusor pressure (p_{ves} or p_{det}), rather than to rely on a "urethral resistance factor." It is common to relate the maximum flow rate to the pressure at maximum flow, but any instant during micturition can be examined in the way proposed.

When presenting data from a group of patients, pressure-flow relationships may be shown on a graph as illustrated in Figure II.5. This form of presentation allows lines of demarcation to be drawn on the graph to separate the results according to the problem being studied. The points shown in the figure are purely illustrative to indicate how the data might fall into groups. The group of equivocal results might include either an unrepresentative micturition in an obstructed or an unobstructed patient, or detrusor insufficiency with or without obstruction. This is the group which invalidates the use of "urethral resistance factors".

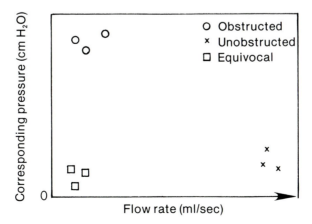

Figure II.5 Recommended presentation of pressure-flow relationships. The points shown are purely illustrative to indicate how the data might fall into groups.

RESIDUAL URINE

Residual urine is defined as the volume of fluid remaining in the bladder immediately following the completion of micturition. The measurement of residual urine forms an integral part of the study of micturition. It is commonly estimated by the following methods:

(1) Palpation.

(2) Catheter or cystoscope: (i) transurethral, (ii) suprapubic.

(3) Radiography: (i) intravenous urography, (ii) micturition cystography.

(4) Ultrasonics: (i) A-scan, (ii) B-scan.

(5) Radioisotopes: (i) clearance, (ii) gamma camera.

Residual urine may result from various causes, such as detrusor insufficiency, infravesical obstruction or psychological inhibition. In the condition of vesicoureteric reflux, urine may re-enter the bladder after micturition and may falsely be interpreted as residual urine. The presence of urine in bladder diverticula following micturition presents special problems of interpretation, since a diverticulum may be regarded either as part of the bladder cavity or as outside the functioning bladder.

The methods mentioned above each have limitations as to their applicability and accuracy in the various conditions associated with residual urine. Therefore it is necessary to choose a method appropriate to the clinical problem.

The absence of residual urine is an observation of clinical value. An isolated finding of residual urine requires confirmation before being considered significant. The absence of residual urine does not exclude the possibility of bladder dysfunction or infravesical obstruction.

In infravesical obstruction there is a variable and poorly understood connection between the occurrence of residual urine and abnormalities in the pressure-flow relationships. In the study of this condition both need to be taken into account and their interrelation could be a fruitful area for future research.

FOURTH REPORT ON THE STANDARDISATION OF TERMINOLOGY OF LOWER URINARY TRACT FUNCTION
Terminology related to neuromuscular dysfunction of the lower urinary tract

Produced by the International Continence Society*

Members: C.P. Bates, W.E. Bradley, E.S. Glen, H. Melchior, D. Rowan, A.M. Sterling, T. Sundin, D. Thomas, M. Torrens, R. Turner-Warwick, N.R. Zinner and T. Hald (Chairman)

This report deals with recommendations on terminology related to neuromuscular dysfunction of the lower urinary tract with particular reference to classification of the neuropathic bladder.

These standards are proposed to facilitate comparison of results by investigators who use urodynamic methods. It is recommended that the acknowledgement of these standards in written publications be indicated by a footnote to the section "Methods and Material" or its equivalent: "Methods, definitions and units conform to the standards proposed by the International Continence Society except where specifically noted".

Lower urinary tract dysfunction

This may be caused by:
(1) Disturbance of the pertinent nervous or psychological control systems.
(2) Disorders of muscle function.
(3) Structural abnormalities.
The term *neuromuscular dysfunction* includes the first 2 categories.

Classifications based on concepts of the cause of a dysfunction, especially on the site of a neurological lesion, may be confusing. A lesion is often difficult to locate with certainty and different lesions may produce identical functional changes in the lower urinary tract.

Therefore such a classification gives little help when considering the management of the end organ abnormality. Without objective information about the function it is impossible to compare results of treatment from different centres. An underlying neurological pathology is, of course, equally important from a prognostic, therapeutic and counselling point of view and must be considered at the same time.

The increasing use of urodynamic methods has made it possible to classify disorders of the detrusor and urethral closure mechanism with some accuracy. However, the range of bladder and urethral abnormalities cannot fully be defined at the present time.

This report presents a basic classification of function. Only neuromuscular function is considered, leaving structural organ changes and complicating factors aside. The lower urinary tract is composed of the *bladder* and *urethra*. They form a functional unit and their interaction cannot be ignored. Each has 2 functions: the bladder to store and void, the urethra to control and convey. When a reference is made to the hydrodynamic function or to the whole anatomical unit as a storage organ—the vesica urinaria—the correct term is the *bladder*. When the specific smooth muscle structure known as the m. detrusor urinae is being discussed, the correct term is the *detrusor*.

For simplicity the bladder/detrusor and the urethra will be considered separately so that a classification based on a combination of functional anomalies can be reached. No attempt has been made to define these in a quantitative way or to consider efficiency. *Sensation* cannot be accurately evaluated, but must be assessed. This classification depends on the results of various objective urodynamic investigations. The number of specific tests may vary from one person to another. Studies of the filling and voiding phases are essential for each patient.

Terms used should be objective, definable and ideally should be applicable to the whole range of abnormality. When authors disagree with the classification presented below, or use terms that have not been defined here, their meaning should be made clear.

From International Continence Society. 1981. Br. J. Urol. **53**:333-335. © British Association of Urological Surgeons.
*Produced following discussion at the International Continence Society Meetings in Manchester, September 1978 and in Rome, October 1979.

DETRUSOR FUNCTION

The detrusor function may be:
1. normal
2. overactive
3. underactive

Activity in this context is related to detrusor contractions interpreted from intravesical (p_{ves}) or detrusor pressure (p_{det}) changes, preferably the latter. Assessment of activity must be made during both filling and voiding, and the classification may change between these 2 phases.

Normal detrusor function

During the filling phase the bladder contents increase in volume without a significant rise in pressure (accommodation). No involuntary contractions occur despite provocation. Normal voiding is achieved by a voluntarily initiated detrusor contraction that is sustained and can be suppressed voluntarily. A normal detrusor so defined may be described as ''stable''.

Overactive detrusor function

Overactive detrusor function is indicated when during the filling phase there are involuntary detrusor contractions, which may be spontaneous or provoked, that the person cannot suppress. Provocation includes rapid filling, alterations of posture, coughing, walking, jumping and other triggering procedures. Voiding may be due to involuntary contractions or to voluntary contractions that cannot be suppressed. Various terms have been used to describe these features and they are defined as follows:

The *unstable detrusor* is one that is shown objectively to contract, spontaneously or on provocation, during the filling phase while the patient is attempting to inhibit micturition. The unstable detrusor may be asymptomatic and its presence does not necessarily imply a neurological disorder.

Detrusor hyperreflexia is defined as overactivity due to disturbance of the nervous control mechanisms. Whether the unstable detrusor is synonymous with detrusor hyperreflexia is unknown at present. Until this controversy is resolved, detrusor hyperreflexia should be confirmed by objective evidence of a neurological disorder.

The use of conceptual and undefined terms such as hypertonic, systolic, uninhibited, spastic and automatic should be avoided. When referring to the volume/pressure relationship in a bladder with a high pressure rise the correct term is a *low-compliance bladder* (*e.g.* a shrunken bladder following radiotherapy).

Underactive detrusor function

In the underactive detrusor there are no contractions during filling. During voiding the contraction may be absent or inadequately sustained. A *noncontractile detrusor* is one which does not contract under any circumstances. *Detrusor areflexia* exists where underactivity is due to an abnormality of nervous control and denotes the complete absence of centrally coordinated contraction. In detrusor areflexia due to a lesion of the conus medullaris or sacral nerve outflow, the detrusor should be described as *decentralised*— not denervated, since the peripheral neurones remain. The bladder function may be described as *autonomous*. In such bladders pressure fluctuations of low amplitude may occur. The use of terms such as atonic, hypotonic, autonomic and flaccid should be avoided. If the volume/pressure relationship of a bladder is referred to as being capacious with little change in pressure, then the correct term is a *high-compliance bladder*.

URETHRAL FUNCTION

The urethral closure mechanism may be:
1. normal
2. overactive
3. incompetent

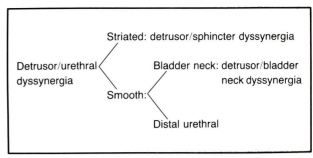

Figure II.6

Normal urethral closure mechanism

The *normal* urethral closure mechanism maintains a positive urethral closure pressure during filling even in the presence of increased abdominal pressure. It may be overcome by detrusor overactivity. During micturition the normal closure pressure decreases to allow flow. The normal closure mechanism is capable of interrupting urination voluntarily.

Overactive urethral closure mechanism

An *overactive* urethral closure mechanism contracts involuntarily against a detrusor contraction or fails to relax at attempted micturition.

Synchronous detrusor and urethral contraction is *detrusor/urethral dyssynergia*. This diagnosis should be qualified by stating the location and type of the urethral muscles (striated or smooth) which are involved (Figure II.6).

Despite the confusion surrounding ''sphincter'' terminology the use of certain terms is so widespread that they are retained and defined here. The term *detrusor/sphincter dyssynergia* describes a detrusor contraction concurrent with an inappropriate contraction of the urethral and/or periurethal striated muscle. In the absence of other neurological features the validity of this diagnosis should be questioned. The term *detrusor/bladder neck dyssynergia* is used to denote a detrusor contraction concurrent with an objectively demonstrated defect of bladder neck opening. No parallel term has been elaborated for possible detrusor/distal urethral (smooth muscle) dyssynergia.

Incompetent urethral closure mechanism

An *incompetent* urethral closure mechanism allows leakage of urine. The negative urethral closure pressure may be persistent (continuous leakage) or due to a rise in abdominal pressure (genuine stress incontinence) or an involuntary fall in intraurethral pressure in the absence of detrusor activity (unstable urethra). Detrusor overactivity is more likely to be accompanied by leakage if there is an involuntary decrease in urethral pressure.

SENSATION

Sensation is difficult to evaluate because of its subjective nature. It is usually assessed by questioning the patient in relation to the fullness of the bladder either during the taking of the clinical history or during cystometry. There are 2 groups of sensory modalities: proprioception, which serves to inform on tension and contraction, and exteroception, which serves to inform on pain, touch and temperature. Sensation can be classified broadly as follows:
1. normal
2. hypersensitive
3. hyposensitive.

Index